Comparative
Health Information
Management

Second Edition

Comparative Health Information Management

Second Edition

Ann H. Peden, MBA, RHIA, CCS

THOMSON

DELMAR LEARNING

Australia Canada Mexico Singapore Spain United Kingdom United States

THOMSON

DELMAR LEARNING

Comparative Health Information Management, Second Edition
by Ann H. Peden, MBA, RHIA, CCS

Vice President, Health Care Business Unit:
William Brottmiller

Editorial Director:
Cathy L. Esperti

Acquisitions Editor:
Rhonda Dearborn

Marketing Director:
Jennifer McAvey

Marketing Channel Manager:
Tamara Caruso

Marketing Coordinator:
Chris Manion

Senior Production Editor
James Zayicek

Editorial Assistant:
Debra S. Gorgos

Developmental Editors:
Bryan Viggiani/Sherry Conners

Library of Congress Cataloging-in-Publication Data

Comparative health information management / [edited by] Ann Peden.—2nd ed.
    p. cm.
   Includes bibliographical references and index.
   ISBN 1-4018-3948-7
   1. Medical records—Management.   2. Medical records—Management—United States.   I. Peden, Ann H.
RA976.C66 2005
362.1'068'4—dc22
2004049399

NOTICE TO THE READER

Publisher does not warrant or guarantee any of the products described herein or perform any independent analysis in connection with any of the product information contained herein. Publisher does not assume, and expressly disclaims, any obligation to obtain and include information other than that provided to it by the manufacturer.

The reader is expressly warned to consider and adopt all safety precautions that might be indicated by the activities described herein and to avoid all potential hazards. By following the instructions contained herein, the reader willingly assumes all risks in connection with such instructions.

The publisher makes no representations or warranties of any kind, including but not limited to, the warranties of fitness for particular purpose or merchantability, nor are any such representations implied with respect to the material set forth herein, and the publisher takes no responsibility with respect to such material. The publisher shall not be liable for any special, consequential, or exemplary damages resulting, in whole or part, from the reader's use of, or reliance upon, this material.

iv

Contents

Preface   xi
Acknowledgments   *xiv*
About the Author   *xvi*

Chapter 1   **Introduction**   1

Ann H. Peden, MBA, RHIA, CCS

The Changing Face of Health Care in America   *1*
Impact on the Role of the Health Information Manager   *15*

Chapter 2   **Hospital-Based Ambulatory Care**   23

Ann H. Peden, MBA, RHIA, CCS

Introduction to Setting   *24*
Regulatory Issues   *27*
Documentation   *27*
Reimbursement   *33*
Information Management   *40*
Quality Improvement and Utilization Management   *44*
Risk Management and Legal Issues   *45*
Role of the Health Information Management Professional   *46*
Trends   *48*

Chapter 3   **Freestanding Ambulatory Care**   **58**

Elizabeth D. Bowman, MPA, RHIA

Introduction to Setting   *59*
Regulatory Issues   *61*
Documentation   *65*
Reimbursement   *79*
Information Management   *82*
Quality Improvement and Utilization Management   *88*
Risk Management and Legal Issues   *89*
Role of the Health Information Management Professional   *91*
Trends   *92*

Chapter 4   **Managed Care**   **103**

Lynn Kuehn, MS, RHIA, CCS-P, FAHIMA

Introduction to Setting   *104*
Regulatory Issues   *109*
Documentation   *112*
Revenue Generation   *113*
Information Management   *117*
Quality Improvement and Utilization Management   *123*
Risk Management and Legal Issues   *125*
Role of the Health Information Management Professional   *127*
Trends   *129*

Chapter 5   **Dialysis**   **135**

Ann H. Peden, MBA, RHIA, CCS

Introduction to Setting   *136*
Regulatory Issues   *139*
Documentation   *140*
Reimbursement   *143*
Information Management   *144*
Quality Improvement and Utilization Management   *151*
Risk Management, Legal, and Ethical Issues   *152*
Role of the Health Information Management Professional   *155*

Chapter 6   Correctional Facilities   162

Barbara Manny, MS, RHIA and Brianna McCloe Rogers, RHIA

Introduction to Setting   164
Regulatory Issues   177
Documentation   179
Reimbursement and Funding   183
Information Management   184
Quality Improvement and Utilization Management   188
Risk Management and Legal Issues   189
Role of the Health Information Management Professional   190
Trends   191

Chapter 7   Mental Health: Long-Term and Acute Services   198

C. Harrell Weathersby, MSW, PhD

Introduction to Setting   199
Regulatory Issues   211
Documentation   213
Reimbursement and Funding   222
Information Management   222
Quality Improvement and Utilization Management   229
Risk Management and Legal Issues   230
Role of the Health Information Management Professional   233
Trends   234

Chapter 8   Substance Abuse   243

Frances Wickham Lee, MBA, RHIA, Kimberly D. Taylor, RHIA
and Melissa King, RHIA

Introduction to Setting   244
Regulatory Issues   254
Documentation   256
Reimbursement and Funding   266
Information Management   267
Quality Improvement and Utilization Management   271
Risk Management and Legal Issues   272
Role of the Health Information Management Professional   275
Trends   280

Chapter 9   **Facilities for Individuals with Mental
Retardation or Developmental Disabilities   290**

Elaine C. Jouette, MA, RHIA, and Judy S. Westerfield, MEd

Introduction to Setting   291
Regulatory Issues   295
Documentation   296
Reimbursement and Funding   297
Information Management   300
Quality Improvement and Utilization Management   316
Risk Management and Legal Issues   316
Role of the Health Information Management Professional   319
Trends   320

Chapter 10   **Long-Term Care   326**

Kris King, MS, RHIA, CPHQ, and Barbara A. Gorenflo, RHIA

Introduction to Setting   327
Regulatory Issues   334
Documentation   336
Reimbursement and Funding   343
Information Management   348
Quality Improvement and Utilization Management   356
Role of the Health Information Management Professional   359

Chapter 11   **Rehabilitation   369**

Terry Winkler, MD, and Ann H. Peden, MBA, RHIA, CCS

Introduction to Setting   370
Regulatory Issues   380
Documentation   384
Reimbursement and Funding   392
Information Management   397
Quality Improvement and Program Evaluation Systems   406
Risk Management and Legal Issues   406
Role of the Health Information Manager   407
Trends   407

Chapter 12   Home Health Care   419

Kim A. Boyles, MS, RHIA, and Gwen D. Smith, RHIA

Introduction to Setting   420
Regulatory Issues   422
Documentation   424
Reimbursement and Funding   428
Information Management   432
Quality Improvement and Utilization Management   433
Risk Management and Legal Issues   437
Role of the Health Information Management Professional   439
Trends   440

Chapter 13   Hospice   446

Karen M. Staszel, RHIA, and Teresa Sherfy, RHIT

Introduction to Setting   447
Regulatory Issues   450
Documentation   455
Reimbursement and Funding   460
Information Management   464
Quality Improvement and Utilization Management   472
Risk Management and Legal Issues   474
Role of the Health Information Management Professional   476
Trends   477

Chapter 14   Dental Care Settings   483

Cheryl L. Berthelsen, PhD, RHIA, Denise D. Krause, MA, MS,
and Francis G. Serio, DMD, MS

Introduction to Setting   484
Regulatory Issues   492
Documentation   493
Reimbursement   499
Information Management   501
Quality Improvement and Utilization Management   507
Risk Management and Legal Issues   508
Role of the Health Information Management Professional   510
Trends   510

Chapter 15   **Veterinary Settings**   **519**

Margaret L. Neterer, MM, RHIA

Introduction to Setting   *520*
Regulatory Issues   *522*
Documentation   *524*
Reimbursement   *529*
Information Management   *530*
Quality Improvement and Utilization Management   *535*
Risk Management and Legal Issues   *536*
Role of the Health Information Management Professional   *542*
Trends   *542*

Chapter 16   **Consulting**   **550**

Karen Wright, MHA, RHIA, RHIT, and Scott Wright, MBA

Introduction to Setting   *553*
Regulatory Issues   *554*
Documentation   *555*
Reimbursement and Compliance   *555*
Role of the Health Information Management Professional   *557*
Trends   *570*

Index   **576**

Preface

Health care is continuing to move from acute care settings into other sites, including ambulatory care and specialized treatment facilities. Today's health information managers are building challenging careers in what were once considered nontraditional sites. Managing the information flow within and among these sites, especially in light of the technologies making electronic health records possible, is a challenge for today's health information managers. *Comparative Health Information Management* was developed to assist health information students meet this challenge. This text includes 15 chapters on diverse settings outside of acute care in which students of health information management may find employment upon graduation, and a sixteenth chapter on consulting, an area that is gaining in popularity as an employment option for today's health information management (HIM) professionals. The contributors come from both the educational and practice arenas and were chosen for their particular expertise in the different content areas.

Content

The text opens with an introductory chapter that describes the recent history of health care in the United States and the changes taking place at the turn of the millennium. The introduction covers such topics as the effect of changes in payment systems on health care, an overview of regulatory and accreditation issues affecting health care, including a section on the Health Insurance Portability and Accountability Act (HIPAA), and the evolution of the electronic health record. This chapter also addresses how these changes affect the HIM professional and lays a foundation of resources that can assist in meeting the challenges of the twenty-first century.

The remaining setting-based chapters follow a consistent template, facilitating a comparison of the different sites by students. Each chapter includes discussions of the following: introduction to setting; regulatory issues; documentation; reimbursement and funding; information management, including data flow, coding and classification, computer systems, and data sets; quality improvement and utilization management; risk management and legal issues; role of the HIM professional; and trends. Although the chapters refer to and build on one another, they can stand alone and may be used out of sequence or as modules.

Chapter 2 discusses HIM issues unique to ambulatory care offered by hospitals. Chapter 3 details a wide variety of ambulatory health care settings and their information management issues. Chapter 4 provides fundamental information on the spectrum of managed care models with which health information managers interact today. Chapter 5 discusses both dialysis providers and the regional networks that monitor them. Chapter 6 explains terms and issues related to health care for incarcerated persons. Chapter 7 discusses both community-based and inpatient mental health care issues. Chapter 8 explains health information issues affecting facilities offering treatment and rehabilitation for chemical dependencies. Chapter 9 describes the unique information maintained in facilities offering care and training for individuals with mental retardation or developmental disabilities. Chapter 10 explains the increasingly sophisticated data management needs of long-term-care settings, including long-term acute care. Chapter 11 explains information management issues in programs designed to improve function for patients who have suffered a debilitating illness or injury. Chapter 12 discusses information management issues, including the new prospective payment system, for organizations caring for the home-bound patient. Chapter 13 outlines requirements for entities providing health care and support for persons who are terminally ill and their families. Chapter 14 provides insight into health information needs for maintaining and improving oral health. Chapter 15 describes the specialized information requirements for animal health care. Chapter 16 provides practical advice to the health information practitioner considering working as a consultant in any of the health care settings described in this book.

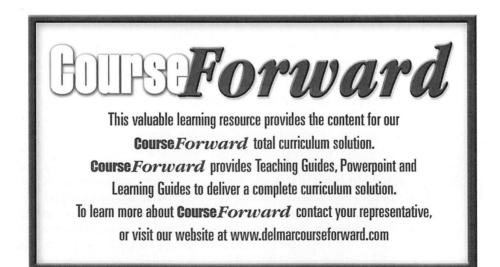

This valuable learning resource provides the content for our
Course*Forward* total curriculum solution.
Course*Forward* provides Teaching Guides, Powerpoint and
Learning Guides to deliver a complete curriculum solution.
To learn more about **Course***Forward* contact your representative,
or visit our website at www.delmarcourseforward.com

Key Features

Chapters 2 through 16 contain the following learning aids to challenge learners:

Learning Objectives   A series of goals for the learner are presented at the beginning of each chapter to help focus study time efficiently. The objectives are outcome-based to provide immediate feedback on progress.

Introduction to Setting   This table gives learners a quick reference to the setting, including common names for the setting, a description, and synonyms.

Summary   Each chapter includes a brief summation of the chapter content, with a focus on key points the learner should retain.

Key Terms   Unfamiliar or critical vocabulary words are listed alphabetically at the end of each chapter and appear in bold on their first use within that chapter. Definitions have also been included within the chapter for quick reference.

Review Questions   A series of knowledge- and application-based review questions challenge learners to apply what they have learned. These may be used for self-study or assigned for class discussion. The answers to the review questions are included in the Instructor's Manual.

Web Activity   A new feature in this edition challenges students to explore information available on the Internet about each setting.

Case Study   A realistic case study based on the chapter content has been included to further challenge learners to apply what they have learned. Each case includes a series of questions to guide learners through the problem-solving process. Cases may be used for in-class discussion or assigned for individual practice. Suggested answers to the cases are included in the Instructor's Manual.

The chapters also include current **References and Suggested Readings** and a listing of **Key Resources**, or organizations and associations pertinent to the chapter topic that will lead the learner to additional information on a particular setting.

New to This Edition

Since the publication of the first edition, Medicare has implemented changes to payment systems in several nonacute settings. Payment system information current as of 2003 is presented in the appropriate chapters, including prospective payment systems implemented in hospital-based ambulatory care, long-term care, home health, and inpatient rehabilitation facilities. The text includes discussion of risk-adjusted systems in managed care, the proposed psychiatric prospective payment system, and other changes in reimbursement affecting nonacute settings.

An overview of the Health Insurance Portability and Accountability Act (HIPAA) is provided in Chapter 1, including standardized code sets and how HIPAA affects the potential adoption of the new coding systems ICD-10-CM and ICD-10-PCS. Setting-specific impacts of HIPAA are described in subsequent chapters, where applicable. For example, Chapter 6 examines the language of HIPAA pertinent to correctional settings, and Chapter 16 describes the necessity of an HIPAA-compliant business associate agreement for the HIM consultant.

A summary of accreditation and regulatory processes has also been added to Chapter 1 to provide a structural framework for the specific agencies and processes presented in subsequent chapters. The Web Activities and Key Resources in each chapter will help students research the latest regulatory information in the ever-changing health care environment. For example, the Web Activity in Chapter 1 invites the students to learn more about the Joint Commission on Accreditation of Health Care Organization's (JCAHO) recently implemented "tracer methodology" for conducting on-site surveys.

Finally, the sequence of chapters has been revised so that human medical and dental health care settings are discussed before attention is turned to animal health care settings. Also, behavioral health care settings are adjacent to one another, as are other similar settings such as long-term care and rehabilitation and home health care and hospice.

Acknowledgments

This book is the result of the efforts of numerous persons. Shirley Anderson had the vision for Delmar's HIM (Health Information Management) series and first suggested this text to the Delmar editorial staff. In 1994, Delmar assembled a focus group of HIM practitioners and educators to plan this text. Accepting the role of editor for this text was much easier given the groundwork that had been laid by the thoughtful contributions of my HIM colleagues.

The author is very grateful for the work of the original contributors, who developed an excellent body of work that the current contributors were able to update, revise, and refine. The names of all contributors, both original and current, are listed at each chapter heading, although some of the original contributors were not able to participate in the second edition. I would like to give these individuals special recognition for their groundbreaking work in the development of this text: Barbara Manny for the correctional chapter, Frances Wickham Lee and Kimberly Taylor for the substance abuse chapter, Elaine C. Jouette for the chapter on individuals with mental retardation and developmental disabilities, Kris King for the long-term care chapter, Kim Boyles for the home health chapter, Karen Staszel for the hospice chapter, and Cheryl Berthelsen for the dental chapter. I owe a tremendous debt of gratitude to these pioneer contributors for bringing the first edition into existence and thus providing much of the substance of the second edition.

The reviewers also played a major role in the development and refinement of this book. Their insights kept us focused on the needs of the readers, and their excellent suggestions have helped make the second edition "new and improved." The author would like to thank the following persons for their role in shaping this text by serving as reviewers during the preparation of the manuscript:

Michelle A. Green, MPS, RHIA
Professor
Department of Physical & Life Sciences
Alfred State College
Alfred, NY

Marjorie McNeill, MS, RHIA, CCS
Interim Director
Division of Health Information Management
School of Allied Health Sciences
Florida A&M University
Tallahassee, FL

Curt Pederson, MBA, PHR
Assistant to the Chair & Director of Student Affairs
Department of Psychology
Wright State University
Dayton, OH

Diane Premeau, RHIT, RHIA
Director Health Information Programs
Chabot College
Hayward, CA

Melanie Schmidt, RMA, RHIA
Program Manager—Health Information Specialist
Arizona College of Allied Health
Glendale, AZ

The chapter authors are also grateful for expert assistance and advice provided to them by others. For Chapter 2: Jim Braden, Mary Palmertree, and Carolyn Gardner for reviewing and supplying figures for the chapter. For Chapter 5: Brenda Dyson, the staff of Network 8, Pam Stephens, Pamela Davis, Derrick Thomas, and Jay Ferchaud for sharing their knowledge of the ESRD networks and dialysis facilities, and for providing photo opportunities and figures. For Chapter 7: Tessie Smith, Ed Payne, Dr. Barbara Carpenter, and Mary Crossman. For Chapter 8: Vernard Jones, A & D Program Coordinator/Clinician at The Pines & Cady Hill Chemical Dependency Programs. For Chapter 11: Staff of Cox Walnut Lawn Rehabilitation Program of Springfield, Missouri, for their assistance in making revisions. For Chapter 15: Various members of the American Veterinary Health Information Management Association (AVHIMA) for providing editorial support.

I would like to thank Melanie Brodnik and Michelle Green for the contacts they provided in locating contributing authors and consultants for the second edition. I want to thank the editorial staff of Delmar Learning for their work on the project, in particular for pulling together the comments from the reviews, for their thoroughness in identifying issues to be addressed, and for their gentle reminders at each stage of the project.

I am very grateful for the support and encouragement I have received from my colleagues at the University of Mississippi Medical Center. I want to thank the administration of the school and Becky Yates, chair of the Health Information Management Department, for creating an environment in the school and department conducive to professional growth and the acceptance of professional challenges. I also thank my fellow faculty members for giving their best to our students and for their support and encouragement. I thank the many guest lecturers and field trip guides who have shared their knowledge of health information management in nontraditional settings with my students and with me. I thank my professors in the Clinical Health Sciences graduate program for what I have learned from them, and I also thank the administration of the graduate program for granting me a much-needed leave of absence to work on this project. I particularly want to thank Lori Evans for the many ways she helped me throughout the project, especially when I was facing numerous time constraints. I also thank my daughter Hope Peden for assisting with some of the technical details of manuscript preparation.

I thank my family, especially my husband, my children and their spouses, my mother and father, my mother-in-law, and also my church family for their encouragement and their prayers. And I thank the One who hears and answers prayer, His Son, who "always lives to make intercession," and His Spirit, who "also helps in our weaknesses."

About the Author

Ann H. Peden, MBA, RHIA, CCS, is associate professor of health information management in the School of Health Related Professions at the University of Mississippi Medical Center in Jackson, Mississippi. She has her MBA from Louisiana Tech University in Ruston, Louisiana, where she also taught in the medical record administration and medical record technology programs. Before teaching, she served as director of medical records at St. Francis Medical Center in Monroe, Louisiana. She completed her undergraduate education at the University of Mississippi. She is presently pursuing her Ph.D. in Clinical Health Sciences at the University of Mississippi Medical Center.

With the support of the University of Mississippi Medical Center, Ann implemented the first Internet discussion group on health information management issues, HIM-L, for which she was awarded the American Health Information Management Association's "Professional Achievement Award." She has received the Mississippi Health Information Management Association's "Distinguished Member Award" and has been honored as "Teacher of the Year" for the University of Mississippi's School of Health Related Professions. Her service to the profession of health information management includes serving as president of the Louisiana Medical Record Association and the Mississippi Health Information Management Association, as well as serving as a member of the nominating committee of the American Health Information Management Association (AHIMA), and as the chair of AHIMA's Coding Policy and Strategy Committee.

About the Contributors

Elizabeth D. Bowman, MPA, RHIA, is a professor in the Department of Health Information Management at the University of Tennessee, Memphis. She is a graduate of Millsaps College and has a Master of Public Administration degree with a concentration in Health Services Administration from the University of Memphis. She obtained a postbaccalaureate certificate in medical record administration from the School of Medical Record Administration at Baptist Memorial Hospital in Memphis. Mrs. Bowman has extensive experience in teaching health information practices in nonacute settings as well as medical terminology, ICD-9-CM and CPT coding, data processing, and statistics.

Barbara A. Gorenflo, RHIA, is the Assistant Administrator of Beechwood Residence and Nursing Home in Getzville, New York. Before her current position, she was the Director of Health Information Management. She has a BS degree in Medical Record Administration from Daemen College, Amherst, New York. She has served as Clinical Instructor for Health Information Technology students at Trocaire and Erie Community Colleges. Mrs. Gorenflo contracts with several long-term care facilities and renal dialysis centers for medical record consulting services. She has done several presentations on medical record documentation issues as well as on HIPAA compliance.

Melissa King, RHIA, is the Information Administrator at Community Counseling Services, a community mental health center in Mississippi. She obtained a bachelor's degree in Health Record Administration from the University of Mississippi Medical Center. She has extensive experience in all aspects of health information management in community mental health, including alcohol and drug treatment programs, reimbursement issues, and information systems planning, implementation, and maintenance.

Denise D. Krause, MA/MS, CNE, MCSE, is an assistant professor in the Department of Periodontics and Preventive Sciences at the University of Mississippi Medical Center. She is a graduate of the University of Kansas and has Master's degrees in International Policy and Russian from the Monterey Institute of International Studies in California, and a Master's degree in Preventive Medicine with a concentration in epidemiology from the University of Mississippi. She has completed professional technical training and has earned specialty certifications as a Certified Novell Engineer and a Microsoft Certified Systems Engineer. Ms. Krause is the director of information technology for the School of Dentistry at the University Medical Center, where she is working on the integration of technology into health information systems and health-related research. She is also a student in the doctoral program in the Department of Preventive Medicine at the University of Mississippi Medical Center.

Lynn Kuehn, MS, RHIA, CCS-P, FAHIMA, is a health care consultant and president of Kuehn Consulting, LLC. She was previously Director of Operations for Children's Medical Group and Operations Administrator for Family Health Plan Cooperative, a staff model HMO, both in Milwaukee, Wisconsin. Ms. Kuehn's technical expertise and experience have led her to co-author *CPT/HCPCS Coding and Reimbursement for Physician Services* for the American Health Information Management Association (AHIMA), now in the fourth edition, and to author *Health Information Management: Medical Record Process in Group Practice* for the Medical Group Management Association (MGMA). She has published numerous articles on health information management issues in many industry publications. In her volunteer role with AHIMA, she has served as a member of the Council on Certification, national chairman and secretary for the Ambulatory Care Section, and national chairman of various committees. Ms. Kuehn holds an M.S. degree in Health Services Administration from Cardinal Stritch University and a B.S. degree in Health Information Administration from Viterbo University.

Margaret L. Neterer, MM, RHIA, is currently manager of the Small Animal Clinical Information Service for the Michigan State University Veterinary Teaching Hospital in East Lansing, Michigan. During her 23 years in this position, Ms. Neterer has also held leadership responsibility at various levels in both veterinary and human health information management professional associations, as well as committee service with the American Veterinary Medical Association. Her areas of expertise include all aspects of management and supervision of veterinary health information services as well as standard-setting in veterinary medical informatics. She is currently creating an online course in medical record maintenance for Michigan veterinarians.

Brianna E. McCloe Rogers, RHIA, is the Supervisor of Clinical Information Services at Aurora Sinai Medical Center in Milwaukee, Wisconsin. She is a graduate of the Health Information Management Systems program from The Ohio State University. Mrs. Rogers previously worked as the Manager of Health Records at the Milwaukee County Jail, where she gained the experience and knowledge to research and revise the chapter on correctional health care.

Francis G. Serio, DMD, MS, FICD, is Professor and Chairman of the Department of Periodontics and Preventive Sciences at the University of Mississippi School of Dentistry. He is also a Diplomate of the American Board of Periodontology. Dr. Serio completed his undergraduate studies at Johns Hopkins University and received his D.M.D. degree from the University of Pennsylvania. He earned his M.S. and certificate in Periodontics at the University of Maryland. He was inducted into the International College of Dentists in 2003. He is currently enrolled in the M.B.A. program at Millsaps College. Dr. Serio previously taught at the University of Maryland. His professional interests include educating predoctoral dental students, the pathogenesis of aggressive periodontitis, periodontal plastic surgery, international volunteer dentistry, and the continuing dental education of general dentists. He has presented more than 100 lectures and continuing education courses in the United States and around the world. He is founder and director of the Dominican Dental Mission Project, which has received both The President's Volunteer Action Award and The Daily Points of Light Award. He has also been actively involved in Dentistry Overseas, a joint project between the American Dental Association and Health Volunteers Overseas, and many other international volunteer dental activities. Dr. Serio has written or co-authored more than 35 scientific articles and three books.

Teresa Sherfy, RHIT, is the Performance Improvement Coordinator at Hospice of Southern Illinois in Belleville, Illinois. She is a graduate of Southwestern Illinois College with an associate degree in Health Information Technology. Mrs. Sherfy has more than eight years of experience working in hospice medical records, performance improvement, compliance, and information systems management.

Gwen D. Smith, RHIA, is a graduate of The College of St. Scholastica Health Information Management program. Having worked for SMDC Home Health, a hospital-based home health agency, she has experience in all aspects of health information management in this setting, including reimbursement and outcomes-based quality improvement. Her expertise also extends to documentation and reimbursement for durable medical equipment utilized in home health.

C. Harrell Weathersby, MSW, PhD, holds a Master's degree in social work and a doctorate in English. He is currently an assistant professor of social work at Southeastern Louisiana University in Hammond, Louisiana. He has served in the past as Executive Director of Region XIV Mental Health Center in Mississippi and Regional Manager for Mental Health Region IX in Louisiana. He has also been employed as Director of the Mississippi State Hospital Division of Community Services, which provides support services to people with severe mental illness who have been discharged from the hospital and as statewide Coordinator of the Community Support Program in the Mississippi Department of Mental Health. He has worked in a variety of human services areas besides mental health, including developmental disability, juvenile justice, and protective services for children. In addition to his ongoing focus on developments in community support treatment modalities for the mentally ill, he has a special interest in the area of cultural diversity as it relates to provision of social services and community development. He was honored with the C. Harrell Weathersby "Father of the Mississippi Alliance for the Mentally Ill" Award, for his assistance in establishing the Alliance for the Mentally Ill chapter in Mississippi. This award is given in his name to an outstanding mental health professional each year at the annual Mississippi AMI Conference for Mental Health Professionals.

Judy S. Westerfield, MEd, is a graduate of Mississippi College and has a Master of Special Education degree from Mississippi State University. Ms. Westerfield has many years of experience in the field of mental retardation and has worked extensively with both institutional and community-based programs serving this population.

Terry Winkler, MD, CLCP, is in private practice in Springfield, Missouri, as a board-certified specialist in physical medicine and rehabilitation and as a subspecialist in spinal cord injury medicine. He is a past medical director of Cox hospital rehabilitation program and medical director of the Curative Rehabilitation Center, a freestanding outpatient rehabilitation program. His practice focuses on spinal cord injury, acquired brain injury, amputations, and life care planning. Dr. Winkler serves on committees reviewing research grants concerning spinal cord injury, and peer reviews articles for publication in the Archives of Physical Medicine and Rehabilitation. Dr. Winkler has numerous publications regarding life care planning and has contributed to every major text in the field of life care planning, contributed to a college text on rehabilitation record systems, has written on the effects of aging with spinal cord injury, and will serve as the medical editor of the new *Guide to Rehabilitation*. Dr. Winkler holds an academic appointment as clinical associate faculty at the University of Florida—Gainesville, where he teaches life care planning. At Southern Missouri State University in Springfield, Missouri, he teaches differential diagnosis to the masters-level physical therapy students. Dr. Winkler's undergraduate training at Louisiana Tech University included a double major in premedical studies and medical record administration. He attended the Louisiana State University School of Medicine and then completed residency training in rehabilitation medicine in Little Rock, Arkansas. Past honors include The Americas Award, Alumnus of the Year at Louisiana Tech University, "Who's Who among Young Americans," and the Jean Claude Belot Award from the Harvard University health sciences program. In addition to his active medical practice, Dr. Winkler is a certified life care planner, serves as a commissioner on the Commission for Health Care Certification, the Foundation of Life Care Planning, and the editorial board of the *Journal of Life Care Planning*.

Karen Wright, MHSA, RHIA, RHIT, has a Master of Health Administration from Ohio University and a bachelor's degree in Health Information Administration from Ohio State University. She has been the coordinator and instructor of Health Information Technology at Hocking College for the past 15 years. In addition to being the transcription supervisor and then director of a medical record department in a 365-bed acute care hospital, Karen has been a consultant at acute care hospitals; nursing, chemical dependency, and behavioral health care facilities; as well as for physician's private practices.

Scott Wright, MBA, has a Masters of Business Administration from Ohio University and has served as the Director of the Small Business Development Center at Ohio University. He is an instructor of Finance at Ohio University, where he has taught for the past 17 years. He has most recently traveled to Germany and Italy directing student consulting projects for various businesses. In addition, Scott has owned and operated many types of businesses.

Chapter 1

Introduction

Ann H. Peden, MBA, RHIA, CCS

Learning Objectives

Upon successful completion of this chapter, you should be able to:

1. Describe important changes affecting health care delivery in the United States.
2. Explain the impact of health care changes on the health information manager.
3. Identify expanding opportunities available to health information managers.

The Changing Face of Health Care in America

U.S. Hospitals and Twentieth-Century Health Care

The twentieth century saw numerous changes in the delivery of health care services. Before the twentieth century, hospitals were perceived as places where people went to die. Antibiotics had not yet been developed, and hospitals offered very little in the way of technology. There was no effective oversight of hospital operations by any outside regulatory authority. However, the twentieth century began a new era for hospitals. For example, in 1910, the **Flexner Report** examined the state of medical education in the United States. The authors of this report, who had been commissioned by the Carnegie Foundation, emphasized the importance of hospital-based training in preparing competent physicians (Litman and Robins, 1991). Shortly after publication of that report, the **American College of Surgeons (ACS)** was founded and began establishing standards for hospitals as part of its mission to improve the quality of care for surgical patients (ACS, 2003). The Flexner Report and the ACS's hospital standardization program inaugurated needed changes that improved the quality of hospital care and increased the American public's expectations of hospitals.

The first health information managers, or "medical record librarians" as they were then called, played an important role in efforts to improve patient care in hospitals. The American College of Surgeons' hospital standardization program emphasized the importance of maintaining medical records, and subsequent accrediting agencies, such as the Joint Commission on Accreditation of Healthcare Organizations (JCAHO), have continued to emphasize the role of accurate and complete health information in providing high-quality patient care.

In 1946, the **Hill-Burton Act** authorized an investigation to determine the need for more hospitals and provided money for their construction. Admissions to hospitals increased dramatically during the mid-twentieth century, as did hospital costs. This period of hospital expansion resulted in increased opportunities for health information practitioners, because at that time a large majority of health information managers practiced in hospital settings.

The latter part of the twentieth century experienced continued changes in health care. Payment issues, technological advances, and changes in society all had an impact on the delivery of health care at the turn of the millennium.

Payment Issues Affecting Health Care Delivery

Payment issues have had a tremendous impact on health care delivery in the United States during the late twentieth and early twenty-first centuries. With an increasing number of patients insured under federal and state health programs, changes in payment mechanisms for these programs have affected all types of health care settings.

Overview of Federal and Federal-State Health Programs

In 1965, Congress enacted as amendments to the Social Security Act, Title XVIII and Title XIX, commonly known as Medicare and Medicaid. **Medicare** (Title XVIII) provides health benefits for social security recipients and other qualified individuals and consists of two parts—Part A, Hospital Insurance, and Part B, Medical Insurance. Part A helps pay for hospital inpatient care, some home health care, skilled nursing care, and hospice care. Part B provides coverage for physician services, hospital outpatient services, some home health care, medical equipment and supplies, and other health services. Medicare beneficiaries pay a monthly premium for the Part B benefit, but not for Part A (CMS, 2003b).

Medicaid (Title XIX) provides medical assistance to lower income individuals and families. Federal and state governments jointly fund the Medicaid program. Because each state establishes and administers its own program, Medicaid services and eligibility requirements vary from state to state (CMS, 2002).

Congress created the **State Children's Health Insurance Program (SCHIP)** as part of the Balanced Budget Act of 1997. SCHIP, also known as Title XXI, allows states to offer health insurance plans for children, up to age 19, who are not already insured.

SCHIP affords families who earn too much to qualify for Medicaid an opportunity to obtain health insurance for their children (CMS, 2003e). The increase in federal and state health insurance programs has made governmental regulations and payment systems important factors in health care delivery.

Payment Changes Affected Hospitals First

When Medicare was implemented in 1966, it paid for health care benefits under a **fee-for-service** plan, which operated in a manner similar to most health insurance plans of the day. Health care providers received a fee for each service provided—each office visit, each day in the hospital, each treatment, and so on. As the costs of this program continued to escalate, the federal government began to look at ways to hold them down, initially by targeting hospital costs. In 1982, enactment of the Medicare inpatient **prospective payment system (PPS)** (a system based on payment amounts determined before services are rendered) forced hospitals into a new way of looking at utilization of their services. This signaled a change in the locations and methods of delivery of health care for the future. Medicare payments to hospitals switched from a **per diem** (per day) basis to a per case basis. Before the prospective payment arrangement, hospitals received payment for each day that the patient stayed in the hospital (per diem). However, prospective payment based any reimbursement primarily on the patient's condition and surgical treatment, regardless of the number of days the patient stayed in the hospital. Under prospective payment, the hospital's cash flow improved if patients were discharged earlier, because costs for extra days in the hospital could not be adequately recovered from Medicare. Hospitals, particularly those with a high volume of Medicare patients, began to have an incentive to encourage shorter inpatient stays and to treat patients in the least costly setting possible. In some states, payers other than Medicare began to implement prospective payment. Increasingly, hospitals began to emphasize programs that shifted care from inpatient settings to alternate care settings, such as outpatient and home care.

Health information managers are crucial to a hospital's success under prospective payment because the data provided by health information services is the basis for inpatient reimbursement under Medicare. Just as the American College of Surgeons' hospital standardization program first brought attention to the role that the then medical record librarians played in the provision of quality patient care in hospitals, Medicare's prospective payment system highlighted the role that health information managers play in the financial health of hospitals. Data transformed into information by health information services continues to be an important factor in numerous decisions hospitals must make in the twenty-first century, such as decisions regarding contracts with managed care organizations.

Managed care organizations (discussed more fully in Chapter 4) became a force during the 1990s, further lowering hospital utilization rates. The earliest so-called prepaid health care models, such as Kaiser Permanente in the western United States, have been in existence since the 1930s (Kaiser Permanente, Online). In the mid-1970s, the federal government stimulated the development of one type of managed care organization, the health maintenance organization (HMO). The name "health maintenance organization" relates to the financial incentive for the health care provider to keep patients healthy. A common method of paying providers in an HMO is the **capitation** model. Under capitation, providers are paid based on the number of patients they agree to treat, rather than on the number of services they provide. Therefore, it is more profitable to the provider if the patient requires fewer services. These types of plans emphasize prevention of disease (health maintenance). When disease occurs, however, treatment is provided in the least costly setting. The number of patients enrolled in various types of managed care programs has increased significantly, continuing the shift of care from the inpatient setting to other less costly health care settings.

Effects of Payment and Financial Changes on Other Settings

Other settings, such as ambulatory care, home health, and long-term care, have been affected both directly and indirectly by payment and other financial changes.

The hospital inpatient prospective payment system (IPPS) obviously affected the delivery of care to hospital inpatients. The IPPS, along with a shift toward managed care, contributed to the increased utilization of ambulatory health care services (services provided in settings where patients generally do not stay overnight). With more patients receiving treatment in ambulatory settings, payers began monitoring ambulatory data and payment more carefully.

Starting with payments to physicians, Congress enacted a law in 1991 creating a professional fee schedule (PFS), which was implemented in 1992 (CMS, 2003d). Before the implementation of the fee schedule, Medicare payments to physicians were based on charges. If the physician's charge was in line with what other physicians in the same specialty usually charged for that service, Medicare would pay its share of the charge. When the fee schedule was implemented, it quantified the physician work, practice expense, and malpractice expense of each service to determine what that service was "worth" relative to other services. Implementation of a payment system based on the "relative value" of services removed from participating physicians the ability to establish their own charges for Medicare patients. Payments under the fee schedule are based on codes representing services performed by physicians and other qualified providers. (More information on the relative value system can be found in Chapter 3.)

In 2000, Medicare began paying hospitals for ambulatory care under an outpatient prospective payment system (OPPS), which is based on codes submitted by the hospital. (See Chapter 2.) As with the hospital IPPS, adequate documentation and accurate coding are extremely important, along with an understanding of the complex regulations governing the PPS. For both physicians and hospitals, greater demands are being placed on the health information systems of ambulatory health care providers. Health information managers are knowledgeable in coding, billing, and clinical documentation—all crucial components in the increasingly complex health data environment facing ambulatory health care.

Medicare payment changes have also affected other health care settings. Skilled nursing facilities came under a prospective payment system in 1998. (See Chapter 10.) The home health prospective payment system became effective in the year 2000. (See Chapter 12.) A prospective payment system for inpatient rehabilitation hospital services (Chapter 11) was implemented in January 2002, followed by implementation of a PPS for long-term care hospitals (Chapter 10) in October of that year (CMS, 2003c). Although the hospital-oriented PPSs are based largely on diagnostic and procedural coding, other PPSs rely on additional types of clinical data that are captured on patient assessment instruments periodically throughout each episode of care. (See Table 1-1 for an overview of Medicare PPSs.) Health information managers with skills in systems analysis can be valuable team members in ensuring a smooth flow of accurate data for any prospective payment system.

Table 1-1   Medicare Prospective Payment Systems

Setting	*Basis for Payment*	*Key Data Collection Instruments*	*Year Implemented*
Hospital Inpatient	Diagnosis Related Groups (DRGs)	Uniform Bill-92 (UB-92)	1982
Skilled Nursing Facilities	Resource Utilization Groups (RUGs)	Minimum Data Set (MDS)	1998
Hospital Outpatient	Ambulatory Payment Classifications (APCs)	Uniform Bill-92 (UB-92)	2000
Home Health	Home Health Resource Groups (HHRGs)	Outcomes and Assessment Information Set (OASIS)	2000
Inpatient Rehabilitation	Case Mix Groups (CMGs)	Inpatient Rehabilitation Facility Patient Assessment Instrument (IRF-PAI)	2002
Long-term Care Hospitals	Long-term Care Diagnosis Related Groups (LTC-DRGs)	Uniform Bill-92 (UB-92)	2002

Source: *Medicare Payment Systems and Coding Files*, Centers for Medicare and Medicaid Services. http://www.cms.hhs.gov/paymentsystems (CMS, 2003)

Other Regulatory and Accreditation Issues Affecting Health Care

Much attention has been focused on health care financing issues in recent years. However, many other challenges face today's health care organizations, ranging from standardization of electronic transactions to implementation of new accreditation processes.

The Health Insurance Portability and Accountability Act of 1996 (HIPAA)

The **Health Insurance Portability and Accountability Act of 1996 (HIPAA)** was enacted to achieve many purposes. As the name implies, one purpose of this legislation was to address the problem of the rising number of uninsured and underinsured Americans by making health insurance portable. For example, HIPAA allows a person with a preexisting medical condition to obtain insurance benefits related to that condition when changing jobs. Another aspect of HIPAA addresses problems of health care fraud and abuse. However, the provisions of HIPAA that have had the greatest impact on health care providers have been its **administrative simplification** provisions. (See Figure 1-1 for an overview of the HIPAA legislation.)

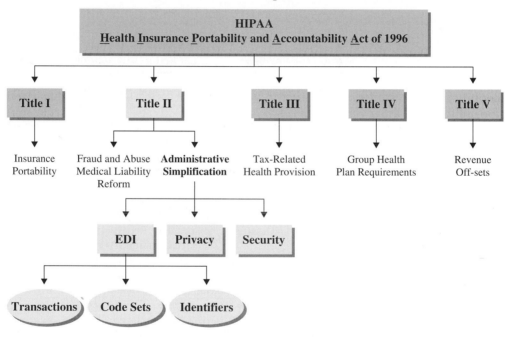

Figure 1-1   How the administrative simplification provisions fit into the overall framework of the Health Insurance Portability and Accountability Act of 1996. Source: *Centers for Medicare & Medicaid Services, Implementing the HIPAA Regulations: A Readiness Workshop for the Small Provider.*

To whom do the administrative simplification provisions apply? **Covered entities (CEs)** under HIPAA are health plans, health care clearinghouses, and health care providers who transmit health information in electronic form (Standards for privacy of individually identifiable health information, 2000).

The rationale for the administrative simplification provisions of HIPAA is that the Unites States spends too much on administrative processes. Consider the following information quoted from the Centers for Medicare & Medicaid Services (CMS):

- Over $1.3 trillion is spent annually in healthcare (more than one-eighth of U.S. economy; close to 14% of GDP; most industrialized nations spend 7% of GDP)
- Over 15% (up to 30%) goes to administration ($200–$400 billion!)
- Lack of e-commerce and electronic exchange of information = higher costs; more fragmented system; poorer quality of care
- Unconnected individuals trying to coordinate care means more, not fewer problems (CMS, 2003a, p. 4)

Although the goals of HIPAA are lofty, achieving them continues to require a substantial investment on the part of health care providers and health plans. Regulations implementing the administrative simplification provisions of HIPAA have been phased in over a period of years. The final rule for transactions was published in 2000, but most covered entities were not required to implement the rule until 2003 because of the two-year regulatory time frame and because of the provision of an additional one-year extension. The HIPAA privacy rule was also published in 2000, updated in 2002, and implemented in 2003 for most covered entities. The security rule was published in 2003, with the compliance deadline for most covered entities established for 2005. This demonstrates the extended time frame required for publication and implementation of the various components of HIPAA.

Health information managers play an important role in the implementation of HIPAA standards. For example, HIPAA's electronic data interchange (EDI) standards include standards for code sets, an arena in which health information managers possess expertise. The August 17, 2000, final rule regarding transactions and standardized code sets for EDI included the following code set standards:

a. *International Classification of Diseases, 9th Edition, Clinical Modification (ICD-9-CM), Volumes 1 and 2*

b. *International Classification of Diseases, 9th Edition, Clinical Modification, Volume 3, Procedures*

c. *National Drug Codes (NDC)*

d. *Code on Dental Procedures and Nomenclature (CDT)*

e. The combination of *Health Care Common Procedure Coding System (HCPCS)* and *Current Procedural Terminology© (CPT)*

(Standards for electronic transactions, 2000).

Will the code sets announced in 2000 continue as HIPAA standards indefinitely? In 2003, the American Health Information Management Association (AHIMA) published a position statement urging the U.S. Department of Health and Human Services (DHHS) to update the code set standards. Specifically, AHIMA called on DHHS to replace ICD-9-CM with ICD-10-CM for diagnoses and ICD-10-PCS for procedures. (ICD-10-PCS is the ICD-10 Procedure Coding System, which would replace Volume 3 of ICD-9-CM.) Both of these systems offer greater detail and more current terminology than ICD-9-CM. ICD-10-CM and ICD-10-PCS also provide greater capacity for future expansion. Furthermore, ICD-10-CM is compatible with ICD-10, the World Health Organization's classification system, which is used by most other countries (AHIMA, 2003). If DHHS publishes a rule making ICD-10-CM and ICD-10-PCS official code set standards under HIPAA, there would be a minimum of two years from the date the rule is published before the new code sets would be implemented.

As long-standing advocates for confidentiality of patient information, health information managers also play a key role in the implementation of the HIPAA privacy rule. The privacy rule established regulations for handling **protected health information (PHI)**, which is any individually identifiable health information. Figure 1-2 lists selected sections of the privacy rule pertaining to PHI.

The privacy rule is quite complex, and only a brief overview of HIPAA privacy is provided here. (The complete rule and other educational materials are available at the CMS Web site, http://www.cms.hhs.gov.) The privacy rule describes how PHI, whether in paper or electronic form, may be used or disclosed. In general, an authorization from the patient or legal representative is required for use or disclosure of PHI. The authorization must contain certain core elements, such as a description of the information to be used or disclosed, who is authorized to make the disclosure, to whom the covered entity may make the requested use or disclosure, the purpose of the requested use or disclosure, an expiration date or event, and the signature of the individual and date. The authorization must also contain certain required statements, such as the individual's right to revoke the authorization in writing. However, a covered entity is permitted to use or disclose PHI for treatment, payment, or health care operations (TPO), within the definitions of the regulation, without a specific authorization for each use or disclosure. HIPAA also requires that each covered entity provide its patients with a written notice of privacy practices (NPP) that explains how the covered entity might use or disclose the individual's health information. The NPP also must contain certain required elements and statements. The privacy rule also explains how the individual may restrict uses and disclosures of PHI as well as the individual's right to access or amend PHI. Furthermore, an individual has a right to receive an accounting of disclosures of PHI made by a covered entity in the six years before the date on which the accounting is requested, with exceptions for certain types of disclosures.

Whereas the privacy rule protects PHI in both paper and electronic formats, the purpose of the security rule is to protect PHI that is maintained in electronic form. Each covered entity must analyze its systems for the electronic maintenance and transmission of PHI to identify and correct security risks. Security risks can be anything from unauthorized "hacking" of information systems to damage caused by natural disasters. There are some required elements in the security standards, but some of the implementation specifications are stated to be "addressable." For addressable implementation specifications, the covered entity must describe how it will implement the

Subpart E—Privacy of Individually Identifiable Health Information

164.500 Applicability.

164.501 Definitions.

164.502 Uses and disclosures of protected health information: General rules.

164.504 Uses and disclosures: Organizational requirements.

164.506 Consent for uses or disclosures to carry out treatment, payment, and health care operations.

164.508 Uses and disclosures for which an authorization is required.

164.510 Uses and disclosures requiring an opportunity for the individual to agree or to object.

164.512 Uses and disclosures for which consent, an authorization, or opportunity to agree or object is not required.

164.514 Other requirements relating to uses and disclosures of protected health information.

164.520 Notice of privacy practices for protected health information.

164.522 Rights to request privacy protection for protected health information.

164.524 Access of individuals to protected health information.

164.526 Amendment of protected health information.

164.528 Accounting of disclosures of protected health information.

164.530 Administrative requirements.

164.532 Transition requirements.

164.534 Compliance dates for initial implementation of the privacy standards.

Authority: 42 U.S.C. 1320d–2 and 1320d–4, sec. 264 of Pub. L. 104–191, 110 Stat. 2033–2034 (42 U.S.C. 1320(d–2(note)).

Figure 1-2   Section numbers and titles of regulations implementing the HIPAA privacy rule with regard to protected health information. Source: Standards for privacy of individually identifiable health information; final rule. (2000, December 28). *Federal Register*, pp. 82461–82829.

required standards in a manner that is appropriate for the environment of the facility (Amatayakul, 2003). To minimize security risks, system users need to be identified and properly authenticated, audit trails and logs should be maintained and reviewed, appropriate backup systems should be in place, the members of the workforce should be educated about system security, and so on. The American Health Information Management Association (AHIMA) and the Healthcare Information and Management Systems Society (HIMSS) are good sources of information for health information managers with regard to HIPAA security issues. (See the Key Resources section at the end of the chapter for AHIMA and HIMSS contact information and Web sites.)

Accreditation Issues Affecting Health Care

Health care organizations generally must be licensed by the state. **Licensure** is a governmental process that requires that a facility meet certain regulations set by the state in order to provide care. Many health care organizations also choose to pursue **accreditation**, which is a voluntary process in which facilities agree to follow a set of standards and receive recognition for having met those standards. The health care settings described in this book may be accredited by a variety of organizations, whose accreditation standards are regularly updated and whose accreditation processes may also change. For example, in 2002, the Joint Commission on Accreditation of Healthcare Organizations (JCAHO) announced a new accreditation process called "Shared Visions—New Pathways," with implementation for all its accreditation programs scheduled for 2004. JCAHO's new process changed the procedures used during an on-site survey, the scoring process, as well as the types of accreditation decisions. Health information managers play an important role in the accreditation process and should stay up-to-date regarding the latest information from the organizations that accredit their facilities. Table 1-2 provides an overview of the settings covered in this textbook and some of the accrediting organizations for each setting. Contact information for these organizations is listed in the Key Resources section of the appropriate chapters.

Other Regulatory Issues Affecting Health Care

Many health care settings are also affected by federal regulations known as *Conditions of Participation* or *Conditions for Coverage*. Health care organizations that want to "participate" in federal programs must be **Medicare certified**, which means they have demonstrated that they meet the standards set forth in the relevant *Conditions of Participation/Coverage*. Routine surveys to determine whether health care organizations meet these standards are conducted by the designated **state agency** for each state. In addition to administering the federal requirements for participation in Medicare and Medicaid programs, the state agency ordinarily administers applicable state licensure requirements as well. Because the state agency conducts its surveys in accordance with federal guidelines, CMS publishes detailed instructions for state surveyors in its *State Operations Manual (SOM)*. The appendices to the *SOM* contain survey forms and other instructions specific to each setting that health information managers may find helpful (see Figure 1-3).

The federal government has granted "deeming" authority to certain voluntary accrediting organizations for some of their programs. This means that a health care provider who is accredited by such an organization is "deemed" to meet the *Conditions of Participation* and does not have to undergo a separate survey process by the state agency. This concept is known as **deemed status**. However, for many of the health care settings described in this book, deemed status is not available, meaning that if these facilities choose voluntary accreditation, they are still required to undergo regular surveys by the state agency as well. (See the Web Activity section at the end of the chapter to locate one accrediting organization's list of deemed status options.)

Table 1-2   Health Care Settings and Examples of Relevant Voluntary Accrediting Organizations
(Note: This list is not exhaustive.)

Chapters	Setting	Organizations
2	Hospital-based Ambulatory Care	American Osteopathic Association Joint Commission on Accreditation of Healthcare Organizations
3	Freestanding Ambulatory Care	Accreditation Association for Ambulatory Health Care Commission for the Accreditation of Freestanding Birth Centers Joint Commission on Accreditation of Healthcare Organizations American Association for Accreditation of Ambulatory Surgery Facilities
4	Managed Care	Accreditation Association for Ambulatory Health Care Joint Commission on Accreditation of Healthcare Organizations National Committee for Quality Assurance
6	Correctional Facilities	American Correctional Association Joint Commission on Accreditation of Healthcare Organizations National Commission on Correctional Health Care
7 and 8	Mental Health and Substance Abuse	Commission on Accreditation of Rehabilitation Facilities Joint Commission on Accreditation of Healthcare Organizations
9	Facilities for Individuals with Mental Retardation or Developmental Disabilities	Commission on Accreditation of Rehabilitation Facilities Council on Quality and Leadership in Supports for People with Disabilities Joint Commission on Accreditation of Healthcare Organizations
10	Long-term Care	Joint Commission on Accreditation of Healthcare Organizations
11	Rehabilitation Facilities	Commission on Accreditation of Rehabilitation Facilities Joint Commission on Accreditation of Healthcare Organizations
12	Home Health Care	Community Health Accreditation Program Joint Commission on Accreditation of Healthcare Organizations
13	Hospice	Joint Commission on Accreditation of Healthcare Organizations
15	Veterinary	American Animal Hospital Association

Technological and Other Issues Affecting the Delivery of Health Care

Although the preceding paragraphs have emphasized financial and payment-related forces affecting health care delivery, several other factors have contributed to the changes in health care delivery. For example, another change that is occurring in health care is a shift from independent institutions and practitioners to networks of health care providers. Hospitals, physicians, and other health care providers have joined together to provide the broad range of services necessary to meet the expectations of the various types of health care plans currently available. Sharing of information among the various providers in such a network can be very limited or quite extensive. The **community**

Appendix	Title
A	Survey Procedures for the Application of Conditions of Participation for **Hospitals**—Interpretive Guidelines
AA	**Psychiatric Hospitals**—Interpretive Guidelines and Survey Procedures
B	Survey Procedures for the Application of Conditions of Participation for **Home Health Agencies**—Interpretive Guidelines
C	Survey Procedures for the Application of Conditions for Coverage for **Independent Laboratories**—Interpretive Guidelines
D	Survey Procedures for the Application of Conditions for Coverage for **Portable X-Ray Service**—Interpretive Guidelines
E	Survey Procedures for the Application of Conditions for Participation for **Outpatient Physical Therapy/Speech Pathology Services**—Interpretive Guidelines
F	Survey Procedures for the Application of Conditions of Participation for **Physical Therapists in Independent Practice**—Interpretive Guidelines
G	Survey Procedures for the Application of Conditions for Coverage for **Rural Health Clinics**—Interpretive Guidelines
H	Survey Procedures for the Application of Conditions for Coverage for **End Stage Renal Disease Facilities**—Interpretive Guidelines
I	Guidelines for Completion of Fire Safety Survey Reports—Interpretive Guidelines for **Life Safety Code** Surveys
J	Survey Procedures and Interpretive Guidelines for **Intermediate Care Facilities for the Mentally Retarded**
K	Interpretive Guidelines for **Comprehensive Outpatient Rehabilitation Facilities (CORFs)**
L	Interpretive Guidelines and Survey Procedures for **Ambulatory Surgical Services**
M	Interpretive Guidelines—**Hospices**
N	Surveyor Procedures for **Pharmaceutical Service Requirements in Long-Term Care Facilities**
P	Survey Protocol for **Long-Term Care Facilities**
Q	Guidelines for Determining Immediate and Serious Threat to **Patient Health and Safety**
R	Resident Assessment for **Long-Term Care Facilities**
S	Interpretive Guidelines for **Screening Mammography**
T	Guidance to Surveyors, **Swing-Bed Hospitals**
V	Interpretive Guidelines and Investigative Procedures for Responsibilities of Medicare Participating **Hospitals in Emergency Cases**
W	Survey Tasks and Interpretive Guidelines for **Rural Primary Care Hospitals**

Figure 1-3 Appendices to CMS Pub 7, *State Operations Manual.* Source: Centers for Medicare & Medicaid Services. http://www.cms.hhs.gov/manuals/pub07pdf/AP-TOC.pdf [2003, December 16].

health information network (CHIN) is one method for providing quick access to clinical data within a network of providers. A CHIN is a computer network that links data provided by various health care providers. For example, a physician in a private clinic would be able to access patient laboratory results provided by a separately operated private laboratory. Sharing of information in this manner can help avoid the expense of duplicate tests and can promote higher quality of care. However, CHINs should be developed in such a way that confidentiality and security of information are maintained. The growth of CHINs presents an opportunity for health information managers to assist with the development of policies and procedures to provide for information security and data integrity (McLendon, 1996).

The practice of **patient-focused care**, which organizes care delivery around the patient rather than around structured departments, has developed in various hospitals. An institution striving for patient-focused care may reorganize many functions once carried out by various departments and assign those functions to a patient-centered team. As health care institutions rethink the way that care is provided, services that were once centralized in a physical location distant from the patient care area have been decentralized and provided by teams nearer to the patient. In some instances, health information functions have been assigned to multiskilled workers on a patient care unit, resulting in a smaller staff in centralized health information services.

Technological advances have also had an important impact on delivery of health care services. As technology has improved, it has become possible to render treatment in other settings that had once required days or weeks of hospital inpatient care. Patients undergo procedures in ambulatory surgery centers and go home after a short (four- to six-hour) waiting period, thus avoiding costs associated with an overnight stay in a hospital. Other treatments once provided only in hospitals are now provided to patients at home, bringing health care practitioners and equipment to the patient's residence. With the advent of **telemedicine**, patients and clinicians separated by hundreds of miles can interact with one another by electronic means. In a telemedicine session, the patient generally is in a remote location from the physician, and medical information is transmitted back and forth between the two locations by video, electronic mail, telephone, satellite, or other electronic means (American Health Information Management Association, 1997). This new technology presents new challenges in health information management with regard to confidentiality and security of information, and maintenance of appropriate licensure and regulatory requirements.

Because patients are treated in a variety of settings, health care professionals have recognized the need for a **longitudinal patient record**, which would maintain health care information throughout the patient's life. Within a given enterprise (which can range from a single facility to a complex integrated health care delivery system), electronic data can be stored in a clinical data repository (CDR). Access to the data in the CDR can be structured to provide clinicians with a view of the patient's data over time through a single point of entry (Soule, 2001). Although this technology produces a longitudinal view of data within the enterprise, lack of data from providers outside the enterprise prevents such a system from maintaining a complete lifetime view of patient data. However, an online personal health record can overcome these limitations. According to the Markle Foundation, a **personal health record (PHR)** is "an Internet-based set of tools that allows people to access and coordinate their lifelong health information and make appropriate parts of it available to those who need it" (2003, p. 2). The Markle Foundation goes on to describe the following attributes of a PHR:

- Each person controls his or her own PHR. Individuals decide which parts of their PHR can be accessed, by whom, and for how long.
- PHRs contain information from one's entire lifetime.
- PHRs contain information from all health care providers.
- PHRs are accessible from any place at any time.
- PHRs are private and secure.
- PHRs are "transparent." Individuals can see who entered each piece of data, where it was transferred from, and who has viewed it.
- PHRs permit easy exchange of information with other health information systems and health professionals (2003, pp. 2–3).

Is there any relationship between a CDR and a PHR? A CDR can contribute toward a PHR in that some CDRs provide personal health record capabilities that allow patients to view their own information and to communicate with their health care providers (Soule, 2001).

CDRs and PHRs are just two aspects of electronic health information management, which is becoming increasingly important. Groups ranging from the Institute of Medicine to the U.S. General Accounting Office have emphasized improvements in the quality of patient care, patient safety, and cost savings that could be achieved through the implementation of information technology. The ultimate information technology goal for many health care organizations is to achieve an **electronic health record (EHR)** that goes beyond merely storing and retrieving data in a repository. EHRs that include capabilities such as generating clinical alerts and reminders and providing readily available decision support can provide patient care benefits in all health care settings.

In addition to technological trends, changes in society are affecting health care providers. The average age of the U.S. population is increasing, and more Americans are suffering from chronic diseases and illnesses associated with advancing age. Long-term care facilities, home health agencies, hospices, and dialysis facilities are important in caring for patients with chronic and sometimes terminal diseases. Both elderly and younger patients benefit from services provided by rehabilitation facilities and mental health services. Societal problems related to addictive behavior have increased the need for substance abuse treatment facilities. Problems in American society have also resulted in a large prison population, increasing the need for health care in correctional institutions. Good health information management practices are important in the care of all of these special populations.

Impact on the Role of the Health Information Manager

Regulatory, technological, and social changes have affected the role of the health information manager. Although the profession of health information management (HIM) originated in the acute care hospital setting, the shift from inpatient to other care settings has expanded opportunities for health information managers beyond this traditional role. In the acute care setting, the skills of the health information manager are vital because quality information is more important than ever to the hospital. In today's hospital, a health information manager is as likely to be found working in the emergency department coordinating the collection of trauma data as in the file area supervising retention and retrieval of records. Although many acute care facilities have reduced the ranks of middle managers, many excellent opportunities are still available in the acute care setting for those who possess the data analysis and information management skills to help a hospital thrive in this increasingly data-driven health care environment. However, the greatest growth in employment opportunities for health information managers is occurring outside the purely acute care setting.

As stated earlier, other issues affecting health care delivery, such as changing patient demographics and societal factors, have increased the number of persons needing certain types of health care services (e.g., long-term care, care in correctional facilities). Health information managers are currently being employed in an ever-widening array of health care facilities. Ambulatory care facilities, health maintenance organizations, home health care agencies, hospices, dialysis facilities, long-term care facilities, rehabilitation organizations, facilities for the mentally retarded or developmentally disabled, mental health facilities, treatment centers for substance abuse, correctional facilities, dental clinics, and veterinary clinics recognize the importance of the skills possessed by the health information manager. Health care providers in a wide variety of settings look to health information managers for expertise as employees or as consultants. Excellent resources for HIM professionals interested in developing and maintaining skills in diverse practice arenas may be found in the communities of practice (CoPs) sponsored by AHIMA. The CoPs provide a forum for information sharing among health information professionals with specialized interests. The communities are dynamic—new communities may be created and inactive communities may be dissolved in response to the needs of the participants. In 2003, CoPs that offered information relevant to topics covered in this text included APCs (Chapter 2, hospital-based ambulatory care), Ambulatory Care Physician Practice (Chapter 3, freestanding ambulatory care), Behavioral Health (Chapters 7–9, mental health, substance abuse, and developmental disability settings), to name only a few. AHIMA members may access the CoPs at AHIMA's Web site. (See the Key Resources section at the end of the chapter.)

The knowledge and talents of health information managers will continue to be important in the vast assortment of individual provider settings and to the health care system as a whole in light of the growing need for high-quality patient information that is accessible within and across settings in a secure and confidential manner.

Summary

Health care in the United States underwent drastic changes in the twentieth century that have continued into the new millennium. The hospital industry flourished as medical science and technology made strides in the improvement of patient care. As health care costs began to become a public concern, the health care field became more diverse, with a much broader range of care settings available to the patient.

Changes in the health care field have affected the profession of health information management, adding more opportunities. The health information manager's skills in data collection, storage, retrieval, and analysis, which have been long appreciated in the inpatient setting, are now needed and valued in other settings as well. Changes in reimbursement methodologies, in the regulatory environment, in patient care delivery, in information technology, in relationships among health care providers, and in society in general have affected health care and the role of the health information manager. The results have been that additional employment and consulting opportunities are available to health information managers today that did not exist in the past.

Key Terms

accreditation   a voluntary process in which facilities agree to follow a set of standards and receive recognition for having met those standards.

administrative simplification   provisions of the Health Insurance Portability and Accountability Act (HIPAA) that address standardization of electronic data interchange, privacy of health information, and security of health data.

American College of Surgeons (ACS)   a professional organization founded in 1913 to "improve the quality of care for the surgical patient by setting high standards for surgical education and practice" (ACS, 2003, p. 1). In the early twentieth century, the ACS established a hospital standardization program that was the forerunner of today's accreditation organizations.

capitation   a method of payment for health care in which the health care provider receives a monthly payment based on the number of persons the provider has agreed to treat, regardless of the number of persons actually treated or the amount of service rendered.

community health information network (CHIN)   a computer network that links health care providers within a community for the purpose of sharing patient-specific clinical information.

covered entity   under HIPAA, a health plan, a health care clearinghouse, or any health care provider that transmits health information in electronic form.

deemed status   the status of a health care provider that is deemed to meet federal *Conditions of Participation* by virtue of accreditation by a federally approved voluntary accrediting organization. With deemed status, the health care provider's accreditation satisfies the *Conditions of Participation*, and routine surveys by the state agency are unnecessary.

electronic health record (EHR) a system in which a health care provider maintains individual patient health records electronically. Fully developed EHRs include capabilities such as generating clinical alerts and reminders and providing readily available decision support.

fee-for-service a method of payment for health care in which the health care provider charges and is paid for each item of service provided.

Flexner Report a report published in 1910 examining the state of medical education in the United States and Canada. The Flexner Report resulted in sweeping changes in the way North American physicians were educated.

Health Insurance Portability and Accountability Act of 1996 (HIPAA) also known as the Kassebaum-Kennedy Act, HIPAA provisions include the portability of health care benefits (for example, upon an individual's changing employment), prevention of fraud and abuse in health care, and simplification of electronic interchange of health care data, while improving the privacy and security of health information.

Hill-Burton Act the "Hospital Survey and Construction Act" enacted by Congress in 1946. This legislation provided federal money to determine the need for more hospitals and to pay for their construction. (Note: Facilities receiving Hill-Burton funds agreed to provide a reasonable volume of service to patients who are unable to pay, an obligation that is still monitored by the federal government today.)

licensure a governmental process in which a facility must meet certain regulations, set by the state, in order to provide care.

longitudinal patient record a record documenting a patient's health status, conditions, and treatments throughout his or her life, and across multiple facilities, providers, and health care encounters.

Medicaid Title XIX of the 1965 Amendments to the Social Security Act, Medicaid is jointly funded by federal and state governments and provides medical assistance to lower income individuals and families.

Medicare Title XVIII of the 1965 Amendments to the Social Security Act, Medicare provides health benefits for social security recipients and other qualified individuals and consists of two parts—Part A, Hospital Insurance, and Part B, Medical Insurance.

Medicare certification process in which a state agency determines that a health care organization meets the standards set forth in the relevant *Conditions of Participation* or *Conditions of Coverage* and is therefore eligible for participation in the Medicare program.

patient-focused care a method of delivering health care that organizes care delivery by patients rather than by departments. An institution striving for patient-focused care may reorganize many functions once carried out by various departments and assign those functions to a patient-centered team.

per diem payment a payment rendered to an institution based on the number of days of service provided.

personal health record (PHR)   "an Internet-based set of tools that allows people to access and coordinate their lifelong health information and make appropriate parts of it available to those who need it" (Markle Foundation, 2003, p. 2).

prospective payment system (PPS)   a payment system in which payment levels for health care services are determined before the services are rendered. In a prospective payment system, the unit of payment is not based solely on the individual services provided, but on payment units that represent general groupings of patient encounters, hospital stays, or episodes of care.

protected health information (PHI)   individually identifiable health information.

state agency   the agency of the state government responsible for administering the federal requirements for participation in Medicare and Medicaid programs. The state agency is ordinarily also charged with administering applicable licensure requirements for the state.

State Children's Health Insurance Program (SCHIP)   also known as Title XXI of the Balanced Budget Act of 1997, SCHIP allows states to offer health insurance plans for children, up to age 19, who are not already insured. SCHIP affords families who earn too much to qualify for Medicaid an opportunity to obtain health insurance for their children.

telemedicine   the practice of medicine in which electronic signals are utilized to transmit clinical information from one site to another. Generally, the patient is in a remote location from the physician, and medical information is transmitted back and forth between the two locations by video, electronic mail, telephone, satellite, or other electronic means.

REVIEW QUESTIONS

Knowledge-based Questions

1. What are some of the changes that have affected hospitals during the twentieth and twenty-first centuries?

2. How have payment issues affected health care delivery?

3. What is fee-for-service payment?

4. What is a per diem payment?

5. As a general rule, what is the basis for payment in a health maintenance organization?

6. Explain the administrative simplification provisions of HIPAA.

7. What is patient-focused care?

8. What impact have the changes in health care had on the health information manager?

9. Into what health care settings other than hospitals have health information managers moved?

Application-based Questions

1. How can the health information manager contribute to improved data quality in a variety of settings?

2. Describe common concerns with regard to health information management in community health information networks, in telemedicine, and in the longitudinal patient record.

3. Select a health care setting other than a hospital. What would you expect the similarities to be between the role of the health information manager in a hospital and in one of the other health care settings? What would you expect the differences to be?

Web Activity

Visit the Joint Commission on Accreditation of Healthcare Organization's Web site at http://www.jcaho.org.

1. Search for information on the "tracer methodology" used by their surveyors under the new JCAHO site visit process. Describe how the tracer methodology works and what its impact might be on health information management.

2. Search for information on "deemed status." Which JCAHO programs offer federal deemed status options?

Case Study

Kerry Kaiser, RHIA, is Getwell Hospital's HIPAA privacy officer and the chair of its HIPAA Compliance Committee. The committee is concerned with all aspects of HIPAA compliance, including transactions, privacy, and security.

1. What items might the committee's agenda include in each of these three areas?

2. Where might Kerry find resources to assist the committee carry out its duties?

References and Suggested Readings

Amatayakul, M. (2003). Translating the language of security (HIPAA on the job series). *Journal of the American Health Information Management Association 74*(6), 16A–16D.

[ACS] American College of Surgeons. (2003, November 12). What is the American College of Surgeons? [Online]. http://www.facs.org/about/corppro.html [2003, December 13].

[AHIMA] American Health Information Management Association. (1997). *Issue: Telemedical Records* [practice brief]. Fletcher, D. M.: Author. [From *Journal of the American Health Information Management Association, 68* (4).]

[AHIMA] American Health Information Management Association. (2003, July 10). Statement in support of prompt adoption of ICD-10-CM and ICD-10-PCS medical code set standards in the United States [Online]. http://library.ahima.org/xpedio/groups/public/documents/ahima/pub_bok1_019951.html [2003, August 6].

Brandt, M. (1993). Roles of health information managers and coders in patient-focused care. *Journal of the American Health Information Management Association, 64* (10), 68–70.

[CMS] Centers for Medicare & Medicaid Services. (2002). *Medicaid: A Brief Summary* [Online]. http://www.cms.hhs.gov/publications/overview-medicare-medicaid/default4.asp [2003, August 5].

[CMS] Centers for Medicare & Medicaid Services. (2003a). *Implementing the HIPAA Regulations: A Readiness Workshop for the Small Provider* [Online]. http://www.cms.hhs.gov/hipaa/hipaa2/events/Updatedslides3.ppt [2003, August 6].

[CMS] Centers for Medicare & Medicaid Services. (2003b). *Medicare and You: 2003* [Online]. http://www.medicare.gov/publications/pubs/pdf/10050.pdf [2003, August 5].

[CMS] Centers for Medicare & Medicaid Services. (2003c). *Medicare Payment Systems and Coding Files* [Online]. http://www.cms.hhs.gov/paymentsystems [2003, August 6].

[CMS] Centers for Medicare & Medicaid Services. (2003d). *Medicare Physician Fee Schedule for 2003* [Online]. http://www.cms.hhs.gov/media/press/release.asp?Counter=712 [2003, August 6].

[CMS] Centers for Medicare & Medicaid Services. (2003e). *State Children's Health Insurance Program (SCHIP)* [Online]. http://www.cms.hhs.gov/schip [2003, August 5].

Health insurance reform: Security standards; final rule. (2003, February 20) *Federal Register,* pp. 8333–8381.

Kaiser Permanente. (Online). Kaiser Permanente: More than 50 Years of Quality. http://www.kaiserpermanente.org/newsroom/history.html [2003, December 13].

Kuehn, L. (Ed.). (1996). *Best of the Brief Encounter: An Ambulatory Care Primer.* Chicago: American Health Information Management Association.

Litman, T., and Robins, L. (1991). *Health Politics and Policy,* 2nd edition. Clifton Park, NY: Thomson Delmar Learning.

Markle Foundation. (2003, July 1). *The personal health working group: Final report* [Online]. http://www.connectingforhealth.org/resources/phwg_final_report.pdf [2003, December 16].

McLendon, K. (1996). Community health information network access. In L. Kuehn (ed.), *Best of the Brief Encounter: An Ambulatory Care Primer* (pp. 121–122). Chicago: American Health Information Management Association.

Prophet, S. (1997). Fraud and abuse implications for the HIM professional. *Journal of the American Health Information Management Association, 68* (4), 52–57.

Soule, D. (2001). What's new in clinical data repositories? *Journal of the American Health Information Management Association 72* (10), 35–39.

Snyderman, R., & Saito, V. Y. (Eds.). (1999). *Integrated Health Delivery Systems: 1999 Duke Private Sector Conference.* Durham, NC: Duke University Health System.

Standards for electronic transactions. (2000, August 17). *Federal Register,* pp. 50311–50373.

Standards for privacy of individually identifiable health information; final rule. (2000, December 28). *Federal Register,* pp. 82461–82829.

Standards for privacy of individually identifiable health information; final rule. (2002, August 14). *Federal Register*, pp. 53181–53273.

Viegas, S. F., & Dunn, K. (1998). *Telemedicine: Practicing in the Information Age.* Philadelphia, PA: Lippincott-Raven Publishers.

Wolterbeek, H., and Wolterbeek, B. (1994). A virtual, longitudinal medical and insurance record. *Journal of the American Health Information Management Association, 65* (9), 50–53.

Key Resources

American College of Surgeons
633 N. Saint Clair St.
Chicago, IL 60611-3211
Phone: 800-621-4111
Fax: 312-202-5001
E-mail: postmaster@facs.org
http://www.facs.org

American Health Information Management Association
233 N. Michigan Avenue, Suite 2150
Chicago, IL 60601-5800
Phone: 312-233-1100
Fax: 312-233-1090
E-mail: info@ahima.org
http://www.ahima.org

The Carnegie Foundation for the Advancement of Teaching
51 Vista Lane
Stanford, CA 94305
Phone: 650-566-5100
http://www.carnegiefoundation.org

Centers for Medicare & Medicaid Services (CMS), Office of Public Affairs
Phone: 202-690-6145
http://www.cms.hhs.gov
For beneficiary questions about Medicare
Phone: 800-MEDICARE
http://www.medicare.gov

Code of Federal Regulations
http://www.gpoaccess.gov/cfr/index.html

Commission on Accreditation of Rehabilitation Facilities
4891 E. Grant Road
Tucson, AZ 85712
Phone: 520-325-1044
Fax: 520-318-1129
http://www.carf.org/

Federal Register
http://www.gpoaccess.gov/fr/index.html

Healthcare Information and Management Systems Society (HIMSS)
230 East Ohio Street, Suite 500
Chicago, IL 60611-3269
Phone: 312-664-4467
Fax: 312-664-6143
http://www.himss.org

Joint Commission on Accreditation of Healthcare Organizations
One Renaissance Blvd.
Oakbrook Terrace, IL 60181
Phone: 630-792-5000
Fax: 630-792-5005
http://www.jcaho.org

Chapter 2

Hospital-Based Ambulatory Care

Ann H. Peden, MBA, RHIA, CCS

Learning Objectives

Upon successful completion of this chapter, you should be able to:

1. Describe types of ambulatory care provided by hospitals.
2. Explain regulatory and accreditation standards that apply to hospital-based ambulatory care.
3. Discuss documentation issues in hospital-based ambulatory care.
4. Describe reimbursement methods for hospital-based ambulatory care.
5. Identify coding and classification systems used in hospital-based ambulatory care.
6. Describe data sets utilized for hospital-based ambulatory care.
7. Cite factors in avoiding legal risk in ambulatory care.
8. Define roles of the health information management professional in hospital-based ambulatory care.

SETTING	DESCRIPTION	SYNONYMS
Hospital Outpatient Unit	An organizational unit of a hospital providing health services to patients who are generally ambulatory and who are not currently inpatients (Glondys, 2000)	Outpatient Department
Hospital Outpatient Clinic	A type of hospital outpatient unit generally organized based on the clinical specialty of the care providers or the types of services needed by the patients (Glondys, 2000)	Clinic
Hospital Emergency Unit	An organizational unit providing medical services needed on an urgent or emergency basis (Glondys, 2000)	Emergency Department
Hospital Observation Unit	An organizational unit for monitoring unstable patients and assessing whether or not they require inpatient admission	Observation Services
Hospital Ambulatory Surgery Unit	An organizational unit for performing elective surgical procedures on patients who generally do not stay at the hospital overnight	Ambulatory Surgery Department
Partial Hospitalization Unit	An organizational unit providing services to behavioral health patients who spend part of the day or night in the hospital setting	Partial Hospitalization Services

Introduction to Setting

Types of Settings

As discussed in Chapter 1, health care delivery continues to shift from acute care settings to other health care settings. Technological advances and changing reimbursement systems have encouraged health care providers to treat many conditions on an outpatient basis. Hospitals, too, have recognized the importance of providing services at less acute levels of service. Statistics bear out the trend toward ambulatory care provided by hospitals. The number of hospital outpatient visits has continued to rise, increasing from 1,681.0 per thousand in the U.S. population in 1997 to 1,890.8 per thousand in 2001. Outpatient surgeries also increased during this period, from 54.8 per thousand to 58.6 per thousand (American Hospital Association, 2003). The percent of hospital revenue contributed by outpatient services grew from 13 percent in the early 1990s to 35 percent at the turn of the millennium (Patrick, 2004). This increased number of outpatient visits has involved a variety of hospital programs, including ambulatory surgery units, hospital clinics, emergency services, observation services, and ancillary services.

Hospital-based **ambulatory surgery**, which began developing in hospitals during the 1970s, is one example of hospital-based ambulatory care that has increased dramatically in recent years. Advances in technology have enabled health care providers to perform many types of surgery on an ambulatory basis that once could be performed only on an inpatient basis. In fact, certain surgical procedures will be reimbursed by third-party payers only when performed in the ambulatory setting (unless a particular patient's condition makes ambulatory surgery unsafe) (Lawrence and Jonas, 1990).

Another type of ambulatory care that has existed in hospitals since the late 1800s is the hospital clinic. Early hospital clinics provided care for the poor and an educational experience for physicians-in-training. With the advent of Medicare and Medicaid, most clinic visits are now reimbursed, which was not always the case before the implementation of these federal programs (Lawrence and Jonas, 1990). Many hospitals still facilitate the teaching function of the clinics by organizing their clinics by medical specialty.

Emergency care is yet another type of ambulatory service provided by hospitals. Most hospitals have an organized emergency department providing a wide range of services. The emergency department may be staffed as a trauma center and be the first area in which an acutely ill patient is treated before hospitalization. In fact, in 1997, 42 percent of the patients admitted to U.S. hospitals were admitted through the emergency department (Mezey, 2002). This chapter, however, focuses on the emergency department as an ambulatory care service, where patients are treated and released. For example, a physician may see his or her private patients in the emergency department to evaluate an acute condition or trauma that occurs outside normal office hours. Other patients present themselves in the emergency department for treatment as outpatients when a primary care physician is not available to them (Lawrence and Jonas, 1990).

One type of outpatient setting that very much resembles the inpatient setting is that of hospital **observation services.** Observation services may be provided in a regular inpatient unit or in a designated observation unit. According to Medicare, observation services are "furnished by a hospital on the hospital's premises, including use of a bed and periodic monitoring by a hospital's nursing or other staff, which are reasonable and necessary to evaluate an outpatient's condition or determine the need for a possible admission to the hospital as an inpatient" (CMS, 2003a, p. 32b.1). The physician should make a determination whether the patient meets criteria for admission as an inpatient within a 24-hour time frame. Some payers have strict rules limiting observation care to 23 hours and 59 minutes, whereas other payers have no strictly enforced limits on observation care. If an observation patient is not admitted to inpatient status, arrangements are made for care in another setting, the patient is discharged or transferred, and the stay is counted and billed as an outpatient encounter.

A **partial hospitalization program (PHP)** is also considered to be a type of hospital outpatient program. Medicare defines partial hospitalization as "a distinct and organized intensive treatment program for patients who would otherwise require inpatient psychiatric care" (CMS, 2003a, p. 32b). In a partial hospitalization program, the patient may receive a variety of services, such as individual or group therapy, occupational therapy, diagnostic services, services of social workers, psychiatric nurses, and other staff, along with other types of services (CMS, 2003a). The patient receives services for a substantial number of hours each day, but is not present at the hospital on a 24-hour basis.

Finally, many settings in the hospital that provide services to inpatients also provide services to outpatients. For example, hospital ancillary services, such as the hospital laboratory or the radiology department, may perform tests on hospital outpatients as well as inpatients.

Types of Patients

Hospital ambulatory care patients come from every walk of life and are treated for a wide range of conditions. Both acute and chronic illnesses can be treated on an ambulatory basis. The following classification of patients is based on the types of services the patients receive rather than on characteristics of the patients themselves (Hanken and Waters, 1994). In general, a **hospital outpatient** is a patient who is evaluated or treated at a hospital facility, but is not admitted to inpatient status. Examples of various categories of hospital outpatients follow:

- **Clinic outpatient:** an outpatient treated in an organized clinic of the hospital in which hospital staff evaluate the patient and manage the patient's care
- **Referred outpatient:** an outpatient who is referred to the hospital for specific services, such as laboratory or radiology examinations. The hospital is responsible only for providing the diagnostic or therapeutic services requested, while the referring physician is responsible for evaluating and managing the patient's care. A related term is *reference laboratory services*, which is used to describe laboratory services performed for other providers. (Note that the term *referral* carries a different meaning when one physician "refers" a patient to another physician. In a physician-to-physician referral, responsibility for evaluating and managing the patient's care *is* often transferred from the referring to the receiving physician.)
- **Emergency outpatient:** an outpatient evaluated and treated in the emergency department of the hospital

Types of Caregivers

Just as there are many different types of hospital ambulatory patients, there are many different types of caregivers who participate in outpatient care. Physicians from every specialty see patients on an outpatient basis. Nurses provide nursing care to outpatients. Other health professionals, such as physical therapists, occupational therapists, clinical laboratory scientists, pharmacists—to name only a few—may provide diagnostic or therapeutic services to hospital outpatients.

One hospital-based ambulatory setting has developed its own specialization. In the hospital emergency department, physicians who are emergency medicine specialists are generally on duty 24 hours a day. Often, other caregivers in the emergency department have received specialized training and certification in basic and advanced life support. Appropriate certifications for hospital emergency department staff are necessary if a hospital wishes to be designated as a regional trauma center (Lawrence and Jonas, 1990).

Regulatory Issues

Licensure

Hospitals must be licensed by the state in which they are located. Licensure requirements vary from state to state. In some states, meeting federal standards or the standards of a voluntary accrediting agency largely fulfills licensing requirements. To obtain the licensure requirements affecting hospital-based ambulatory care for a given state, a health information manager would contact the agency in that state responsible for licensure of hospitals.

Federal Regulations

To be eligible to receive payment from Medicare, the ambulatory services provided by hospitals must meet the federal requirements contained in the *Conditions of Participation for Hospitals* (2002) or be "deemed" to meet these requirements by virtue of voluntary accreditation by an approved agency. Accreditation by either the Joint Commission on Accreditation of Healthcare Organizations (JCAHO) or the American Osteopathic Association (AOA) provides "deemed" status for hospitals with regard to the *Conditions of Participation* (CMS, 2002a).

To meet federal program requirements, each state's own certifying agency surveys nonaccredited hospitals, comparing their practices to standards in the *Conditions of Participation for Hospitals*. In addition, both state-surveyed and voluntarily accredited hospitals may be randomly selected for validation surveys conducted by the Centers for Medicare & Medicaid Services (CMS).

Whether or not a hospital undergoes surveys by JCAHO, AOA, the state, or a validation agency, the ambulatory care services are further surveyed in conjunction with the inpatient services by that surveying organization.

Accreditation

Hospitals voluntarily seek accreditation to demonstrate to their patients, to their communities, to insurers, to managed care organizations, and to others that their organizations are providing quality care. As with federal requirements, the ambulatory care services provided by a hospital seeking voluntary accreditation are surveyed along with the inpatient services as a part of the routine accreditation process. As previously mentioned, both the JCAHO and the AOA are voluntary accrediting organizations whose standards are "deemed" to be in compliance with the federal *Conditions of Participation*. The majority of U.S. hospitals are JCAHO-accredited.

Documentation

The fundamentals of good patient documentation apply in the hospital ambulatory care setting as in all settings. Several accrediting and regulatory guidelines that apply to inpatient documentation also apply to ambulatory care documentation. The extent of documentation in a hospital ambulatory care record will depend in part on the type of services received. For example, the most extensive ambulatory care records are generally the records of ambulatory surgery patients. This type of record will resemble an inpatient record, including a history and physical examination report, an operation report, anesthesia records, postoperative recovery notes, and, when appropriate, pathology reports. On the other hand, the least extensive hospital outpatient records will usually be those of referred outpatients, sometimes consisting only of a set of orders and test results. However, because there must be a physician order documented for every test the hospital performs, these records are frequently audited by third-party payers. Another important documentation element that must be obtained from the physician when the test is ordered is clinical information that describes the reason for the test. Without information on the diagnoses or symptoms that prompted the physician to order the test, the hospital lacks the information needed to demonstrate that the test was medically necessary and risks losing reimbursement.

JCAHO Documentation Requirements

As the body that surveys most hospital-based ambulatory care providers, the JCAHO's standards regarding documentation merit attention. Some of JCAHO's information management (IM) standards that apply both to inpatients and outpatients are quoted as follows (JCAHO, 2003a):

- The hospital initiates and maintains a medical record for every individual assessed or treated (p. 252).
- Only authorized individuals make entries in medical records (p. 252). . . .
- The medical record thoroughly documents operative or other procedures and the use of sedation or anesthesia (p. 253).
- A preoperative diagnosis is recorded before surgery by the licensed independent practitioner responsible for the patient (p. 253).
- Operative reports dictated or written immediately after surgery record the name of the primary surgeon and assistants, findings, technical procedures used, specimens removed, and postoperative diagnosis (p. 253). . . .
- When the operative report is not placed in the medical record immediately after surgery, a progress note is entered immediately (p. 253). . . .

JCAHO (2003a) also has established documentation standards specifically for ambulatory care patient records. One such requirement applies to the records of patients receiving "continuing ambulatory care services" (p. 253) (e.g., clinic outpatients). Medical records of these outpatients must contain a "summary list of known significant diagnoses, conditions, procedures, drug allergies, and medications" (p. 253). Furthermore, this summary list must be made part of the outpatient's record by the third visit. The summary list is updated as appropriate on each visit (see Figure 2-1). Although the description of the summary list brings to mind a form in a paper

THE UNIVERSITY HOSPITALS AND CLINICS
Jackson, Mississippi

PEDIATRIC PATIENT DATA
SUMMARY LIST

Addressograph

ALLERGIES	DATE	ALLERGY	DATE	ALLERGY	DATE	ALLERGY

DATE	SIGNIFICANT DIAGNOSIS	DATE	PROCEDURES
		DATE	ASSISTIVE DEVICES

IMMUNIZATION RECORD

VACCINE	DATE GIVEN	M.D./CLINIC	VACCINE	DATE GIVEN	M.D./CLINIC
DtaP #1			HIB #1		
DtaP #2			HIB #2		
DtaP #3			HIB #3		
DtaP #4			HIB #4		
DtaP #5					
Td-ADULT			HBV #1		
			HBV #2		
OPV/IPV 1			HBV #3		
OPV/IPV 2					
OPV/IPV 3			MMR #1		
OPV/IPV 4			MMR #2		
OPV/IPV 5					
			PNEUMOVAX		
OTHER			VARICELLA		

FORM #   , Revised 12/01   Page 1 of 2

Figure 2-1   Sample summary list form for ambulatory care patient records. (Courtesy of the University of Mississippi Medical Center, Jackson, MS.)

THE UNIVERSITY HOSPITALS AND CLINICS
Jackson, Mississippi

PEDIATRIC PATIENT DATA
SUMMARY LIST

Addressograph

DATE	MEDICATIONS	DATE	MEDICATIONS

FORM #   , Revised 12/01   Page 2 of 2

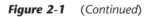

Figure 2-1   *(Continued)*

record, this information does not necessarily have to be maintained in paper format. The needed information can be extracted from a computerized database.

There are also JCAHO standards that pertain to records of emergency patients. Some of these IM requirements are listed as follows (JCAHO, 2003a):

- When emergency, urgent, or immediate care is provided, the time and means of arrival are also documented in the medical record (p. 253).

- The medical record notes when a patient receiving emergency, urgent, or immediate care left against medical advice (p. 253).

- The medical record of a patient receiving emergency, urgent, or immediate care notes the conclusions at termination of treatment, including final disposition, condition at discharge, and instructions for follow-up care (p. 253).

Other Factors in Ambulatory Care Documentation

Documentation in the ambulatory care setting is under increased scrutiny because of the role it plays in determining the level of physician service provided. The level of service determines the appropriate code, which determines the physician's reimbursement. (Reimbursement to the *hospital* is discussed in the Reimbursement section of this chapter.) This issue is particularly important in teaching hospitals in which **residents**, as part of their graduate medical education, participate with teaching physicians in caring for patients. The *Code of Federal Regulations* contains the basic rules that regulate Medicare payments to teaching physicians (Physician services in teaching settings, 2002). How these rules are applied is explained in the *Medicare Carriers Manual*, along with specific examples of acceptable and unacceptable documentation (CMS, 2003b).

Most teaching hospitals pay residents a salary, to which Medicare contributes through indirect medical education allowances. In this situation, services performed by residents are not paid on a fee-for-service basis, but a teaching physician who is present during the performing of the services may bill Medicare. For evaluation and management services, the teaching physician's documentation must make it clear that the teaching physician was present during the key portion of the service and that the teaching physician evaluated and participated in the management of the patient. Merely countersigning the resident's note is insufficient documentation to justify payment (CMS, 2003b).

Figure 2-2 provides examples of Medicare's rules regarding fee payments for services of teaching physicians. These rules are excerpted from the *Code of Federal Regulations* and are relevant to a discussion of hospital-based ambulatory care because teaching hospitals are major providers of hospital-based ambulatory care. They apply to documentation in Medicare records in all states, and in some states, to Medicaid records also.

There is an "outpatient exception" to the rules provided in Figure 2-2. However, not all outpatient care will fall under the outpatient exception, so the "general" rules

---

Section 415.172 Physician fee schedule payment for services of teaching physicians.

(a) General rule. If a resident participates in a service furnished in a teaching setting, physician fee schedule payment is made only if a teaching physician is present during the key portion of any service or procedure for which payment is sought.

(1) In the case of surgical, high-risk, or other complex procedures, the teaching physician must be present during all critical portions of the procedure and immediately available to furnish services during the entire service or procedure.

(i) In the case of surgery, the teaching physician's presence is not required during opening and closing of the surgical field.

(ii) In the case of procedures performed through an endoscope, the teaching physician must be present during the entire viewing.

(2) In the case of evaluation and management services, the teaching physician must be present during the portion of the service that determines the level of service billed. (However, in the case of evaluation and management services furnished in hospital outpatient departments and certain other ambulatory settings, the requirements of Section 415.174 apply.)

(b) Documentation. Except for services furnished as set forth in (the exceptions) . . . , the medical records must document the teaching physician was present at the time the service is furnished. The presence of the teaching physician during procedures may be demonstrated by the notes in the medical records made by a physician, resident, or nurse. In the case of evaluation and management procedures, the teaching physician must personally document his or her participation in the service in the medical records. . . .

Figure 2-2   Examples of Medicare rules regarding fee payments for services of teaching physicians. (Excerpted from 42 CFR 415.172)

will apply in those instances. Figure 2-3 provides another excerpt from the *Code of Federal Regulations* that explains the outpatient exception.

The Office of the Inspector General (OIG) of the U.S. Department of Health and Human Services audited records at several teaching hospitals. The purpose of this initiative, also known as PATH (Physicians at Teaching Hospitals), was to require the teaching hospital or their faculty practice plans to reimburse Medicare for payments not substantiated by documentation in the hospital's records. The first hospitals to be audited were required to repay millions of dollars to the federal government for payments made to teaching physicians for services at levels that could not be substantiated in the documentation. Although the PATH initiative is no longer a part of the OIG work plan, the aggressive enforcement action initiated by PATH has caused teaching hospitals to conduct their own regular audits of teaching physician documentation to ensure compliance with CMS regulations.

Section 415.174 Exception: Evaluation and management services furnished in certain centers.

(a) In the case of certain evaluation and management codes of lower and mid-level complexity . . . carriers may make physician fee schedule payment for a service furnished by a resident without the presence of a teaching physician. For the exception to apply, all of the following conditions must be met:

   (1) The services must be furnished in a center that is located in an outpatient department of a hospital or another ambulatory care entity in which the time spent by residents in patient care activities is included in determining intermediary payments to a hospital. . . .

   (2) Any resident furnishing the service without the presence of a teaching physician must have completed more than 6 months of an approved residency program.

   (3) The teaching physician must not direct the care of more than four residents at any given time and must direct the care from such proximity as to constitute immediate availability. The teaching physician must—

      (i) Have no other responsibilities at the time;

      (ii) Assume management responsibility for those beneficiaries seen by the residents;

      (iii) Ensure that the services furnished are appropriate;

      (iv) Review with each resident during or immediately after each visit, the beneficiary's medical history, physical examination, diagnosis, and record of tests and therapies; and

      (v) Document the extent of the teaching physician's participation in the review and direction of the services furnished to each beneficiary.

   (4) The range of services . . . includes . . . acute care . . . chronic care . . . coordination of care . . . comprehensive care. . . .

   (5) The patients seen must be an identifiable group of individuals who consider the center to be the continuing source of their health care and in which services are furnished by residents under the medical direction of teaching physicians. . . .

Figure 2-3   Explanation of Medicare's outpatient exception. (Excerpted from 42 CFR 415.174)

Reimbursement

There are various mechanisms for reimbursing hospital outpatient care. Reimbursement concepts related to managed care are discussed in Chapter 4, but other reimbursement mechanisms, including ambulatory payment classifications (APCs), are discussed here.

Hospital Chargemaster or Charge Description Master (CDM)

For most outpatient ancillary services such as laboratory and radiology, the hospital usually maintains a computerized data file called the **chargemaster** or **charge description master (CDM)**, which lists appropriate codes for the service and the hospital's charge for that service. Unlike ambulatory surgery procedures, which require human intervention to assign a code based on documentation in the patient record, chargemaster procedures are automatically coded by a computer program when the charge for the service is entered. Therefore it is important to properly maintain the chargemaster file, making sure that it reflects current codes and reasonable charges.

Medicare

Medicare is a federal program that pays for health care for older Americans and disabled persons. Payments to hospitals fall under Part A of Medicare, whereas payments for physician's services fall under Part B. CMS contracts with private organizations that handle the claims processing and payments for the Medicare program in a given region. The claims processing organization for Medicare Part A is called the **fiscal intermediary (FI).** The organization that processes Medicare Part B claims is known as the **Medicare carrier**. Although the issues related to documentation by teaching physicians earlier in this chapter are Part B issues, the information provided in this section relates to hospital reimbursement, or Part A of Medicare.

Diagnosis Related Group (DRG) Payment Window

As described in Chapter 1, Medicare reimburses hospitals for inpatient care under a prospective payment system that pays the hospital on a "per case" basis according to the diagnosis related group (DRG) assigned to each patient's stay. When a hospital provides services to a Medicare patient as an outpatient within 72 hours before a related inpatient admission, charges for those outpatient services must not be billed separately. Instead, the outpatient diagnoses and procedures must be coded and submitted with the inpatient bill. Because some hospital admissions occur unexpectedly within 72 hours after outpatient treatment, hospitals have inadvertently submitted both inpatient and outpatient bills to Medicare in these cases, in violation of the 72-hour rule. Medicare requires hospitals to implement systems to avoid submitting separate bills for outpatients admitted to inpatient status within the 72-hour window. Failure to comply with the 72-hour rule may result in financial penalties to the hospital. The Office of the Inspector General's (OIG's) work plan for 2003 included a review of the DRG payment window to determine whether it would be appropriate to expand the time frame of the window to as much as 14 days (OIG, 2002), but this idea did not receive further attention in 2004. Included in the 2004 work plan, however, was a review to determine whether Medicaid programs could save money by implementing a DRG payment window (OIG, 2003).

The Hospital Outpatient Prospective Payment System (OPPS)
and Ambulatory Payment Classifications (APCs)

The basic units of payment in Medicare's **Hospital Outpatient Prospective Payment System (HOPPS or OPPS)** are known as **ambulatory payment classifications (APCs).** The APC system, implemented in the year 2000, established groups of outpatient procedures and services that have similar clinical characteristics and similar costs. One major difference between the APC and DRG systems is that an outpatient may be assigned more than one APC per encounter, whereas an inpatient is assigned only one DRG per hospital admission. Consider the case of an emergency department patient whose visit includes evaluation and management, x-rays, and a procedure. In such a case, as many as three APCs may be generated—one APC for the evaluation and management services, a second APC for the x-rays, and a third APC for the procedure. APCs are based on Healthcare Common Procedural Coding System (HCPCS) codes assigned by the hospital. The hospital's reimbursement from Medicare is the dollar amount associated with each APC as updated by CMS on an annual basis. See Figure 2-4 for excerpts from the APC table for the calendar year 2003.

Notice that in Figure 2-4 each APC is assigned a **status indicator,** which is an alphabetic character that indicates the APC type and whether or how that APC is paid under the OPPS. The four status indicators that appear in the excerpt in Figure 2-4 are "S," "T," "P," and "V." A status indicator of "T" means that the associated APC represents a significant procedure that is **discounted** (paid at less than the full amount) when other procedures are performed with it. The "S" status indicator represents a significant service that is *not* discounted when more than one APC is present on a claim. The "P" status indicator means that the associated APC is a partial hospitalization service. The "V" status indicator represents a medical visit with its associated evaluation and management services. All four of the status indicators in Figure 2-4 are paid under the OPPS. Status indicators "S," "T," and "V" are paid as separate APCs, and status indicator "P" is paid on a per diem APC basis. In 2003, there were 15 different status indicators. See Figure 2-5 for a list of the 2003 status indicators, the services they represent, and their payment status.

As indicated in Figure 2-4, medical visits in a hospital clinic or emergency department (ED) are classified according to one of three levels of service—low level, midlevel, or high level—based on evaluation and management (E&M) coding. In determining the level of service of an encounter, hospitals have historically developed their own criteria for assigning the E&M codes and have not followed the same guidelines that physicians follow. The American Hospital Association (AHA) and the American Health Information Management Association (AHIMA) developed a joint recommendation to adopt a uniform methodology for E&M code assignment for all hospitals that would be distinct from the E&M coding rules for physicians. If CMS adopts this recommendation, hospital medical visits will utilize a set of codes that are different from the E&M codes used by physicians (AHA & AHIMA, 2003).

When the OPPS was initiated in 2000, observation services were not separately reimbursable. However, in 2002, Medicare resumed payment for observation services

ADDENDUM A—LIST OF AMBULATORY PAYMENT CLASSIFICATIONS (APCs) WITH STATUS INDICATORS, RELATIVE WEIGHTS, PAYMENT RATES, AND COPAYMENT AMOUNTS CALENDAR YEAR 2003

APC	Group title	Status indicator	Relative weight	Payment rate	National unadjusted copayment	Minimum unadjusted copayment
0001	Level I Photochemotherapy	S	0.3779	$19.71	$7.09	$3.94
0002	Fine needle Biopsy/Aspiration	T	0.5911	$30.83		$6.17
0003	Bone Marrow Biopsy/Aspiration	T	1.2306	$64.18		$12.84
0004	Level I Needle Biopsy/ Aspiration Except Bone Marrow	T	1.7441	$90.96	$23.47	$18.19
0005	Level II Needle Biopsy / Aspiration Except Bone Marrow	T	3.1201	$162.72	$71.59	$32.54
0006	Level I Incision & Drainage	T	1.7926	$93.49	$24.12	$18.70
0007	Level II Incision & Drainage	T	10.0191	$522.51	$108.89	$104.50
0008	Level III Incision and Drainage	T	16.1430	$841.87		$168.37
0009	Nail Procedures	T	0.6298	$32.84	$8.34	$6.57
0010	Level I Destruction of Lesion	T	0.6589	$34.36	$10.08	$6.87
0011	Level II Destruction of Lesion	T	1.8507	$96.52	$27.88	$19.30
0012	Level I Debridement & Destruction	T	0.7849	$40.93	$11.18	$8.19
0013	Level II Debridement & Destruction	T	1.0756	$56.09	$14.20	$11.22
0015	Level III Debridement & Destruction	T	1.5407	$80.35	$20.35	$16.07
0016	Level IV Debridement & Destruction	T	2.6162	$136.44	$57.31	$27.29
0017	Level VI Debridement & Destruction	T	15.8233	$825.20	$227.84	$165.04
0018	Biopsy of Skin/Puncture of Lesion	T	0.9399	$49.02	$16.04	$9.80
0019	Level I Excision/ Biopsy	T	3.7693	$196.57	$71.87	$39.31
0020	Level II Excision/ Biopsy	T	7.1898	$374.96	$113.25	$74.99
0021	Level III Excision/ Biopsy	T	13.9338	$726.66	$219.48	$145.33
0022	Level IV Excision/ Biopsy	T	17.3930	$907.06	$354.45	$181.41
0023	Exploration Penetrating Wound	T	2.5193	$131.38	$40.37	$26.28
0033	Partial Hospitalization	P	4.6026	$240.03	$48.17	$48.01
0339	Observation	S	7.2188	$376.47		$75.29
0600	Low Level Clinic Visits	V	0.8430	$43.96		$8.79
0601	Mid Level Clinic Visits	V	0.9690	$50.53		$10.11
0602	High Level Clinic Visits	V	1.4631	$76.30		$15.26
0610	Low Level Emergency Visits	V	1.4147	$73.78	$19.57	$14.76
0611	Mid Level Emergency Visits	V	2.5290	$131.89	$36.47	$26.38
0612	High Level Emergency Visits	V	4.3410	$226.39	$54.14	$45.28

Figure 2-4 Excerpts from Addendum A—List of ambulatory payment classifications (APCs). (Source: *Federal Register*, November 1, 2002.)

ADDENDUM D—Payment Status Indicators for the Hospital Outpatient Prospective Payment System

Indicator	Service	Status
A	Durable Medical Equipment, Prosthetics and Orthotics (excluding implanted DME and prosthetics)	DMEPOS Fee Schedule
A	Physical, Occupational and Speech Therapy	Physician Fee Schedule
A	Ambulance	Ambulance Fee Schedule
A	EPO for ESRD Patients	National Rate
A	Clinical Diagnostic Laboratory Services	Laboratory Fee Schedule
A	Physician Services for ESRD Patients	Physician Fee Schedule
A	Screening Mammography	Physician Fee Schedule
C	Inpatient Procedures	Not Payable under OPPS; Admit Patient; Bill as Inpatient
D	Deleted Code	Deleted Effective Beginning of Calendar Year
E	Non-Covered Items and Services, Codes not Reportable in Hospital Outpatient Settings	Not Paid Under Medicare or When Performed in a Hospital Outpatient Setting
F	Corneal tissue acquisition; orphan drugs	Paid at Reasonable Cost
G	Drug/Biological Pass-Through	Paid Under OPPS; Separate APC Payment Includes Pass Through Amount
H	Device Category Pass-Through	Paid Under OPPS; Separate Cost Based Pass Through Payment
L	Influenza Vaccine; Pneumococcal Pneumonia Vaccine	Paid reasonable cost; not subject to deductible or coinsurance
K	Non Pass-Through Drug/Biological, Certain Brachytherapy seeds	Paid Under OPPS; Separate APC
N	Items and Services Packaged into APC Rate	Paid under OPPS; Payment Is Packaged Into Payment for Other Services
P	Partial Hospitalization	Paid under OPPS; Per Diem APC
S	Significant Procedure, Not Discounted When Multiple	Paid Under OPPS; Separate APC
T	Significant Procedure, Multiple Procedure Reduction Applies	Paid Under OPPS; Separate APC
V	Visit to Clinic or Emergency Department	Paid Under OPPS; Separate APC
X	Ancillary Service	Paid Under OPPS; Separate APC

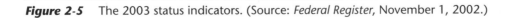

Figure 2-5   The 2003 status indicators. (Source: *Federal Register*, November 1, 2002.)

with certain restrictions. Only cases with diagnoses of chest pain, asthma, or congestive heart failure are eligible for reimbursement under the OPPS. Furthermore, for each diagnosis, certain tests must be performed to qualify for the observation APC (Prophet-Bowman, 2003). The required diagnostic tests are as follows:

- For chest pain, at least two sets of cardiac enzymes and two sequential electrocardiograms
- For asthma, a breathing capacity test or pulse oximetry
- For congestive heart failure, a chest x-ray and an electrocardiogram and pulse oximetry (CMS, 2003c)

Finally, an E&M code or the code for direct admission to observation must accompany the observation code, and the length of observation services billed should be at least eight, but no more than 48 hours (Prophet-Bowman, 2003).

The OPPS allows additional payments to cover the costs of innovative medical devices, drugs, and biologicals. Called "pass-through payments," these categories provide separate payments in addition to regular APC payments. Payments for a given drug, device, or biological can be made on a pass-through basis for two to three years (CMS, 2002b).

Hospital-based clinics are considered to be "provider-based clinics" under the OPPS. When a Medicare patient is seen in a hospital-based clinic, the clinic receives an APC payment and the physician receives a reduced payment for his or her services (because there is no practice expense—it has been shifted to the hospital). The total of the two payments is greater than the full fee schedule payment that a physician in a freestanding clinic would receive. Therefore, CMS scrutinizes applications for provider-based status from clinics that had not claimed any hospital affiliation before the implementation of the OPPS.

It is important to remember that details of the OPPS change annually. To obtain the most current information, the health information manager should consult the latest regulations at the CMS or *Federal Register* Web sites.

Other Payers

Other payers may pay for hospital outpatient care under a variety of systems. Traditional indemnity insurance plans pay the usual, customary, and reasonable charges of the hospital. However, fewer patients are enrolled in a pure indemnity type of plan. Generally, there are incentives for patients to use the services of a provider who has agreed not to exceed certain limits on charges. For more information on the wide range of payment mechanisms for ambulatory care, see Chapter 4.

Billing

The Uniform Bill (UB-92 or CMS 1450) is the standard form for submitting information to third-party payers when filing claims for hospital services (see Figure 2-6). The National Uniform Billing Committee (NUBC) has been working on an updated

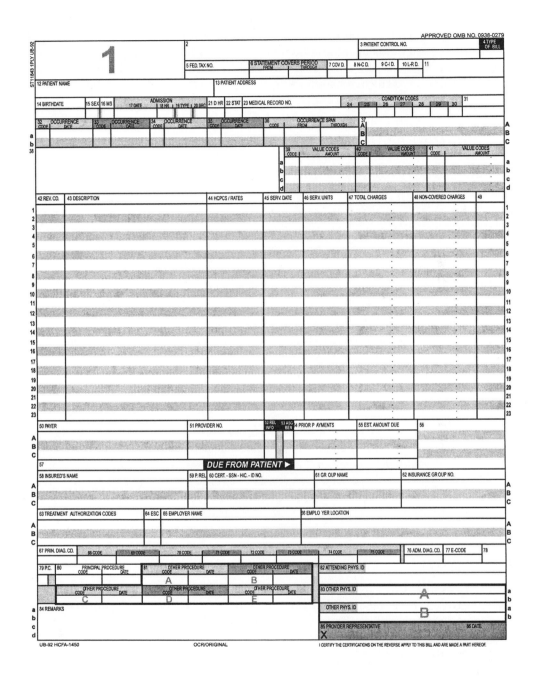

Figure 2-6 The UB-92 (CMS 1450) Uniform Bill.

version of the Uniform Bill. This draft version is called the UB-02 and contains expanded fields to accommodate longer codes in the event that ICD-10-CM and ICD-10-PCS become official coding standards (NUBC, 2002). Under HIPAA, physicians use the CMS 1500 form for submitting claims. Electronic transmission of claims is the norm for both hospital and physician claim submission.

Information Management

Coding and Classification

Coding of diseases and procedures serves several purposes in hospital-based ambulatory care. Hospitals can use coded data to study patterns in the services they render or to assist in the evaluation of the outcomes of care. Accurate coding is also crucial to receiving appropriate reimbursement for hospital-based ambulatory care.

International Classification of Diseases, 9th Revision, Clinical Modification (ICD-9-CM)

ICD-9-CM, developed by the National Center for Health Statistics, is the classification system used for coding the patient's condition, diagnosis, or reason for encounter. The UB-92 was designed to capture ICD-9-CM codes in the diagnoses fields. Because ICD-9-CM is used in billing, it is also generally used as the coding system for the hospital's internal disease databases.

Healthcare Common Procedural Coding System (HCPCS)

HCPCS is the system required by CMS (formerly HCFA) for coding services provided to Medicare patients. CMS adopted the American Medical Association's *Current Procedural Terminology©* as the coding system comprising the bulk of HCPCS. The CPT codes are designated by CMS as "Level I" codes. The codes that CMS developed are known as HCPCS "Level II" or national codes. These are alphanumeric codes, consisting of a letter (A–V) and four numerical digits. (Note: HCPCS Level III or local codes were discontinued in 2003.)

Revenue Codes

Revenue codes are reported on the UB-92 to indicate the general nature of the service provided. To file a valid claim, the revenue code must be appropriate to the HCPCS code listed with it. Therefore, to avoid rejection of claims, the appropriate revenue codes are usually included in the chargemaster file along with the HCPCS code for the service being billed.

Coding Edits

Fiscal intermediaries (FIs) process hospital outpatient claims using the Outpatient Code Editor (OCE), which identifies coding errors on hospital outpatient bills that can cause the claim to be rejected. National Correct Coding Initiative (NCCI or CCI) edits also apply to the APC system. The purpose of the CCI edits is to prohibit unbundling of procedures, a practice that results in excessive payment to the provider when multiple codes are reported instead of a combination code. The CCI edits are voluminous and are updated quarterly, making it difficult to keep abreast of them using manual methods. Most hospitals use code-editing software to flag codes that contain possible OCE or CCI errors. Identifying and correcting errors before the bill is submitted results in more efficient claims processing and a better cash flow for the hospital.

Data and Information Flow

Most hospitals begin the ambulatory patient's record with an outpatient registration procedure. Information necessary to identify the patient is gathered and recorded. Generally, this identifying information is entered into a computerized database, or master patient index system, and may also be printed out or manually recorded for immediate reference. As various assessments, diagnostic procedures, and treatments are completed, the results are incorporated into the patient's record, along with diagnostic impressions or conclusions and plans for future care.

To meet accreditation requirements, the hospital must be able to quickly assemble all components of the patient's record when a patient is seen in any hospital setting. Many hospitals achieve this goal by maintaining all components of the paper record together in a unit record. In this scenario, all records of inpatient, clinic, emergency, or any other type of hospital encounter would be maintained in a single record, centralized in the health information services area of the hospital. The advantage of this system is that there is only one record for the patient, and it is not necessary to assemble scattered components of the record when the patient is seen. However, in a large facility with numerous clinics that may not be physically close to one another, maintaining a single paper record is much more challenging. In this situation, certain clinics may maintain their own records. When a patient has more than one record in various clinics, JCAHO requires that "each record notes that there is additional information elsewhere" (JCAHO, 2003, Intent of IM.7.4 and IM.7.4.1).

Computer systems are solving the problem of making the record quickly available in any setting. As hospitals move toward the electronic health record, more components of the patient's clinical record are maintained online. An electronic patient record can be accessed by diverse providers throughout the hospital as the patient arrives at various departments for different services.

Computer Systems

As with many areas of health care, the first computer applications in hospital-based ambulatory care were related to billing functions. However, the importance of maintaining clinical information electronically has been emphasized repeatedly by groups such as the Institute of Medicine (IOM), which devoted an entire chapter to the benefits of information technology in its 2001 publication, *Crossing the Quality Chasm: A New Health System for the 21st Century.* In response to a request from the U.S. Department of Health and Human Services in 2003, the IOM wrote a letter report outlining the key capabilities of an electronic health record (EHR) system. Both hospitals and ambulatory care are specifically addressed in this report, which lists the following core functionalities of an electronic health record system:

- Health information and data
- Results management
- Order entry/management
- Decision support
- Electronic communication and connectivity
- Patient support
- Administrative processes
- Reporting and population health management (p. 7)

The IOM report listed specific functions needed and a projected time frame by site of care for each of the areas outlined. For example, under "Health information and data," the IOM specified that by 2004–2005, EHRs for both hospitals and ambulatory care settings should be capable of capturing problem lists, procedures, diagnoses, medication lists, allergies, demographics, diagnostic test results, radiology results, and so on. An EHR with the capabilities described in the IOM report offers numerous advantages both to the patient and to the clinicians who care for the patients. Because in a given day, an ambulatory patient may receive evaluation and treatment in several different hospital departments, an EHR that is readily available to all who see the patient can improve patient care. Patient safety can be enhanced through the use of computerized order entry by linking to decision support systems that warn of possible drug interactions or wrong dosages and by alerting prescribing clinicians to patient allergies. An EHR can also generate reminders of services that are needed by a patient. These are just a few of the ways in which an EHR can benefit ambulatory patient care in a hospital setting.

One method of capturing data for use in an EHR is already in use in many hospital emergency departments—voice recognition technology. With a voice recognition system, the emergency physician can dictate reports directly to the computer. The computer converts the spoken word into a report without the labor of a transcriptionist typing the report. The report can also be electronically signed by the physician who generated the report.

Data Sets

Standardization Efforts

The **Uniform Ambulatory Care Data Set (UACDS)** was one of the first attempts to standardize ambulatory data collection efforts. The National Committee on Vital and Health Statistics (NCVHS) approved the most recent revision of this 16-item data set in 1989. However, the trend in data set development since the mid-1990s has been to make provision for both inpatient and outpatient data in the same data set. This is only logical because the most commonly used forms and processes for reporting patient data (e.g., UB-92, CMS-1500) are designed to handle both inpatient and outpatient data. In 1996, the NCVHS developed a set of 42 core health data elements that could be used in either the inpatient or outpatient setting (NCVHS, 1996).

The greatest impetus toward collection of standardized data in ambulatory and all other health care settings has been provided by the Health Insurance Portability and Accountability Act (HIPAA). The HIPAA electronic data interchange (EDI) provisions require the adoption of standards for transactions, code sets, and identifiers. CMS (formerly HCFA) delegated development and maintenance of the EDI standards to the following designated standards maintenance organizations (DSMOs):

1. Accredited Standards Committee X12
2. Dental Content Committee of the American Dental Association
3. Health Level Seven
4. National Council for Prescription Drug Programs
5. National Uniform Billing Committee
6. National Uniform Claim Committee (CMS, 2000)

Data Elements for Emergency Department Systems (DEEDS) is an example of one data set that is specific to the ambulatory setting. Version 1.0 of DEEDS included more than 150 data elements in the following eight categories:

- Patient identification data
- Facility and practitioner identification data
- ED payment data
- ED arrival and first assessment data
- ED history and physical examination data
- ED procedure and result data
- ED medication data
- ED disposition and diagnosis data (NCIPC, 1997)

The Accredited Standards Committee X12 has incorporated DEEDS into its preliminary standard for EDI of attachments (Washington Publishing Company, No date).

Common Working Files

For Medicare beneficiaries, CMS contracts for the maintenance of nine regional databases throughout the United States. A file, called the **common working file (CWF),** is maintained for each beneficiary. Information from both Part A and Part B claims are maintained in these files, which are used by fiscal intermediaries and Medicare carriers for coordination of benefits, claims validation, and for tracking utilization patterns.

Quality Improvement and Utilization Management

Quality Improvement (QI)

JCAHO requires that accredited hospitals implement hospital-wide performance improvement programs. Therefore ambulatory care services would be included when the quality of the hospital's services are analyzed. JCAHO's approach to performance improvement emphasizes designing processes, collecting data related to performance, analyzing the data collected (including comparing the hospital's performance to a standard or to that of peer hospitals), establishing priorities for processes to be improved, developing improvements for the priorities identified, and evaluating the degree of improvement achieved and sustained (JCAHO, 2003b). The flowchart in Figure 2-7 provides a graphic illustration of this approach.

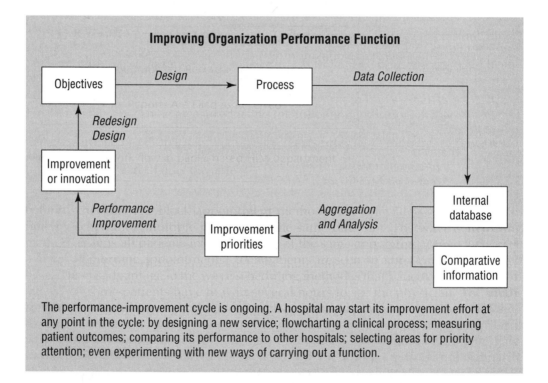

Improving Organization Performance Function

The performance-improvement cycle is ongoing. A hospital may start its improvement effort at any point in the cycle: by designing a new service; flowcharting a clinical process; measuring patient outcomes; comparing its performance to other hospitals; selecting areas for priority attention; even experimenting with new ways of carrying out a function.

Figure 2-7 Flowchart illustrating JCAHO's process for improving performance and outcomes. (Joint Commission on Accreditation of Healthcare Organizations. (2003). *Joint Commission 2003 Automated Comprehensive Accreditation Manual for Hospitals.* Oakbrook Terrace, IL: Author. Copyright © 2003 JCAHO. All rights reserved. Reprinted by permission.)

Utilization Management (UM)

Utilization management focuses on the appropriateness, efficiency, and cost-effectiveness of health care. In the current climate of managed care and with a prospective payment system for Medicare in place, it is more important than ever for hospitals to be sure they are rendering ambulatory services efficiently. In the past, hospitals were reimbursed based either on their costs or their charges. Now both Medicare and private insurers limit the charges and costs they will pay. With the implementation of a prospective payment system, some items and services are packaged with others and are not reimbursed separately. To operate efficiently in such an environment requires a team effort from physicians, hospital staff, and administration.

Risk Management and Legal Issues

Many hospitals have risk management departments, whose role is to protect the organization from financial loss that could occur as a result of **potentially compensable events (PCEs)**, which are occurrences that may result in litigation against the health care provider or that may require the health care provider to compensate an injured party. Almost all hospitals have occurrence (or incident) reporting systems that allow risk managers to track PCEs and to identify risk areas within the organization that can be targeted for improvement. Some hospitals have moved from paper-based occurrence reporting to electronic systems that allow risk managers to receive, review, and analyze occurrence reports online. The specific challenges for risk management in hospital ambulatory care are described in the following paragraphs.

The increase in outpatient utilization presents new challenges for hospital risk managers. Financial incentives to treat patients on an outpatient rather than an inpatient basis should be balanced with policies that encourage inpatient admission when appropriate in a given situation. Also, the limited duration of face-to-face contact between caregivers and patients in the outpatient setting requires extra attention to patient relations and documentation (Eubanks, 1990).

Because telephone contact often precedes or follows an outpatient visit, documentation of these calls is important. Both what the patient tells the caregiver and what the caregiver tells the patient should be recorded. A follow-up telephone call is routine after many ambulatory surgery procedures. Proper documentation verifies that the patient was given correct instructions and provides evidence of the patient's condition after surgery. A follow-up phone call can be a good public relations tool as well, which is also an important element in risk management (Eubanks, 1990). Phone calls should be HIPAA-compliant. When the patient is not available, messages containing clinical information (e.g., test results) should not be left on answering machines or with persons other than the patient.

The emergency department is an area in which the hospital is particularly at legal risk. Patients and family members being treated in the emergency room are often under extreme stress and are sometimes less likely to be understanding of the stresses that the emergency department staff may be facing. Emergency department staff must be well-versed, not only in clinical assessment and treatment, but also in customer service and in legal aspects of emergency care. An example of a law with which the emergency department staff should be familiar is the **Emergency Medical Treatment and Active Labor Act (EMTALA)**, which imposes a legal duty on hospitals to screen and stabilize, if necessary, any patient who arrives in the emergency department (Curran, Hall, Bobinski, & Orentlicher, 1998). The purpose of EMTALA is to prevent the "dumping" of patients who may not be able to pay for emergency department services. Therefore an appropriate screening cannot be delayed to inquire about insurance status or method of payment. If the patient is found to have an emergency medical condition, the hospital is required to stabilize the patient before attempting to transfer the patient elsewhere. In the case of a woman in active labor, stabilization generally means that delivery is completed before transfer (Special responsibilities of Medicare hospitals in emergency cases, 2002).

Role of the Health Information Management Professional

The health information management (HIM) professional can play a variety of roles in hospital-based ambulatory care. A health information manager may take a traditional type of role in centralized health information services or may work in one of the outpatient settings. Most hospitals now have compliance departments, and the skills of health information managers are vital in promoting compliance with both billing and HIPAA regulations. Many hospitals are also employing health information managers as chargemaster coordinators. The specifics of each of these positions will vary from institution to institution, but a general idea of what could be expected in each is provided in the following sections.

Centralized Health Information Services

A centralized health information services department deals with both inpatient and outpatient issues. A large facility with many outpatient clinics may or may not have certain positions in the central department devoted to outpatient services. Whether or not separate outpatient positions exist in the department, those in leadership positions in health information services must be familiar with JCAHO requirements that affect the patient record and must provide training for others in the department as appropriate.

The most common outpatient specialization within centralized health information services is that of outpatient coding specialist. Because HCPCS/CPT codes are not required on inpatient bills, health information services will often assign certain coders to code all outpatient services. This arrangement allows coders to develop a specialization in outpatient coding rules, which are different from inpatient coding rules. Such specialization can lead to greater accuracy in outpatient coding.

Some hospitals may also have a supervisory-level position designated to handle issues related to outpatient clinics or other outpatient services. Because of the challenges in filing and retrieving a large number of records that may be requested at very short intervals for continuing outpatient care, someone on the health information services staff may be assigned to serve as a liaison or team member with the hospital's ambulatory services.

Specialized Outpatient Areas

Depending on size, activity, and organizational structure, any of the outpatient areas discussed in this chapter could benefit from the knowledge and skills of a full-time HIM professional. Sometimes, because of the physical location of hospital-based ambulatory facilities, it is necessary to maintain outpatient records in a satellite or decentralized location. In this situation, a health information professional can help with any of the information management functions of the satellite facility. The health information manager could plan and implement record storage, retention, and retrieval strategies for the outpatient unit. Depending on the organizational structure, the health information manager could also direct coding and billing activities in a specialized outpatient unit. In fact, all of the so-called traditional functions of health information management—release of information, data collection and analysis, management and supervision, and so on—could be directed by a health information manager in a satellite outpatient unit.

Compliance Officer

Most hospitals appoint full-time compliance officers who manage the compliance program. A health information manager possesses skills ideally suited for this position. For example, a billing compliance director must have expert knowledge of documentation and coding guidelines. The person in this position must also be able to educate others about the compliance program as well as the federal guidelines. Another important aspect of the compliance program would be to audit records against codes submitted and to develop plans for corrective action when problems arise (Physician's Payment Update, 1996). HIPAA compliance is another area in which the health information manager can provide expertise. An HIM professional can provide HIPAA training; develop policies, procedures, and forms; or monitor the hospital's ongoing compliance with the HIPAA privacy, security, and/or EDI regulations. Because developing an effective compliance program is a team effort involving many departments and health care professionals, good leadership skills are vital. In many hospitals, the compliance program has developed into a distinct department. Health information managers may lead the compliance department and/or work in specialized compliance areas within the department.

Chargemaster Coordinator

Because much of the coding for an ambulatory patient's bill is generated automatically by the hospital's chargemaster, it is important that someone with a knowledge of coding be involved in chargemaster maintenance. Some hospitals bring in health information managers as consultants to review their chargemasters. A number of hospitals have employed health information managers on a full-time basis to supervise chargemaster maintenance.

The person in charge of chargemaster maintenance would ensure that HCPCS codes are added, changed, or deleted and are properly listed in the chargemaster. The chargemaster coordinator would also verify that the codes being used in the chargemaster accurately reflect the procedures that are being performed. Therefore, developing and maintaining an accurate chargemaster requires communicating with leaders in the various departments whose charges are included in the chargemaster. Another duty of the chargemaster coordinator would be to work with the various departments to help set appropriate prices for services included in the chargemaster.

Another department with which the chargemaster coordinator would work closely is the patient accounts or billing department. When claims are rejected, the chargemaster coordinator should be notified to determine whether the cause of the rejection lies with the chargemaster. Also, when patients call with questions about their bills, the patient accounts department can contact the chargemaster coordinator for assistance in explaining the charges. Under the OPPS, maintenance of an accurate and efficient chargemaster is crucial. Leadership skills are increasingly important to develop the necessary teamwork needed to maintain an effective chargemaster and accompanying processes.

Trends

Hospitals continue to merge with other health care facilities and to incorporate formerly freestanding ambulatory care services into their systems. The JCAHO has recognized this trend and now offers accreditation for provider networks. Health information managers will experience increasing opportunities and challenges as they address the information needs of more complex networks of providers.

Summary

Hospitals offer a variety of services on an ambulatory basis. These include services performed in ambulatory surgery units, hospital clinics, emergency services, observation services, partial hospitalization, and ancillary services. Patients treated in these ambulatory programs are generally termed "hospital outpatients." Three specific types of outpatients often served by hospitals are clinic outpatients, referred outpatients, and emergency outpatients.

Many different types of health care professionals participate in outpatient care. Physicians, nurses, physical therapists, occupational therapists, clinical laboratory scientists, pharmacists, and others may provide diagnostic or therapeutic services to hospital outpatients. Specialists in emergency medicine work in many hospital emergency departments.

Hospital regulations require that all hospitals be licensed by the state in which they are located. Other regulations to which hospital outpatient services may be subject are found in the federal *Conditions of Participation for Hospitals* and in the accreditation standards of a voluntary group, such as the Joint Commission on Accreditation of Healthcare Organizations (JCAHO) or the American Osteopathic Association (AOA).

Documentation requirements for hospital outpatients depend on the type of services received. Requirements for documentation in outpatient records can be found in the regulations and standards of governmental and voluntary accreditation agencies. An example of a specific requirement for outpatient records is JCAHO's requirement for documentation of an outpatient "summary list."

Factors other than regulatory and accreditation requirements play a role in ambulatory care documentation. Documentation audits by third-party payers to determine whether services billed are appropriately documented in the patient record are increasingly common. Health care providers lose reimbursement for services not properly documented. Rules have been promulgated clarifying what documentation is necessary to justify services billed by teaching physicians.

Reimbursement methodologies for hospital outpatient care include managed care contracts, fee schedule payments, and a prospective payment system, APCs.

The major coding and classification systems used in the hospital outpatient setting are ICD-9-CM and HCPCS (whose major component is CPT). Medicare requires that diagnoses be reported on the UB-92 as ICD-9-CM codes. Outpatient procedures must be reported with HCPCS and a corresponding revenue code.

Data and information flow into the patient record from each significant contact the outpatient has with a member of the health care team. The hospital must be able to quickly assemble all components of the patient's record when a patient is seen in any hospital setting. In a large enterprise using paper records, maintaining a comprehensive, yet readily accessible record is a challenge. Computer systems can help solve the problem of making the record quickly available to any outpatient unit. An electronic health record can be accessed by diverse providers throughout the hospital as the patient presents to various departments for different services. However, safeguards must be built into any health care computer system to protect the confidentiality of the patient's clinical information and to ensure that only those with a legitimate need access this information.

HIPAA is now the driving force determining the standards for the data elements that should be maintained for every ambulatory care patient. A data set for each Medicare beneficiary is also found in the common working file.

Measuring and improving the quality of care is important in hospital-based ambulatory care. JCAHO requires that accredited hospitals implement hospital-wide performance improvement programs, which would include ambulatory care. Utilization management programs analyze the appropriateness, efficiency, and cost-effectiveness of patient care. Risk management focuses on improving care, documentation, and patient satisfaction to reduce the possibility of legal liability.

The HIM professional can play a variety of roles in hospital-based ambulatory care. A health information manager may take a traditional type of role in centralized health information services or may work in one of the outpatient settings. The position of compliance officer is a position for which health information managers are particularly well-suited. Many hospitals are also employing health information managers as chargemaster coordinators and team leaders.

Key Terms

ambulatory payment classifications (APCs)   groupings of outpatient services (based on the HCPCS code assigned) that determine the payment the hospital receives under the Hospital Outpatient Prospective Payment System (HOPPS).

ambulatory surgery (also called "same-day" surgery)   surgery in which it is planned that the patient will arrive at the facility, have surgery, recover from any anesthesia, and be ready for discharge in a single day, thus avoiding an overnight stay in the health care facility.

chargemaster or charge description master (CDM)   a computer file that contains a list of the Healthcare Common Procedural Coding System codes and associated charges for services provided to hospital patients.

clinic outpatient   an outpatient treated in an organized clinic of the hospital in which hospital staff evaluate the patient and manage the patient's care.

common working file   a file maintained on each Medicare beneficiary in one of nine regional databases. This file contains claims history information from both Part A and Part B claims and data on utilization patterns of Medicare beneficiaries.

discounting   reducing the payment for additional procedures or ambulatory patient groups so that these other items are not paid at the full rate, as they would be if they had been the only services performed in a given encounter.

Emergency Medical Treatment and Active Labor Act (EMTALA)   a federal law that imposes a legal duty on hospitals to screen and stabilize, if necessary, any patient who arrives in the emergency department. The purpose of EMTALA is to prevent the "dumping" of patients who may not be able to pay for emergency department services.

emergency outpatient   an outpatient evaluated and treated in the emergency department of the hospital.

fiscal intermediary (FI)   an organization with a contract with the CMS to process and pay Part A Medicare claims.

hospital outpatient　a hospital patient who receives care at the hospital, but who is not admitted to inpatient status.

Hospital Outpatient Prospective Payment System (HOPPS or OPPS)　Medicare's payment system for hospital outpatient services. Implemented in the year 2000, the basic unit of payment in the OPPS is the ambulatory payment classification (APC) of each service provided.

Medicare carrier　an organization having a contract with the CMS to process and pay Part B Medicare claims.

observation services　"services furnished by a hospital on the hospital's premises, including use of a bed and periodic monitoring by a hospital's nursing or other staff, which are reasonable and necessary to evaluate an outpatient's condition or determine the need for a possible admission to the hospital as an inpatient" (CMS, 2003a, p. 32b.1).

partial hospitalization program (PHP)　an intensive treatment program in which patients receive services for part of each day. These patients would otherwise require inpatient psychiatric care (CMS, 2003a).

potentially compensable event (PCE)　an occurrence that may result in litigation against the health care provider or that may require the health care provider to financially compensate an injured party.

referred hospital outpatient　an outpatient who is referred to the hospital for specific services, such as laboratory or radiology examinations. The hospital is responsible only for providing the diagnostic or therapeutic services requested, while the referring physician is responsible for evaluating and managing the patient's care.

resident　primarily, a licensed physician, dentist, or podiatrist who participates in an approved graduate medical education (GME) program. The term "resident" may also be applied to "a physician who is not in an approved program, but who is authorized to practice only in a hospital, for example, individuals with temporary or restricted licenses, or unlicensed graduates of foreign medical schools" (Physician services in teaching settings, 2002, p. 661).

revenue codes　used on the UB-92 to indicate the general nature of the services provided. Revenue codes must be appropriate to any HCPCS codes listed with them.

status indicator　an alphabetic character that indicates the type of each APC and whether or how that APC is paid under the Hospital Outpatient Prospective Payment System (OPPS).

Uniform Ambulatory Care Data Set (UACDS)　one of the first attempts to standardize ambulatory data collection efforts. The National Committee on Vital and Health Statistics (NCVHS) approved the most recent revision of this 16-item data set in 1989. Since that time, the NCVHS has focused its efforts on core data elements that could be used in either the inpatient or outpatient setting.

REVIEW QUESTIONS

Knowledge-based Questions

1. What has been the trend in the utilization of hospital-based ambulatory services? What factors help account for this trend?

2. List and describe five different types of outpatient services.

3. List and describe three different types of hospital outpatients.

4. What organization accredits the majority of hospitals in the United States?

5. What are the key issues in documentation of ambulatory surgery?

6. What are the key issues with regard to documentation of services rendered by teaching physicians?

7. What is the hospital chargemaster or charge description master?

8. What are APCs and what is their impact on hospital reimbursement?

9. What coding systems are used in hospital-based ambulatory care?

10. What is EMTALA?

11. What factors should be considered to avoid legal risk in ambulatory care?

12. Describe various roles of the HIM professional in hospital-based ambulatory care.

Application-based Questions

1. If JCAHO requires that "the hospital initiates and maintains a medical record for every individual assessed or treated," what factors allow a hospital to maintain only test results in the case of some referred outpatients?

2. Obtain a recent edition of JCAHO's *Accreditation Manual for Hospitals* and locate standards that would be particularly relevant to ambulatory surgery.

Web Activity

Visit the Web site of the Health Care Compliance Association at http://www.hcca-info.org.

Locate information about the "CHC" certification offered by this group. Find the Healthcare Compliance Certification Board (HCCB) handbook, and look at the detailed content outline for their certification examination. In which content areas do you feel you could demonstrate skill as a result of your health information management training? Which content areas would require more training on your part?

Case Study

Melba Hinkle is the team leader for ambulatory care health information services at Anywhere Medical Center. The medical center has had difficulty in maintaining an up-to-date summary list of "known significant diagnoses, conditions, procedures, drug allergies, and medications" in each ambulatory patient's record as required by the JCAHO. Although an appropriate form has been designed for recording this information, responsibility for recording the information has not been consistently assigned throughout all outpatient departments. Therefore, the physicians are reluctant to rely on the information found in the summary list out of concern that important data may have been omitted.

Anywhere Medical Center is in the process of moving toward an electronic health record. Some of the information needed for the summary list is already maintained in the hospital's computer system. Melba is interested in developing a computerized summary list that would meet JCAHO requirements and meet the needs of the medical staff for reliable information.

1. What data elements would need to be included in a computerized summary list?

2. What are the possible sources for each data item? At what point would each data element be entered into the computer system?

3. What are the possible methods for providing the summary list information to the physician and other health care providers at the time of each outpatient encounter? What factors would determine the successful implementation of each of these methods?

References and Suggested Readings

American Health Information Management Association. (1992). *Professional Practice Standards for Health Information Management Services in Ambulatory Care.* Chicago: American Health Information Management Association.

American Hospital Association. (2003). *Hospital Statistics.* Chicago: Health Forum LLC.

[AHA & AHIMA] American Hospital Association & American Health Information Management Association. (2003). Recommendation for standardized hospital evaluation and management coding of emergency department and clinic services [Online]. http://www.hospitalconnect.com/aha/advocacygrassroots/advocacy/agencyletters/2003/FedAg0306 27EMcoding.html [2003, August 3].

American Medical Association. (2003). *Current Procedural Terminology.* Chicago: American Medical Association.

Association of American Medical Colleges. (1996). A synopsis of the new Medicare rules on payment for teaching physicians. Washington, DC: AAMC.

Build an effective coding compliance program. (1996). *Physician's Payment Update,* October, 156–157.

[CMS] Centers for Medicare & Medicaid Services. (2002a). Chapter 1: Program background and responsibilities. *State Operations Manual* [Online]. http://cms.hhs.gov/manuals/pub07pdf/part-01.pdf [2003, July 31].

[CMS] Centers for Medicare & Medicaid Services. (2002b). Outpatient prospective payment system (OPPS) fact sheet [Online]. http://www.cms.hhs.gov/regulations/hopps/changecy2003.asp [2003, August 3].

[CMS] Centers for Medicare & Medicaid Services. (2002c, November 1). Hospital outpatient prospective payment system (2003 CY). *Federal Register*, pp. 66717–67046.

[CMS] Centers for Medicare & Medicaid Services. (2003a). Chapter II: Coverage of hospital services. *Hospital Manual* [Online]. http://cms.hhs.gov/manuals/10_hospital/ho00.asp [2003, July 31].

[CMS] Centers for Medicare & Medicaid Services. (2003b). Chapter XV—Fee schedule for physicians' service, Section 15016, Supervising physicians in teaching settings. *Medicare Carriers Manual, Part 3—Claims Process* [Online]. http://cms.hhs.gov/manuals/14_car/3b15000.asp [2003, August 2].

[CMS] Centers for Medicare & Medicaid Services. (2003c, January 3). Transmittal A-02-129—2003 Update of the Hospital Outpatient Prospective Payment System (OPPS). [Online]. http://www.cms.hhs.gov/manuals/pm_trans/A02129.pdf [2003, August 2].

Conditions of Participation for Hospitals, *Code of Federal Regulations*, Title 42, Pt. 482, 2002 ed.

Curran, W. J., Hall, M. A., Bobinski, M. A., & Orentlicher, D. (1998). *Health Care Law and Ethics*. New York: Aspen Law & Business.

Eubanks, P. (1990). Outpatient care: A nationwide revolution. *Hospitals*, August 5, 28–35.

Feste, L. K. (1989). *Ambulatory Care Documentation*. Chicago: American Medical Record Association.

Glondys, B. (2000). Glossary of healthcare services and statistical terms. In K. G. Youmans, *Basic healthcare statistics for health information management professionals* (pp. 139–175). Chicago: American Health Information Management Association

Hanken, M. A., and Waters, K. A. (1994). *Glossary of Healthcare Terms*. Chicago, IL: American Health Information Management Association.

[HCFA] Health Care Financing Administration. (2000, August 17). Announcement of designated standard maintenance organizations. *Federal Register*, p. 50373.

Institute of Medicine. (2001). *Crossing the Quality Chasm: A New Health System for the 21st Century*. Washington, D.C.: National Academy Press.

Institute of Medicine. (2003). *Key capabilities of an electronic health record system: Letter report*. [Online]. http://books.nap.edu/html/ehr/NI000427.pdf [2003, December 18].

[JCAHO] Joint Commission on Accreditation of Healthcare Organizations. (2003a). *Hospital Accreditation Standards*. Oakbrook Terrace, IL: Author.

[JCAHO] Joint Commission on Accreditation of Healthcare Organizations. (2003b). *Joint Commission 2003 Automated Comprehensive Accreditation Manual for Hospitals*. Oakbrook Terrace, IL: Joint Commission on Accreditation of Healthcare Organizations.

Korttila, K. (1990). Recovery period and discharge. In P. F. White (Ed.), *Outpatient Anesthesia* (pp. 369–396). New York: Churchill Livingstone.

Kovner, A. R. & Jonas, S. (Eds.). (2002). *Health Care Delivery in the United States*, 7th edition. New York: Springer Publishing Company.

Kovner, A. R. (1990b). Hospitals. In A. R. Kovner (Ed.), *Health Care Delivery in the United States*, 4th edition (pp. 141–176). New York: Springer Publishing Company.

Kuehn, L. (1994). *Learning Guide for Ambulatory Care*. Chicago, IL: American Health Information Management Association.

Lawrence, R. S., and Jonas, S. (1990). Ambulatory care. In A. R. Kovner (Ed.), *Health Care Delivery in the United States*, 4th edition (pp. 106–140). New York: Springer Publishing Company.

Lefkowitz, R., and Topor, I. (Eds.). (1989). *Comparative Medical Record Keeping in Health Care Facilities*. Owings Mills, MD: National Health Publishing.

Mezey, A. P. (2002). Ambulatory care. In A. R. Kovner & S. Jonas (Eds.), *Health Care Delivery in the United States*, 7th edition (pp. 173–198). New York: Springer Publishing Company.

[NCIPC] National Center for Injury Prevention and Control. (1997). Data elements for emergency department systems, release 1.0 [Online]. Atlanta, GA: Centers for Disease Control and Prevention. http://www.cdc.gov/ncipc/pub-res/pdf/deeds.pdf [2003, August 4].

[NCVHS] National Committee on Vital and Health Statistics. (1996). Core health data elements: Report of the National Committee on Vital and Health Statistics [Online]. http://www.ncvhs.hhs.gov/ncvhsr1.htm#Future [2003, August 4].

[NUBC] National Uniform Billing Committee. (2002, August 22). Highlights of changes contained in the draft UB-02 [Online]. http://www.nubc.org/public/whatsnew/ub02draft1.pdf [2003, August 4]

[OIG] Office of the Inspector General, U.S. Department of Health and Human Services. (2002). Centers for Medicare and Medicaid Services Work Plan for Fiscal Year 2003 [Online]. http://oig.hhs.gov/reading/workplan/2003/2-CMS%20FY03.pdf [2003, December 18].

[OIG] Office of the Inspector General, U.S. Department of Health and Human Services. (2003). Centers for Medicare and Medicaid Services Work Plan for Fiscal Year 2004 [Online]. http://oig.hhs.gov/publications/docs/workplan/2004/2-CMS%20FY04.pdf [2003, December 18].

Orkin, F. K. (1990). Economic and regulatory issues. In P. F. White (Ed.), *Outpatient Anesthesia* (pp. 87–105). New York: Churchill Livingstone.

Patrick, S. (2004). Hospitals see growth in outpatient services. *Dallas Business Journal* [Online]. http://www.bizjournals.com/dallas/stories/2004/03/01/newscolumn7.html [2004, May 12].

Physician services in teaching settings. *Code of Federal Regulations*, Title 42, Part 415, Subpart D, 2002 ed.

Prophet-Bowman, S. (2003). Observation services present compliance challenges. *Journal of the American Health Information Management Association, 74*(3), 60, 62–65.

Roizen, M. F., and Rupani, G. (1990). Preoperative assessment of adult outpatients. In P. F. White (Ed.), *Outpatient Anesthesia* (pp. 181–200). New York: Churchill Livingstone.

Special responsibilities of Medicare hospitals in emergency cases. *Code of Federal Regulations*, Title 42, Part 489, Section 24, 2002 ed.

Washington Publishing Company. (No date). Implementation guides adopted for use under HIPAA [Online]. http://hipaa.wpc-edi.com/HIPAA_40.asp [2003, August].

Key Resources

American Health Information Management Association
(See Chapter 1 for contact information.)

American Hospital Association
One North Franklin
Chicago, IL 60606-3421
Phone: 312-422-3000
http://www.aha.org

American Osteopathic Association
142 East Ontario Street
Chicago, IL 60611
Phone: 800-621-1773 or 312-202-8000
Fax: 312-202-8200
http://www.aoa-net.org

American Society for Healthcare Risk Management (ASHRM)
1 N. Franklin Street
Chicago, IL 60606
Phone: 312-422-3980
Fax: 312-422-4580
http://www.hospitalconnect.com/ashrm/aboutus/aboutus.html

Association of American Medical Colleges
2450 N Street, NW
Washington, DC 20037
Phone: 202-828-0400
Fax: 202-828-1125
http://www.aamc.org

Centers for Medicare & Medicaid Services
7500 Security Boulevard
Baltimore, MD 21244
Phone: 877-267-2323
http://www.cms.hhs.gov

Health Care Compliance Association
5780 Lincoln Drive, Suite 120
Minneapolis, MN 55436
Phone: 888-580-8373
Fax: 952-988-0146
http://www.hcca-info.org

Healthcare Financial Management Association
Two Westbrook Corporate Center, Suite 700
Westchester, IL 60154-5700
Phone: 800-252-HFMA (4362)
Fax: 708-531-0032
http://www.hfma.org

Joint Commission on Accreditation of Healthcare Organizations
(See Chapter 1 for contact information.)

Medical Group Management Association
104 Inverness Terrace East
Englewood, CO 80112-5306
Phone: 303-799-1111
http://www.mgma.com

Office of the Inspector General
Department of Health and Human Services
Room 5541, Cohen Building
330 Independence Avenue, SW
Washington, DC 20201
Phone: 202-619-1343
http://oig.hhs.gov

Chapter 3

Freestanding Ambulatory Care

Elizabeth D. Bowman, MPA, RHIA

Learning Objectives

Upon successful completion of this chapter, you should be able to:

1. List the types of freestanding ambulatory centers and differentiate among them regarding the kinds of programs and services they offer.
2. Define basic terms related to freestanding ambulatory care facilities.
3. List the major agencies or organizations that set standards for the facility and interpret their standards.
4. Discuss pertinent record completion, filing, quality assessment, coding and indexing, and computer systems for freestanding ambulatory care facilities.
5. Discuss payment systems for freestanding ambulatory care.

SETTING	DESCRIPTION	SYNONYMS/ EXAMPLES
Public Health Department	Organization that provides services to promote the health of the community as a whole, such as immunizations and disease screenings	Community Health
Neighborhood Health Centers	Ambulatory setting developed in the 1960s to provide ambulatory care to the indigent of a particular neighborhood	
Industrial Health Centers	Ambulatory setting in which care is provided to employees at their place of work or at an employer-contracted site	Industrial Clinic
Ambulatory Surgery Centers	Setting provided for surgery on an ambulatory basis	Surgicenter
Urgent Care Centers	Ambulatory care setting in which patients are seen on a walk-in basis without appointments	Minor Emergency Center Walk-in Clinic
Physician Private Practices	Setting in which physicians practice independently rather than being employed by an organization such as an urgent care center or clinic	Doctor's Office Solo Practice Group Practice
University Health Centers	Ambulatory setting in which care is provided to students while they are in college, as well as faculty and staff in some cases	Student Health University Health Employee Health
Birth Centers	Ambulatory setting that provides labor and delivery services for uncomplicated deliveries	Birthing Centers

Introduction to Setting

Care Settings

How is **freestanding ambulatory care** different from hospital-based ambulatory care? The obvious difference is that freestanding sites are not located within the hospital. There are a variety of types of freestanding settings, and freestanding ambulatory care is the setting in which most people receive care. The type of ambulatory care facility determines the types of patients seen, the type of caregivers, and, therefore, the type of information collected.

A large portion of freestanding ambulatory care is provided by **physician private practices** where physicians open an office to see ambulatory patients. Physicians may practice alone, called solo practice, or in a group. A group practice usually involves three or more physicians, either all of the same specialty or of different specialties. Physicians practicing together usually share records, equipment, and offices and have an arrangement to divide the profits of the practice. Historically, such practices have been the most common setting in which ambulatory care is provided.

Other types of ambulatory care have been developed to meet the needs of patients. **Public health departments**, for example, provide a variety of services to improve the health of the community as a whole, in addition to health care for individuals. An emphasis is placed on preventive services such as immunizations, screenings, and notifying contacts of patients with infectious conditions such as tuberculosis and syphilis to prevent further spread of the condition throughout the community.

Neighborhood health centers were a result of the federal social legislation in the 1960s. Their purpose was to meet the medical needs of people who, because of their location and their inability to pay, were not receiving the care they needed in the traditional physician's office or clinic. In addition, these centers were created to provide training and employment to those living near the center (Patton, 1990).

Urgent care centers arose to meet the need for care outside regular physicians' office hours, traditionally provided in expensive hospital emergency departments. Urgent care centers usually see patients on a walk-in basis without appointments and provide basically the same services as physicians' offices.

Ambulatory surgery centers (ASCs) arose to meet the need for a less expensive setting than the hospital for low-risk surgical procedures. Their growth was fed by the Omnibus Reconciliation Act of 1980 that set up a Medicare payment system specifically for ASCs (Wong, 1990). Although some physicians perform minor surgical procedures in their offices, the main difference in a freestanding ASC is that it usually has at least one full operating room, is often licensed by the state, and provides surgical privileges to doctors in the community, not just in one practice (Duggar, 1990).

Occupational/Industrial health centers provide care to employees at their place of work. Services range from providing care for minor injuries sustained on the job to providing physical examinations when employees are hired or when they are returning to work following an accident. They often provide screenings such as auditory tests for employees at risk of hearing loss or exposure-level tests for employees working with hazardous substances.

University health centers provide care to students while they are enrolled in college, as well as to faculty and staff in some cases. Some centers provide only minor services, whereas others provide the full scope of care. The extent of their services often depends on the size of the university and the range of services available to students outside the university community.

Birth centers and **family planning centers** arose to counteract what was felt to be a rigidity by hospitals in providing birthing and family planning options. They provide a homelike atmosphere for deliveries and provide contraceptive and other family planning services. Hospitals historically would not allow family or other support persons within the labor and delivery suites. Alternative caregivers such as midwives were also not allowed to perform deliveries. Freestanding birth centers and family planning centers were developed to provide the homelike environment requested by patients along with a variety of caregivers providing support.

Types of Patients

The type of freestanding ambulatory facility is the first factor to consider in developing health information management services. The second important factor is the type of patients seen in the setting. As can be seen from the types of settings providing ambulatory care, a variety of patients are included. Patients seen in the ambulatory setting are not critically ill. Care may be provided to well patients, such as well-baby care and the health screenings provided in industrial health settings. Most of the patients, however, are the ambulatory sick who may have minor acute problems, such as sore throats and earaches, or chronic conditions, such as heart disease and diabetes. All ages of patients are included. Some facilities see only a certain type of patient. Birth centers, for example, see pregnant women. Ambulatory surgery centers see patients with surgically treatable diseases. The types of patients seen by a facility affect the information that must be maintained. In a pediatric clinic, for example, information on immunizations and growth and development is necessary. Birth centers need to provide information on labor and delivery.

Types of Caregivers

The next information to find out is what types of caregivers are seeing patients in the facility. Different types of caregivers provide different types of documentation, which affect the information available (see Figure 3-1). Because physician practices provide most ambulatory care services, physicians are the main caregivers. They may be in private practice, or they may be employees of settings such as university health or urgent care centers.

Other professionals such as **nurse practitioners (NPs)** also provide care in the ambulatory setting. A nurse practitioner is a registered nurse who has had additional training in areas such as family or pediatric care. NPs are often the primary caregivers in settings such as industrial clinics and neighborhood health centers. **Certified nurse midwives (CNMs)** often practice in birth and family planning centers. **Physician assistants (PAs)** may be seen in settings similar to those employing nurse practitioners. PAs are not nurses but have received training to use independent judgment in treating patients. Other practitioners that may be seen include dentists, nutritionists, and counselors (Benson et al., 1987).

Regulatory Issues

Determining types of caregivers in a facility identifies both who is entering information into the health information system and who are the internal users of information. The regulations that a facility must follow determine the external users of information

Ambulatory Caregivers	Type of Service Provided
Physician	MD or DO providing complete medical care
Nurse Practitioner (NP)	Advanced practice RN providing care independently within a certain area of practice such as family care or pediatrics
Certified Nurse Midwife (CNM)	Advanced practice RN providing care during pregnancy, labor, and delivery in uncomplicated cases
Physician Assistant (PA)	Non-RN using independent judgment in providing care
Dentist	DDS or DMD specializing in care of the teeth and gums
Nutritionist	Practitioner providing advice and planning for patients' nutritional needs
Counselor/therapist	Practitioner providing care for behavioral and mental problems
Psychologist	Ph.D. providing care for behavioral and mental problems
Social Worker	Practitioner assisting patients with social and environmental problems
Chiropractor	Practitioner providing manipulation, usually of the spine, to improve health
Podiatrist	Practitioner providing care of the feet

Figure 3-1   Caregivers in freestanding ambulatory care.

and standards for what information should be maintained. Regulations and standards are usually determined by accreditation, certification, and licensure bodies.

Licensure

The requirements for licensure vary by the type of facility. Because licensure standards are set by the state, often through the state department of health, they are different in every state. Laws governing which facilities must be licensed differ from state to state. In most states, physicians' offices do not require licensure. Ambulatory surgery centers and birth centers, however, usually have to meet licensure standards. Most licensure standards include rules for what information must be maintained by the facility in its health records. They are, therefore, an excellent source of information on what must be included in the information system.

Medicare Certification

As noted in Chapter 1, certain types of health care facilities must be Medicare-certified according to *Medicare Conditions of Participation* or *Conditions of Coverage* before they can participate in the Medicare program. *Conditions of Coverage/Participation* exist for ambulatory surgical services and for rural health clinics. In the case of rural health clinics (RHCs), Medicare certification confers a special status that permits cost-based reimbursement from Medicare and Medicaid. The goal of the rural health clinic program is to increase access to primary care in medically underserved rural areas by using PAs, NPs, and CNMs in physician shortage areas (Rural Assistance Center, 2003).

The *Conditions of Coverage* require ambulatory surgery centers to "maintain complete, comprehensive, and accurate medical records," including documentation of patient identification information, medical history and results of physical examination, preoperative diagnostic studies performed, findings and techniques of the operation, including a pathologist's report on tissue removed, allergies and abnormal drug reactions, anesthesia administration entries, informed consent documentation, and discharge diagnosis (42CFR416.47).

Medicare standards for rural health clinics include a requirement that records be maintained for each patient and that a designated professional staff member be assigned the responsibility for maintenance of the records. Included in the requirements for record content are identification and social data, consent forms, history, summary of the visit, disposition and instructions to the patient, physical examinations, laboratory and other diagnostic results, consultant's findings, physician's orders, reports of treatment, and medications. In addition, the standards require that medical records be retained for at least six years from the date of the last entry in the record unless a longer retention period is required by state law (42CFR491.10).

Accreditation

Unlike licensure, which must be undertaken if required by the state, accreditation is a voluntary process. Accreditation is not as common in ambulatory care as in hospitals, for several reasons. First, it is not required for reimbursement as it is in hospitals. Second, the variety of facilities makes developing standards for all settings difficult (Avery and Imdieke, 1984). Much of ambulatory care is provided in private physicians' offices, too, and accreditation has not been a high priority because this process is an added expense. (See Figure 3-2 for the accreditation organizations commonly found in ambulatory care.)

The Joint Commission on Accreditation of Healthcare Organizations (JCAHO) is the best-known health care accreditation agency. It has developed the *Accreditation Manual for Ambulatory Health Care* that includes standards for freestanding ambulatory care settings. When freestanding ambulatory facilities are accredited, it is more common, however, for them to be accredited by the Accreditation Association for Ambulatory Health Care Inc. Its standards are published in the *Accreditation Handbook for Ambulatory Health Care*. Both organizations primarily accredit organized clinic settings. Other accreditation agencies accredit only a particular type of ambulatory care. One example is the American Association for Accreditation of Ambulatory Surgery Facilities, Inc., which accredits only single or multispecialty surgical facilities owned or operated by board-certified surgeons. Another specialty accreditation organization is the Commission for the Accreditation of Birth Centers with its *Standards for Birth Centers*.

Accreditation Organization	*Standards*
Joint Commission on Accreditation of Healthcare Organizations	*Accreditation Manual for Ambulatory Health Care* *Accreditation Manual for Office-Based Surgery*
Accreditation Association for Ambulatory Health Care Inc.	*Accreditation Handbook for Ambulatory Health Care*
Commission for the Accreditation of Birth Centers	*Standards for Birth Centers*
American Association for Accreditation of Ambulatory Surgery Facilities, Inc.	*Standards and Checklist Booklet Resource Manual*

Figure 3-2   Accreditation organizations in freestanding ambulatory care.

Although many facilities do not choose to be accredited, accreditation standards can still provide health information managers with a set of benchmarks for the information system within their facility. HIM professionals should be aware of accreditation standards in setting up new systems and evaluating existing ones to establish that the best possible methods and policies are followed.

Other Regulations: Compliance

The **Office of the Inspector General (OIG)** in the Department of Health and Human Services is charged with checking the compliance of providers with the laws and regulations covering reimbursement for federal programs such as Medicare. This office has identified large sums of money that were received by providers through error or fraud. The Department of Justice has recouped billions of dollars under laws such as the Federal False Claims Act and the Health Insurance Portability and Accountability Act (HIPAA).

To avoid such penalties, providers are encouraged to develop a compliance plan that ensures conformity to federal requirements. The OIG has published model **compliance plans** to provide guidance for a variety of health settings including Individual and Small Group Physician Practices (OIG, 59434) in developing internal controls. These plans include seven components as follows:

- Conducting internal monitoring and auditing
- Implementing compliance and practice standards
- Designating a compliance officer or contact
- Conducting appropriate training and education
- Responding appropriately to detected offenses and developing corrective action
- Developing open lines of communication
- Enforcing disciplinary standards through well-publicized guidelines

When conducting internal monitoring and auditing, practices are urged to audit both standards and procedures as well as claims submission. The claims audit may be retrospective (looking at previous claims) or prospective (looking at claims before submission). When a Medicare overpayment is discovered in a retrospective audit, the health care provider is required to disclose and refund the overpayment. One advantage of conducting a prospective audit is that errors can be caught before claim submission, allowing the practice to avoid the additional paperwork resulting from overpayment refunds. From a baseline audit, problem areas can be identified, and periodic audits must then be carried out at least once a year. Monitoring should be an ongoing process.

Once the risk areas have been identified, practice standards and procedures must be developed to deal with those risks. Suggestions from the OIG include "(1) Developing a written standards and procedures manual; and (2) updating clinical forms periodically to make sure they facilitate and encourage clear and complete documentation of patient care" (OIG, 59438). The main risk areas to be addressed include coding, billing, reasonable and necessary services, documentation, improper inducements, kickbacks, and self-referrals.

Ideally one person should be designated as a compliance officer or contact. The role of this person would be to oversee the adherence of the practice/facility to the compliance plan that it has developed.

Targeted training and education programs should emphasize providing training for staff members most in need of training and the areas of most risk. However, general training should cover all risk areas and include all staff members who could participate in or identify an error or a violation of the compliance program. Training must be ongoing and must address any changes in the laws, regulations, and coding systems that affect compliance.

When offenses are detected, a corrective action plan must be developed. There is a Provider Self-Disclosure Protocol, developed by the OIG, which should be followed in such cases. Open lines of communication are necessary to ensure that everyone is aware of how to report what they believe to be fraudulent or in error. Finally, disciplinary procedures must be in place to deal with violations of the compliance plan.

Documentation

Documentation involves the process of recording information about the care being provided in the ambulatory care center. Many factors influence what must be documented, including those factors already discussed: type of facility, type of patients, types of caregivers, and internal and external users of information. It is easiest to think about documentation by going through the care process with the patient to see what items of data must be maintained (see Figure 3-3).

Registration/Demographic Information

The first contact the patient usually has with any ambulatory care setting is the **registration** process. During this step, demographic information, such as the patient's

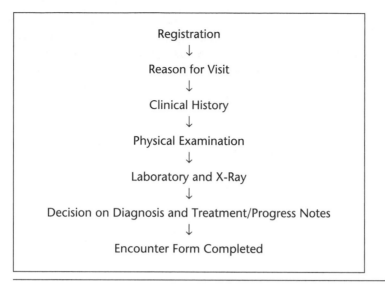

Figure 3-3   Flow of care and documentation.

name and address, and financial information, such as responsible party and insurance coverage, are collected. Often this information is first documented by having the patient complete a form upon arrival at the facility (see Figure 3-4). This information is then entered into the patient's record by clerical personnel either on an information form or in a computerized demographics/finance screen. Usually the form completed by the patient does not become a part of the official record.

History and Physical

Once basic information has been received from the patient, the actual care process begins. The first step is finding out why the patient is being seen, or the **reason for visit**, and obtaining a history of the illness. The nurse often begins this process by asking the patient for the reason for visit and a brief history. Sometimes the patient may complete a history form, either manually or on the computer. The comprehensiveness of the history depends on the patient's reason for visit. A visit for a sore throat, for example, would require only minimal information. A visit for shortness of breath would require a more exhaustive inquiry into the patient's past history and family and social history. The caregiver, either the physician, nurse practitioner, or physician assistant, then completes the physical. Like the history, the physical varies in completeness depending on the patient's reason for visit.

Laboratory and X-Ray Reports

The history and the physical examination begin the fact-finding process to gain the information needed to make a diagnosis and to determine a plan of treatment.

Patient Data

_____
MEDICAL RECORD NO

THIS IMPORTANT INFORMATION IS CONFIDENTIAL. PLEASE BE HONEST. ANSWER THE QUESTIONS AS BEST YOU CAN. IF YOU NEED ASSISTANCE, ASK YOUR PROVIDER.

Patient's   Name:_____   _____/_____/_____
             (last)   (first)   (middle)   Social Security Number

Previous   Names   Used:_____

Address:_____/_____/_____/_____
             (street)   (city)   (state)   (zip)   (county)

Home Phone: (   )_____Sex:___Race: ___Marital Status: M__S__Sep__D__W__

Birth   Date:_____ Age:_____ City:_____State/Country   of   Birth:_____

Mother's   Maiden   Name:_____
                            (last)   (first)

Father's   Name:_____
                     (last)   (first)

No. in Family:_____   Head of Household:_____Guardian:_____

Other Family   **LAST**   **FIRST**   **DATE OF BIRTH**   **SEX**   **RELATIONSHIP**
       Members: _____
                  _____
                  _____
                  _____
                  _____
                  _____

Person to Contact in Case of Emergency:_____
                                           (last)   (first)
       Relationship: _____   Phone No:(   )_____
       Address:_____
                    (street)   (city)   (state)   (zip)
Nearest Relative: _____
                            (last)   (first)
       Relationship: _____   Phone No:(   )_____
       Address:_____
                    (street)   (city)   (state)   (zip)

Previous Visits to The Regional Medical Center of Memphis (The Med)? No__Yes__ Please Explain:
_____

Patient's   Occupation:_____

Employment Status: Full-Time_ Part-Time_ Unemployed_ Retired_ Student_ Military_ Other_

Employer: _____ Business Phone:(   ) _____ Ext:_____

Address:_____
                (street)   (city)   (state)   (zip)
Religion: _____

Do you have any communication barriers for which you might require additional assistance?
       No_ Yes_: Language__ Please identify_____ Unable To Read__ Deaf___
                      Blind_____ Other:_____

Printed in **THE MED** Print Shop

Figure 3-4   Registration form. (Courtesy of Memphis Family Care Center.)

Sometimes additional information is needed, such as clinical laboratory tests and X-rays. Simple tests may often be provided in the office or clinic, but more complicated procedures may require that the patient be referred elsewhere. Results of the tests may be kept in a computerized printout or may be recorded on a reporting slip or typed for entry in the record.

Progress Notes

Once all the needed information has been collected, the caregiver usually records diagnoses or major problems in narrative form along with plans for treatment such as medications prescribed. In some settings, the documentation for the entire encounter may take the format of a long note, which may be handwritten or typed.

Encounter Form

At the end of the visit, an **encounter form** or **superbill** is usually generated (Figure 3-5). This form includes information on the patient's diagnoses and treatments along with disease and procedure codes and charges. Usually completed, at least in part, by the caregiver, the encounter form may become a part of the patient's record. It may, however, be stored separately because its main purpose is to provide information for billing and insurance processing rather than documenting the care process.

Copies of Hospital Records

If the patient has been hospitalized, copies of forms from the hospital, such as the operative report and discharge summary, are often sent to the facility. These are usually filed in the patient's record.

Problem List

In facilities that see patients regularly, a **problem list** is often used (Figure 3-6). The problem list is a numbered list of the patient's diagnoses or problems, often including allergies and medications taken. It should appear in a conspicuous place in the record, usually at the front, and must be updated regularly. The problem list, therefore, serves as a table of contents for the record by summarizing the patient's care over time.

Special Requirements

The process just outlined is universal for most ambulatory care encounters. Some types of facilities or encounters may have more specialized documentation requirements

Memphis FamilyCare Center Encounter Form

Patient's Name	Chart #	Diagnoses: (List Primary Dx as #1)

Patient's Name _____ Chart # _____

Patient's SSN _____ Encounter # _____
Date _____ Age _____

Insurance Type (circle below)

New Patient   Yes   No   TennCare   Com   Self Pay   Other

Diagnoses: (List Primary Dx as #1)
1
2
3
4
5
6

DX #	DESCRIPTION	KEY 1	DX #	DESCRIPTION	KEY 1	DX #	DESCRIPTION	KEY 1
	OFFICE VISITS			**MEDICATIONS con't.**			**LAB: OUTSIDE (con't.)**	
	New Pt. Problem (10)	99201		MMR	90707		Bilirubin: Direct	82251
	New Pt. Expanded (20)	99202		Phenergan	J2550		Blood Count (Reticulocyte)	85044
	New Pt. Detailed (30)	99203		Pneumovac	90732		Calcium	82310
	New Pt. Comprehensive (45)	99204		Polio (OPV)	90712		Carbon Dioxide (Bicarb.)	82374
	New Pt. Comprehensive (60)	99205		PPD (Intradermal)	86580		CPK	82550
	Est. Pt. Simple (5)	99211		Procardia	J9999		Culture: Bacterial-Routine	87070
	Est. Pt. Problem (10)	99212		Rocephin (250 mg.)	J0696		Culture: Blood	87040
	Est. Pt. Expanded (15)	99213		Tetanus	90703		Culture: Chlamydia	87110
	Est. Pt. Detailed (25)	99214		Tetramune	90720		Culture: GC	87081
	Est. Pt. Comprehensive (40)	99215		Toradol	J3490		Culture: Herpes	87252
	New Pt.-Well Child; 0-1 yr	99381		Other			Culture: Throat	87060
	New Pt.-Well Child; 1-4 yr	99382		Other			Culture: Urine (Quantat)	87086
	New Pt.-Well Child; 5-11 yr	99383					Culture/Sens. - Urine	87088
	New Pt.-Well Child; 12-17 yr	99384					Dilantin	80185
	New Pt.-Well Pt.; 18-39 yrs	99385		**LAB: IN-HOUSE**			Drug Screen (Indicate Drug)	80100
	New Pt.-Well Pt.; 40-64 yrs	99386		Accu - Check (Glucometer)	82948		Estrogen: Total	82672
	New Pt.; over 65 yrs	99387		Albumin	82040		FANA	86255
	Est. Pt.-Well Child; 0-1 yr	99391		Alk. Phos.	84075		Folic Acid	82746
	Est. Pt.-Well Child; 1-4 yr	99392		ALT (SGPT)	84460		GC Probe	87178
	Est. Pt.-Well Child; 5-11 yr	99393		AST (SGOT)	84450		GGTP	82977
	Est. Pt.-Well Child; 12-17 yr	99394		Bilirubin - TOTAL	82250		Hemoglobin: Glycosylated	83036
	Est. Pt.-Well Pt.; 18-39 yrs	99395		BUN	84520		Hepatitis A Antibody	86296
	Est. Pt.-Well Pt.; 40-64 yrs	99396		CBC/Diff. (Automated)	85025		Hepatitis B Surface Anti.	86291
	Est. Pt.-Well Pt.; over 65 yrs	99397		Chlamydia	86631		Hepatitis C Antibody	86302
	Consultation	99243		Cholesterol	82465		Hepatitis Panel	80059
	Development Assessment	99178		Creatinine	82565		HGB	85018
	Other			Glucose	82947		HIV Antigen	86311
	Other			GTT	82951		Iron	83540
				HCG - Serum (Pregnancy)	84703		Isoenzymes	82552
				HCG - Urine (Pregnancy)	84702		Lead Level	83655
				HDL	83718		Lipase	83690
	PROCEDURES			Hematocrit	85014		Lithium (Quantitative)	80178
	Administering Vaccine	Q0124		Hemoccult	82270		Magnesium	83735
	Aerosol Trtmt: Initial	94664		KOH	87220		Pap Smear	88150
	Aerosol Trtmt: F/U	94665		Mono Spot	86308		Phenobarb Level	82205
	Chem. Destruct. Lesion: Female	56501		Panels:			PKU	84030
	Chem. Destruct. Lesion: Male	54050		Arthritis	80072		Prostate Specific Antigen	84153
	EKG	93000		Exec (General Health)	80050		Protime	85610
	Hearing Screening	V5008		Lipid	80061		Sensitivity, Antibiotic	87181
	Insert Implant Contracept. Cap	11975		Liver	80058		Thyroid Panel w/TSH	80092
	Remove Foreign Body Ear(s)	69200		Potassium	84132		Thyroid Panel w/o TSH	80091
	Rem Impact. Cerumen One or Both	69210		Protein - Total	84155		TIBC	83550
	Remove Implant Contracept. Cap.	11976		Rheumatoid (RA)	86430		T-3 (Triiodothyronine)	84480
	Skin Biopsy	11100		Sed Rate - Automat.	85651		T-4 (Thyroxine): Total	84336
	Suture (specify length & site)			Serum Ketone	82009		Vol. Measure/Timed Coll. each	81050
	Other			Sickle Screen	85660		Other	
	Other			Sodium	84295		Other	
				Strep Screen	86403			
	MEDICATIONS			Triglyceride	84478			
	Bicillin up to 600,000	J0530		Uric Acid	84550		LAB Handling Fee	99000
	Bicillin up to 1,200,000	J0540		Urinalysis	81000		ACE Bandage	A4460
	Bicillin up to 2,400,000	J0580		VDRL/RPR/ART	86592		Other	
	B12	J3420		WBC	85048		Other	
	Demerol/Meperdine up to 50 mg.	J2175		Wet Mount	87210			
	Depo - Medrol 20mg	J1020		Other				
	Depo - Medrol 40mg	J1030		Other				
	Depo - Medrol 80mg	J1100					**REFERRALS**	
	Depo - Provera 150 mg	J1055					Dental	
	Depo - Testosterone	J1090					Dermatology	
	DPT	90701					OB/GYN	
	HBV (Hepatitis B Vac.)	90731		**LAB: OUTSIDE**			Other	
	HIB (H Influenza B Vac.)	90737		Amylase	82150		Other	
	Influenza	90724		B12	82607			

Comments:

Provider's Signature _____   Appt. Date _____

Figure 3-5 Encounter form. (Courtesy of Memphis Family Care Center.)

PROBLEM LIST

NO.	DIAGNOSED	PROBLEM DESCRIPTION / COMMENTS	TYPE	RESOLVED

Figure 3-6   Problem list. (Courtesy of Memphis Family Care Center.)

because of the specialized care provided, as shown in Figure 3-7. In designing documentation methods for a facility, the type of facility and the care provided must be carefully considered.

Type of Setting	Special Documentation Requirements
Ambulatory Surgery Center	Surgical Consent Operative Report Anesthesia Report Recovery Room Report Pathology Report Discharge Instructions
Birth Centers	Prenatal Record Labor and Delivery Record Physical Assessment of Newborn Follow-up Plan
Pediatric Care	Growth and Development Charts Immunization Record
Industrial Health	New-Hire Physical Return-to-Work Physical Transfer/Promotion and Annual Physical Health Monitoring Auditory and Vision Records

Figure 3-7 Special documentation requirements.

Ambulatory Surgery Centers

Ambulatory surgery centers add surgical documentation to the basic documentation just discussed. Necessary testing is often done before the day of surgery and must be present in the record before the surgery is done. Another important item of documentation is the consent for treatment. The surgeon is responsible for explaining the risks and alternatives associated with the surgery and for obtaining the patient's consent to the procedure. This consent process is often documented on a consent for surgery form that includes the name of the surgery, the name of the surgeon, the alternatives to the surgery, and the risks involved. The record should be checked to see that preoperative documentation is available. Intraoperative documentation includes data about the surgery. Each caregiver has a role in documenting the care given. The anesthesiologist must document the anesthesia given, any fluids given, and the patient's pulse, respiration, and blood pressure throughout the procedure. The surgeon must document the preoperative and postoperative diagnoses, the findings of the surgery, and the methods used. When the patient leaves the surgical suite, the care given during the recovery period must also be documented, including vital signs and recovery from general anesthesia. If tissue was removed during the surgery, a pathology report describing the gross and microscopic findings is also included. Finally, instructions to the patient must be documented to ensure that the patient knows postoperative wound care, complications to watch for, and when to return for follow-up, if necessary.

Birth Centers

In birth centers, labor and delivery is the process that must be documented. Such documentation usually begins with the prenatal record, which starts when the woman comes for initial care during the pregnancy. Because this care usually occurs in the physician's or midwife's office throughout the pregnancy, a copy of the office prenatal record must be sent to the birth center at regular intervals late in the pregnancy so that it is available at the time of the delivery. Prenatal documentation includes prenatal history and physical, weight gain, prenatal testing, gestational stage of the pregnancy, and any pregnancy complications.

Labor and delivery records provide documentation of the labor process including the onset of labor, length of labor, labor monitoring, pain management during the labor process, and the method of delivery.

Physical assessment of the newborn is also entered in the birthing center record including the Apgar score (a rating based on certain physical functions at one minute and five minutes after birth), an overall scoring of the physical condition of the newborn, weight, and other physical assessments.

Finally, a follow-up plan must be included that documents follow-up instructions such as when the mother and baby should return to the caregiver for evaluation.

Pediatric Preventive Health Services

For children, **immunizations** must be documented so that the caregiver can tell at a glance whether an immunization is needed on a particular visit (see Figure 3-8). **Growth and development charts** are also included that record height and weight to monitor growth patterns (see Figure 3-9).

Industrial Health Services/Occupational Medicine

Many different types of documentation are included in industrial health records, depending on the type of service provided. The record frequently includes physical examinations. Examinations may be done after hiring but before placement on the job. They provide a basis for assessing the employee's health at the time of hire versus various times later during the employment period. **Return-to-work physicals** are done for employees injured on the job who must be judged fit to work before returning to the workplace. Transfer or promotion and annual physicals are frequently provided for executive personnel. Health monitoring for exposure to hazardous or toxic substances or other health threats such as loud noise is also a common part of the industrial record. Vision records may be included for work settings where vision is an important factor in job performance such as for pilots. Finally, if care is provided

MEMPHIS FAMILYCARE CENTER
IMMUNIZATION RECORD

PATIENT NAME: _____ BIRTH DATE: _____ CLINIC MR #: _____

I have read the information contained in the "Important Information" form(s) about the disease(s) and the vaccine.
I have had an opportunity to ask questions which were answered to my satisfaction.
I believe I understand the benefits and risks of the vaccine(s) and request that the vaccine(s) indicated below be given
to me or to the person named in the identification space on the form for whom I am authorized to make this request.

VACCINE	DATE GIVEN M/D/Y	AGE	SITE	VACCINE MANUFACTURER	VACCINE LOT NUMBER	HANDOUT PUB. DATE	NURSE INITIALS	SIGNATURE OF PARENT/GUARDIAN
DTP1								
DTP2								
DTP3								
DTP/DTaP4								
DTP/DTaP5								
DT								
DTP/Hib1								
DTP/Hib2								
DTP/Hib3								
DTP/Hib4								
Td								
OPV/IPV1								
OPV/IPV2								
OPV/IPV3								
OPV/IPV4								
MMR1								
MMR2								
Hib1								
Hib2								
Hib3								
Hib4								
HepB1								
HepB2								
HepB3								

Figure 3-8 Immunization record. (Courtesy of Memphis Family Care Center.)

in the clinic for illness or accident treatment, the usual documentation of the care process must be included.

When selecting the documentation requirements for a particular facility, the HIM professional should begin with the universal components such as history and physical, progress notes, and laboratory and X-ray data. Then the particular needs of the site should be determined by looking at the specific type of care provided, which

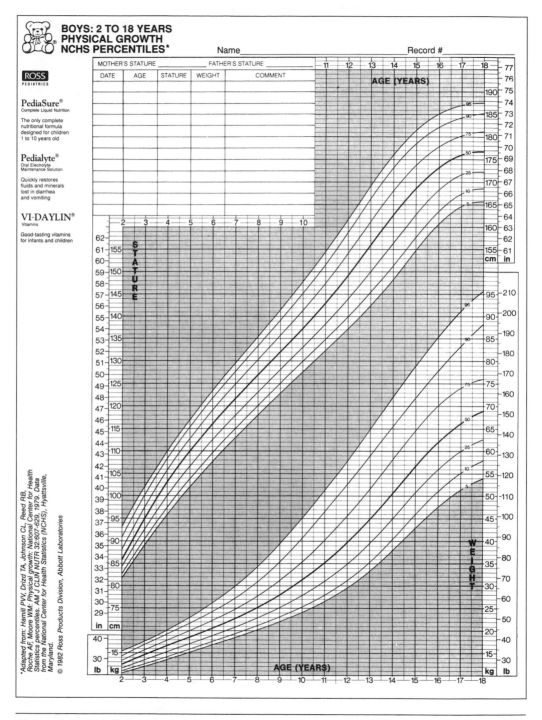

Figure 3-9 Height/weight record. (Courtesy of Memphis Family Care Center.)

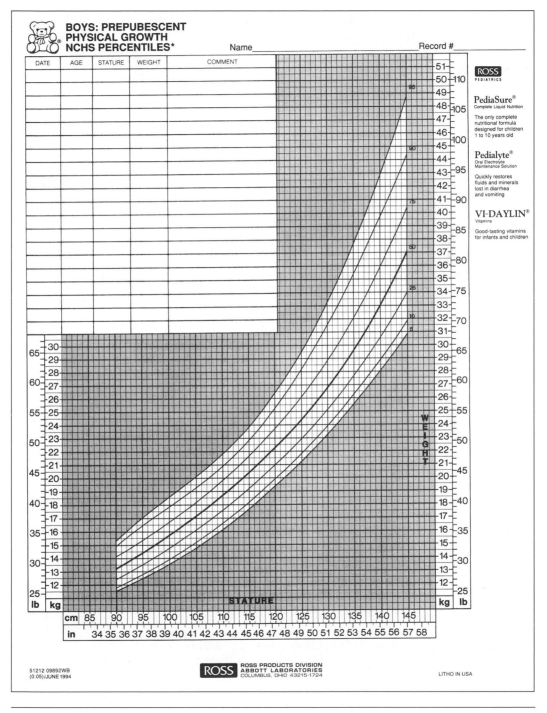

Figure 3-9   *(Continued)*

must be documented. Accreditation and licensure standards for the specific type of facility also help define the content of the documentation.

Record Format

The organization of data and information is defined as the record format (see Figure 3-10). The traditional format is called **source oriented**, with the information presented according to its source such as laboratory, X-ray, physician, nursing, and so forth. This format has the advantage of being familiar to caregivers, but it makes the process of reading the record and integrating data from the different sources more difficult.

Format	Characteristics
Source Oriented	Arranged according to source (e.g., laboratory, nursing, etc.)
Integrated	Chronological
Problem Oriented	Problem list Keyed to problem number
Computer Based	Electronic

Figure 3-10   Record formats.

In physicians' offices, the **integrated format** is frequently used. In this format, all information is entered in chronological order with each visit listed. Other events such as telephone calls are listed chronologically between visits. Test results and copies of hospital records are entered as they are received. This method makes it easy to look at each episode of care. However, it is more difficult to look at the patient's care across time or, especially, to monitor a particular data element over time. For example, it is often desirable to look for trends in laboratory values. This is more difficult with the integrated format because the laboratory results are scattered throughout the record rather than grouped into one location.

The **problem-oriented medical record (POMR)** is a third format that is occasionally used. The problem-oriented medical record was developed by Dr. Lawrence Weed to provide a more systematic method of record keeping. The key component of the POMR is the problem list. As was discussed previously, this is a list of the patient's problems and diagnoses and serves as a quick overview of the patient's health. In a true problem-oriented record, all parts of the record are indexed to the problem list. First, the clinical database consisting of the history, physical, and laboratory and X-ray findings is developed. Then a list of problems is developed and numbered. A plan indexed to the problem list is then generated with a plan for each problem identified by problem number. Each order and progress note is also indexed to the problem number so that it can be seen at a glance what problem is being addressed. Although the POMR is a systematic record-keeping process, it has not gained wide usage in ambulatory care. Generally, it is more likely seen in larger clinics with more caregivers and a greater need for coordination of care.

The **electronic health record (EHR)** is the format that is slowly gaining greater acceptance. With the EHR, patient demographic and clinical information is entered into a computer system. It can be retrieved either sequentially by encounter or through a querying process to access particular pieces of data.

The choice of record format depends primarily on the preference of the caregivers. The main principle that must be followed, however, is that all caregivers within a facility must use the same format. Without this uniformity, it is very difficult to find data in records documented by different caregivers. Committees are often formed to suggest a format and should consider the variety of users in making the decision.

Patient Identifier/Filing Methods

Patient identifier refers to how the patient is identified in a health information system, whether paper based or computer based, and how information about that patient is found (see Figure 3-11). In small settings, the patient's name is the primary identifier. If a paper-based filing system is used in such a setting, the records are filed alphabetically by the patient's name. In a computerized system, the patient's record may be accessed through the patient's name. Such a system quickly becomes cumbersome

Patient Identifier	*Advantage*	*Disadvantage*
Patient Name	Easily obtained No need for master patient index	Misspellings Many patients with same/similar names Need for secondary identifier to verify Cumbersome with a large number of records
Patient Number— unit or serial	Unique to each patient Uniform in length Confidentiality	Requires patient index to locate record
Patient Number— Social Security number	Most patients have Social Security number	Some patients do not have Social Security number Threat to privacy
Family Numbering	Availability of information for all family members together Useful for billing Useful in mailings	Frequent changes in family structure require changes in identification system

Figure 3-11 Patient identifiers used in ambulatory care.

because patients frequently have the same name. In a computerized system, a whole list of patients may be found if the name is the primary patient identifier. A secondary piece of information must frequently be used with this method to verify that the correct patient has been found. Common secondary identifiers are the Social Security number, birth date, or mother's maiden name.

When a system is too large to use an alphabetical system, a number is usually assigned to identify the patient. If a number is used, there must be a master patient index file by patient name to provide the patient's number. In an EHR, the patient's record could be found by searching the database using the patient's name or number.

A variety of methods are used to assign these numbers. One way is first to decide the number of digits to be used in the number and then to start at zero and assign the numbers. A six-digit number is frequently used to allow an adequate amount of numbers for the patient population. A decision would have to be made on whether the patient would keep the same number for all visits (a unit system) or would receive a new number for each visit to enable the facility to distinguish among visits by the number (serial system). Most ambulatory care facilities use the unit numbering system.

Some facilities use the Social Security number to identify patients. This method is useful because most Americans have a Social Security number. It is difficult, however, because some patients, such as babies, do not have a number and other patients may be using an incorrect one. In cases where the patient does not have a Social Security number, a pseudo-number (false number) must be assigned. Using the Social Security number also raises issues of privacy because the government maintains information about individuals using the Social Security number as an identifier.

A **family numbering system** is used in some facilities. With this numbering system, the family is assigned a number. All members of the family use the same number with a suffix specifying their unique identifier within the family. The family number might be 425687, with the father being 425687-1, the mother 425687-2, and the child 425687-3. One advantage of this system is for settings in which the whole family is treated and when social and medical information about the entire family might be helpful in treating individuals. Family numbering can also be useful for billing purposes and mailings to family members. With the frequent changes in family structure through divorce and other family breakups, however, keeping up with the family unit and changing the record system to match it is a frustrating and frequently impossible task.

In selecting a patient identifier, the needs of the facility must be the primary consideration. In a facility where the patient may be seen once and never again, such as an ambulatory surgery center, it would be foolish to use a family numbering system. Industrial settings might use the Social Security number because all of their employees have this number in their personnel files. A small facility would be best served by an alphabetical system. With an alphabetical system, a separate master patient index to identify the patient's number would not be needed. Again, the facts of facility type, caregivers, and patient type should determine the decision.

Reimbursement

Fee for Service

How is care paid for in freestanding ambulatory care settings? (see Figure 3-12). The traditional method is called **fee for service**. In this system, the patient pays according to the type and amount of service provided. Usually, for example, there is a basic fee for the visit. Separate fees are assigned for laboratory tests, X-rays, or other services provided beyond the basic visit. In some facilities treating low-income patients, the fee for service may be charged based on a sliding scale, with the amount determined by the patient's income. The problem with fee for service has been that payers feel it offers an incentive to provide more service. A variety of systems have been devised to change the incentives from providing more service to providing only what is absolutely required by the patient's condition.

Payment System	Setting
Fee for Service	Any setting
Physician Fee Schedule	Physicians/Medicare part B
ASC System	Ambulatory surgery/Medicare
Capitation	Any setting

Figure 3-12   Payment methods in freestanding ambulatory care.

Medicare Physician Fee Schedule

For physician reimbursement, Part B of Medicare now pays using the **Medicare Physician Fee Schedule (MPFS) or (PFS)**, which is based on the **resource-based relative value scale (RBRVS)**. Medicare Part B includes physician payment and payment for services for limited-license practitioners who treat only particular types of problems or parts of the body, such as dentists, oral and maxillofacial surgeons, optometrists, podiatrists, and chiropractors. Other services included are diagnostic tests other than clinical diagnostic lab tests, diagnostic and therapeutic radiology services, and physical and occupational therapy services (independent practice only) (Summary of Final RBRVS Regulations, 1992). Nonphysician care givers such as physician assistants, nurse practitioners, certified Registered Nurse Anesthetists, certified nurse midwives, clinical psychologists, and clinical social workers also are paid at a rate tied to the RBRVS (Summary of Final RBRVS Regulations, 1992). Services provided to a patient by nurse practitioners or physician assistants when the physician is on site are termed **"incident to"** services and are fully reimbursed at the physician's rate provided by the fee schedule. **Locum tenens** physicians are those temporarily working in place of another physician. The regular physician bills for the services provided by the locum tenens physician. The fee schedule is based on the *Healthcare*

Common Procedure Coding System (HCPCS). For each HCPCS code, there are three main components or relative value units (RVUs) influencing payment. These include an amount for physician work, an amount for overhead expenses, and an amount for malpractice expenses. These three amounts are specific for each HCPCS code (Summary of Final RBRVS Regulations, 1992). Each of these RVUs is adjusted by a geographic factor for the area in which the practice is located. The sum of the amounts from the three RVUs adjusted for geographic location is then multiplied by a uniform conversion factor, which is a fixed dollar amount, to determine the fee (Summary of Final RBRVS Regulations, 1992). The fee schedule is revised to include new HCPCS codes and is published annually in the *Federal Register*.

Ambulatory Surgery Center Groups

Freestanding ambulatory surgery centers are paid by Medicare under a system based on the HCPCS code. This method provides facility payment, not physician payment. In this system, the HCPCS codes are listed (called the **ASC list**) and divided into groups (called **ASC groups**; see Figure 3-13). An amount of payment is assigned for each group. The freestanding ambulatory surgery facility, therefore, receives a payment based on the patient's surgery grouping according to the HCPCS code.

Ambulatory Payment Classification (APCs)

When Congress passed the legislation that created the Medicare outpatient prospective payment system, its intent was for the system to apply to freestanding ambulatory surgery centers as well as hospital-based outpatient services. Although the

Group 1	$340
Group 2	$455
Group 3	$520
Group 4	$643
Group 5	$731
Group 6	$840*
Group 7	$1015
Group 8	$989*
Group 9	$1366

*Includes $150 allowance for intraocular lens.

(CMS, 2003)

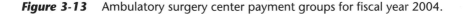

Figure 3-13 Ambulatory surgery center payment groups for fiscal year 2004.

system was implemented in hospital-based ambulatory care, there was a delay in implementing APCs as the payment system for freestanding ambulatory surgery centers. At this writing, no announcement has been made regarding a date for bringing freestanding ambulatory surgery centers under a system based on the ambulatory payment classification system.

Capitation

RBRVS and ASC group payments were efforts to change the incentives from paying more when more care was given to paying a fixed amount. **Capitation** is a method of payment that carries this effort even further. Under capitation, caregivers receive a fixed amount of payment per month for everyone under their care enrolled in a particular health care plan. For this fixed amount of payment, all necessary health services must be provided. The incentive is, therefore, to provide only care that is absolutely necessary to avoid losing money.

Knowing the reimbursement methods affecting the facility is important for the HIM professional. Documentation of the patient's care must support the level of billing from the facility. For PFS and ASC payments based on HCPCS codes, it is important that the documentation support the codes selected. More third-party payers are auditing ambulatory documentation to ensure that reimbursement matches the care documented.

Medicaid—Early and Periodic Screening, Diagnostic, and Treatment (EPSDT) Service

The **Early and Periodic Screening, Diagnostic, and Treatment (EPSDT)** service is a program of Medicaid for children younger than 21. It ensures that these services are provided and paid for whether or not they are normally included under the state's Medicaid program. Screening services include history and physical, appropriate immunizations, health education, vision, hearing, and dental services. Problems identified under the screening provisions must then also be fully diagnosed and treated.

Reimbursement Resources

The Centers for Medicare and Medicaid Services (CMS) has a variety of manuals and materials that provide information about reimbursement under the Medicare and Medicaid programs. **Program manuals** provide the basic instructions for the two programs. **Program transmittals** are periodically issued to provide a revision for a specific manual. **Program memoranda**, on the other hand, provide guidance and changes in the programs but are not tied to a specific program manual. These manuals, transmittals, and memoranda must be maintained to ensure that the facility is following the latest guidance. Claims for Medicare ambulatory care under Part B are filed with a carrier, a contractor for claims in a particular state or region. Carriers publish **Local Medical Review Policies (LMRPs)** or **Local Coverage Determinations (LCDs)**, which must be consistent with federal guidelines but provide further guidance for providers in the area served by a particular carrier. LMRPs/LCDs are important references for coders because they list diagnosis codes that indicate the medical necessity of certain procedures and services.

Information Management

Once the basic facts about the setting have been determined, the health information manager is able to evaluate or develop systems to meet the needs of the facility. All of the pieces of the puzzle come together in the HIM system.

Coding and Classification

Most facilities use some method to code diagnoses and procedures. This process involves assigning a number to the diagnoses and procedure according to an established classification method (see Figure 3-14). Coding is done in ambulatory care primarily to expedite the reimbursement process because most third-party payers require codes for the diagnoses and procedures submitted on bills. Most computer systems can more easily use numbers rather than verbal descriptions of the patient's diagnoses and procedures. The main factor usually considered in choosing coding systems for ambulatory care, therefore, is what systems are required by the third-party payers. Most ambulatory care settings do not want to code with one system for reimbursement and another for other classification purposes.

The *International Classification of Diseases, Ninth Revision, Clinical Modification (ICD-9-CM)* is the system most often used for coding diagnoses in ambulatory care. This system also includes procedure codes that are not used in ambulatory care settings. The disease classification in ICD-9-CM is maintained by the National Center for Health Statistics of the U.S. government and is revised semi-annually. These

Coding System	Use	Organization Responsible
International Classification of Diseases, Ninth Edition, Clinical Modification	Coding diagnoses	National Center for Health Statistics
Healthcare Common Procedure Coding System (HCPCS)	Coding procedures	
Level I *Current Procedural Terminology*		American Medical Association
Level II National Codes		Centers for Medicare and Medicaid Services (CMS)

Figure 3-14 Most common coding systems used in freestanding ambulatory care.

updates take effect in April and October of each year and require that ambulatory facilities update their coding, especially the preprinted codes included on encounter forms or superbills. A new edition of the International Classification, *International Classification of Diseases, 10th Revision, Clinical Modification* (ICD-10-CM) has been developed, and discussion is under way for ICD-10-CM to replace ICD-9-CM. No exact implementation date has been announced.

The **Healthcare Common Procedural Coding System (HCPCS)** is used in coding procedures in ambulatory care. Two levels of codes make up the HCPCS system. Level I consists of CPT codes developed by the American Medical Association (AMA). This coding system is revised by the AMA, and a new version of the codebooks is published each year. As with the revised ICD-9-CM codes, changes in the CPT system must be included in encounter and superbill forms. Level I codes generally reflect physician services. Level II codes in HCPCS are called national codes and are developed by the Centers for Medicare and Medicaid Services (CMS) of the U.S. government. Level II codes usually classify nonphysician services such as dental care and ambulance services. Types of injections can also be specified using Level II codes. [Level III codes were local codes developed by the Medicare carrier or intermediary. Level III local codes were eliminated by the Health Insurance Portability and Accountability Act (HIPAA) as of December 31, 2003.] Most third-party payers require reporting of diagnoses using ICD-9-CM and procedures using HCPCS.

Other coding systems may occasionally be seen in ambulatory settings. The **International Classification of Primary Care (ICPC)**, for example, is a coding system developed by the World Organization of National Colleges, Academies, and Academic Associations of General Practitioners/Family Physicians (WONCA). It includes chapters arranged by body systems with components that describe the reason why the patient is being seen for care at the primary care level.

Data and Information Flow

Many health information professionals are most familiar with the work flow within the hospital HIM department. The work begins with the patient's discharge, and staffing requirements are often determined based on the number of discharges to be processed each day. In ambulatory care, on the other hand, the visit is the driving force in determining the work flow and staffing requirements (Figure 3-15). The visit creates the need for the patient's record to be located so that past care can be reviewed and the care process during the visit recorded.

The work flow begins when an **appointment** is scheduled for the patient. Standard scheduling and block appointment methods such as wave scheduling and modified wave scheduling are typical appointment scheduling patterns. In **standard scheduling**, patients are scheduled continuously throughout the day with appointment times at specific intervals (e.g., every 15 minutes). This method can sometimes result in wasted physician time when visit lengths are shorter than expected or when patients are "no-shows." Standard scheduling does not eliminate patient waiting time because some visits run longer than the time allotted, putting all subsequent visits

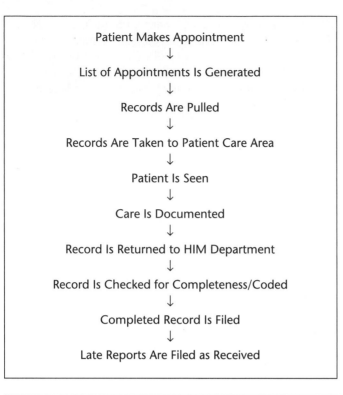

Patient Makes Appointment
↓
List of Appointments Is Generated
↓
Records Are Pulled
↓
Records Are Taken to Patient Care Area
↓
Patient Is Seen
↓
Care Is Documented
↓
Record Is Returned to HIM Department
↓
Record Is Checked for Completeness/Coded
↓
Completed Record Is Filed
↓
Late Reports Are Filed as Received

Figure 3-15 Work flow in paper-based HIM department.

behind schedule. The block appointment methods help alleviate wasted physician time by scheduling multiple patients for the same time slot. The **wave scheduling** method assigns all patients in a large block at the same appointment time (e.g., 9:00 a.m. for all morning appointments), then patients are seen on a first-come, first-served basis. The disadvantage to the wave scheduling method is that patient satisfaction suffers when some patients have to wait several hours to see the physician. The **modified wave scheduling** method protects both patient and physician time by scheduling the first two patients in each hour at the same time and allowing a catch-up period at the end of each hour in which no patients are scheduled. Although some patients have to wait when the modified wave method is used, the wait periods are not ordinarily any longer than with standard scheduling, and physician time is better utilized (Chung, 2002).

The HIM department commonly receives a list of appointments several days before the patient's scheduled appointment. In a paper-based system, records for established patients are then pulled and made available on the day that the patient is to be seen. A computer-based system provides the patient's information immediately through the computerized system. For new patients, the record must be initiated at the time of the patient's appointment. Usually this process is begun by the reception-ist or admissions clerk, who will see that identifying information is entered into the paper-based system or into the computer, and basic record forms are provided in a new record for a paper-based system. Each encounter must then be documented dur-ing the patient's visit. **Walk-ins** are frequently a problem. Walk-ins are patients who arrive without an appointment or who receive an appointment at the last minute. In paper-based systems, methods must be established for ensuring that medical records are available for these patients.

After the visit, the paper-based record must be returned to the HIM department and checked in to assure that it was received. In some facilities, the paper record is then filed. Others, however, review the record to confirm that the documentation has been completed and the sections of the record are placed in the correct order before the record is filed.

The patient identifier has an influence on how paper records are filed. When the patient's name is the primary identifier, the records are obviously placed in alpha-betical order by patient last name. In systems using a number as a primary identifier, the record may be filed in straight numerical order. Large systems, however, are often set up in **terminal digit** order, in which the record is filed first by the last two digits of the number. For example, if the patient's number is 93-02-78, it would first be filed in the 78 section. Then it would be put in order by the middle digits, 02, and finally in numerical order by the first two digits, 93. This system allows for the files to expand evenly rather than having most of the activity at the end of the numbers assigned, as is found in a straight numerical system. If several clerical personnel perform the fil-ing function, terminal digit has the additional advantage of spreading them through-out the filing area.

Paper-based records are usually kept in file folders. These may be plain manila filing folders marked with the patient's identifier. Often, however, in either an alpha-betical or a numerical system, a method of **color coding** is used on the folder. Each set of numbers or a group of letters is assigned a color on the folder. It is then easy to look at the files and to identify misfiles by the presence of a different color in a block of records of the same color. Paper records may be kept in a variety of equipment. File cabinets with file drawers are sometimes used, although these take up more space. Open-shelf filing is also commonly chosen. Sometimes motorized filing units are selected to house the records.

The addition of late reports is another function of the HIM department. Labora-tory and X-ray results are often sent to the HIM department after the visit and must be filed in the proper record.

Record Linkage to Other Sites/Facilities

Many freestanding ambulatory care centers have multiple sites and must find a way to provide patient information among the various sites. This task is easiest with an electronic health record that can be accessed from all sites. In such a system, any of the locations can access the patient's information through the computer.

In paper-based systems, the record can only be in one site at a time. Facilities use a variety of ways to maintain the location or home base of the record. In some sites, the patient designates a home facility where he or she is usually seen, and the record is routinely kept at that location. Other facilities keep the record in the last site where the patient was seen. In either case, if the patient is seen in a site other than the record's home base, a method must be chosen to have information available at another site when the patient is seen there. For scheduled visits, a courier is often used to transport the record to the site of the visit. For unscheduled visits, the pertinent parts of the record may be faxed to the other site from the home base. It is important, in either case, to have policies and procedures to ensure the safety of the record. If a courier is used, locked courier pouches may be used to hold the record during transport and to avoid unauthorized viewing. Facilities that fax information between sites must ensure that the fax is being attended when the material is sent to avoid unauthorized access to the copies. Care must also be taken that the facsimile copies are properly disposed of.

Computer Systems

Ambulatory care centers often use computers to assist in the operation of the facility (see Figure 3-16). A scheduling system, for example, is often an important part of such a system for the HIM department. The patient's scheduled visit is entered into the computer, and a list of records needed for a particular day can then be automatically generated from the schedule.

Computer Applications	*Functions*
Scheduling or Appointment System	System used to set up patient appointments
Patient Registration System	System used to enter demographic and financial information about the patient
Financial System	System used to maintain information on services billed, insurance coverage, and billing and collections
Electronic Health Record (EHR) System	System in which the patient record is kept in electronic form in a computer-based system
Decision Support System	System that aids the caregiver in making a diagnosis or treatment decision
Reminder System	System that reminds the caregiver of preventive services that should be scheduled on a regular basis such as annual mammograms

Figure 3-16 Computer applications commonly seen in freestanding ambulatory care settings.

A **patient registration** or **appointment system** is also vital to keep up with basic identifying information about the patient. In such a system, basic information about the patient including name, address, insurance, and responsible party is collected when the patient is first seen. It is important that this information be updated at each visit to maintain an accurate file. The registration system provides a master patient index for the HIM department, including the patient's record number, which is a vital identifier to enable the department to locate the patient's records.

Financial systems maintain information on services billed, insurance coverage determination, payment received from patients and insurance companies, and collections efforts. Some systems provide for electronic data interchange (EDI) so that bills are sent electronically to third-party payers rather than using paper bills. Financial systems often tie in with the encounter form to show the services that the patient received during the visit. The HIM department may use data from the financial system to retrieve information for activities such as utilization management and quality assessment. In the financial system, there is also information on items billed such as medications, diagnostic tests, and procedures.

Electronic health records (EHRs) are in use in some freestanding ambulatory care settings. Currently many facilities also keep paper records in addition to the EHR, possibly because of state laws requiring records to be kept in paper form for a certain period. It may also be because care providers want to use the paper record rather than the EHR. Many care providers do not want to input data into the EHR themselves, thus leaving HIM departments to provide this data entry function. Some physicians' offices and other ambulatory care settings are leading the way toward an electronic health record because the ambulatory record is less complex and easier to computerize than the hospital record. In other facilities, there is still a total dependence on the paper-based record. The computer is still primarily used for administrative tasks.

Some advantages of an electronic health record extend beyond just having the information on the computer where it can be accessed by multiple users across broad geographic areas. One of these functions is decision support. In **decision-support systems**, information about the patient's signs and symptoms, laboratory and other diagnostic tests is used with an artificial intelligence system to help the physician in selecting a diagnosis. Automated online reminders can also be built into the system to remind physicians that patients need certain services such as immunizations for children, yearly mammograms, or routine monitoring.

Other technologies are affecting ambulatory care. Handheld computers or personal digital assistants (PDAs) provide caregivers with a pocket-sized device that can be used to access information on topics such as drugs. The device can also be connected to the ambulatory care center computer system through a cradle or wireless network to allow parts of the electronic medical record to be downloaded from or uploaded to the main system. A main issue with PDAs is security because they are small enough to be lost or easily stolen. Input of large amounts of data is also difficult. Speech recognition technology will greatly enhance the functionality of PDAs when it is more reliable.

Another technology that is receiving some use by caregivers is electronic mail. Patients can query the caregiver about problems or ask for refills on medication. Once again, security can be an issue because unauthorized persons may access the e-mail if appropriate safeguards are not in place. It is also important that e-mail communications be entered into the patient's medical record so that a record is kept (Wager, 1999, p. 46).

There is some use of the Internet for remote accessing of information, too. Once again, security is the biggest issue, and means must be included in the system to ensure data security and integrity. Who may access information through the Internet must also be addressed. In some cases, patients wish to access their own records through the Internet, and policies must be devised to define what information they may access.

COSTAR (computer-stored ambulatory record) is an example of an electronic health record system currently in use in the United States. (Somand, 1988). COSTAR was developed at the Harvard Community Health Plan in Boston and provides a completely computer-stored medical record and clinic system. Core modules include patient registration, scheduling, medical data capture and reports, financial and accounts receivable, a quality assurance system, and query language to enable users to retrieve information in a variety of formats (Anderson, 1992).

Data Sets

In many settings, minimum data sets have been developed to provide guidance on what information should be kept in patient records. A second function that these data sets serve is to provide standard definitions for the data set items collected. In ambulatory care, the uniform ambulatory care data set has been developed to serve that purpose. This data set includes three main types of data: patient data, provider data, and encounter data. Patient data provides basic identifying information about the patient. Provider data includes information about the provider such as a unique provider identifier and location. **Encounter** data includes the date, reason for encounter, services received, and disposition (Hanken and Waters, 1994). The minimum data set provides an excellent source for the HIM professional to determine the minimum data that must be kept for each encounter. In addition, definitions for terms such as *encounter* can help the HIM professional in developing statistical measures. It is important that the statistics measure the indicated items uniformly.

Quality Improvement and Utilization Management

Quality Improvement

A major use of health information in ambulatory care is the assessment of the quality of care provided by the facility. The quality assessment and improvement process in ambulatory care follows the same methods used in other care settings. Problems or processes must be chosen for study; data must be collected to measure these processes; data must be assessed; and a method for improvement must be developed. The major difference in ambulatory care is that many factors affecting the quality of care are not within the sole control of the ambulatory facility. The patient's contact with the facility is usually brief, and the patient's outcome depends in large part on the patient's compliance with the care plan developed (Norman et al., 1995). The patient's continuity of care may depend on factors in the patient's, not the facility's, control, such as missed appointments and consistent use of a primary provider to coordinate care. Methods to improve compliance must be included in the quality assessment process because they affect the patient's outcome. Patient satisfaction is also an important part of the quality assessment process in ambulatory care because the patient's compliance may be closely tied to satisfaction with the care received. The ability to determine the quality of care within a facility is highly dependent on the quality of data collected within the health record.

Utilization Management

Utilization management is the process of determining the medical necessity of services and treatment provided to the patient (Michelson, 1989). In the hospital setting, this process often focuses on whether the patient requires hospitalization. In ambulatory care, utilization management is more likely to focus on the necessity of a service such as referral to a specialist or use of an expensive procedure such as a magnetic resonance imaging study or the appropriateness of referrals for hospitalization. Emphasis should be on services that are either high volume or high cost because not all services can be examined. Standards or criteria that are credible and specific should be set.

There are two basic approaches to utilization management. One is **prospective review/precertification** in which the service is examined before it is provided. Data is collected, usually by a nurse, from the patient and the physician. The facts of the individual case are compared to the appropriateness criteria. If the standards are met, the nurse can usually approve the service. If the standards are not met, a physician advisor may be asked to review the case and make a determination. Types of activities typically undergoing prospective review include authorization for referral, authorization for a procedure, preadmission review before hospitalization, and second surgical opinion (Mittman, 1995).

The second major approach is **retrospective review**. In this methodology, care is looked at after it is given. Usually a sample of cases is selected. Data is then collected from medical records, and the information from the record is compared to the appropriateness standards. Feedback is then given to the appropriate caregiver regarding inappropriate care provided (Michelson, 1989).

Risk Management and Legal Issues

Many legal and risk management issues that arise in freestanding ambulatory care relate to the fact that much of the care is not provided by the caregiver but by the patient and the family (see Figure 3-17). Communication is a vital part of ensuring that the care is given as prescribed. Care recommendations, for example, are often provided through telephone calls. It is important that telephone calls be documented in

---

Risk Management Issues

Documenting Telephone Calls

Documenting Missed and Cancelled Appointments

Documenting Written Discharge Instructions

Documenting Provider Signatures

Documenting Informed Consent Process

Documenting Changes Since Last Visit

Documenting Noncompliance

Documenting Incidents

Figure 3-17   Risk management issues in freestanding ambulatory care.

the record so that some report exists of care recommendations. Prescribed medications must especially be documented, including the name of medication, when prescribed, and the pharmacy that received the called-in prescription (Complete Documentation for Ambulatory Care Is a Center's Best Form of Risk Management, 1990). Failure to document such care can lead to a situation of the caregiver's word versus the patient's on whether needed advice was given and followed.

Documenting missed and canceled appointments is also vital because patients can have adverse effects from not keeping an appointment as scheduled. Documenting that the appointment was missed or canceled provides additional information on the patient's responsibility in such a situation (Complete Documentation for Ambulatory Care Is a Center's Best Form of Risk Management, 1990).

Freestanding ambulatory sites, particularly ambulatory surgery centers, often provide written instructions for patients to take home to help patient compliance and understanding (Complete Documentation for Ambulatory Care Is a Center's Best Form of Risk Management, 1990). Such instruction sheets should be included in the medical record. If they are not, a statement should be included in the record that a particular instruction sheet was given to the patient, and copies of the different instruction sheets should be kept on file in the facility.

Determining which caregivers provided care can be enhanced, particularly years later in the case of a legal suit involving the facility, if a notebook of provider signatures is maintained indicating the provider, the specialty or profession, and a sample of the usual signature (Complete Documentation for Ambulatory Care Is a Center's Best Form of Risk Management, 1990). With this notebook, the record can be reviewed and a determination quickly made regarding the caregivers involved in the case.

Documentation of the physician's discussion regarding informed consent is especially important in ambulatory surgery settings but must be furnished for any invasive procedure, whatever the setting. A consent form signed by the patient should contain the substance of the items discussed including alternatives to the procedure and any risks involved. Narrative progress notes should include further detail about the discussion regarding the procedure or service to be provided (Complete Documentation for Ambulatory Care Is a Center's Best Form of Risk Management, 1990).

Caregivers should be advised to include documentation of changes since the patient's last visit and any evidence of noncompliance (Complete Documentation for Ambulatory Care Is a Center's Best Form of Risk Management, 1990). Such facts could be vitally important if a legal case should result.

Legibility is also a risk management issue. If prescriptions are illegible, for example, there is a risk that the medication will be dispensed incorrectly, potentially causing the patient harm. Some organizations have implemented systems in which providers use PDAs to generate and print prescriptions to address this patient safety concern. Illegibility is also a problem in the area of compliance. If an auditor cannot read a provider's records, the documentation cannot be used to support the services billed, which could lead to legal issues with the OIG.

It is extremely important that abnormal test results be reviewed by the ordering physician. Each facility should develop a procedure to ensure that the physician sees the results and documents actions taken on the basis of the results. For example, physicians may be asked to initial the laboratory report and document in the progress notes section of the record that the patient was contacted and advised of what to do about abnormal results.

Many facilities use **incident** or **occurrence reports** as internal documentation of unusual events such as falls, incorrect medications given or taken, or other untoward occurrences. The purpose of the incident/occurrence report is to provide documentation of events so that facilities can take steps to avoid such events in the future. The report usually goes to the facility's attorney and is thus protected by the attorney–client privilege. A copy of the incident report should not be placed in the record, but details about the event should be recorded there (Complete Documentation for Ambulatory Care Is a Center's Best Form of Risk Management, 1990).

Role of the Health Information Management Professional

The role of the HIM professional in freestanding ambulatory care is to provide expertise concerning information, regulations, computerization, and management. Information management and supervision of personnel are currently the main functions of the HIM professional because the primary role of the HIM department in a paper-based ambulatory care setting is chart location and control. These tasks require that the information be organized and stored in a way that makes it easy to retrieve, either through computerized or paper-based storage. With a paper-based system, personnel are needed to file and retrieve records and to make sure that loose sheets such as laboratory reports are placed in the correct record. These employees must be trained in filing methods and in confidentiality and security so that information is not released improperly. This training function may also include instruction of employees and caregivers outside the HIM department in proper documentation, use of the record, and confidentiality.

The role of the health information manager has been affected by the move to the EHR in freestanding ambulatory care. As facilities decide to implement EHRs, health information managers are involved in the implementation of these new systems and may serve as project directors. The implementation of an electronic record system changes the role of the HIM professional from one of managing the filing and retrieval of the paper record to one of managing the data contained in the record and the electronic record process. HIPAA also adds new roles for the HIM professional who may serve as the privacy and/or security officer for the facility.

In smaller ambulatory care settings, HIM professionals may often undertake roles outside those usually identified with health information management. In some settings, for example, HIM professionals have duties in areas such as purchasing or patient registration.

The HIM field is not as well known in ambulatory care as it has been in the hospital area. HIM professionals must also serve as marketers for their skills and have the flexibility to assume a variety of responsibilities.

Trends

Several trends are evident in freestanding ambulatory care. The first is the continuing shift of care to the ambulatory setting. As government programs such as diagnosis related groups (DRGs) have attempted to hold down hospital costs, a shift has taken place to the less-expensive ambulatory setting. This movement will continue, and the role of ambulatory care settings in the health care arena will be enhanced.

Another trend will be increased integration of freestanding ambulatory care sites with other health care facilities. Health care is increasingly provided by networks, including all facets of health care from primary care to specialized hospital care. Ambulatory care settings will increasingly find themselves part of this continuum of care and, therefore, part of bigger health care corporations. Such a shift will provide more support for individual ambulatory care settings but will also be expected to provide increased regulation and standardization of the health care process. It should be expected that new reimbursement methods for ambulatory care will be developed, resulting in additional scrutiny of the documentation of that care.

In health information management there will be an increased use of computerization in ambulatory care. Because the ambulatory care process is less complex and less regulated than that in the hospital, ambulatory care centers have an excellent opportunity to become leaders in the process of computerizing the medical record. HIM professionals should have excellent opportunities to participate in this trend.

Summary

The HIM professional must be aware of many factors about a facility before providing information management services. The type of facility determines the types of caregivers and the types of patients seen, thus setting out the documentation that must be provided. Accreditation and licensing standards as well as the reimbursement systems applicable to the setting also serve as benchmarks for documentation and storage and retrieval methods. HIM professionals looking at quality of care and utilization must be aware of the role that the patient takes in whether the plan of care is followed and, thus, in the outcome achieved. Patients' participation in their care, or the lack of such participation, is also a risk management factor that affects documentation requirements. Knowledge of all these elements provides the HIM practitioner with the tools necessary to offer exceptional service to meet the needs of the ambulatory facility.

Key Terms

ambulatory surgery center (ASC) a setting provided for surgery on an ambulatory basis. Centers usually have at least one full-time operating room and provide surgical privileges to physicians in the community.

appointment or scheduling system a system by which appointments are scheduled for patients.

ASC groups/ASC list a Medicare reimbursement system for ambulatory surgery in which the HCPCS codes are listed (ASC list) and then divided into groups (ASC groups), with the payment depending on the group assigned.

birth center ambulatory setting that provides labor and delivery services in uncomplicated deliveries.

capitation a method of reimbursement in which the physician or facility receives a fixed amount each month for each patient enrolled in the plan, regardless of the amount of care that the patient receives.

color coding a system that helps prevent the misfiling of records by assigning colors to numbers or letters and displaying those colors on the record folder so that misfiled records are easily spotted by their mismatched color patterns.

compliance plan a plan for ensuring that a facility/practice is complying with all laws and regulations regarding reimbursement under the Medicare and Medicaid System.

computer-stored ambulatory record (COSTAR) an example of an electronic health record system currently in use in ambulatory settings.

Current Procedural Terminology **(CPT)** a coding system for procedures that is used extensively in ambulatory care and that forms a part of HCPCS.

decision-support system a computerized system that assists physicians in deciding on a diagnosis or treatment.

Early and Periodic Screening, Diagnostic and Treatment (EPSDT) a program of Medicaid for children younger than 21 that ensures that these services (screening, diagnostic, and treatment) are provided and paid for whether or not they are normally included under the state's Medicaid program.

electronic health record   a record format in which the patient information is kept in electronic form.

encounter   face-to-face contact between the patient and the provider (Uniform ambulatory care data set).

encounter form   a form used for billing purposes including the services the patient received, the charges, and the diagnosis and procedure codes.

family numbering system   a numbering system in which the family is given a number and each individual receives that number with a suffix indicating his or her position within the family.

family planning center   an ambulatory setting that provides family planning services.

fee for service   a reimbursement system in which the payment is based on the type and amount of service provided.

financial system   a computer system that maintains information on services billed, insurance determination, payment received, and collection efforts.

freestanding ambulatory care   care provided to patients who do not stay overnight in a setting not located within a hospital.

growth and development chart   a graphic recording of a child's height and weight over time.

Healthcare Common Procedural Coding System (HCPCS)   a system used by ambulatory care facilities to code procedures and services.

immunization record   record that maintains a list of immunizations that a child has received and often indicates when additional immunizations will be required.

incident report   internal documentation of an unusual event such as a fall, incorrect medications given or taken, or some other untoward occurrence. (See also *occurrence report*.)

incident to   services provided to a patient by nurse practitioners or physician assistants when the physician is on site.

industrial health center   an ambulatory setting where care is provided to employees at their place of work.

integrated format   a record format in which the information is entered in chronological order.

International Classification of Diseases, Ninth Revision, Clinical Modification (ICD-9-CM)   a classification system used by ambulatory care facilities for coding diagnoses.

International Classification of Diseases, 10th Revision, Clinical Modification **(ICD-10-CM)**   a revision of the International Classification of Diseases that will replace ICD-9-CM.

International Classification of Primary Care (ICPC)   a coding system developed by the World Organization of National Colleges, Academies, and Academic Associations of General Practitioners/Family Physicians (WONCA). It includes chapters arranged by body systems with components that describe the reason why the patient is being seen for care at the primary care level.

Local Medical Review Policies (LMRPs) or Local Coverage Determinations (LCDs)   guidance published by Medicare carriers that includes information on codes that indicate medical necessity of services.

locum tenens   an arrangement by which one physician temporarily works in place of another physician.

modified wave scheduling   an appointment scheduling method that schedules the first two patients in each hour at the same time and provides a catch-up period at the end of each hour in which no patients are scheduled.

neighborhood health center   an ambulatory setting developed in the 1960s to provide ambulatory care to the indigent of a particular neighborhood.

nurse midwife   a nurse practitioner who handles pregnancy, labor, and delivery.

nurse practitioner (NP)   a registered nurse who has additional training and credentials that allow for limited independent practice.

occurrence report   internal documentation of an unusual event such as a fall, incorrect medications given or taken, or some other untoward occurrence. (See also *incident report*.)

Office of the Inspector General (OIG)   the office in the Department of Health and Human Services responsible for monitoring compliance with reimbursement laws and regulations.

patient identifier   an item of data that identifies the patient in the health information management system, such as the patient's name or medical record number.

patient registration system   a computer system that contains demographic and financial information for every patient.

physician private practice   a setting in which physicians practice in their own business rather than working for an organization such as a clinic or urgent care center.

physician assistant   a professional who is not a nurse but has received training to use independent judgment in treating patients.

problem list   a numbered list of the patient's problems over time that serves as a table of contents for the problem-oriented medical record.

problem-oriented medical record (POMR) format   a record format in which the parts of the record are keyed to the problem number listed on the problem list.

Program Manuals for Medicare and Medicaid   basic instructions for the two programs developed by the Centers for Medicare and Medicaid Services.

program memoranda   provide guidance and changes in the Medicare and Medicaid programs but are not tied to a specific program manual.

program transmittals   periodically issued by CMS to provide a revision for a specific program manual.

prospective review/precertification   one of two basic approaches to utilization management, prospective review determines whether services are needed before they are provided.

public health department   an organization that provides services to promote the health of the community as a whole, such as immunizations and disease screenings; usually an agency of state or local government.

reason for visit   the reason provided by the patient for why care is requested.

registration   the process by which basic demographic and financial information is obtained from the patient and entered into the health information system.

resource-based relative value scale   a reimbursement system used by Medicare Part B to reimburse physicians. It is based on the relative value of the services provided.

retrospective review   one of two basic approaches to utilization management, retrospective review examines care after it has been given to identify inappropriate care and provide feedback to the caregiver.

return-to-work physical   a physical done before an employee may return to the job after an injury or illness.

source-oriented format   a record format in which the information is organized according to the source of the information, such as laboratory, nursing, etc.

standard scheduling   a method in which appointments are scheduled continuously throughout the day with appointment times at specific intervals (e.g., every 15 minutes).

superbill   a form used for billing purposes that includes the services the patient received, the charges, and diagnosis and procedure codes.

terminal digit filing   a filing system in which records are filed first by the last two digits of their numbers, allowing files to expand evenly.

university health center   an ambulatory setting in which care is provided to university staff and students.

urgent care center   an ambulatory care setting in which patients are seen on a walk-in basis without appointments. These centers provide service for longer hours than most private physician practices.

walk-ins   patients who arrive without an appointment or who receive an appointment at the last minute.

wave scheduling   an appointment scheduling method that assigns all patients in a large block for the same appointment time (e.g., 9:00 a.m. for all morning appointments) then patients are seen on a first-come, first-served basis.

REVIEW QUESTIONS

Knowledge-based Questions

1. List and describe three types of freestanding ambulatory care settings.
2. Define the following terms used in ambulatory care: encounter, nurse practitioner, reason for visit, superbill.
3. Name the two main organizations that accredit ambulatory care.
4. List the major types of documentation that are basic to all ambulatory care encounters and settings.
5. What types of patient identifiers are used in ambulatory care?
6. What types of data are included in the uniform ambulatory care data set and how does this affect the content of the ambulatory record?
7. What are ASC groups, and how are they used in Medicare reimbursement?

Application-based Questions

1. Compare and contrast the fee-for-service and PFS/RBRVS reimbursement systems.
2. How does documentation in an industrial health center differ from that in a physician's practice and why?
3. How is quality assessment in ambulatory care similar to and different from quality assessment in the acute inpatient setting?

Web Activity

LMRPs/LCDs can be reviewed at the Medicare Coverage Database at the CMS Web site: http://www.cms.hhs.gov/mcd/search.asp.

When you arrive at the site, select "Local Coverage." After Local Coverage has been selected, you will be permitted to select a state or Medicare carrier and a keyword, code, or topic as search criteria. Make appropriate selections and then click the "Search Now" button. (Hint: You will get more "hits" if you search on "All States.") Select one of the items from the list produced and review the document. What type of information does the document contain? How might this information be useful to a freestanding ambulatory care provider?

Case Study

Judy Jordan has just begun working as the health information manager in a very large physicians' group practice. The patient's name is the primary patient identifier used, and the records are filed alphabetically. Misfiles are a frequent problem, and in the large practice patients frequently have similar names. The records are not kept in a uniform format. Many of the doctors use an integrated format, but three of the physicians use the POMR. In reviewing the encounter forms, Judy finds codes that are no longer currently valid. Judy questions the staff and finds that no one can remember when the encounter form had been updated. Bills are frequently returned for invalid codes. Patient registration and appointment systems have been computerized, but the staff also keeps a manual appointment log. A computerized list of appointments is given to the HIM clerk on the day prior to the appointments so that the records can be pulled and available when the patients arrive. Many appointments that are entered in the manual log are not also entered in the computerized appointment system. The HIM clerk, therefore, spends extensive time each day pulling records for those appointments that were not on her computerized list. Judy has been asked to make suggestions for making the office run more smoothly.

1. What are the main problems that she should identify?
2. Develop a plan to solve each of the problems identified above.

References and Suggested Readings

Accreditation Clinic. (1995). *Joint Commission Perspectives, 15* (4), 13–14.

Ambulatory Care Section. (1993). *A Learning Syllabus for Ambulatory Care.* Chicago: American Health Information Management Association.

Ambulatory Care Section. (2001). *Documentation for Ambulatory Care: Revised Edition.* Chicago: American Health Information Management Association.

Anderson, J. G. (1992). Computerized medical record systems in ambulatory care. *Journal of Ambulatory Care Management, 15* (3), 67–75.

Avery, M., and Imdieke, B. (1984). *Medical Records in Ambulatory Care.* Rockville, MD: Aspen Systems Corporation.

Bazzoli, Fred. (2002). Free-Ranging Physicians. *Health Data Management, 40* (11), 56–58, 60.

Benson, D. S., Gartner, C., Anderson, J., Schweer, H., and Kirchgessner, R. (1987). The ambulatory care parameter: A structured approach to quality assurance in the ambulatory care setting. *Quality Review Bulletin, 13* (2), 51–55.

Benson, D. S., Van Osdol, W., and Townes, P. (1988). Quality ambulatory care: The role of the diagnostic and medication summary lists. *Quality Review Bulletin, 14* (6), 192–197.

Berthelsen, C. L. (2001). Personal Digital Assistants: The Healthcare Matter at Hand. *Journal of the American Health Information Management Association, 72* (9), 40–42, 44, 46, 48.

Briggs, B. (2001). Doctors Sound Off on I.T. Concerns. *Health Data Management, 9* (1), 38–40, 42, 44, 46.

Briggs, B. (2002). Web-Based Technology Closing Gap with Physicians. *Health Data Management, 10* (10), 42–44, 46, 48, 50, 52, 54.

Burgess, B. (1999). An EMR Education for a Student Health Center. *Journal of the American Health Information Management Association, 70* (6), 42–44.

[CMS] Centers for Medicare & Medicaid Services. (2003, August 8). Update of rates and wage index for ambulatory surgical center (ASC) payments effective October 1, 2003. Transmittal AB-03-116. http://www.cms.hhs.gov/manuals/pm_trans/AB03116.pdf [2003, December 30].

Chiama, E. T., Morisse, R. F., and Nawrocki, B. A. (1991). Becoming chart smart the academic way. *Medical Group Management Journal, 38* (5), 40–45.

Chung, M.K. (2002). Tuning up your patient schedule. *Family Practice Management, 9* (1): 41–45.

Complete documentation for ambulatory care is a center's best form of risk management. (1990). *Medical Records Briefing, 5* (10), 10–11.

Douglas, J. T. (1994). Group practice computing: The road to managing information. *Medical Group Management Journal, 41* (4), 15–16, 18, 42.

Duggar, B. C. (1990). Ambulatory surgery facilities definition and identification. *Journal of Ambulatory Care Management, 13* (1), 1–9.

Edelson, J. T. (1995). Physician use of information technology in ambulatory medicine: An overview. *Journal of Ambulatory Care Management, 18* (3), 9–19.

Ferris, A. K., and Wyszewianski, L. (1990). Quality of ambulatory care for the elderly: Formulating evaluation criteria. *Health Care Financing Review, 12* (1), 31–38.

Fleming, N. S., and Jones, L. F. (1991). The use of dedicated software to customize ambulatory care reporting. *Journal of Ambulatory Care Management, 14* (1), 47–57.

Forms will help doctors with new RBRVS documentation. (1992). *Medical Records Briefing, 7* (2), 4–5.

Georgoulakis, J. M., et al. (1990). A comparison of ambulatory classification systems: A preliminary report. *Journal of Ambulatory Care Management, 13* (3), 39–49.

Gillespie, G. (2002). PDAs are Willing, But Will They be Able?. *Health Data Management, 10* (12), 20–22, 26, 28.

Glass, B. L., and Mitchell, S. (1992). The ambulatory care medical record: An administrative nightmare. *Medical Group Management Journal, 39* (5), 58–64.

Goldfield, N. (1993). A quality improvement process for ambulatory prospective payment. *Journal of Ambulatory Care Management, 16* (2), 50–60.

Goldfield, N. (1995). The Measurement and Management of the Quality of Ambulatory Services: A Population-Based Approach. In Vahe Kazandjian and Elizabeth Sternberg, *The Epidemiology of Quality,* pp. 171–193. Gaithersburg, MD: Aspen Publications.

Hanken, M. A., and Waters, K. A. (Eds.). (1994). *Glossary of Healthcare Terms.* Chicago: American Health Information Management Association.

The Health Information Management Handbook: Non-Acute Care Edition. (2000). Marblehead, MA: Opus Communications.

Hodgkins, M. L. (1995). Are you ready for the computer-based patient record? *Journal of Ambulatory Care Management, 18* (3), 1–8.

Ingersoll, S., and Personnett, J. D. (1990). Simplified approach to the ambulatory care diagnostic summary list. *Quality Review Bulletin, 16* (3), 127–129.

Jones, J. M., and Matherlee, K. (1990). Medicare's prudent approach to paying for ambulatory surgery services. *Journal of Ambulatory Care Management, 13* (1), 25–32.

Jones, M. (1992). RBRVS is still evolving: Seven issues of interest to physicians and health information professionals. *Journal of the American Health Information Management Association, 63* (9), 44–48.

Kalata, M. (1998). An HIM Metamorphosis. *Journal of the American Health Information Management Association, 69* (9), 55–57.

Kinsinger, L. S., Harris, R. P., and Kaluzny, A. D. (1999). CQI in Primary Care. In *Continuous Quality Improvement in Health Care: Theory, Implementation, and Applications,* 2nd ed. Gaithersburg, MD: Aspen Publications.

Lee, F. W. (2000). Adoption of Electronic Medical Records as a Technology Innovation for Ambulatory Care at the Medical University of South Carolina. *Topics in Health Information Management, 21* (1), 1–20.

Lee, F. W. (1992). Using database software for quantitative review and active caseload lists in a community health setting. *Topics in Health Information Management, 13* (1), 35–44.

Licari, J. R., and Sklade, S. A. (1993). Freestanding ambulatory surgery centers: A survey of health record practices and utilization of credentialed health information professionals. *Journal of the American Health Information Management Association, 64* (6), 91–94.

Lloyd, D. J. (1994). Commentaries on "A Short Story . . ." *Medical Group Management Journal, 41* (4), 36.

McCormack, J. (2000). The Internet Reroutes Electronic Records. *Health Data Management*, 8 (5), 50–51, 54, 56, 58, 60, 62.

Majerowicz, A. F. (1990). Selection and implementation of a bar-code-based management system in ambulatory care. *Journal of the American Medical Record Association*, 61 (5), 28–36.

Manger, B. J. (2001). *Documentation Requirements in Non-Acute Care Facilities and Organizations.* New York: The Parthenon Publishing Group, 2001.

Manning, F. F. (1994). A short story: It is possible, are you ready for it? *Medical Group Management Journal*, 41 (4), 32, 34–35, 38–40.

Matson, T. A., and McDougall, M. D. (Eds.). (1990). *Information Systems for Ambulatory Care.* Chicago: American Hospital Publishing, Inc.

Michelson, L. D. (1989). Utilization review for ambulatory care: Eliminating unnecessary care. *Journal of Ambulatory Care Management*, 12 (4), 7–14.

Miller, C. J. (1992). Physicians need your help. *Journal of the American Health Information Management Association*, 63 (9), 37–38.

Miller, S. T., and Flanagan, E. (1993). The transition from quality assurance to continuous quality improvement in ambulatory care. *QRB: Quality Review Bulletin*, 19 (2), 62–65.

Mittman, C. (1995). Utilization management for medical groups: Using information to achieve collaboration. *Medical Group Management Journal*, 42 (1), 46, 48–52.

Montoya, I. D., and Richard, A. J. (1995). The case for a code of ethics in an ambulatory care setting. *Journal of Ambulatory Care Management*, 18 (3), 68–76.

More women using new birth-site options. (1991). *Hospitals*, 65 (20), 14.

Norman, L. A., and Hardin, P. A. (1990). A multipurpose, computer-assisted program to improve ambulatory medical care: A preliminary report. *Quality Review Bulletin*, 16 (10), 365–372.

Norman, L. A., et. al. (1995). Computer-assisted quality improvement in an ambulatory care setting: A follow-up report. *Journal on Quality Improvement*, 21 (3), 116–131.

OIG Compliance Program for Individual and Small Group Physician Practices. (2000). *Federal Register*, 65 (194) 59434–59452.

Orkin, F. K., et. al. (1992). An information system for quality and utilization management in ambulatory surgery. *Journal of Ambulatory Care Management*, 15 (4), 24–29.

Parks, C. L., et al. (1991). Quality of care in a chain of walk-in centers. *QRB: Quality Review Bulletin*, 17 (4), 120–125.

Pasternak, D. P., et al. (1991). Critical issues surrounding the evolution of ambulatory surgery. *Journal of Ambulatory Care Management*, 14 (1), 24–33.

Patton, L. T. (1990). Community health centers at 25: A retrospective look at the first 10 years. *Journal of Ambulatory Care Management*, 13 (4), 13–21.

Professional Practice Standards for Health Information Services in Ambulatory Care (1992). Chicago: American Health Information Management Association.

RBRVS regulations bring good and bad news. (1992). *Medical Records Briefing*, 7 (1), 1, 3.

Re, R. N., and Krousel-Wood, M. A. (1990). How to use continuous quality improvement theory and statistical quality control tools in a multispecialty clinic. *Quality Review Bulletin*, 16 (11), 391–397.

Riley, W. A., et al. (1991). The Maryland experience and a practical proposal to expand existing models in ambulatory primary care. *Journal of the American Medical Association, 266* (8), 1118–1122.

Ripps, A. S. (1997). Ambulatory Care Computerized Patient Record Systms: Benchmark Security Features and Safeguards. *Jounal of the American Health Information Management Association, 68* (5), 32–34.

Rizk, K. H. (1992). The billing process: Improving efficiency and effectiveness. *Journal of Ambulatory Care Management, 15* (2), 11–18.

Rural Assistance Center. (2003, November 07). Rural health clinics: Frequently asked questions [Online]. http://www.raconline.org/info_guides/clinics/rhcfaq.php [2003, December 26].

Schoenfelt, S. (1999). Next Generation: How Internet Technology Propels the Electronic Medical Record. *Journal of the American Health Information Management Association,* 70 (8), 31–36.

Smith, W. R., et al. (1992). Developing a computerized ambulatory medical record to document health promotion and disease prevention activities during the clinic encounter. *Journal of Ambulatory Care Management, 15* (4), 9–17.

Sullivan, K. W., and Meier, E. M. (1992). Quality improvement: A race with no finish. *Medical Group Management Journal, 39* (1), 12–14, 16–18, 46–48, 50–54.

Summary of final RBRVS regulations. (1992). *Medical Records Briefing, 7* (1), 7–9.

Waegemann, C. P., and Tessier, C. (2002). Documentation Goes Wireless: A Look at Mobile Healthcare Computing Devices. *Journal of the American Health Information Management Association,* 73 (8), 36–39.

Wager, K., et al. (1999). Working Smarter, Not Harder, in a Family Practice. *Journal of the American Health Information Management Association,* 70 (6), 44–46.

With one form, doctors track phone consultations, and documentation is never lost. (1990). *Medical Records Briefing, 5* (10), 11–12.

Wojcik, C. (1993). Coding, documentation and dollars. *Journal of the American Health Information Management Association, 64* (6), 74–82.

Wong, H. C. (1990). The evolution of freestanding ambulatory surgical care. *Journal of Ambulatory Care Management, 13* (1),11–20.

Zender, A. (1999). Building a Better CPR in Ambulatory Care. *Journal of the American Health Information Management Association,* 70 (3), 42–43.

Zirul, D. L. (1992). Accepting the challenge of physician practice. *Journal of the American Health Information Management Association, 63* (9), 40–42.

Zuvekas, A. (1990). Community and migrant health centers: An overview. *Journal of Ambulatory Care Management, 13* (4), 1–12.

Key Resources

Accreditation Association for Ambulatory Health Care, Inc. (AAAHC)
3201 Old Glenview Rd.
Wilmette, IL 60091-2992
Phone: 847-853-6060
http://www.aaahc.org

American Association for Accreditation of Ambulatory Surgery Facilities, Inc.
1202 Allanson Rd.
Mundelein, IL 60060
http://www.aaaasf.org

American Health Information Management Association
(See Chapter 1 for contact information.)

Commission for the Accreditation of Freestanding Birth Centers
3121 Gottschall Road
Perkiomenville, PA 18074-9604
Phone: 215-234-0564
http://www.BirthCenters.org/naccinaction/commission.shtml

Department of Health and Human Services
Office of Inspector General
Fraud Prevention and Detection
http://www.oig.hhs.gov/fraud.html

Joint Commission on Accreditation of Healthcare Organizations
(See Chapter 1 for contact information.)

Medical Group Management Association (MGMA)
104 Inverness Terrace East
Englewood, CO 80112-5306
Phone: 303-799-1111
http://www.mgma.com

Rural Assistance Center
PO Box 9037
Grand Forks, ND 58202
Phone: 1-800-270-1898
Fax: 1-800-270-1913
E-mail: info@raconline.org
http://www.raconline.org

Chapter *4*

Managed Care

Lynn Kuehn, MS, RHIA, CCS-P, FAHIMA

Learning Objectives

Upon successful completion of this chapter, you should be able to:

1. Identify the various forms of managed care organizations and compare how they are structured.
2. Explain why the term *member* is used to refer to individuals in this setting.
3. Determine the accreditation organization most appropriate for each form of managed care organization.
4. Describe the types of reimbursement that a managed care organization receives and the various methods of reimbursing providers of care.
5. Describe the concept of coordination of benefits and explain why it is important to a managed care organization.
6. Explain why the structure of the managed care organization affects the way health care documentation is managed.
7. Identify the basic requirements for a managed care computer system.
8. Explain why the health plan employer data and information set (HEDIS) is helping improve the quality of health care delivery in managed care.

SETTING	DESCRIPTION	SYNONYMS/ EXAMPLES
Health Maintenance Organization (HMO)	An insurance entity that provides or arranges for health services for a covered population after prepayment of a fixed premium.	Staff Model HMO Group Model HMO Network Model HMO IPA Model HMO Mixed Model HMO
Preferred Provider Organization (PPO)	An insurance entity that contracts with providers to create a preferred network. The insured population is allowed to use any provider but using network providers results in a lesser cost to the patient.	Preferred Provider Network Preferred Provider Option
Point-of-Service (POS) Plan	An insurance plan that combines the health maintenance and preferred provider concepts, creating several levels of out-of-pocket cost options for the insured. The insured makes the choice at the time of service.	Point-of-Sale Plan Open-Ended HMO Open Access HMO
Managed Indemnity Plan	An insurance plan that reimburses the insured for expenses incurred, but incorporates some managed care principles to help control costs.	Modified Indemnity Insurance
Integrated Delivery System (IDS)	A group of facilities contracted together to provide the comprehensive set of services that any patient may need. They are owned, leased, or grouped together by long-term contracts and are recognized by the public as a combined operating entity.	Integrated Delivery Network (IDN)

Introduction to Setting

Defining the managed care industry is like shooting at a moving target. Just when you think you've got it figured out, someone thinks the market needs a different twist on a familiar theme. Managed care is the provision of comprehensive health care services, coordinated through a primary care provider (PCP) with emphasis on preventive care after the patient formally enrolls in a health care plan. Managed care is based on a preventive model and ensures convenient access by effective coordination of care, with a reduction in inappropriate utilization and costs. The PCP is a physician serving as a **gatekeeper** who coordinates all of the patient's health care and decides what, if any, additional care or testing is required.

Managed care began as an alternative delivery system in the mid-1980s but now is regarded more as the industry standard. The use of this type of health care has grown and will continue to grow as employers, the government, and other purchasers of health care want to provide higher-quality care at a lower cost.

The major types of **managed care organizations (MCOs)** are health maintenance organizations (HMOs), preferred provider organizations or networks (PPOs), and indemnity insurance that has incorporated some managed care features. Each of these is unique, and this dynamic industry also contains hybrid combinations of all of these.

The terms *managed care* and *health maintenance organization* are not synonymous, although they are often misused interchangeably. HMOs use managed care techniques and are, therefore, MCOs. However, not all managed care organizations are HMOs, for example, PPOs and managed indemnity plans. The definitions, structure, operation, and information needs of all of these various types of organizations are the subject of this chapter.

Types of Managed Care Organizations

The types of managed care organizations found in the industry today are health maintenance organizations, preferred provider organizations, managed indemnity plans, and point-of-service plans.

Health Maintenance Organizations

Health maintenance organizations (HMOs) are business entities that either arrange for or provide health services to an enrolled population after prepayment of a fixed sum of money, called a premium. By receiving this premium, the HMO is paid to keep its patients healthy. Once the patient becomes ill, the prepayment serves as an incentive for the patient to seek early treatment and for the caregiver to provide care with the greatest efficiency and best possible outcome.

HMOs are found in a variety of different forms, each named by its organizational structure. Regardless of the structure, "the entity must have three characteristics to call itself an HMO:

1. An organized system for providing health care or otherwise assuring health care delivery in a geographic area

2. An agreed upon set of basic and supplemental health maintenance and treatment services

3. A voluntarily enrolled group of people." (A Glossary of Terms: The Language of Managed Care and Organized Health Care Systems, 1994)

Staff Model

The **staff model HMO** is the most tightly organized HMO structure. The HMO entity owns the facilities and arranges for health care through employed physicians, who are allowed to see only the particular HMO patients. All profits accrue to the HMO, rather than to the physicians, and the physicians are paid salaries. Some staff model HMOs own only the clinic facilities and contract with local providers for the remainder of the services, such as hospital and ambulatory surgery services. Other staff model HMOs own a comprehensive group of facilities that provide all of the services under the same ownership. The staff model is the only model where the HMO actually owns the facilities where care is provided. Most staff model HMOs changed their structures into another model during the 1990s, with two large noteworthy exceptions: Kaiser Permanente and Group Health Cooperative (CMS, 2003).

Group Model

The **group model HMO** has an exclusive contract with one multispecialty medical group that provides all physician services. Other facilities necessary to provide the comprehensive health care package are contracted using the same methods as other models. The contract with the multispecialty group may contain a year-end reconciliation clause, where the multispecialty group may receive a percentage of any unused premiums at year-end. This provides significant incentive for proper patient care and financial management. The existence of this model is rare in the marketplace in the 21st century.

Network Model

The **network model HMO** contracts with more than one physician group, hospital, and other facilities to provide a comprehensive health care package. The physicians may share in some of the profit or loss of the HMO according to contract terms but are not required to provide care only to the patients of a particular HMO. The HMO portion of their business may vary from low to high participation.

Independent Practice Association Model

The **independent practice association (IPA) model** was developed primarily as a way for the solo practice physician to participate in the managed care market. This model has two varieties: the physician initiated and the insurance entity initiated. In the model initiated by physicians, the HMO is formed by the physicians who are placing their own resources as the start-up funds. The HMO contracts with each physician and the other facilities necessary to make up the HMO. In this variety of IPA, the physicians are highly at risk for the resources they use to back the HMO. They may also purchase large amounts of reinsurance, or stop-loss insurance, to provide insurance after expenses of a given amount have been paid per enrollee, such as after $50,000 or $100,000 per enrollee has been paid per year.

Insurance entities also develop IPA model HMOs because of their ease of development. A comprehensive group of providers and facilities, plus financial resources, are the only ingredients necessary to develop an IPA model—things readily available through most insurers. Either of these IPA models provides a wide choice of physicians from which enrollees may choose. However, financial viability has been difficult to achieve as the independent physicians have little incentive to change their practice patterns, which is necessary to maintain profitability.

Mixed Model

The **mixed model HMO** operates within two or more different types of organizational structures to provide flexibility to members, diversity of income to the HMO, and attractive pricing to the employers. Mixed models can also be created during mergers and acquisitions.

Preferred Provider Organizations

In an effort to guide enrollees to more cost-effective providers, the **preferred provider organization (PPO)** was developed by the insurance industry. The providers that participate in the PPO agree to provide services to PPO patients at a discounted rate in return for the promise of a higher volume of patients. The patients who use the PPO providers pay little or no out-of-pocket expenses, whereas those who use other providers pay significantly higher portions of the providers' charges. Although the patient is not limited to a certain list of providers, there is a strong financial incentive to choose providers included in the PPO.

Managed Indemnity Plans

Indemnity insurance is the industry term for traditional health insurance, where the insured patient is reimbursed for expenses after the care has been given. This traditional insurance often has **deductible** and **coinsurance** responsibilities for the insured. A deductible is the amount of expenses the insureds must pay each year from their own pockets before the plan will make payments. Coinsurance is the portion of the cost for which the insured has financial responsibility, usually based on a fixed percentage. This coinsurance becomes effective on expenses above the deductible amount.

Traditional indemnity insurance places financial responsibility on the insureds, but also gives them total freedom to use any provider of care they wish, at whatever price. Before the development of managed care, insurance companies thought that these deductible and coinsurance features would encourage insureds to purchase health care wisely. In reality, these features had little effect on purchasing decisions while the costs of health care and health care premiums continued to rise out of control.

Managed indemnity plans were created to provide insureds with the freedom to choose their health care provider, but also to control both premium levels and health care costs. The managed indemnity plans work the same as traditional insurance with the addition of some cost-control measures. The most common cost-control measures included in these plans are preauthorization of expensive tests, surgical procedures, and inpatient hospitalizations, under the assumption that many of these may be unnecessary.

Critics say that managed indemnity plans are just an indemnity insurance company impersonating as managed care. This is said with good reason. To truly qualify as an MCO, the plan needs to have direct involvement in how medicine is practiced. Simply preauthorizing certain services probably does not qualify. For the purposes of this discussion, however, managed care is left "to the eye of the beholder" and all types are included here.

Point-of-Service Plans

A point-of-service plan can incorporate any or all of the above managed care strategies. By enrolling in a point-of-service plan, insureds choose the type of provider to use and how much out-of-pocket expense they are willing to pay in return for that ability to choose. As an example, at the point-of-service (day of care), the patient can choose the HMO physician with no out-of-pocket cost, the PPO in-network provider at a 10-percent coinsurance cost, or a PPO out-of-network provider at a 20-percent coinsurance cost. Some point-of-service plans still require the PPO out-of-network provider to receive preauthorization for certain services, as in managed indemnity plans. With this point-of-service plan, the patient has a great freedom of choice.

With all of the managed care options included here, there are advantages and disadvantages to both providers and patients. The greater the freedom to choose a provider, the higher the out-of-pocket expense to the patient, and the stricter the HMO control over practice patterns, the less at risk the provider income becomes. The individual patients and providers choose the amount of freedom or control with which they are willing to live and work.

Types of Patients

Patients within a managed care organization are referred to as **members**. They have chosen a particular health plan, usually for a period of one year, and become members of the organization for that period of time. Some plans also refer to members as **subscribers** if they are the individuals who are the primary recipients of the insurance benefit, and as **dependents** if they are the spouse or child of the primary recipient. Families, or *insured units*, are also referred to as *contracts*, because the primary recipient makes the insurance decision for the entire family. If the subscriber of the insurance makes the decision to change managed care plans, the contract is lost to another managed care organization. Managed care organizations also refer to the number of individuals holding coverage with their company as the number of covered lives.

All people eligible to receive care within the MCO are still referred to as patients while they are accessing the health care system. Because managed care organizations arrange for or provide care using a network of facilities, the patients are the same types of patients as seen in the individual facilities.

Types of Caregivers

The caregivers encountered in managed care are the traditional caregivers mentioned throughout this text. These caregivers provide illness-related care. In addition, managed care uses health educators to educate patients in preventive measures that can help them retain good health and case managers to administer disease management and chronic illness programs.

Illness

The primary care component of managed care uses physician extenders to provide illness-related care more than other settings in health care. Physician assistants (PAs) and nurse practitioners (NPs) both assist the primary care physicians by performing preventive services such as patient teaching and routine physical examinations, and by performing assessments of acute, but non-life-threatening, conditions for the physician. PAs and NPs are trained to perform tasks that might otherwise be completed by a physician but do not require the same level of education.

PAs must practice under the direction of a physician and have their documentation reviewed and countersigned by the physician. NPs are licensed registered nurses who have received master's-level training in areas of specialty such as adult, family, or pediatric practice. NPs can work independent of a physician but most frequently work as part of a team of primary care practitioners.

Wellness

Preventive care and wellness are a central focus of a health maintenance organization and most managed care organizations. Wellness coordinators or health educators are used in health plans to assist primary care providers in this portion of the mission.

No formal educational preparation is specifically required for the role of health educator. This role is filled by other health professionals who enjoy the teaching portion of health care. Nurses and dietitians function in a preventive role in managed care. Some organizations may also employ an exercise physiologist or physical therapist for cardiopulmonary rehabilitation and strengthening of members. A frequent role for the health educator is teaching chronic disease management for conditions such as asthma or diabetes. Specialized nurse educators extend the care provided by primary providers when they teach prenatal classes or write educational material for the members.

Regulatory Issues

Managed care is concerned with two types of regulatory organizations: governmental agencies and voluntary accrediting associations.

Governmental Regulation

Governmental regulation takes place at the federal and state levels. The federal regulation is concerned with care provided to enrollees of government programs and the state regulation is concerned with the managed care organization's insurance license.

The Centers for Medicare and Medicaid Services (CMS)

Medicare entered the managed care arena as a direct purchaser through the Balanced Budget Act of 1997, with a plan called Medicare+Choice (M+C), which states: "To participate in M+C, beneficiaries must be eligible for Part A and have elected Part B benefits. M+C plans receive capitated payment for providing Part A and Part B services to beneficiaries which replace the amount Medicare would have paid under Part A and B. M+C enrollees are responsible for both the Medicare Part B premium ($58.70 per month for 2003), which is retained by the Medicare program and any additional premium collected by the M+C plan. M+C plans may offer additional benefits, such as prescription drugs, eye exams, hearing aids, or routine physical exams" (CMS, 2003) but, at a minimum, must provide the exact coverage that Medicare would provide.

Enrollment in M+C plans in 2002 was estimated at 5.6 million beneficiaries, or 11 percent of the Medicare population, but enrollment has been declining. In 2004, CMS changed the name of this program to **Medicare Advantage** and increased payments to participating health plans, in anticipation of improving their attractiveness.

The Medicare Managed Care Manual (found on the Internet at http://cms.hhs.gov/manuals/116_mmc/mc86toc.asp) provides information on participation, including information on the Quality Assessment and Performance Improvement requirements for Medicare managed care plans.

Clinical Laboratory Improvement Amendments of 1988

The Clinical Laboratory Improvement Amendments of 1988 (CLIA) were originally developed in response to concerns about potentially preventable deaths caused by poor Pap smear testing. This law was effective on September 1, 1992, and refers to all laboratories, including those operated in HMOs and physician practices within managed care networks.

The basic items that CLIA addresses are testing complexity, personnel standards, proficiency testing requirements, quality control standards, patient test management, cytology testing, inspections, and fees. The regulations of CLIA require that every laboratory possess a certificate to operate and that sanctions are given to a laboratory that fails to meet the operational standards or proficiency testing guidelines. MCOs require proof of CLIA compliance during the laboratory contracting process. (Requirements are found on the Internet at http://www.cms.hhs.gov/clia/.)

State Regulation

Although many MCOs providing services to Medicare and Medicaid beneficiaries are regulated by the CMS Office of Managed Care, many MCOs are not. MCOs with only commercial enrollees are regulated solely by their individual state insurance laws. These laws vary throughout the United States and are administered by the insurance commissioner's office or HMO regulatory agency in each state to ensure that the MCO is financially able to operate as an insurance company.

Voluntary Accreditation

Voluntary accreditation takes three approaches with managed care. The MCO can decide on any of these approaches:

- National Committee for Quality Assurance (NCQA) accreditation
- Joint Commission on Accreditation of Healthcare Organizations (JCAHO) accreditation or Accreditation Association for Ambulatory Health Care (AAAHC) accreditation
- Both NCQA and JCAHO or AAAHC accreditation

National Committee for Quality Assurance

The **National Committee for Quality Assurance** (**NCQA**, pronounced NIK-QWA) has been accrediting managed care organizations since 1979. The Washington, D.C.– based organization was established by the Group Health Association of America (GHAA) and the American Association of Foundations for Medical Care, which is now the American Managed Care and Review Association (AMCRA), both trade organizations for the HMO industry. NCQA originally did governmental reviews for federally qualified HMO status in the 1980s. In the early 1990s, NCQA received a grant from the Robert Wood Johnson Foundation to develop a new set of standards separate from the trade associations.

The current standards include six sections: Quality Assurance, Credentialing, Utilization Management, Members' Rights and Responsibilities, Preventive Health Services, and Medical Records. The accreditation process involves a two- to four-day site visit by three members of a survey team. Accreditation is granted for a provisional one year or a full three-year status, with any accreditation status being very difficult to obtain. While the survey is all-encompassing, the central focus is on the insurance aspects of the MCO.

NCQA manages the Health Plan Employer Data and Information Set (HEDIS), the performance measurement tool used by more than 90 percent of the nation's health plans. (See Data Sets later in this chapter for additional information.) HEDIS performance measurement data are the basis for NCQA's Health Plan Report Card, a tool designed to help consumers learn more about their health plan options and the quality of care that the health plans provide. The Health Plan Report Card is available on the NCQA Web site and reports quality based on a star system, from one to four stars being assigned in five categories: Access and Service, Qualified Providers, Staying Healthy, Getting Better, and Living with Illness. Accredited HMOs and PPOs are rated against regional and national averages and benchmarks. Viewing this report card data allows consumers to make health plan enrollment choices based on both quality and cost.

Joint Commission on Accreditation of Healthcare Organizations

The Joint Commission on Accreditation of Healthcare Organizations (JCAHO) performs accreditation surveys for networks of many types using the *Comprehensive Accreditation Manual for Health Care Networks*. These networks include all of the types of managed care organizations discussed in this chapter, except managed indemnity plans, which are not a comprehensive network for delivery of care.

During the JCAHO survey, the survey team assesses the network's ability to function as a whole. The network is made up of many diverse facilities. This accreditation process is especially valuable to network model HMOs, IPA model HMOs, and PPOs, in which multiple facilities under different management need to function as a cohesive unit.

Accreditation Association for Ambulatory Health Care

The Accreditation Association for Ambulatory Health Care (AAAHC) accredits the health care delivery portion of staff model, group model, and network model HMOs. AAAHC uses the *Accreditation Handbook for Ambulatory Health Care* to survey the physician office and clinic portions of these HMOs. The survey consists of an on-site visit by at least two surveyors for a minimum of two days and is aimed at the health care delivery rather than the insurance aspects of the HMO or MCO. Figure 4-1 summarizes the voluntary accreditation associations and the organizations they accredit.

Documentation

Documentation methods for different types of managed care organizations are determined by the structure of the organization, such as whether a clinic is owned by the MCO or contracts with the MCO.

Staff Model

Documentation requirements for staff model HMOs are set directly by the HMO. Documentation of services provided by all caregivers is found in the centralized record for the member, which is kept at the member's clinic. The primary care provider (PCP) functions as the gatekeeper and writes orders for all diagnostic and therapeutic procedures that the PCP cannot perform. Copies of the results of these

Accreditation Association	Applicability
National Committee for Quality Assurance (NCQA)	All HMO, PPO, and POS plans
Accreditation Association for Ambulatory Health Care (AAAHC)	Staff model HMOs at each clinic site, but not as an HMO Group model HMOs at the physician group, but not as an HMO Network model HMOs at the clinic site, but not as an HMO
Joint Commission on Accreditation of Healthcare Organizations (JCAHO) Network Standards	Integrated delivery system (IDS) in its ability to function as a single entity. Each part of the entity may be individually accredited by JCAHO or other organization

Figure 4-1   Voluntary accreditation associations.

procedures are sent to the PCP for review. Courtesy copies from inpatient admissions are also sent to the PCP for review and future reference.

The content of the clinic documentation is guided by appropriate accreditation association standards. The structure of the staff model HMO, with the physician as an employee, determines that the record is the property of the HMO.

Group Model Through Managed Indemnity Plans

The structure of these MCOs places all documentation under the control of the physician group or physician serving as the primary care provider, rather than the MCO. The MCO does not actually maintain any medical documentation but ensures that the primary care providers will, by requiring it in their managed care contracts. Contract requirements are written to ensure that enough information is maintained to comply with the appropriate AAAHC, JCAHO, or NCQA standards.

Revenue Generation

The MCO produces its revenue by selling an insurance product, which is the ability to provide quality health care to the member. In turn, the MCO must reimburse the providers of care for the services they provide to the members on behalf of the MCO.

Managed Care Organization Revenue

Premium payments are received from multiple sources in MCOs. Employers pay the premiums for a large percentage of members, but some members pay their own premiums because of changes in employment or self-employment. Some MCOs also contract with the government to insure Medicare and Medicaid patients, and the MCO receives the premium directly from CMS or the individual states on behalf of these members.

The amount of premium payment can be determined in several ways. Community rating is a method of determining premiums based on actual or anticipated costs for members in a specific geographic location (city, metropolitan area, or state). Age/sex rating is a method of structuring premiums based on enrollee/membership statistics of age and sex. Composite rating is a method of determining premiums in which one uniform premium applies to all subscribers regardless of the number of claimed dependents, or the same flat rate per member. Experience rating determines premiums based on the actual utilization of individual subscriber groups. This method is not acceptable in a federally qualified HMO but is the most frequently used method in traditional indemnity insurance.

Any premium rate can be structured to a lower amount by requiring a **copayment** from the member at the time of care. A copayment is usually a flat amount, such as $10 per visit.

Reimbursement to the Provider of Care

Salary

In a staff model HMO, providers of care are actual employees of the HMO. Providers work under contract but receive a monthly or bimonthly salary payment, regardless of whether their patient **panel** is full. A provider's panel is the group of patients who have chosen the provider as their primary care provider. The size of the panel is HMO-specific, either by raw numbers of members, such as 1,600 members, or stratified by age group, such as 400 children, 1,000 adults, and 200 seniors.

Capitation (Per Member Per Month)

Capitation is the payment of a fixed dollar amount for each covered person, for the provision of a predetermined set of health services for a specific period of time. Providers are responsible for providing all of the care needed to each of the patients for whom they receive a capitation. With this capitation arrangement, the provider assumes the risk for the cost and for the frequency of the services provided. As an example, the provider may receive $40 per month for each patient assigned to him or her, whether or not the patient receives care or makes multiple visits. This capitation payment is usually made monthly, based on the monthly patient panel, or assigned group of patients. This rate is known as per member per month, or PMPM. Out of this capitation payment, providers must pay support staff and office expenses. Claims are sent to the MCO for information purposes only and not for payment processing. Providers who practice effectively can make money under this arrangement, whereas those who do not manage their resources well are financially at risk.

Per Diem

Per diem means paid by the day or at a daily rate. These rates are negotiated with centers such as hospitals and skilled nursing facilities (SNFs). The per diem covers the nursing care plus room and board charges. Special procedures or surgical services are charged separately. This amount is the only payment the facility receives for the care.

Fee Schedule, Negotiated

The MCO and the provider can negotiate a fee schedule for a flat rate per procedure, visit, or service. This allows any provider willing to negotiate to be part of the MCO network, even those where no historical data are available on use and cost. This method is normally used when services are needed on a less frequent basis, but the cost varies widely from case to case. Negotiating a fee schedule allows more consistent budgeting of payment dollars by the MCO.

Fee Schedule, Resource-Based Relative Value Scale

Another way to negotiate a fee schedule is to use the resource-based relative value scale (RBRVS) unit value as the base and negotiate the conversion factor (the dollar amount per unit) that provides appropriate reimbursement. As an example, if the RBRVS unit value for a procedure is 2.5 and the negotiated conversion factor is $45 for all procedures, the fee paid to the provider in this case would be $112.50.

Discounted Charges

In this method, the provider agrees to see MCO patients and charge the MCO the regular fee-for-service rate. The MCO discounts the rate by a certain amount, usually a percentage, before the payment is made. The negotiation of this payment method is the easiest to accomplish, offers the greatest financial risk to the MCO, and gives little financial incentive to the provider to practice more cost-effectively. The total charge may be limited by a maximum allowable threshold for a particular service.

With all of these reimbursement mechanisms, the providers receive the reimbursement from the MCO. Except when copayments are required as a provision of the health plan contract, any remaining balance cannot be billed to the member. Those balances become the "cost of doing business" for the provider and cannot be billed to any other party. Figure 4-2 summarizes the advantages and disadvantages of the different reimbursement methods.

Coordination of Benefits

Coordination of benefits (COB) means determining who is the primary insurance payer and ensuring that no more than 100 percent of the charges are paid to the provider and/or reimbursed to the patient.

Method	Provider	Advantage	Disadvantage
Salary	Physicians	Predictable revenue for the provider, regardless of number of patients in panel	Efficient providers cannot ask for a payment larger than the maximum panel size, limiting their total salary.
Capitation	Primarily physician services	Predictable expenses for the MCO and predictable revenue for providers	Works only when some patients do not seek care and a significant portion are not "sicker" than average.
Per Diem	Primarily inpatient facilities	Flat rate regardless of type of care given	Good historical data is required to negotiate an appropriate rate.
Fee Schedule, Negotiated	Any noninpatient facility or physicians	Allows per-unit billing but at a controlled and predetermined cost per unit	Can be negotiated without good historical data or for less frequently used providers.
Fee Schedule, RBRVS Based	Physician services	As above, but can be related to Medicare reimbursement	Not all procedures have an RBRVS value assigned to them.
Discounted Charges	All providers	Easiest to establish, but provides no incentive for cost-effectiveness by providers	Provides the greatest flexibility of charges for the provider and the greatest financial risk for the MCO.

Figure 4-2   Reimbursement to providers of care.

Dual Insurance Coverage

Some patients have two insurers because both spouses receive coverage through their employer or because they have purchased an HMO policy to supplement the deficiencies of a basic policy, such as Medicare. It is in the best interest of an MCO to determine and record who the primary insurance carrier is for each member so that the coordination of benefits rules can be applied correctly. In some cases, the MCO may be a secondary payer.

The method of determining the primary payer in dual-coverage cases is different from state to state. The most popular method used in determining the primary payer when both spouses carry insurance on the family is the "birthday rule." The spouse with the birthday earliest in the calendar year is the primary insurer for the children, with each spouse's insurance being primary for themselves. Determining whose insurance is primary for the family is important to the MCO, because for a dual-covered family, the MCO may be the primary carrier for the subscriber only and not for the other family members. If the subscriber's spouse carries the primary insurance for the family, the MCO is responsible for the full benefit level for the subscriber and only the unpaid balance, usually 20 percent or less, on the other family members. HMOs must follow the rules for determining when Medicare is the secondary payer.

The MCO that owns health care facilities can bill other primary payers for the care provided in its facilities or by its salaried or capitated providers, thus offsetting the expense of care. When paying claims, the MCO can direct claims to other payers if it is not the primary payer.

Workers' Compensation, Motor Vehicle Accidents, and Personal Injury Cases

Many MCO members are injured at work, in a motor vehicle accident, or by another individual. In these cases, the member may prefer to receive care from his or her PCP. It may, in fact, be better for the patient's overall health and wellness to see the PCP who knows his or her medical history. In these situations, the MCO can submit a claim to the workers' compensation, motor vehicle, or personal injury carrier and receive reimbursement for the care provided. This diverts the expense to the appropriate insurance carrier, while the MCO's overhead and/or capitation remains the same.

Information Management

The information management system in a managed care organization is determined by the structure of the organization. If the managed care organization owns facilities that are part of the organization, the health information management system would be similar to the systems described in other chapters of this book.

The information gathered and maintained in the insurance portion of the organization is maintained using procedures and systems similar to those used in the medical insurance industry.

Coding and Classification Systems

The two basic coding and classification systems used to collect and manage data in managed care are the ICD-9-CM diagnosis system and the CPT procedure system. Other systems may be used as the individual needs of an organization dictate.

ICD-9-CM Diagnosis Codes

The *International Classification of Disease, Ninth Revision, Clinical Modification* (ICD-9-CM) was implemented in 1979 and is the classification system for diagnoses required by CMS on all health care claims received. The ICD-9-CM coding system is the only system used throughout the health care industry to describe diagnoses, and these codes are collected on all claims for all services in managed care.

ICD-9-CM diagnosis codes also have another use in Medicare Advantage plans—as a component of a system for adjusting capitation payments to health plans based on the patient's health status. Traditionally, Medicare adjusted its payments to health plans based on geographic and demographic factors associated with each enrollee (e.g., age, gender, Medicaid eligibility, and institutional status) (Tully & Rulon, 2000). In 1998, the **Principal In-Patient Diagnostic Cost Group (PIP-DCG)** model was proposed as an initial mechanism for adjusting payments to Medicare managed care organizations based on patient diagnoses. When an enrollee was hospitalized, the principal diagnosis code determined into which PIP-DCG the patient would fall in most instances (Health Care Financing Administration, 1998). The PIP-DCG in turn determined the amount of added risk of requiring more costly health care services that the enrollee represented. The numerical risk factor associated with each PIP-DCG was a component in determining the amount by which payment to the MCO would be increased. The PIP-DCG risk-adjusted payment model began to be phased in during the year 2000 (Pope et al., 2000). In 2004, CMS implemented a more comprehensive model that considers all sites of service, not just inpatient hospitalization. The new model uses selected ICD-9-CM codes to place patients into groups known as **Hierarchical Condition Categories (HCCs)**. The CMS-HCC model is additive, meaning that if a patient falls into more than one HCC, additional risk will be calculated and the payment to the organization will be increased further (CMS, 2004).

CPT Procedure Codes and HCPCS Codes

Current Procedural Terminology (CPT) is an American Medical Association (AMA) publication that describes physician diagnostic and therapeutic procedures and their codes. CMS incorporated the CPT codes into its Healthcare Common Procedural Coding System (HCPCS) used to describe physician services for reimbursement. CPT and the full HCPCS coding systems are the basis for the resource-based relative value scale (RBRVS) system. CPT codes are routinely collected on all claims except for facility charge claims. Using CPT and HCPCS codes allows the MCO to compare services used and costs across delivery sites.

Special Uses of Coded Data

ICD-9-CM Procedure Codes

The ICD-9-CM classification system contains a separate volume of codes used to describe medical procedures. These codes best describe procedures from a facility perspective and are mainly used to describe hospital-based services. MCOs collect these codes on UB-92 claims, the standard facility charge claim form.

Diagnosis Related Groups

Diagnosis related groups (DRGs) were implemented in the early 1980s for use in describing inpatient services. The classification system groups inpatients who are medically related by diagnosis, treatment, and length of stay. Patients are grouped into major diagnostic categories (MDCs) and further subgrouped into a specific DRG. Only one DRG is assigned per stay.

Many MCOs collect the DRG number or determine the number by entering the ICD-9-CM diagnosis and procedure codes into a special computer program called a "grouper." Medicare pays a flat rate per inpatient stay, based on the DRG for that stay. This allows Medicare to more accurately predict the expenses for the insured population and forces the inpatient facility to share a large portion of the risk. The hospital receives a set payment, regardless of how many days the patient stays and how large the bill might actually be. This payment method is also used by some MCOs to pay inpatient claims for similar reasons.

UB-92 Revenue Codes

Revenue codes are collected on all claims submitted on a UB-92 claim form. Normally these forms contain facility and service charges from hospitals, skilled nursing facilities, and home care agencies. Revenue codes define a specific accommodation type, ancillary service, or billing calculation. They are three-digit numbers that are grouped into categories of numbers having similar meaning.

Data and Information Flow

Data Collection and Transfer

Data is collected differently depending on the structure of the MCO. Staff model and group model HMOs are able to collect encounter data on the patients they see in their clinics. All types of HMOs are able to collect referral data after a referral has been issued, and all types of MCOs are able to collect claims data from providers requesting payment.

Encounter Data

An **encounter** is "contact between a patient and a provider who is responsible for the assessment and evaluation of the patient at a specific contact, exercising independent judgment" (Abdelhak, 2001). Encounter data is collected at the time of the service and reported in its raw form, rather than in the form of claims (billing) data.

Referral Data

A **referral** is an authorization to receive a specific health service from a specific health provider that will be paid for by the HMO. All HMOs issue referrals before specialty care can be given. PPOs and managed indemnity plans do not issue referrals because patients are allowed to see other providers if they are willing to pay the additional cost. Referral data is collected at the time the referral is given by all organizations that issue referrals.

Most MCOs process referrals by online request systems or telephone voice and data recognition systems to speed the processing. Authorization for care ahead of time in the form of a referral allows the MCO to direct patients to appropriate providers in the network and to record the estimated future expense that will be incurred for the care.

Claims Data

Claims data is collected as a by-product of the claims payment process. IPA model HMOs, PPOs, and managed indemnity plans can access service data in the form of claims data. For facilities such as hospitals, the data available is from the UB-92 claim form. Data for physicians and similar providers is from their billing form, the CMS 1500.

Statistical Data

All available data, including encounter, referral, and claims data, is combined and organized to provide useful management statistics. The two major ways that statistics are divided in MCOs are by member and by contract. HMOs frequently work with statistical data by member, and PPOs and managed indemnity plans work with their data by contracts, although MCOs may use both methods.

By Per Member Per Month (PMPM)

Frequency of service utilization and the cost of procedures is evaluated and displayed by employer purchasing group, by provider or facility site, and by provider panel, based on the number of members in the MCO for that month.

By Per Contract Per Month (PCPM)

Frequency and cost are evaluated and displayed in the same way based on the number of total contracts the MCO has for the month.

Computer Systems

A computer system that is able to perform the functions necessary for managed care is vital to the profitability of the MCO. The requirements for a basic computer system are much different than for either a hospital or physician office practice, even though MCOs may include these facilities in their networks. All computer functions are designed to assist care providers and staff to appropriately utilize resources.

Basic System Requirements

Eligibility/Enrollment

Enrollment is the process of placing a person into the database of covered individuals of the MCO. **Eligibility** refers to whether the person is allowed to receive care under the MCO contract and the dates of coverage. The enrollment database is similar to the master patient index found in health care facilities and includes dates of enrollment and disenrollment, demographic information, and the party responsible for paying the premium.

Benefit Levels

The benefit level may not be the same for all members of an MCO. Most managed care organizations sell a variety of insurance packages, some that allow more services than others, or that allow certain benefits at a higher payment level than others. Benefit levels must be tracked for each individual member because many members have dual insurance coverage or different benefit packages, even within the same family or contract. A system that only tracks this information for the subscriber may miss the detail necessary to divert claims to another more appropriate payer.

Patient Registration and Scheduling

Hospitals within an MCO require a patient registration system and all service providers require some form of scheduling software to manage their health care environment.

Authorization and Referral Management

Managed care organizations provide preauthorization for admissions and procedures and issue referrals for care that cannot be provided by the PCP. This information must be maintained in the computer system and must be accessible to the PCP. The best systems include practice guidelines that are accessible and allow the PCP to review and document clinical decisions in real time within the computer.

Utilization Management/Case Management

Computer software should identify cases that are appropriate for case management through evaluation of encounter data, referral data, or claims data. This allows the utilization management staff to assist the PCP in managing the multiple resources needed to properly care for complicated cases. The best systems provide accessible information about clinical practice guidelines for both inpatient and outpatient management.

Billing/Claims Production

Staff model and group model HMOs require software to create claims for another primary insurer for patients with dual insurance coverage. In addition, this software should have the ability to post payments to these charges and maintain accounts receivable information for tracking purposes.

Payment/Claims Processing

The claims processing software allows the MCO to pay claims for authorized services and should verify the eligibility/enrollment files, benefit levels, and referral data before the payment is processed. Capitated visits should be recorded in the claims database even though no actual payment is processed. Without this capitated data, there is no information to manage the financial aspects of the MCO that are covered under capitation.

Cost Accounting

The cost accounting portion of the computer system should tie together the accounts payable portion of the business and the accounts receivable portion from premiums. In staff model HMOs, coordination of benefits (COB) income must also be tracked. COB income is received when the staff model bills another primary insurer for services it provided in its clinics.

Advanced System Requirements

Electronic Health Record (EHR)

The answer to collecting patient health information and having it available throughout the network of facilities is ultimately the electronic health record. Without the EHR, the MCO is still a combination of different facilities that try their best to achieve effective communication in real time.

Kaiser Permanente, a staff model HMO based in California, has developed a homegrown product in collaboration with a major information technology vendor. Plans are underway to implement the same product nationwide to increase efficiency and improve the quality of patient care (Rollins, 2003).

Executive Decision Making

Data from any or all of the computer systems may be needed to determine where and when decisions are needed and to help in the decision-making process.

Purchased Mainframe Systems

Because of the complexity and variability of MCO structure, any purchased software system must be extremely flexible to meet the needs of any managed care organization. The most effective purchased systems have a great number of parameters that may be customized according to the needs of the client MCO.

Data Sets

Health Plan Employer Data and Information Set

The **health plan employer data and information set (HEDIS)** is a core set of performance measures for managed care plans. HEDIS was designed in 1991 by NCQA to help employers compare health plans, understand the value of what their health care premium is purchasing, and hold the health plan accountable for performance against these measures. HEDIS provides a consistent measure of five key performance areas: Quality, Access and Patient Satisfaction, Membership and Utilization, Finance, and Health Plan Management. These five areas contain more than 40 measures, such as the number of pregnant enrollees receiving prenatal care within the first trimester and the number of enrollees assigned to a primary care physician. A list of HEDIS measures is available at the NCQA Web site.

Employer-Specific Data Sets

Some national employers, such as IBM and Xerox, are asking for data specifically on their enrollees, either using HEDIS indicators or by identifying their own issues for tracking.

Quality Improvement and Utilization Management

The accreditation associations, CMS, and many employer purchasing groups require an active quality improvement program within managed care organizations to ensure that care is delivered in a cost-effective manner with consistently appropriate outcomes.

Quality Improvement

The components of a quality improvement program for a managed care organization are detailed as follows. They include an oversight committee that uses a comprehensive plan and the use of quality indicators to identify trends.

Oversight Committee Using a Comprehensive Plan

To ensure that quality improvement is a continuous process, MCOs use an oversight committee that is guided by a comprehensive quality plan. The quality plan is developed by the senior staff and approved by the board of directors, at least annually. The oversight committee receives and reviews reports and project requests from subcommittees within the organization. The committee structure is designed to provide a place for each area of the business to report its quality issues and findings.

Quality Indicators

Quality indicators are a quantitative measuring tool for monitoring and evaluating performance. These indicators are important to an MCO because it is very difficult to manage what has not been measured. Quality in an MCO has several aspects, including medical outcomes, operational effectiveness, patient satisfaction, and financial stability.

Operational Indicators

The operational effectiveness indicators measure how well the MCO is performing in comparison to preset goals. These can also include patient satisfaction level goals about how well the "customer" or patient feels the MCO is performing. Examples include:

Telephone call turnaround time

Percentage of telephone calls answered in under thirty seconds

Appointment availability—all service areas

Percentage of rescheduled appointments—administrative reasons

Pharmacy refill turnaround time

Lobby wait times

Claims processing turnaround time

Medical Indicators

Medical indicators are also referred to as outcome measures because they express the MCO's ability to obtain a successful outcome from the care that is delivered. Some examples are:

Percentage of members receiving prenatal care in the first trimester

Percentage of babies born at or above an appropriate birth weight

Percentage of operative patients without wound infection

Unanticipated emergency room visits within 24 hours after surgery

Unplanned emergency department visits after primary care visit on same day

Rates of mammograms, Pap smears, immunizations, or physicals

Financial Indicators

Financial stability can be measured using the following indicators:

Days in Claims Payable (calculated as the reverse of Days in Accounts Receivable), or

$$\frac{\text{Ending \$ in Claims Payable}}{\text{\$ in Claims Payable for the period}} \div \text{Days in the Period}$$

Hospital bed days per 1,000 members

Number of avoidable hospital days

Hospital **bed days** are equivalent to the inpatient statistic known as inpatient service days. The measurement of bed days per 1,000 members is a standard MCO measurement that can be compared among MCOs nationwide. Avoidable hospital days are defined through the utilization management program and include such items as performing an ambulatory diagnostic workup as an inpatient, delay in obtaining or failure to appropriately use home care services, or delay in receiving consultation, testing, or procedures. These types of indicators measure the MCO's overall ability to act as a unit for successful patient care and financial outcomes.

Utilization Management

Utilization management is part of the quality improvement function of an MCO because data about underutilization and overutilization can provide insight into possible quality issues within the MCO.

Preauthorization and/or Concurrent Review

Using clinical practice guidelines on potentially expensive or difficult cases can provide consistent quality of care and can save the MCO money by performing the correct test or procedure at the correct time in the treatment plan. Preauthorization of expensive procedures can also perform the same function and can assist the MCO in locating the best possible facility for performing the procedure.

Written Utilization Protocols and Coordination of Care

Written utilization protocols help providers deal with basically uncomplicated but common cases, and can help avoid unnecessary hospitalizations and provide quicker recovery for the patient. Coordination of care staff helps ensure that the patient receives care at the correct point from the correct providers. In addition, coordination of care staff helps the PCP manage chronic disease patients more effectively.

Risk Management and Legal Issues

Risk management in managed care is more comprehensive because of the wide variety of services provided under the managed care concept. Each of the facilities included in the managed care organization, both owned and contracted, monitors for potential risks that are particular to their own settings.

Documentation of care coordination between these settings is very important in managed care because patients feel that "managed care" means that care happens, or should happen, seamlessly across many facilities. If this does not happen, patients may see their care as less than optimal and consider litigation.

Identifying Unusual Events

Unusual events are reported and tracked within the MCO. Unusual events represent a primary source of litigation for MCOs, similar to other health care providers. Unusual events can be the delay or denial of services that are later determined to have been necessary or emergent, failure to direct a patient to the proper source of care, or any medical incident normally tracked elsewhere, such as an incorrect medication administration.

Informed Consent for Procedures

The providers within the MCO use the same procedures as other providers when they obtain informed consent from patients or their legal representatives before performing procedures. In addition to individual liability on the part of the physician or facility, the MCO is also at risk for being a party to a malpractice suit.

Credentialing

Credentialing is "a process of review to approve a provider who applies to participate in a health plan. Specific criteria and prerequisites are applied in determining initial and ongoing participation in the health plan" (A Glossary of Terms: The Language of Managed Care and Organized Health Care Systems, 1994). The MCO performs its own investigation because external efforts may not have been valid. The prerequisites that are evaluated include the credentialing elements verified traditionally by hospitals. These elements include:

1. Current competence in the field
2. Work history
3. Physical and mental health status
4. Challenges to licensure and registrations
5. Limitation or termination of clinical privileges
6. Pending professional liability actions
7. Felony convictions
8. Federal Drug Enforcement Administration Registration
9. National Practitioner Data Bank information

Provider's Office Evaluation

In addition to personal credentialing of the provider, the provider's office is also evaluated to assess whether the office is organized and managed appropriately for inclusion in the MCO network.

Structured Review

The provider's office is evaluated, before the signing of a contract, for such items as acceptable facilities, available staff, accessibility of care, and systems for medical management including computerization appropriate for the size of the office or facility.

Record Review

A health record review is completed to determine if the records are accessible, standardized in format, legible, properly secured to the folder, signed and dated, and contain the patient's name on each page. Other items may be evaluated based on the applicability of the Accreditation Association for Ambulatory Health Care (AAAHC), Joint Commission on Accreditation of Healthcare Organizations (JCAHO), or National Committee for Quality Assurance (NCQA) record content standards.

Economic Credentialing

Economic credentialing is performed to ensure that the provider is not underutilizing services and compromising the health of the member or overutilizing services and creating unnecessary expense. The MCO uses statistical data such as the number of inpatient admissions per 1,000 members and charges per HCPCS code or DRG to evaluate financial performance. Economic credentialing results in the exclusion of a provider only in the rarest of situations and primarily for severe underutilization of services.

Recredentialing

Providers are recredentialed every two years to be sure that no new information is ignored. A tickler system is used to help reevaluate providers on time, checking such items as medical quality indicator results, malpractice claims experience, overall patient satisfaction rating, and the number of member complaints.

Contract Management

The MCO is built on contracted relationships. An index of contracts, including expiration dates and any proposed contract changes, is maintained to be sure all contracts remain valid and at an optimal level of reimbursement.

Role of the Health Information Management Professional

Developing and Implementing Information Plan Based on Organizational Needs

The health information management (HIM) professional in managed care is found mainly in the staff model, group model, and network model HMO performing the traditional role of health information manager. These HMO settings require the HIM professional to maintain security and confidentiality of records. In addition, the HIM professional performs data collection and coding of encounter data. The HIM professional is concerned with record storage, appropriate information technology within the facilities, and personnel management. As in other facilities, this person normally participates highly in, or leads, the preparation for an accreditation survey visit.

Specialized Functions

The HIM professional receives a unique mix of education and training, which allows an individual to perform other functions that are less traditional within an MCO.

Enrollment Management

The enrollment database in an MCO is a highly detailed version of a master patient index, an index traditionally maintained by the HIM professional. The HIM professional's knowledge of data management and patient identification systems provides some of the best foundation possible for performing or supervising this function.

Clinical Data Specialist

The role of clinical data specialist is best filled by an HIM professional because this person "concentrates on data management functions including clinical coding, outcomes management, specialty registries and research databases" (Abdelhak, 2001, p. 51). This specialist would also use knowledge of medicine, management, and data display to interpret, summarize, and display information found in the claims, encounter, and enrollment databases.

Claims Processing/Management

The largest database maintained in most MCOs is the claims database. In addition to management of the claims database, the claims processing supervisor helps determine whether claims are coded properly and are acceptable for payment. The HIM professional's medical knowledge, combined with financial experience or ability, can prepare him or her well for the role of claims processing supervisor.

Quality Management

Specialization in quality management performance improvement by the HIM professional is likely in a managed care organization. Knowledge of all areas of health care provides an excellent foundation for performing the quality management function.

Risk Management

HIM professionals frequently fill the role of risk manager. "Risk management activities are intended to achieve the following goals: 1) minimize the potential for injuries occurring, 2) respond promptly and appropriately to injured parties, and 3) anticipate and plan for ensuing liability when injuries occur" (Abdelhak, 2001, p. 407–408). The HIM professional's study of medicine, management, and the legal system provides an excellent background for performing the duties of risk manager.

Chief Information Officer

The information technology knowledge of the HIM professional can easily be used to perform the role of chief information officer (CIO) for a managed care organization.

Trends

Integrated Delivery Systems/Networks

Integrated delivery systems/networks (IDS/Ns) are a group of facilities, contracted together, to provide the comprehensive set of services that a patient may need. These facilities and services are owned, leased, or grouped together through long-term contracts and are recognized by the public as being a combined operating entity.

Integrated delivery systems are not the same as managed care organizations because they do not always contain an insurance provision. However, because an MCO requires a full network of providers, the IDS/N is a natural place to look when contemplating an MCO contract.

The Changing Role of the PCP

The primary care provider is playing less of a role in gatekeeping than ever before in many MCOs. Although most Medicare and Medicaid HMOs still retain the PCP gatekeeper function, other HMOs are abandoning the concept and reallocating the funds into stronger disease management and chronic care management programs. Evidence points toward this trend continuing as resources are funneled to the proper management of the sickest patients in the HMO.

In addition, the population will continue to transition to less restrictive MCO models, PPOs, and POS products without the gatekeeper function, if premiums remain comparable.

Summary

The structure of MCOs continues to change to meet market demand, with more MCOs changing to open network styles. Quality improvement and data management are two key areas within the managed care environment, both of which are excellent employment opportunities for HIM professionals. The managed care field will continue to change and grow, to meet the needs of purchasers and in an attempt to control health care expenses.

Key Terms

bed day   an inpatient service received by one member for one 24-hour period.

capitation   payment of a fixed dollar amount to a provider for each patient assigned to that provider, regardless of the amount of care the patient receives.

Clinical Laboratory Improvement Amendments of 1988 (CLIA)   federal legislation that provides for regulation of all clinical laboratories, including those operated in HMOs and physician practices within managed care networks.

coinsurance the amount of expense that is the responsibility of the insured under an indemnity insurance policy, usually 20 percent.

coordination of benefits determining which insurance is the primary payer and ensuring that no more than 100 percent of the charges are paid to the provider and/or reimbursed to the patient.

copayment a flat-rate payment, such as $10 per visit, made by the covered individual for a specific service at the time of the service.

deductible the amount of expenses the insureds must pay each year from their own pockets before the plan will reimburse them.

dependent the spouse or child of the primary insurance recipient.

eligibility whether a person is able to receive benefits under an insurance policy.

encounter contact between a patient and a provider who is responsible for the assessment and evaluation of the patient at a specific contact, exercising independent judgment.

gatekeeper the primary care provider who coordinates all of the patient's health care and decides what, if any, additional care is required.

group model HMO a rarely seen model in which the HMO has an exclusive contract with one multispecialty medical group that provides all physician services and contracts with other facilities as necessary to provide comprehensive services.

health maintenance organization (HMO) a business entity that either provides or arranges for health services for a covered population after prepayment of a fixed premium.

health plan employer data and information set (HEDIS) a core set of standard performance measures for managed care in the areas of quality, access and patient satisfaction, membership, utilization, finance, and health plan management.

Hierarchical Condition Categories (HCCs) disease groupings based on ICD-9-CM codes from both inpatient admissions and outpatient visits in Medicare Advantage organizations. HCCs are used to risk-adjust payments to MCOs.

indemnity insurance traditional health insurance where the insured is reimbursed for expenses after the care has been given.

independent practice association (IPA) model an HMO model that was developed primarily as a way for the solo practice physician to participate in the managed care market.

integrated delivery systems/network (IDS/N) a group of facilities contracted together to provide the comprehensive set of services that any patient may need. They are owned, leased, or grouped together by long-term contracts and are recognized by the public as a combined operating entity.

managed care organization (MCO) an organization that provides comprehensive health services, coordinated through a primary care provider who acts as a gatekeeper, after the patient formally enrolls in the organization.

managed indemnity plans indemnity insurance plans that do not limit the insured's choice of health care providers, but do include cost-control measures, such as preauthorization of expensive tests, surgical procedures, and inpatient hospitalization.

Medicare Advantage a program by which eligible Medicare beneficiaries may choose to receive their health care through a qualified managed care plan, which in turn receives capitation payments from Medicare for each enrollee.

mixed model HMO an HMO that operates within two or more different types of organizational structures to provide flexibility to members.

member a patient who is enrolled in a managed care organization.

National Committee for Quality Assurance an accreditation association that accredits only managed care organizations.

network model HMO an HMO that contracts with multiple physician groups, hospitals, and other facilities to provide a comprehensive health care package.

panel the group of patients who have chosen a particular provider as their primary care provider.

per diem a reimbursement methodology where the payment is based on the number of days of care.

preferred provider organization (PPO) an insurance entity that contracts with providers to create a preferred network. The insured population is allowed to use any provider, but using network providers results in a lesser cost to the patient.

Principal In-Patient Diagnostic Cost Groups (PIP-DCGs) the first risk adjustment model that Medicare used to adjust capitation payments made to M+C plans based largely on the principal diagnoses of hospitalized enrollees.

referral an authorization to receive a specific health service from a specific health provider that will be paid for by the HMO.

staff model HMO the most tightly organized HMO structure. The HMO entity owns the facilities and arranges for health care through employed physicians, who are allowed to see only the particular HMO patients.

subscriber primary recipient of the insurance benefit.

REVIEW QUESTIONS

Knowledge-based Questions

1. What coding systems would be used to code a hospital claim submitted to an MCO for payment? What systems would be used for a physician claim?

2. What three characteristics are required for an organization to qualify as an HMO?

3. How does an MCO perform coordination of benefits?

4. What does the abbreviation PMPM mean, and why is it important in managed care?

5. What two benefits will the MCO realize from using online referral processing?

6. Explain the difference between coinsurance and copayment.

Application-based Questions

1. Why wouldn't a managed indemnity plan collect referral data?

2. Why could the discounted charges reimbursement mechanism seem attractive to both the physician and the MCO?

3. Why would an MCO want to reimburse hospitals by a DRG payment?

4. An HMO with 50,000 members had 13,024 inpatient service days for last month. What formula would you use to determine bed days per 1,000, and what was this HMO's rate for last month?

Web Activity

Visit the NCQA Web site at http://www.ncqa.org and locate the latest list of HEDIS measures. (Hint: Select "Programs," then "HEDIS Programs," then the latest version of HEDIS, then "List of Measures.") If you were a health information manager in a pediatric clinic and were planning to present HEDIS results to your medical staff, which of the measures listed would you select for your report?

Case Study

The senior management team of Efficient Network HMO is evaluating the year-end data related to emergency room (ER) expenses. One physician group within the network had ER expenses that were three times the rate of any other group within the network. Senior management has studied group operations and theorizes that three factors are influencing the high rate of expense. The group does not utilize triage nurses, does not have after-hours urgent care services, and has limited office hours from 8:30 to 11:30 a.m. and 1:30 to 5:00 p.m. An answering service, not staffed by nurses, relays calls during the remainder of the hours.

The physician group is willing to work on the problem but is asking for detailed, comparative information from the HMO's senior management team before it implements any changes. How would you, as the clinical data specialist for the HMO, answer the following questions:

1. What information would be useful to senior management of the HMO and the physician practice in evaluating the ER expenses?

2. What data sources would you use to obtain data?

3. How could the reports be structured to provide meaningful information?

References and Suggested Readings

Abdelhak, M. (Ed.). (2001). Health Information: Management of a Strategic Resource, 2nd edition. Philadelphia, PA: W.B. Saunders Company.

A Glossary of Terms: The Language of Managed Care and Organized Health Care Systems (revised ed.). (1994). Minnetonka, MN: United HealthCare Corporation.

Centers for Medicare and Medicaid Services (CMS). (2003). Health Care Industry Market Update – Managed Care. Baltimore, MD: Department of Health and Human Services. http://www.cms.hhs.gov/marketplace

CMS. (2004). 45 Day Notice for 2004 M+C Rates. [Online]. http://www.cms.hhs.gov/health-plans/rates/2004/45day-section-a.asp [2004, April 23].

Health Care Financing Administration. (1998, September 8). Medicare program: Request for public comments on implementation of risk adjusted payment for the Medicare+Choice program and announcement of public meeting. *Federal Register, 63* (173), 47506–47513.

Health Data Management—The Magazine of Electronic Health Care Networking. New York: Faulkner and Gray Publishing. (various issues)

Health Plan Employer Data and Information Set 2003, Volumes 1–7. (2003). Washington, DC: National Committee for Quality Assurance.

Kongstvedt, P. R. (1993). *The Managed Health Care Handbook, Second Edition*. Gaithersburg, MD: Aspen Publishers, Inc.

National Committee for Quality Assurance. (2003). *Standards for the Accreditation of Managed Care Organizations*. Washington, DC: Author.

Pope, G. C., Ellis, R. P., Ash, A. S., Liu, C., Ayanian, J. Z., Bates, D. W., Burstin, H., Iezzoni, L. I., and Ingber, M. J. (2000). Principal inpatient diagnostic cost group model for Medicare risk adjustment. *Health Care Financing Review, 21* (3), 93–118.

Rollins, G. (2003). Turning a physician practice on its head: Kaiser leader reveals the challenges, benefits of EHR. *Journal of the American Health Information Management Association, 74*, (3), 32–33.

Tully, L., and Rulon, V. (2000). Evolution of the uses of ICD-9-CM coding: Medicare risk adjustment methodology for managed care plans. *Topics in Health Information Management, 21* (2), 62–67.

Key Resources

Accreditation Association for Ambulatory Health Care, Inc. (AAAHC)
(See Chapter 3 for contact information.)

American Health Information Management Association (AHIMA)
(See Chapter 1 for contact information.)

Clinical Laboratory Improvement Amendments of 1988
www.cms.hhs.gov/clia/

CMS Medicare Advantage Plans
http://www.cms.hhs.gov/healthplans/

Joint Commission on Accreditation of Healthcare Organizations (JCAHO)
(See Chapter 1 for contact information.)

Medicare Managed Care Manual
http://www.cms.hhs.gov/manuals/116_mmc/mc86toc.asp

National Committee for Quality Assurance (NCQA)
1350 New York Avenue, NW
Suite 700
Washington, DC 20005
Phone: 202-628-5788
www.ncqa.org

U.S. Government Printing Office
Phone: 202-783-3238
www.access.gpo.gov

Chapter *5*

Dialysis

Ann H. Peden, MBA, RHIA, CCS

Learning Objectives

Upon successful completion of this chapter, you should be able to:

1. Describe the care given to patients with end-stage renal disease (ESRD).
2. Describe how and by whom dialysis facilities are surveyed for compliance with various regulations and standards.
3. List key documentation requirements for dialysis patient records.
4. State the source of payment for most dialysis treatment in the United States.
5. Explain the role of the ESRD networks in the collection and aggregation of data on dialysis patients.
6. Describe quality improvement activities in ESRD organizations.
7. Describe the role of the health information management professional in organizations dealing with ESRD.

SETTING	DESCRIPTION	SYNONYMS
End-Stage Renal Disease (ESRD) Facility	A facility where patients receive dialysis treatments	Limited Care Unit Dialysis Facility Dialysis Unit Dialysis Center
ESRD Network	One of 18 organizations with contracts with the Centers for Medicare and Medicaid Services (CMS) assessing the quality of care rendered to ESRD patients and collecting and analyzing ESRD data	Network

Introduction to Setting

Dialysis is a procedure necessary to maintain the life of a person whose kidneys have failed. **Chronic renal failure**, a condition in which an individual's kidneys are no longer able to perform the job of excreting the body's wastes or promoting homeostasis, usually results from other medical conditions that damage the kidneys. When the chronic renal failure is irreversible, the person has **end-stage renal disease (ESRD)** and requires some type of **renal replacement therapy (RRT)** (dialysis or a kidney transplant) to survive.

There are numerous organizations involved in caring for dialysis patients and in monitoring the quality of care rendered to dialysis patients. The two settings discussed in this chapter are ESRD facilities and **ESRD networks**. Of these two general types of settings, only the ESRD facility actually provides patient care. The ESRD networks process and analyze data provided by the ESRD facilities and provide other types of services, such as patient education.

There are several synonyms for ESRD facilities. The federal government uses the term *ESRD facility* for a facility offering dialysis services. The Joint Commission on Accreditation of Healthcare Organizations (JCAHO) uses the terms *dialysis center* and *dialysis unit* for this type of facility. None of these terms is universally preferred over the others. This chapter uses the terms interchangeably.

Types of Patients

Patients requiring treatment in a dialysis unit generally are persons experiencing chronic renal failure who have not yet undergone a kidney transplant or who for some reason are not candidates for a transplant. Because the kidneys of these patients are unable to filter out wastes, the end products of metabolism must be removed from their bodies by artificial means. Dialysis is the process of removing these wastes and maintaining the body's proper fluid, electrolyte, and acid–base balance by the process of diffusion.

There are two types of dialysis: hemodialysis and peritoneal dialysis. In **hemodialysis**, the patient's blood circulates outside the body (extracorporeally) through an artificial kidney (dialyzer) that removes metabolic wastes and helps maintain homeostasis. When a patient is expected to be on long-term hemodialysis, surgery is generally performed to create an easy means of vascular access, such as creation of an arteriovenous fistula. To keep the body free of excessive waste products, the patient generally dialyzes three times per week for three to five hours per session. Patients may obtain hemodialysis treatment in freestanding dialysis facilities, in the dialysis unit of a hospital, or in their own homes. In 2001, almost 90 percent of dialysis patients in the United States received hemodialysis on-site in an ESRD facility, in either a freestanding unit or in a unit affiliated with a larger health care organization.

The most common type of ESRD facility is the freestanding ESRD facility. As noted previously, the ESRD facility provides dialysis care on-site for most of its patients. After training, some patients are able to perform their own hemodialysis at home with the aid of a friend or relative. However, these home hemodialysis patients and the peritoneal dialysis patients described as follows still present themselves at the ESRD facility at least monthly for evaluation. About 0.5 percent of dialysis patients perform home hemodialysis.

Peritoneal dialysis uses the patient's own abdominal cavity to filter out wastes. A tube is inserted through an incision into the patient's abdomen, and the dialysis solution **(dialysate)** is introduced into the peritoneal space. The dialysate draws the urea and other toxins out of the blood across the peritoneal membrane. Other products from the dialysate diffuse across the membrane into the blood.

In **continuous ambulatory peritoneal dialysis (CAPD)**, the patient is able to perform his or her own dialysis almost anywhere, because very little special equipment is required. The CAPD patient dialyzes three or four times a day, at home or at work. Approximately 4 percent of ESRD patients in the United States are on CAPD.

Continuous cycling peritoneal dialysis (CCPD) utilizes a machine to perform peritoneal dialysis once each day while the patient sleeps rather than three or four times throughout the day as in CAPD. Like the CAPD patients, CCPD patients generally come to the ESRD facility only for training and for monthly evaluations or when a complication arises. About 5 percent of dialysis patients in the United States use CCPD.

The type of dialysis treatment used is largely the patient's choice. CAPD patients generally choose this method because they can incorporate it into their routine and do not have to rely on others to assist with their dialysis. CCPD is a popular choice for children because they can continue their daily routine and dialyze at night while sleeping. The disadvantage of both forms of peritoneal dialysis is the increased risk of infection. Also, any type of self-administered dialysis requires a patient who is motivated and capable of performing and documenting self-care. (See Table 5-1 for a summary of the prevalence of each modality.)

Table 5-1 U.S. Prevalence of Various Dialysis Modalities December 31, 2001. (In-Center Peritoneal Dialysis includes patients in training for home modalities.) (CMS, No date b).

Modality	In-Center Hemodialysis	In-Center Peritoneal Dialysis (PD)	Home Hemodialysis	Home CAPD	Home CCPD	Home, Other PD
Number	246,230	296	1,367	11,722	14,933	29
Percentage	89.68%	0.11%	0.50%	4.27%	5.44%	0.01%

Types of Caregivers

A multidisciplinary team cares for patients in a dialysis unit. The caregivers who have the most contact with the patient on each visit are registered nurses and licensed practical nurses who are assisted by technicians. Nurses and technicians are employees of the dialysis facility and are present with the dialysis center patients on a daily basis.

Other professionals maintain a regular schedule of visits to the dialysis unit, although they do not ordinarily practice at the dialysis center on a daily basis. In a moderately large freestanding dialysis unit, these professionals are on-site several times a month to see patients. For example, physicians see patients on a regular basis and play a primary role in determining the patient's treatment regimen. Dietitians educate patients on the importance of following the prescribed diet and also monitor nutritional status. Social workers discuss psychosocial issues with patients and address problems that relate to family support, transportation, and other environmental factors that could affect the patient's compliance with the program of treatment. These other professionals usually see individual patients on a monthly basis and often more frequently.

ESRD personnel evaluate home hemodialysis and peritoneal dialysis patients' conditions on a regular basis, usually monthly. At one of these patient's regular visits to the dialysis unit, a nurse may examine the dialysis log sheets kept by the patient that contain information about each dialysis session. Health care workers check the patient's blood pressure, weight, medications, and review the results of monthly lab tests. A nurse checks the patient's dialysis access sites for signs of infection. In addition, these monthly evaluations include visits with the social worker, dietitian, and physician.

One other caregiver, the transplantation surgeon, may see the dialysis patient only infrequently. The transplantation surgeon periodically evaluates dialysis patients to determine whether they are eligible for transplant. Usually one transplantation surgeon sees many dialysis patients from numerous dialysis facilities in a given geographic area.

Regulatory Issues

The most important regulations for dialysis facilities are the federal regulations for ESRD facilities. Almost all dialysis facilities offer dialysis services to Medicare patients, so almost all dialysis facilities are subject to federal regulations. This is true whether the facility is freestanding or affiliated with a hospital or other organization.

A dialysis unit in a hospital accredited by the JCAHO is also subject to JCAHO standards in addition to federal standards. However, the federal regulations are more detailed than the JCAHO standards, so a hospital dialysis facility that meets federal standards should have no problems meeting JCAHO standards.

Individual states may also have their own regulations for dialysis facilities. However, these are usually modeled on federal standards, so again, the predominant regulatory issues in most states are found in the federal guidelines.

Surveys

Dialysis units are surveyed to determine if they are in compliance with both state and federal guidelines by each state's own surveying agency. For example, a survey team from the state department of health usually visits a dialysis facility annually and compares the facility's performance to federal regulations (and any state regulations that may apply). These surveys are usually unannounced, so the facility must be ready for a survey at any time.

In addition, federal surveyors may conduct an unexpected **validation survey** to determine whether the state agencies to whom the regular surveys have been delegated are appropriately evaluating facilities according to federal regulations. Even though the primary purpose of the validation survey is to serve as a check on the state surveying agency, any deficiencies noted in the validation survey must still be corrected by the dialysis facility.

Federal Regulations

Federal regulations affecting ESRD facilities are found in the *Conditions for Coverage of Suppliers of End Stage Renal Disease (ESRD) Services* (42 CFR Part 405 Subpart U, 2002). These regulations are comprehensive and apply to every aspect of the facility's operation. Relevant information from federal regulations is interspersed throughout this chapter, under topics such as "Documentation" and "Data and Information Flow." Of particular interest to health information management professionals is the requirement found in 42 CFR 405.2102 that the ESRD facility obtain the services of a "medical record practitioner." A registered health information administrator (RHIA) or a registered health information technician (RHIT) who has contracted with the dialysis facility to visit the dialysis unit periodically as a consultant will meet the requirement for a qualified medical record practitioner. Other regulations pertaining to medical record personnel are found in 42 CFR 405.2139. This section states that a member of the facility's staff must be designated to serve as supervisor of medical records. This medical record "designee" will usually have other responsibilities at the facility but is the person who is responsible for the day-to-day activities involving the medical record. This staff member's duties are to be sure that the medical records are properly documented, completed, and preserved.

Joint Commission on Accreditation of Healthcare Organizations

Hospital-based acute and chronic dialysis facilities may also be accredited on a voluntary basis by the JCAHO. Dialysis units are specifically mentioned in JCAHO standards on "Care of Patients," "Education," and "Management of the Environment of Care" (JCAHO, 2003). Although dialysis units are not specifically mentioned in the "Management of Information" standards, JCAHO's general requirements regarding patient information (discussed in Chapter 2) apply to hospital dialysis units just as they apply to other patient care units.

ESRD Networks

ESRD networks were established by federal law to monitor quality and appropriateness of care provided to ESRD patients. The Omnibus Reconciliation Act (OBRA) of 1986 reorganized the ESRD program and set up 18 network areas across the United States to assess the quality of care given to ESRD patients (see Figure 5-1). These networks perform their work under contract with the Centers for Medicare and Medicaid Services (CMS). In addition to their quality assessment activities, the networks also collect and analyze data on ESRD patients in their regions. The networks profile patient status changes and deal with patient grievances. They also publish an annual report of these and other activities. Some of these roles of the ESRD networks are discussed later in the chapter.

Documentation

Documentation in an ESRD facility may be paper based, computer based, or a combination of both. When only paper records are kept in a dialysis facility, they can be voluminous because a patient can remain in dialysis treatment for decades and because the treatments and evaluations are so frequent. Maintaining portions of the record in a computer system is an increasingly common practice. Regardless of the method of maintaining patient records, the facility must be careful to document all required items.

Federal regulations require the ESRD facility to maintain complete medical records on all patients. A summary of specific federal requirements from 42 CFR 405.2139 is presented in outline form in Figure 5-2.

Federal regulations (42 CFR 405.2137) require the development of a "written long-term program and a written patient care plan to ensure that each patient receives the appropriate modality of care and the appropriate care within that modality" (Conditions for Coverage, 2002, p. 147). Both of these documents are

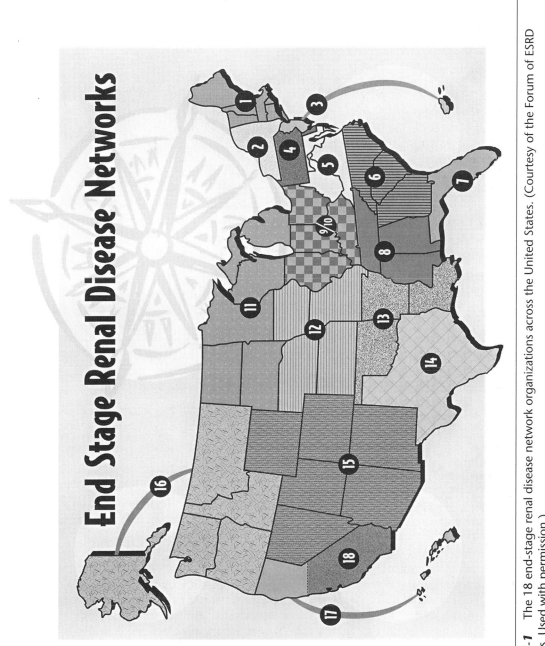

Figure 5-1 The 18 end-stage renal disease network organizations across the United States. (Courtesy of the Forum of ESRD Networks. Used with permission.)

Each patient's medical record contains sufficient information to:
- identify the patient clearly
- justify the diagnosis and treatment
- document the results accurately

All medical records contain the following general categories of information:

Documented evidence
- of assessment of the needs of the patient
- of whether the patient is treated with a reprocessed hemodialyzer
- of establishment of an appropriate plan of treatment
- of the care and services provided
- that the patient was informed of the results of the assessment of suitability for transplantation and home dialysis
- identification and social data
- signed consent forms
- referral information with authentication of diagnosis
- medical and nursing history of patient
- reports of physician examination(s)
- diagnostic and therapeutic orders
- observations and progress notes
- reports of treatments and clinical findings
- reports of laboratory and other diagnostic tests and procedures
- discharge summary including final diagnosis and prognosis

Figure 5-2   Medical record requirements adapted from 42 CFR 405.2139 (a) *Standard: medical record.*

developed by a multidisciplinary team. Both documents are personalized for the individual patient. The long-term program emphasizes the selection of the treatment modality (dialysis or transplantation) and the setting in which dialysis takes place (home, self-care, or on-site at a dialysis facility). The patient care plan "reflects the psychological, social, and functional needs of the patient" and the care needed to reach long-term and short-term goals (Conditions for Coverage, 2002, pp. 147–148).

The Forum of ESRD Networks' Quality Assurance Committee has also described a medical record model to improve the quality of the dialysis medical record. Improving the quality of the medical record improves the team's ability to provide care and encourages a consistent approach. The medical record model presents a format for medical records that should contain the information necessary for continuity of patient care and qualitative review. The medical record model is more detailed than federal regulations and can provide more specific guidance for facilities seeking to improve their documentation. For example, the federal regulations simply require documentation of "observations and progress notes," whereas the medical record model provides recommendations regarding the contents and frequency of progress notes. To demonstrate this detail, for example, the following excerpts regarding progress notes are taken from the Forum of ESRD Networks' medical record model.

Progress Notes

"Progress notes should provide an accurate picture of the progress of the patient that reflects changes in patient status, plans and results of changes in treatment regimen, diagnostic testing, consultations, unusual events, etc. Either single discipline or integrated multidisciplinary progress notes may be utilized.

The following are minimal entries:

Each discipline, physician(s), nurse(s), social worker(s) and dietitian(s) should record the progress of the patient at regular intervals:

Monthly—unstable patients
Quarterly—stable patients

Patient condition and response to treatment noted on daily treatment record." (Forum of ESRD Networks, 1992).

Reimbursement

A person with ESRD generally is eligible for Medicare coverage on the basis of the ESRD diagnosis if the patient, a spouse, or a parent has made sufficient contributions to the Social Security system. At present, more than 90 percent of dialysis patients receive benefits through Medicare's ESRD program. However, because Medicare is the secondary payer during the first 30 months of ESRD-based eligibility, dialysis facilities also frequently deal with other third-party payers (USD-HHS, No date). Even after Medicare has begun paying, many patients also receive some benefits from other insurance programs, such as an employer's group insurance policy.

Medicare Part A pays the dialysis facility a composite rate per treatment based on three treatments per week for each patient on chronic dialysis. However, no payment is made for patients who miss treatments (no-shows). This composite rate includes payment for some of the other services the patient receives, such as some of the routine laboratory tests. However, certain types of tests, such as bone density monitoring and nerve conduction studies, are paid separately. Some treatments, such as erythropoietin administration, are separately reimbursable.

In general, a physician receives a monthly payment from Medicare Part B based on the number of visits for each patient. Physicians may receive additional payments for other services, such as evaluation and management services rendered to inpatients.

Information Management

Coding and Classification

The ESRD facility codes diagnoses using the International Classification of the Diseases, 9th revision, Clinical Modification (ICD-9-CM). Coding in an ESRD facility is mainly used for reimbursement. For Medicare, the code submitted to the ESRD network and ultimately to CMS when dialysis is first initiated must be an ICD-9-CM code that CMS recognizes as end-stage renal disease.

Physicians who see ESRD patients must also code their encounters with the patient for reimbursement purposes. For physician reimbursement, diagnoses are coded with ICD-9-CM and the services performed by the physician are coded with the Healthcare Common Procedural Coding System (HCPCS).

At the national level, CMS maintains coded data submitted by dialysis providers that can be used for research and purposes other than reimbursement. This is discussed more completely in the sections on "Data and Information Flow."

Data and Information Flow

Data and information flow can be viewed at the level of the individual patient and at the aggregate level of many patients in a given area.

Individual Patient Data

At the level of the individual patient, the initial information on a dialysis patient is gathered when the patient is admitted to the dialysis facility. Information flows into the patient record from many sources. The caregivers document their interactions with, and assessments of, the patient. The patient contributes to portions of the record, such as the plan of care. The facility also receives copies of portions of the patient's hospital record whenever the patient is admitted to the hospital. Information from reference laboratories and other facilities that have treated or tested the patient are also included in the patient's record.

When a dialysis patient is transferred to another facility, the transfer of information between the two facilities is very important. Federal regulation 42 CFR 405.2137 specifically requires that a copy of the patient's long-term program and patient care plan be sent with the patient or within one working day whenever the patient is transferred to another facility. A transfer agreement between the dialysis facility and a local hospital can facilitate the transfer of information when a dialysis patient is admitted or discharged from one location to another.

Because hemodialysis patients should dialyze three times per week, planning a vacation or an extended trip out of town involves the ESRD facility. The local dialysis facility must contact another facility in the city to which the patient is traveling. The distant facility must agree to treat the patient while the patient is in that location. The transfer of referral information back and forth between the distant and the local facility is important in providing quality patient care.

Aggregate Data

As previously mentioned, the ESRD networks are responsible for collecting and analyzing data on ESRD patients in their areas. The facilities treating patients are responsible for completing various federal forms. These forms are forwarded to the ESRD network. The network enters data from the forms into its computer system on a daily basis. Then, on a monthly basis, data from the forms is electronically transmitted to CMS, where it is aggregated on a national scale. One form completed annually is the ESRD Facility Survey. (See Figure 5-3 for an excerpt from this form.) This data is also processed by the networks for CMS.

Using this data and other beneficiary-specific data, CMS has developed a comprehensive database called the End-Stage Renal Disease (ESRD) Program Management and Medical Information System (PMMIS). The ESRD PMMIS includes medical and demographic information for the Medicare ESRD population. CMS uses the data for program analysis, policy development, and epidemiologic research. (CMS, 2002).

Computer Systems

To plan a successful dialysis treatment program, the physicians and nurses need data on the patient's condition and response to treatment. Because of the large amount of clinical information collected on dialysis patients, dialysis facilities have been among the first to adopt computerized clinical records (see Figure 5-4).

By keeping medication records and data from each dialysis session in computer storage, clinicians can track the patient's response to treatment. The computer can generate reports showing the patient's weight, blood pressure, and so forth, before and after each treatment and can compute monthly averages for various clinical data elements. These simple reports can be used to educate the patient and to encourage compliance with the prescribed diet and medication regimen. The caregivers also learn more about each patient from studying the accumulated data available in computer-generated reports.

Even though this important clinical information is often kept online, most dialysis facilities find it necessary to maintain a paper record as well. Consents, referral information, and so forth, are nearly always in paper format. As in most health care facilities, computer systems are also used for billing and accounting purposes.

Data Sets

There are several data sets for dialysis patients. The "End Stage Renal Disease Medical Evidence Report: Medicare Entitlement and/or Patient Registration" form (CMS

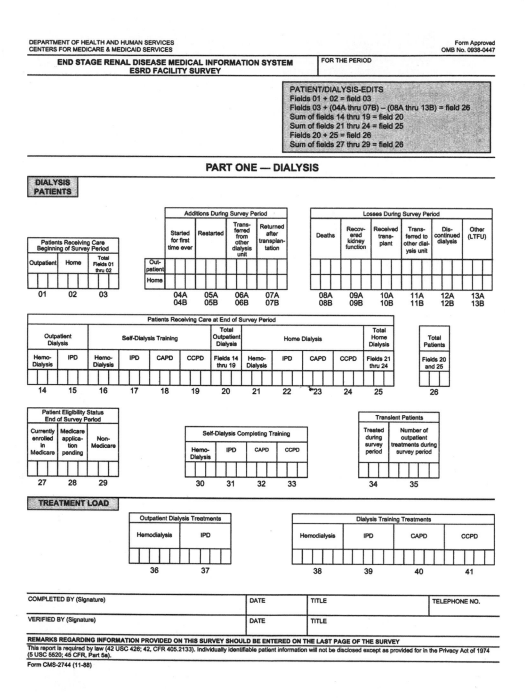

Figure 5-3 Excerpt from the ESRD Facility Survey form (CMS 2744).

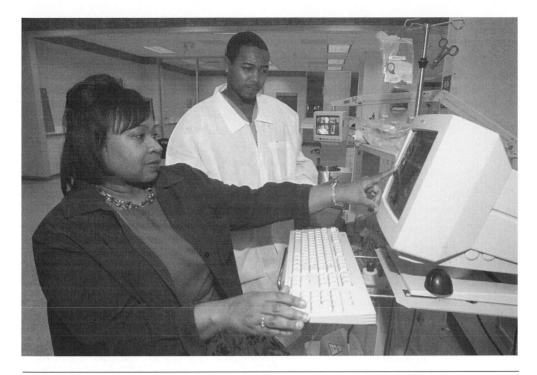

Figure 5-4   Chairside data entry in a dialysis facility. (Photo courtesy of the University of Mississippi Medical Center Department of Public Affairs. Reprinted with permission.)

2728) contains data that is completed by the dialysis facility for each new dialysis patient and forwarded to the ESRD network and then to CMS (see Figure 5-5).

The "ESRD Death Notification" form (CMS 2746) is completed for each ESRD patient who expires, and the data from this form is also transmitted to the ESRD network and to CMS (see Figure 5-6).

The ESRD networks also collect bimonthly census data from each dialysis facility. They maintain a status file on each patient, a master patient index file, a follow-up file, and a transplant file.

Data on kidney transplants is available from the United Network for Organ Sharing (UNOS). Under a contract with the Health Resources and Services Administration of the U.S. Department of Health and Human Services, UNOS manages the Organ Procurement and Transplantation Network (OPTN). One of the most important functions of OPTN is facilitating the matching of donor organs and transplant recipients. This is accomplished by means of a computer system and an Organ Center that operates 24 hours a day. However, OPTN also collects and manages data about organ donation and transplantation for kidney, pancreas, liver, intestine, heart, and lung procedures. Most candidates on the UNOS waiting list for organs are waiting for kidney donations (UNOS, 2003).

U.S. DEPARTMENT OF HEALTH & HUMAN SERVICES
CENTERS FOR MEDICARE & MEDICAID SERVICES

FORM APPROVED
OMB NO. 0938-0046

END STAGE RENAL DISEASE MEDICAL EVIDENCE REPORT
MEDICARE ENTITLEMENT AND/OR PATIENT REGISTRATION

A. COMPLETE FOR ALL ESRD PATIENTS

1. Name *(Last, First, Middle Initial)*

2. Health Insurance Claim Number	3. Social Security Number

4. Full Address *(Include City, State, and Zip)*	5. Phone Number ( )
	6. Date of Birth ___/___/___ MM DD YYYY

7. Sex ☐ Male   ☐ Female

8. Ethnicity ☐ Hispanic: Mexican   ☐ Hispanic: Other   ☐ Non-Hispanic

9. Race *(Check one box only)*
☐ White
☐ Black
☐ American Indian/Alaskan Native
☐ Asian
☐ Pacific Islander
☐ Mid-East/Arabian
☐ Indian sub-Continent
☐ Other, specify _____
☐ Unknown

10. Medical Coverage *(Check all that apply)*
a. ☐ Medicaid
b. ☐ DVA
c. ☐ Medicare
d. ☐ Employer Group Health Insurance
e. ☐ Other Medical Insurance
f. ☐ None

11. Is Patient Applying for ESRD Medicare Coverage? *(if YES, enter address of Social Security office)*
☐ Yes   ☐ No

CITY	STATE	ZIP

12. Primary Cause of Renal Failure *(Use code from back of form)*	13. Height INCHES OR CENTIMETERS	14. Dry Weight POUNDS OR KILOGRAMS

15. Employment Status *(6 mos. prior and current status)*

Prior / Current
☐ ☐ Unemployed
☐ ☐ Employed Full Time
☐ ☐ Employed Part Time
☐ ☐ Homemaker
☐ ☐ Retired due to Age/Preference
☐ ☐ Retired (Disability)
☐ ☐ Medical Leave of Absence
☐ ☐ Student

16. Co-Morbid Conditions *(Check ALL that apply currently or during last 10 years)* *See instructions
a. ☐ Congestive heart failure
b. ☐ Ischemic heart disease, CAD*
c. ☐ Myocardial infarction
d. ☐ Cardiac arrest
e. ☐ Cardiac dysrhythmia
f. ☐ Pericarditis
g. ☐ Cerebrovascular disease, CVA, TIA*
h. ☐ Peripheral vascular disease*
i. ☐ History of hypertension
j. ☐ Diabetes (primary or contributing)
k. ☐ Diabetes, currently on insulin
l. ☐ Chronic obstructive pulmonary disease
m. ☐ Tobacco use (current smoker)
n. ☐ Malignant neoplasm, Cancer
o. ☐ Alcohol dependence
p. ☐ Drug dependence*
q. ☐ HIV positive status   ☐ Can't Disclose
r. ☐ AIDS   ☐ Can't Disclose
s. ☐ Inability to ambulate
t. ☐ Inability to transfer

17. Was pre-dialysis/transplant EPO administered?
☐ Yes   ☐ No

18. Laboratory Values Prior to First Dialysis Treatment or Transplant *See Instructions.

LABORATORY TEST	VALUE	DATE	LABORATORY TEST	VALUE	DATE
a. Hematocrit (%)			e. Serum Creatinine (mg/dl)		
b. Hemoglobin (g/dl)*			f. Creatinine Clearance (ml/min)*		
c. Serum Albumin (g/dl)			g. BUN (mg/dl)*		
d. Serum Albumin Lower Limit (g/dl)			h. Urea Clearance (ml/min)*		

B. COMPLETE FOR ALL ESRD PATIENTS IN DIALYSIS TREATMENT

19. Name of Provider	20. Medicare Provider Number

21. Primary Dialysis Setting ☐ Hospital Inpatient ☐ Dialysis Facility/Center ☐ Home	22. Primary Type of Dialysis ☐ Hemodialysis ☐ IPD ☐ CAPD ☐ CCPD ☐ Other
23. Date Regular Dialysis Began ___/___/___ MM DD YY	24. Date Patient Started Chronic Dialysis at Current Facility ___/___/___ MM DD YY
25. Date Dialysis Stopped ___/___/___ MM DD YY	26. Date of Death ___/___/___ MM DD YY

CMS-2728-U3 (6-97)

Figure 5-5   CMS 2728.

C. COMPLETE FOR ALL KIDNEY TRANSPLANT PATIENTS

27. Date of Transplant	28. Name of Transplant Hospital	29. Medicare Provider Number for Item 28
___/___/___ MM DD YY		

Date patient was admitted as an inpatient to a hospital in preparation for, or anticipation of, a kidney transplant prior to the date of actual transplantation.

30. Enter Date	31. Name of Preparation Hospital	32. Medicare Provider Number for Item 31
___/___/___ MM DD YY		

33. Current Status of Transplant

☐ Functioning   ☐ Non-Functioning

34. If Nonfunctioning, Date of Return To Regular Dialysis	35. Current Dialysis Treatment Site
___/___/___ MM DD YY	☐ Hospital Inpatient ☐ Dialysis Facility/Center ☐ Home

D. COMPLETE FOR ALL ESRD SELF-DIALYSIS TRAINING PATIENTS (MEDICARE APPLICANTS ONLY)

36. Name of Training Provider	37. Medicare Provider Number of Training Provider

38. Date Training Began	39. Type of Training
___/___/___ MM DD YY	☐ Hemodialysis ☐ IPD ☐ CAPD ☐ CCPD

40. This Patient is Expected to Complete *(or has completed)* Training and Will Self-dialyze on a Regular Basis. ☐ Yes ☐ No	41. Date When Patient Completed, or is Expected to Complete, Training ___/___/___ MM DD YY

I certify that the above self-dialysis training information is correct and is based on consideration of all pertinent medical, psychological, and sociological factors as reflected in records kept by this training facility.

42. Printed Name and Signature of Physician Personally Familiar with the Patient's Training	43. UPIN of Physician in Item 42

E. PHYSICIAN IDENTIFICATION

44. Attending Physician *(Print)*	45. Physician's Phone No. ( )	46. UPIN of Physician in Item 44

PHYSICIAN ATTESTATION

I certify, under penalty of perjury, that the information on this form is correct to the best of my knowledge and belief. Based on diagnostic tests and laboratory findings, I further certify that this patient has reached the stage of renal impairment that appears irreversible and permanent and requires a regular course of dialysis or kidney transplant to maintain life. I understand that this information is intended for use in establishing the patient's entitlement to Medicare benefits and that any falsification, misrepresentation, or concealment of essential information may subject me to fine, imprisonment, civil penalty, or other civil sanctions under applicable Federal laws.

47. Attending Physician's Signature of Attestation *(Same as Item 44)*	48. Date ___/___/___ MM DD YY

49. Remarks

F. OBTAIN SIGNATURE FROM PATIENT

I hereby authorize any physician, hospital, agency, or other organization to disclose any medical records or other information about my medical condition to the Department of Health and Human Services for purposes of reviewing my application for Medicare entitlement under the Social Security Act and/or for scientific research.

50. Signature of Patient *(Signature by Mark Must Be Witnessed.)*	51. Date ___/___/___ MM DD YY

G. PRIVACY ACT STATEMENT

The collection of this information is authorized by section 226A of the Social Security Act. The information provided will be used to determine if an individual is entitled to Medicare under the End Stage Renal Disease provisions of the law. The information will be maintained in system No. 09-70-0520, "End Stage Renal Disease Program Management and Medical Information System (ESRD PMMIS)", published in the Privacy Act Issuance, 1991 Compilation, Vol. 1, pages 436–437, December 31, 1991, or as updated and republished. Collection of your Social Security number is authorized by Executive Order 9397. Furnishing the information on this form is voluntary, but failure to do so may result in denial of Medicare benefits. Information from the ESRD PMMIS may be given to a congressional office in response to an inquiry from the congressional office made at the request of the individual; an individual or organization for a research, demonstration, evaluation, or epidemiologic project related to the prevention of disease or disability, or the restoration or maintenance of health. Additional disclosures may be found in the *Federal Register* notice cited above. You should be aware that P.L. 100-503, the Computer Matching and Privacy Protection Act of 1988, permits the government to verify information by way of computer matches.

H. FOR ESRD NETWORK USE ONLY IN CASES REFERRED TO ESRD MEDICAL REVIEW BOARD

52. Network Confirmed as ESRD	53. Authorized Signature	54. Date	55. Network Number
☐ Yes ☐ No		___/___/___ MM DD YY	

CMS-2728-U3 (6-97)

Figure 5-5   *(Continued)*

DEPARTMENT OF HEALTH AND HUMAN SERVICES
CENTERS FOR MEDICARE & MEDICAID SERVICES

FORM APPROVED
OMB NO. 0938-0448

ESRD DEATH NOTIFICATION
END STAGE RENAL DISEASE MEDICAL INFORMATION SYSTEM

According to the Paperwork Reduction Act of 1995, no persons are required to respond to a collection of information unless it displays a valid OMB control number. The valid OMB control number for this information collection is 0938-0448. The time required to complete this information collection is estimated to average 17 minutes per response, including the time to review instructions, search existing data resources, gather the data needed, and complete and review the information collection. If you have any comments concerning the accuracy of the time estimate(s) or suggestions for improving this form, please write to: CMS, 7500 Security Boulevard, N2-14-26, Baltimore, Maryland 21244-1850.

1. PATIENT'S LAST NAME	FIRST	MI	2. HEALTH INSURANCE CLAIM NUMBER

3. PATIENT'S SEX
a. ☐ Male   b. ☐ Female

4. PATIENT'S STATE OF RESIDENCE

5. DATE OF BIRTH
MONTH DAY YEAR

6. DATE OF DEATH
MONTH DAY YEAR

7. PROVIDER NAME AND ADDRESS (CITY AND STATE)

8. PROVIDER NUMBER

9. PLACE OF DEATH (Check one)
a. ☐ Hospital b. ☐ Dialysis c. ☐ Home d. ☐ Other

10. WAS AN AUTOPSY PERFORMED?
a. ☐ Yes   b. ☐ No

11. CAUSES OF DEATH (Enter code form List of Causes below.)
a. Primary Cause [   ]
b. Were there Secondary Causes? ☐ No ☐ Yes, Specify
(1)[   ] (3)[   ]
(2)[   ] (4)[   ]

LIST OF CAUSES

CARDIAC
23 Myocardial infarction, acute
24 Hyperkalemia
25 Pericarditis, incl. cardiac tamponade
26 Atherosclerotic heart disease
27 Cardiomyopathy
28 Cardiac arrhythmia
29 Cardiac arrest, cause unknown
30 Valvular heart disease
31 Pulmonary edema due to exogenous fluid

VASCULAR
35 Pulmonary embolus
36 Cerebrovascular accident including intracranial hemorrhage
37 Ischemic brain damage/Anoxic encephalopathy
38 Hemorrhage from transplant site
39 Hemorrhage from vascular access
40 Hemorrhage from dialysis circuit
41 Hemorrhage from ruptured vascular aneurysm
42 Hemorrhage from surgery (not 38, 39 or 41)
43 Other hemorrhage (not Codes 38-42, 72)
44 Mesenteric infarction/ischemic bowel

INFECTION
49 Septicemia, due to vascular access
50 Septicemia, due to peritonitis
51 Septicemia, due to peripheral vascular disease, gangrene
52 Septicemia, other
53 Pulmonary infection (bacterial)
54 Pulmonary infection (fungal)
55 Pulmonary infection (other)
56 Viral Infection, CMV
57 Viral Infection, Other (not 64 or 65)
58 Tuberculosis
59 A.I.D.S.
60 Infections, other

LIVER DISEASE
64 Hepatitis B
65 Other viral hepatitis
66 Liver-drug toxicity
67 Cirrhosis
68 Polycystic liver disease
69 Liver failure, cause unknown other

GASTRO-INTESTINAL (see also 50)
72 Gastro-intestinal hemorrhage
73 Pancreatitis
74 Fungal peritonitis
75 Perforation of peptic ulcer
76 Perforation of bowel (not 75)

OTHER
80 Bone marrow depression
81 Cachexia
82 Malignant disease, patient ever on immunosuppressive therapy
83 Malignant disease (not 82)
84 Dementia, incl. dialysis dementia, Alzheimer's
85 Seizures
86 Diabetic coma, hyperglycemia, hypoglycemia
87 Chronic obstructive lung disease (COPD)
88 Complications of surgery
89 Air embolism
90 Accident related to treatment
91 Accident unrelated to treatment
92 Suicide
93 Drug overdose (street drugs)
94 Drug overdose (not 92 or 93)
98 Other identified cause of death, please specify: _____
99 Unknown

12. FOR ALL DEATHS INDICATE YES/NO
Renal replacement therapy discontinued prior to death: ☐ Yes ☐ No
If Yes, check one of the following:
a. ☐ Following HD and/or PD access failure
b. ☐ Following transplant failure
c. ☐ Following chronic failure to thrive
d. ☐ Following acute medical complication
e. ☐ Other

13. IF DECEASED RECEIVED A TRANSPLANT
a. Date of most recent transplant [   ] MONTH DAY YEAR
b. Was kidney functioning (patient not on dialysis) at time of death? ☐ Yes ☐ No ☐ Unknown
c. Did transplant patient resume chronic maintenance dialysis prior to death? ☐ Yes ☐ No

14. REMARKS

15. NAME OF PHYSICIAN	16. SIGNATURE OF PERSON COMPLETING THIS FORM	DATE

This report is required by law (42, U.S.C. 426; 20 CFR 405, Section 2133). Individually identifable patient information will not be disclosed except as provided for in the Privacy Act of 1974 (5 U.S.C. 5520; 45 CFR Part 5a).

Form CMS-2746-U3 (8-96)

Figure 5-6   CMS 2746.

Quality Improvement and Utilization Management

Quality improvement and utilization management are major responsibilities of the ESRD networks. Federal regulation 42 CFR 405.2112 charges the ESRD networks with:

(a) Developing network goals for placing patients in settings for self-care and transplantation

(b) Encouraging the use of medically appropriate treatment settings most compatible with patient rehabilitation and the participation of patients, providers of services, and renal disease facilities in vocational rehabilitation programs.

(c) Developing criteria and standards relating to the quality and appropriateness of patient care and, with respect to working with patients, facilities, and providers of services, for encouraging participation in vocational rehabilitation programs.

(d) Evaluating the procedures used by facilities in the network in assessing patients for placement in appropriate treatment modalities

. . . .

(g) Evaluating and resolving patient grievances

(h) Appointing a network council and a medical review board (each including at least one patient representative) . . .

(i) Conducting on-site reviews of facilities and providers as necessary, as determined by the medical review board or CMS . . .

(j) Collecting, validating, and analyzing data . . . (ESRD Network Organizations, 2002, p. 141).

Quality Improvement

Each dialysis facility is required by CMS to conduct its own internal quality monitoring program. Examples of areas of care likely to be studied in a quality monitoring program are the facility's water treatment system, infection control procedures, the proper functioning of the dialysis equipment, and the adequacy of the dialysis treatments themselves.

The ESRD networks also perform quality improvement activities for their regions. For example, the ESRD Clinical Performance Measures (CPM) Project collects clinical data on a statistically significant sample of ESRD patients. According to the *Medicare ESRD Network Organizations Manual*, the networks are responsible for developing and conducting quality improvement projects based on the CPMs for "adequacy of dialysis, anemia management, and vascular access, or other CPMs developed or adopted by CMS" (CMS, 2003a, p. 2). The form depicted in Figure 5-7 is an excerpt from the 2003 CPM data collection form. This excerpt focuses on performance measures related to anemia management. In addition to developing local quality improvement projects, the networks are also required to participate in national quality improvement initiatives. For example, in 2003, the national project focused on vascular access improvement.

Clinical practice guidelines represent another quality improvement mechanism. The National Kidney Foundation (NKF) has developed evidence-based guidelines as a component of a project called the Kidney Disease Outcomes Quality Initiative (K/DOQI). The NKF has already published four sets of clinical practice guidelines— for hemodialysis adequacy, for peritoneal dialysis adequacy, for vascular access, and for treatment of anemia of chronic kidney disease—with more guidelines under development (NKF, 2001). One evidence of the importance and impact of the K/DOQI guidelines is that CMS incorporated outcome measures from the first four K/DOQI guidelines into their clinical performance measures projects (CMS, 2002).

Utilization Management (UM)

In the individual dialysis facility, a multidisciplinary team develops a plan of care for each individual dialysis patient. In developing a long-term program for a patient, the team considers a transplant as a possibility. Patients who have kidney transplants generally have higher survival rates, a better quality of life, and lower overall medical costs than patients on dialysis. Therefore, one aspect of utilization management in a dialysis program is the determination of whether a given patient would benefit from a kidney transplant. A transplant surgeon is a member of the team that determines the patient's long-term plan of care. The patient is a vital member of that team as well. In addition, the patient's nephrologist, a registered dietitian, a qualified social worker, and a registered nurse participate with the patient in determining the type of treatment that would be best for him or her.

Data submitted to the ESRD networks is also used by the networks and CMS to study overall utilization patterns. For example, the networks may examine laboratory values submitted on the CMS-2728 form to evaluate trends in their regions regarding the appropriateness of initiation of dialysis.

Risk Management, Legal, and Ethical Issues

Many of the legal issues in a dialysis facility are the same as in any other health care facility. The patient must give consent to treatment, must authorize the release of medical information, and has the right to expect that the confidentiality of clinical information will be protected. Records must also be protected against loss or destruction (42 CFR 405.2139). Dialysis facilities are "covered entities" under the Health Insurance Portability and Accountability Act of 1996 (HIPAA) and so must comply with all of HIPAA's privacy, security, and transactions standards. Dialysis treatment facilities may release protected health information to the ESRD networks as public policy disclosures required by law for health oversight. However, because the facilities must be able to provide an accounting of disclosures to its patients as mandated by HIPAA, facilities should maintain records of their disclosures to the ESRD networks and other regulatory authorities.

IN-CENTER HEMODIALYSIS (HD) CLINICAL PERFORMANCE
MEASURES DATA COLLECTION FORM 2003

[Before completing please read instructions at the bottom of this page and on pages 4, 5 and 6]

PATIENT IDENTIFICATION	MAKE CORRECTIONS TO PATIENT INFORMATION ON LABEL IN THE SPACE BELOW

Place Patient Data Label Here

12. If the above patient information is incorrect make corrections in space above then continue to question 13. Please verify patient's race and answer question 13 below. If patient unknown or was not dialyzed in the unit at any time during OCT 2002 – DEC 2002 return the blank form to the Network.

13. Patient's Ethnicity (Check appropriate box). ❑ non-Hispanic ❑ Hispanic, Mexican American (Chicano) ❑ Hispanic, Puerto Rican ❑ Hispanic, Cuban American ❑ Hispanic, Other ❑ Unknown

14. **Patient's height (MUST COMPLETE):** _____inches OR _____centimeters

15. **Did patient have limb amputation(s) prior to Dec. 31, 2002:** ❑ Yes ❑ No

16. Has the patient ever been diagnosed with any type of diabetes? ❑ Yes (go to 17) ❑ No (go to 18) ❑ Unknown (go to 18)

17. If question 16 was answered **YES**, was the patient taking medications to control the diabetes during the study period? ❑ Yes ❑ No If **YES**, was the patient using insulin during the study period? ❑ Yes ❑ No

Individual Completing Form **(Please print):**

First name: _____ Last name: _____ Title: _____

Phone number: (_____) _____ - _____ Fax number: (_____) _____ - _____

INSTRUCTIONS FOR COMPLETING THE IN-CENTER HEMODIALYSIS CLINICAL PERFORMANCE MEASURES DATA COLLECTION FORM 2003

The label on the top left side of this form contains the following patient identifying information (#'s 1-11). If the information is incorrect make corrections to the right of the label.

1. LAST and first name.
2. DATE of birth (DOB) as MM/DD/YYYY.
3. SOCIAL Security Number (SSN).
4. HEALTH Insurance Claim Number (HIC), (same as Medicare number).
5. SEX (1=Male; 2=Female; 9=Unknown).
6. RACE (1=American Indian/Alaska Native; 2=Asian; 3=Black; 4=White; 5=Unknown; 6=Pacific Islander; 7=Mid East Arabian; 8=Indian Subcontinent; 9=Other Multiracial).
7. PRIMARY cause of renal failure by CMS-2728 code.
8. DATE, as MM/DD/YYYY, that the patient began a regular course of dialysis.
9. ESRD Network number. Do not make corrections to this item.
10. Facility's Medicare provider number.
11. The most RECENT date this patient returned to hemodialysis following: transplant failure, an episode of regained kidney function, or switched modality.

12. Review the patient and facility-specific information contained on the pre-printed label. Please verify the patient's race, item 6 above. If any of the information is incorrect write corrections in the space to the right of the label. If the patient is unknown or if the patient was not dialyzed in the unit at any time during OCT 2002 through DEC 2002, send the blank form back to the ESRD Network office. Provide the name and address of the facility providing services to this patient on December 31, 2002, if known.

13. Patient's Ethnicity. Please verify the patient's ethnicity with the patient and check appropriate box.

14. Enter the patient's height in inches or centimeters. HEIGHT MUST BE ENTERED, do not leave this field blank. You may ask the patient his/her height to obtain this information. If the patient had both legs amputated, record pre-amputation height and check YES for item 15.

15. For the purpose of this study, check NO if this patient has had toe(s), finger(s), or mid-foot (Symes) amputation; but **check YES if this patient has had a below-knee, below-elbow, or more proximal (extensive) amputation prior to Dec. 31, 2002.**

16. Check either "Yes", or "No", or "Unknown" to indicate if the patient has ever been diagnosed with any type of diabetes. If **YES**, proceed to question 17.

17. If the answer to question 16 is **YES**, please check either "Yes" or "No" to indicate if the patient was taking medications to control the diabetes during the study period. If the answer to 17 is **YES**, please check either "Yes" or "No" to indicate if the patient was using insulin during the study period. Study period is OCT 2002-DEC 2002.

PLEASE COMPLETE ITEM 18 ON PAGE 2 OF THIS DATA COLLECTION FORM, ITEMS 19 AND 20 ON PAGE 3, 21 AND 22 ON PAGE 4.
INSTRUCTIONS FOR COMPLETING THESE ITEMS ARE ON PAGES 4, 5 AND 6.

CMS – 820 (Rev.02/19/03)

Figure 5-7   Excerpt from Clinical Performance Measures Data Collection Form, 2003.

2

IN-CENTER HEMODIALYSIS (HD) CLINICAL PERFORMANCE MEASURES DATA COLLECTION FORM 2003 (CONTINUED)			
18. ANEMIA MANAGEMENT: For each lab question below, enter the lab value obtained from the monthly lab draw for each month: OCT, NOV, DEC 2002. Enter NF/NP if the lab value cannot be located.			
	OCT 2002	**NOV 2002**	**DEC 2002**
A. Pre-dialysis laboratory hemoglobin (Hgb) from the monthly lab draw:	___ ___ . ___ g/dL	___ ___ . ___ g/dL	___ ___ . ___ g/dL
B.1. Was there a prescription for Epoetin during the seven days immediately before the Hgb in 18A was drawn or a prescription for Darbepoetin (Aranesp™) during the month immediately before the Hgb in 18A was drawn?	Epoetin: ❏ Yes (go to 18B.2) ❏ No (go to 18C) Darbepoetin: ❏ Yes (go to 18B.2) ❏ No (go to 18C)	Epoetin: ❏ Yes (go to 18B.2) ❏ No (go to 18C) Darbepoetin: ❏ Yes (go to 18B.2) ❏ No (go to 18C)	Epoetin: ❏ Yes (go to 18B.2) ❏ No (go to 18C) Darbepoetin: ❏ Yes (go to 18B.2) ❏ No (go to 18C)
B.2. What was the PRESCRIBED Epoetin dose in units for each treatment during the 7 days immediately BEFORE the Hgb in 18A was drawn or the PRESCRIBED Darbepoetin dose in micrograms for the MONTH immediately BEFORE the Hgb in 18A was drawn? (See instructions on page 4)	Epoetin: _____ units/tx _____ units/tx _____ units/tx Darbepoetin: _____ mcg/month	Epoetin: _____ units/tx _____ units/tx _____ units/tx Darbepoetin: _____ mcg/month	Epoetin: _____ units/tx _____ units/tx _____ units/tx Darbepoetin: _____ mcg/month
B.3. How many times per week was Epoetin prescribed or how many times per month was Darbepoetin prescribed?	Epoetin: _____ x per week Darbepoetin: _____ x per month	Epoetin: _____ x per week Darbepoetin: _____ x per month	Epoetin: _____ x per week Darbepoetin: _____ x per month
B.4. What was the prescribed route of administration? (Check all that apply)	Epoetin: ❏ IV ❏ SC Darbepoetin: ❏ IV ❏ SC	Epoetin: ❏ IV ❏ SC Darbepoetin: ❏ IV ❏ SC	Epoetin: ❏ IV ❏ SC Darbepoetin: ❏ IV ❏ SC
C. Serum ferritin concentration from the monthly lab draw:	___ ___ ___ ___ ng/mL	___ ___ ___ ___ ng/mL	___ ___ ___ ___ ng/mL
D. % transferrin (iron) saturation from the monthly lab draw:	___ ___ ___ %	___ ___ ___ %	___ ___ ___ %
E. Was iron prescribed at any time during the month?	❏ Yes ❏ No (go to 19)	❏ Yes ❏ No (go to 19)	❏ Yes ❏ No (go to 19)
F. If yes, what was the prescribed route of iron administration? (Check all that apply).	❏ IV ❏ PO	❏ IV ❏ PO	❏ IV ❏ PO
G. If the patient was prescribed IV iron, what was the total dose of IV iron **administered** during the month?	_____ mg/month	_____ mg/month	_____ mg/month

Figure 5-7   (*Continued*)

The retention period for clinical information on dialysis patients, according to federal statute, is five years following the patient's discharge or, in the case of a minor, three years after the patient comes of age according to state law, whichever is longer. Of course, when the requirements of state law are more stringent than the federal regulations, the state retention statutes must be followed.

Because the success of dialysis treatment depends largely on patient compliance, it is especially important that clinical professionals document patient education. They should also record action taken when the patient is not complying with the treatment regimen.

As a long-term life-sustaining treatment, renal replacement therapy has been a focal point for numerous ethical issues. For example, a disruptive, abusive patient can create unsafe conditions for other patients in a dialysis facility. An ethical and legal dilemma in this situation arises in determining whether or how the health care provider may transfer or discharge such a patient, given that the patient's life depends on continued dialysis. Kidney transplant is also a type of renal replacement therapy, and, unlike many other types of transplants, a kidney may be obtained from a living donor. This brings its own unique set of ethical issues, ranging from the competency of the prospective donor to the suitability of the prospective recipient (Friedman, 2000). As with other life-saving measures, there are also ethical issues surrounding the initiation of and withdrawal from dialysis. The Renal Physicians Association and the American Society of Nephrology have addressed this subject through the development of a comprehensive clinical practice guideline and toolkit entitled, *Shared Decision-Making in the Appropriate Initiation of and Withdrawal from Dialysis* (RPA/ASN, 2000).

Role of the Health Information Management Professional

Health information management (HIM) professionals practice in a variety of roles in ERSD health care. Because ESRD facilities are required by federal regulations to obtain the services of a medical record practitioner, a health information manager may work either full-time or as a consultant to an ESRD facility. In this role, the HIM professional is concerned with procedures related to the documentation, storage, retrieval, and security of individual patient records. The consultant provides advice on the development of systems to provide timely, appropriately accessible patient information to caregivers and administrators. A consultant visits the dialysis unit periodically to review a sample of records and to discuss procedures for record maintenance with the employee who serves as medical record supervisor. Some facilities employ a HIM professional full-time in the medical record supervisor role. Often several dialysis units are owned by a single entity, such as a corporation. In this type of arrangement, the company headquarters may employ an HIM professional on a full-time basis to assist all of the units with HIM issues.

The ESRD networks also employ health information professionals. Health information managers may work as data coordinators, quality improvement coordinators, quality managers, and even as executive directors in some networks.

Summary

Dialysis facilities treat patients who are experiencing chronic renal failure. The two types of dialysis are hemodialysis and peritoneal dialysis. Hemodialysis is usually administered by nurses and technicians in a dialysis facility, but may also be self-administered by the patient at home. Peritoneal dialysis is usually self-administered by the patient at home.

Multidisciplinary teams of registered and licensed nurses, technicians, physicians, dietitians, and social workers, along with the patient, plan and administer the dialysis treatment regimen. The services of a qualified medical record practitioner are also required, at least on a consulting basis, to ensure that the patient records are properly documented and preserved.

Most freestanding dialysis units must meet the federal guidelines for ESRD facilities, because Medicare is the chief source of funding for these facilities. Therefore, the federal documentation requirements represent the minimum guidelines for quantity and quality of documentation for dialysis patient records.

Information management for dialysis facilities requires the implementation of systems to meet a variety of needs. Not only must information be coded and transmitted for reimbursement purposes, but data must be submitted to the ESRD networks for quality improvement and utilization management. Also, computer systems are being increasingly utilized for online storage of clinical information and for portions of the patient record itself.

A health information manager can play several roles in the dialysis health care system. HIM professionals provide services both in treatment settings (ESRD dialysis units) and in regulatory settings (ESRD networks). HIM professionals work in positions extending from medical record supervisor to executive director.

Key Terms

chronic renal failure (CRF)   a condition in which an individual's kidneys are no longer able to perform the job of excreting the body's wastes or promoting homeostasis.

continuous ambulatory peritoneal dialysis (CAPD)   a form of peritoneal dialysis in which the patient is able to dialyze him or herself three or four times per day without special assistance and a minimum amount of equipment.

continuous cycling peritoneal dialysis (CCPD)   a form of peritoneal dialysis in which the patient uses a cycler machine to dialyze once a day for nine or ten hours, generally while sleeping.

dialysate   a solution used to filter products across a semipermeable membrane by the process of diffusion. Waste products filter into the dialysate from the blood, while certain other products, such as bicarbonates, filter into the blood from the dialysate.

dialysis   "the process of artificially removing metabolic end products and water across a semipermeable membrane by diffusion" (McAfee, 1987). The two most common types of dialysis are hemodialysis and peritoneal dialysis. (See also *peritoneal dialysis*.)

end-stage renal disease (ESRD)   irreversible chronic renal failure. When a patient is in end-stage renal disease, he or she requires either dialysis or a kidney transplant to maintain life.

ESRD networks   eighteen organizations that have contracted with the Centers for Medicare and Medicaid Services (CMS) to assess the quality of care rendered to ESRD patients and to collect and analyze ESRD data.

hemodialysis   cleansing of the blood as it circulates through an artificial kidney machine outside the patient's body.

peritoneal dialysis   filling of the patient's abdominal cavity with a solution (dialysate), and the semipermeable membrane across which the products diffuse is the patient's own peritoneal membrane. The fluid containing the wastes is later withdrawn from the peritoneal cavity.

renal replacement therapy (RRT)   a treatment that replaces kidney function. The treatment may be some type of dialysis or it may be kidney transplantation.

validation survey   a survey conducted by a regional office of the CMS to determine whether the surveys being conducted by state agencies (or other groups) are appropriately assessing the facility's operations.

REVIEW QUESTIONS

Knowledge-based Questions

1. Explain the following types of care given to end-stage renal disease patients: hemodialysis, CAPD, and CCPD.
2. Who performs regular surveys of dialysis facilities? Who performs validation surveys of dialysis facilities?
3. What items of information should be documented for each dialysis patient?
4. What is the source of payment for most patients who have been on dialysis for more than 30 months?
5. What role do the ESRD networks play in the collection and aggregation of data on dialysis patients?
6. What types of QI activities take place in dialysis facilities?
7. What is the role of the health information manager in organizations dealing with end-stage renal disease?

Application-based Questions

1. Compare and contrast ESRD Networks with quality improvement organizations.
2. What resources would a health information consultant find helpful in consulting for ESRD facilities?

Web Activity

In 2003, CMS proposed a new form to replace CMS 2728. Visit the CMS "forms" Web site at http://www.cms.hhs.gov/forms to determine whether this new form has been adopted. Upon arriving at the Web site, scroll down (or use the "Find" feature of your Web browser) to locate CMS 2728 in the list of forms. Click on the CMS 2728 hyperlink to see what the current form looks like. Is it identical to the form depicted in Figure 5-5 or has the form been changed? Are any other proposed new forms listed on this page? If so, what are they?

Case Study

Kay Carnes has begun consulting for a dialysis facility that began computerization of its patient records approximately six months ago. On her first consultation visit, she examined both the computerized and paper portions of the medical record. She found that certain portions of the record, which had not yet been computerized, were maintained in sturdy three-ring binders. These binders were labeled on the spine with the patient's name and the patient's treatment schedule (e.g., John Doe, M-W-F, or Mary Smith, T-T-S). The paper-based portion of the record included signed consent forms, assessment forms by various disciplines, outside lab reports, history and physical examination reports from the patient's physician or last hospital visit, identification data, CMS data collection forms, and the patient care plans. The computer-based portion of the record included data from each dialysis treatment and progress notes from the nurses, the dietitian, and the social worker. On some of the older records in which all of the progress notes were handwritten, Kay noticed that the physicians had recorded monthly progress notes. However, there were no progress notes from the physicians in the computer-based portion of the record that covered the past six months. Kay asked the unit director, a registered nurse, about this. The director answered that all of the other disciplines were entering their own progress notes into the computerized record during or after each patient contact. However, the physicians were accustomed to handwriting their progress notes and, therefore, did not use the computer. The physicians had continued to see each patient on a monthly basis, but there was very little documentation in the chart to indicate this after the computer-based record had been implemented.

1. What issues should Kay address in her consultation report to this facility?
2. What recommendations would you make if you were in her place?

References and Suggested Readings

Brandt, M. (1995). Medicare *Conditions of Participation* outline additional standards for healthcare providers. *Journal of the American Health Information Management Association, 66* (8), 20–26.

[CMS] Centers for Medicare & Medicaid Services. (2002). *2002 Annual Report: ESRD Clinical Performance Measures Project*. Baltimore, MD: Department of Health and Human Services, Centers for Medicare & Medicaid Services, Center for Beneficiary Choices.

[CMS] Centers for Medicare & Medicaid Services. (2002, June 17). Report of modified or altered system. *Federal Register, 67* (116), 41244–41250.

[CMS] Centers for Medicare & Medicaid Services. (2003a). Chapter 5—Quality improvement. *Medicare ESRD Network Organizations Manual* [Online]. http://cms.hhs.gov/manuals/ 114_eno/eno114index.pdf [2003, July 29].

[CMS] Centers for Medicare & Medicaid Services. (2003b). *Medicare Renal Dialysis Facility Manual* [Online]. http://cms.hhs.gov/manuals/29_rdf/rd0-fw.asp [2003, July 29].

[CMS] Centers for Medicare & Medicaid Services. (No date a). Appendix H—Survey procedures and interpretive guidelines for end-stage renal disease facilities. *State Operations Manual.* [Online]. http://cms.hhs.gov/manuals/pub07pdf/AP-D-I.pdf [2003, July 30].

[CMS] Centers for Medicare & Medicaid Services. (No date b). *Summary Report of the End Stage Renal Disease (ESRD) Networks' Annual Reports 2001* [Online]. http://www.cms.hhs.gov/ esrd/2i.pdf [2003, July 26].

Conditions for Coverage of Suppliers of End Stage Renal Disease (ESRD) Services. *Code of Federal Regulations*, Title 42, Part 405, Subpart U, 2002 ed.

ESRD network organizations. *Code of Federal Regulations*, Title 42, Part 405, Section 405.2112, 2002 ed.

Forum of ESRD Networks, Quality Assurance Networks. (1992, May). Medical Record Model.

Friedman, E. A. (2000). *Legal and Ethical Concerns in Treating Kidney Failure: Case Study Workbook.* Dordrecht, The Netherlands: Kluwer Academic Publishers.

[JCAHO] Joint Commission on Accreditation of Healthcare Organizations. (2003). *Joint Commission 2003 Automated Comprehensive Accreditation Manual for Hospitals*. Oakbrook Terrace, IL: Joint Commission on Accreditation of Healthcare Organizations.

McAfee, L. (1987). A consultant's guide to renal dialysis units. *Journal of the American Medical Record Association, 58* (7), 44–46.

Medical Media Publishing, Inc. (1992*a*). Module I: Today's dialysis environment: An overview. *Core Curriculum for the Dialysis Technician: A Comprehensive Review of Hemodialysis*, 20–30.

Medical Media Publishing, Inc. (1992*b*). Module II: The person with renal failure. *Core Curriculum for the Dialysis Technician: A Comprehensive Review of Hemodialysis*, 23–26.

Merck Manual (16th ed.). (1992). Rahway, NJ: Merck Research Laboratories.

[NKF] National Kidney Foundation. (2001). *Executive Summary—K/DOQI Clinical Practice Guidelines* [Online]. http://www.kidney.org/professionals/doqi/guidelines/doqi_upex.html [2003, July 29].

[RPA/ASN] Renal Physicians Association & American Society of Nephrology. (2000). *Shared Decision-Making in the Appropriate Initiation of and Withdrawal from Dialysis.* (Clinical Practice Guideline No. 2). Washington, DC: Authors.

Spath, P. L. (1990, August/September). Assessing the quality of renal dialysis services. *Long-Term Care Spectrum, 3* (4), 13–15.

The Travelers. (1994, September). OBRA 93 on ESRD. *Medicare Newsletter,* 5.

The Travelers. (1994, December). Implementation instructions for the 1995 physician fee schedule policy changes. *Medicare: Special Bulletin*, 5.

[UNOS] United Network for Organ Sharing. (2003). *U.S. Transplantation Data*. [Online]. http://www.unos.org/data/default.asp?displayType=usData [2003, July 26].

[USDHHS] U.S. Department of Health and Human Services. (No date). *Medicare Coverage of Kidney Dialysis and Kidney Transplant Services*. [Online]. http://www.medicare.gov/publications/pubs/pdf/esrdcoverage.pdf [2003, July 26].

Zysman, F. (1990, August/September). Providing consultation for dialysis units. *Long-Term Care Spectrum*, 3 (4), 12–13.

Key Resources

American Association of Kidney Patients
3505 E. Frontage Rd., Ste. 315
Tampa, FL 33607
Phone: 800-749-2257
Fax: 813-636-8122
http://www.aakp.org

American Nephrology Nurses Association
P. O. Box 56
Pitman, NJ 08071
Toll Free: 888-600-ANNA (2662)
Telephone: 856-256-2320
Fax: 856-589-7463
http://anna.inurse.com

American Society of Nephrology
1725 I Street, NW, Suite 510
Washington, DC 20006
Phone: 202-659-0599
Fax: 202-659-0709
http://www.asn-online.org

American Society of Transplantation
17000 Commerce Pkwy, Suite C
Mt. Laurel, NJ 08054
Phone: 856-439-9986
Fax: 856-439-9982
http://www.a-s-t.org

American Society of Transplant Surgeons
1020 North Fairfax Street, Suite 200
Alexandria, VA 22314
Phone: 888-990-2787
http://www.asts.org/index.cfm

Association of Organ Procurement Organizations
1364 Beverly Road, Suite 100
McLean, VA 22101
http://www.aopo.org

Forum Clearinghouse
Forum of End-Stage Renal Disease Networks
1527 Huguenot Road
Midlothian, VA 23113
Phone: 804-794-2586
http://www.esrdnetworks.org

National Association for Nephrology Technicians/Technologists
P. O. Box 2307
Dayton, OH 45401-2307
Phone: 937-586-3705
Toll free: 877-607-6268
Fax: 937-586-3699
http://www.dialysistech.org

National Renal Administrators Association
1904 Naomi Place
Prescott, AZ 86303-5061
Tel: 928-717-2772
Fax: 928-441-3857
http://www.nraa.org

Renal Physicians Association
1700 Rockville Pike, Suite 220
Rockville, MD 20852
Phone: 301-468-3515
Fax: 301-468-3511
http://www.renalmd.org

United Network for Organ Sharing
700 North 4th Street
P.O. Box 2484
Richmond, Virginia 23218
Phone: 804-782-4800
http://www.unos.org

Chapter 6

Correctional Facilities

Barbara Manny, MS, RHIA
Brianna McCloe Rogers, RHIA

Learning Objectives

Upon successful completion of this chapter, you should be able to:

1. Identify the types of correctional facilities that exist and the responsible authority for each.
2. Identify the various health care delivery models that may exist in correctional institutions.
3. Distinguish between the various types of licensure and certification available for correctional professionals.
4. Recognize the different accrediting organizations and the strengths and weaknesses of each.
5. Identify the role of HIPAA in correctional facilities.
6. Identify situations where the application of technology can help reduce costs and increase access to health care.

SETTING	DESCRIPTION	SYNONYMS/EXAMPLES
Prisons	Individual facilities operated by a unit of a state or the federal government for the confinement of adults 18 years or older, convicted of a felony whose sentence exceeds one year (Anno, 1992).	There are three different classifications for prisons: maximum, medium, and minimum security.
Jails	Institutions administered by local units of government (i.e., cities or counties) with the authority to detain adults for a period of 48 hours or longer and for the confinement of adults convicted of misdemeanors whose sentence does not exceed one year. Also used to hold individuals awaiting trial. Police lock-ups are not included in the definition of correctional facilities.	In various locations these facilities may also be known as detention centers, county prisons, or workhouses (ACA, 1985).
Juvenile Detention Facilities	Facilities operated by a unit of government for the confinement of individuals younger than 18 years of age.	
Bureau of Immigrations and Customs Enforcement (ICE)	May be considered a type of correctional facility, although correction and rehabilitation are not part of their mission. ICE detention centers are used to hold immigrants or aliens during periods of investigation into their legal status or during resolution of a deportation order after they are convicted and have met their sentencing obligations.	
Correctional facilities operated by the Army, Navy, Air Force, or Marines	All branches of the U.S. military operate their own correctional facilities in the United States and overseas.	
Shelters or Halfway Houses	Incarcerated individuals often use these facilities as a means of completing their sentences or making the transition back to society.	

As crime rates have increased steadily since the mid-1970s, the correctional industry in the United States has undergone dramatic changes and is experiencing enormous growth in the **inmate** population. The greatest increase in the prison population occurred between 1980 and 1990, when the total prison population increased more than 200 percent (ACA, 1993). According to the Bureau of Justice Statistics, approximately 1,962,220 prisoners are held in prisons and jails nationwide, as reported on December 31, 2001 (BJS, 2001).

U.S. correctional institutions are complex organizations. Their purpose is to enhance public safety by keeping separate those persons deemed a threat to individuals or their property. Each level of government—federal, state, county, and city—is responsible for the operation of some type of correctional facility. The various levels of government operate independently of each other. Even the operation of facilities within the same system varies. This chapter provides students of health information management with a general understanding of the nature of correctional institutions, and specifically, the role of health information management in the delivery of health care in correctional settings.

Introduction to Setting

The operation of correctional institutions and, more specifically, the delivery of health care to inmates was not of great concern to many individuals or organizations until fairly recently. It was not until the early 1970s, when civil rights advocates and health professionals began taking a serious look at the lack of health care services available to inmates, that the conditions under which inmates lived became widely known.

Before 1970, few efforts were made to identify and change the status of health care delivery in correctional facilities. A common misconception was that **prisons** provided better health care than **jails**. Jails typically lacked the funds necessary to maintain an infirmary, so treatment was often provided by the emergency departments of community hospitals, but prison inmates were rarely sent outside the system for care because prisons were more likely to have some type of medical care available on-site. Prison health care staff were not likely to be as well trained as their peers working in private or public institutions. The health staff practicing in correctional institutions were often physicians with institutional licenses or unlicensed foreign medical graduates. Support staff often included untrained medical corpsmen and untrained inmate "nurses" (Anno, 1992).

Both federal and state laws affect prisoners' rights. In general, prisoners lose some of their civil rights, such as the right to vote, when they are incarcerated. However, the Eighth Amendment to the U.S. Constitution prohibits cruel and unusual punishment, which means that prisons must provide a minimum standard of living for prisoners. Also, the Fourteenth Amendment's Equal Protection Clause protects prisoners against unequal treatment on the basis of race, sex, and creed. Prisoners also have limited rights to speech and religion. Other Constitutional rights that apply to prisoners include due process in the right to administrative appeals and a right of access to the parole process (Legal Information Institute, 2002).

In 1976, the landmark case *Estelle v. Gamble* created a "right" to health care for inmates. The case applied a two-prong test to determine the extent of the medical care duty owed to inmates. Correctional institutions would be in violation of inmates' constitutional rights if (1) correctional officials showed a "deliberate indifference" to inmates' medical needs and (2) the inmates' needs were "serious." The vagueness of the language used in the court's ruling and the creation of a "right" to health care has created enormous difficulties for correctional institutions, including a continuous rise in inmate petitions claiming violations of their "right" to health care (Posner, 1992).

Today inmates receive treatment for AIDS (acquired immune deficiency syndrome), cardiovascular disease, and even rehabilitation services. The physical settings have changed substantially and can range from small infirmaries to large medical facilities with specialty clinics. Critics of correctional health care seek the availability of even more extensive and expensive treatment and facilities.

Organizational structure and methods of administration vary depending on the level of government operating a facility, corresponding laws and court orders, and characteristics of the incarcerated populations. Health information management students and professionals should fully understand the structure of the correctional facility and government in which they intend to work.

There is still relatively little empirical data available about the correctional health care delivery systems in operation around the United States. Several organizations have conducted studies and continue to examine the state of correctional health care delivery systems, but large-scale research efforts are needed to provide current, accurate information about the state of correctional health care.

State Departments of Correction

The traditional organizational model places responsibility for health services with wardens. In this model, health professionals must report directly to the warden, which does not promote consistency in the policies and procedures used to operate a health care delivery system. It can also be a source of conflict and ethical concern for health care professionals if the warden is not sympathetic to the health care needs of inmates. The placement of a health services program within a state **department of correction (DOC)** may be an indication of the perceived importance of health services (Anno, 2001).

The use of a statewide **health services director (HSD)** is common. An HSD is responsible for overseeing the health care delivery system, developing statewide policies and procedures, and approving the health services budget. An ideal arrangement would have an HSD as head of a separate division with direct access to the head of the DOC. To be hired, an HSD must have had clinical and administrative experience (Anno, 1992).

In the late 1980s, several state DOCs still used the traditional organizational model, meaning they had no one at the central office with full-time responsibility for overseeing health services, and the health professionals reported to the warden. Historically there might have been an individual responsible for "programs," which could include anything from food service to mental and medical health care. The problem with health professionals reporting to wardens is not just that the wardens are nonmedical personnel and might not understand the need for expensive equipment. If the wardens are not progressive correctional administrators, the focus of the health staff could be shifted away from providing adequate care (Anno, 1992).

A survey conducted in 1999 by the **National Commission on Correctional Health Care (NCCHC)** received responses from 28 (54%) of the 52 prison systems surveyed. Because of the low response rate, no definitive conclusions can be drawn about the extent to which states have abandoned the traditional model. However, all but one of the 28 prison systems had at least one full-time person operating a central health office for the DOC, and some systems had more than 75 persons employed in the DOC central health office. Twenty-one of the 28 systems operated health services with contracted staff instead of or in addition to DOC employees. Only seven prison systems operated their DOC health services solely with their own employees (Anno, 2001).

Operation by State versus Contracted Firms

Correctional facilities have used contracted services for many years, mainly for ancillary services. The first such contract occurred in 1978 at a state correctional facility. Some correctional facilities have begun contracting all health services, including mental health, dental, and clinical services. Supporters of contract firms claim cost reductions to the state and improvements in the efficiency and quality of care. Critics claim state-operated services can be cost-effective, and savings realized by firms are done at the expense of inmates (Anno, 2001).

Critics argue that for-profit correctional facilities have no incentive to spend money on adequate health services or appropriate facilities and that it is the responsibility of the government alone to punish criminals. Supporters of private enterprise cite profit as their motive for providing inmates with adequately equipped facilities and appropriate medical care, thus reducing their risk of litigation. Profit is also their incentive for using proactive policies and programs to hold costs down, something government bureaucracies have been reluctant and unable to do.

Prisons

A prison confines, houses, feeds, clothes, educates, and polices its population. Responsibility for the operation of most prisons falls under the authority of a state DOC. Within a state system, individual prisons are run by wardens or superintendents. Wardens have more or less complete control over the operation of their prison, so administrative policies and procedures may differ greatly from facility to facility.

Prisons are classified by their level of security. *Maximum security prisons* have heavily armed guards and high fences and walls, and very restrictive rules for controlling the movement of inmates. These facilities house the inmates who have the longest sentences. *Medium security prisons* have slightly less restrictive rules and facilities. Individuals convicted of misdemeanors—offenses less serious than felonies—are kept in medium security prisons. *Minimum security prisons* offer the least restrictive rules and facilities. They house individuals convicted of nonviolent crimes such as forgery and obstruction of justice.

The physical structure of prisons is determined in part by the population and the security measures required for their confinement. Common configurations include structures that resemble a wheel hub and spokes. The hub usually houses a main security center and the spokes contain the cells. Other common designs resemble a long pole with intersecting shorter poles with cells, or a campus resembling small groups of apartment buildings (*World Book Encyclopedia*, 1996). Figure 6-1 is an example of one type of prison design.

The **Federal Bureau of Prisons (FBP)** was established in 1930 by an act of Congress and operates under the direction of the U.S. Department of Justice. There are more than 100 federal facilities operated by the FBP including penitentiaries, prison camps, and metropolitan correctional/detention centers. The FBP encourages inmates to participate in a range of programs that will help them live crime-free upon their release (USDOJ, Online). Federal prisons house individuals charged and convicted of crimes against the United States such as kidnapping. The FBP is headquartered in Washington, D.C., but the administration of facilities is divided into six regions across the country (ACA, 1996). Figure 6-2 shows one of these facilities.

An individual awaiting trial in federal courts may be free on bond or may be detained by the U.S. Marshals Service. A person who has not been sentenced, but is

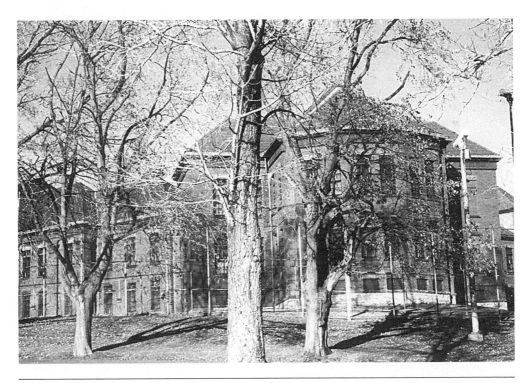

Figure 6-1   Fishkill Correctional Facility, Beacon, New York. (Photo courtesy Linda Manny.)

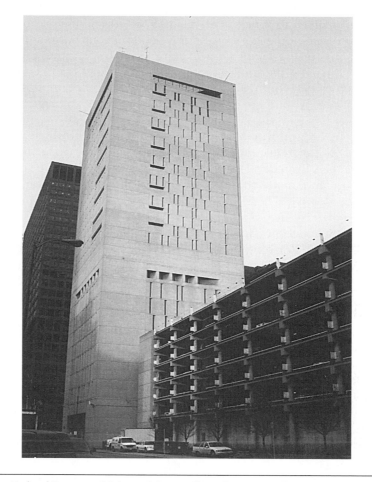

Figure 6-2 Federal Bureau of Prisons Metropolitan Correctional Center, Chicago, Illinois. (Photo courtesy Barbara Manny.)

incarcerated while awaiting trial is a *detainee*, whereas a *prisoner* has been tried and sentenced to a period of incarceration. The U.S. Marshals Service must place detainees in custody in an appropriate facility, but cannot place detainees in a federal prison. The U.S. Marshals Service ordinarily contracts with local jails, which must meet certain criteria, to house detainees.

Initial health screenings of inmates are done within 24 hours of admission to correctional facilities. This screening begins the inmate's health record. The treatment available to inmates during their confinement varies greatly by the type and location of the facility. Variations in levels of care may result from financial considerations, characteristics of the inmate population, or availability of resources. Some correctional institutions have little more than an examination room and a visiting physician, whereas others have on-site hospitals with mental health, rehabilitation, and substance abuse services.

Jails

Jails are generally the responsibility of local governments. Most of the jails in operation are administered by sheriffs who are elected officials. Reporting to the sheriff is a county administrator or a board of county commissioners. A police chief reports to the administrator or board and oversees law enforcement while a corrections director oversees administration of the jails. In some areas, a DOC may have been developed to administer county and/or municipal jails. The FBP has its own jails in several cities that hold individuals awaiting trial in federal courts. Some areas of the United States have federal courts but no federal detention facility. For these areas, the FBP contracts with the local jail to house the federal pretrial prisoners.

The three primary purposes for jails are (1) to detain those awaiting trial after arrest; (2) to hold those being transferred to a state or federal prison or mental facility; and (3) to punish a minor crime (misdemeanor) for those serving a sentence of less than one year. There are three types of jails: detention, sentenced, and detention sentenced. A *detention jail* is solely for the confinement of those awaiting trial. *Sentenced jails* are for those serving misdemeanor sentences, and *detention-sentenced jails* house both detainees and individuals who have been sentenced (Miller, 1978).

Occasionally jails are used to house inmates in an effort to alleviate overcrowding in prisons. Typically a prison will have a contractual agreement with a jail for a specific number of beds. As soon as space becomes available at the prison, the inmates are transferred out of the jail. Housing prisoners in jails is only a temporary solution to the problem of overcrowding in prisons.

The provision of health services in jails is the responsibility of the sheriff. Some jurisdictions require screening upon intake for communicable diseases, such as tuberculosis and venereal diseases, but all jails perform medical examinations after booking procedures have been completed. Some courts have required the screening of intoxicated persons and continuous monitoring throughout the detoxification period. This is an important precaution because intoxication often masks symptoms of fractures, diabetes, and illnesses that could be mistaken for drunkenness. Most jails do not have on-site medical facilities. Those that do usually have only an examination room and an office. Most large urban jails have a separate infirmary with beds that are used for inmates who are too ill to remain in their cells but not ill enough to be transferred to a hospital. Inmates can be isolated in an infirmary bed to prevent the spread of communicable diseases and sometimes when their treatment includes devices that could be used as weapons, such as crutches.

Juvenile Facilities

Before the nineteenth century, juveniles were confined with adults and, in some jails, this still occurs. Today, there are two main types of **juvenile detention facilities**, short term and long term. Responsibility for juvenile facilities belongs either to the state department of corrections or the local county.

Short-term facilities include detention centers, shelters, and reception and diagnostic centers. *Detention centers* are similar to county jails in appearance and function. These centers are used to hold juveniles awaiting jurisdictional or dispositional hearings. *Shelters* are used for dependent and neglected juveniles and are usually not secure buildings. Public shelters typically house only children waiting an order of the court or those confined by a public welfare agency. *Reception* and *diagnostic centers* are basically way stations for juveniles moving from short- to long-term facilities. Juveniles received are screened, diagnosed, and sent to an appropriate facility based on the diagnosis. Facilities are often part of state-operated juvenile systems (Klempner, 1981).

Long-term facilities include training schools, ranches, group homes, and halfway houses. *Training schools* are typically located in rural areas. The primary purpose of training schools is the reeducation and development of juvenile offenders. Juveniles learn vocational skills and can complete their high school equivalency examination (GED). *Ranches*, *camps*, and *farms* are also in rural settings and tend to offer fewer academic and vocational programs. *Group homes* are generally found in urban environments and house approximately 15 to 30 juveniles. These facilities are not secure, and residents usually attend school or have jobs. *Halfway homes* are similar to group homes. They are generally used for first-time offenders, those almost ready for release, and sometimes for juveniles with no other available living arrangements (Klempner, 1981).

Responsibility for health services at juvenile facilities rests with the authority responsible for their operation. Some juvenile facilities are within the jurisdiction of the state DOC, and others are run by a county authority. Health care services in juvenile facilities are similar to those found in other types of correctional institutions. Depending on the size of the facility, characteristics of the inmate population, and budgetary resources, the health care services may be extensive or almost nonexistent. Accredited facilities generally have disease prevention and health promotion programs that address issues such as sexually transmitted and bloodborne diseases as well as the use of tobacco products and family planning services. Counseling and mental health services are considered critical by advocates of the juvenile justice system.

Bureau of Immigration and Customs Enforcement

The United States has operated some form of immigration control since 1882. From 1940 until 2003, the Immigration and Naturalization Service (INS) was the agency responsible for enforcing immigration laws. In 2003, the border and security functions of the former INS were transferred into the Directorate of Border and Transportation Security within the Department of Homeland Security and reorganized as a part of the **Bureau of Immigration and Customs Enforcement (ICE)** (BICE, Online). INS immigration service functions were placed into a separate **Bureau of Citizenship and Immigration Services (BCIS)** (BCIS, Online). Generally, a person applying to become a naturalized citizen of the United States must have been a person of good moral character for the given statutory period. An applicant is permanently barred from naturalization if he or she has been convicted of murder or of an aggravated felony (USAIS, 2002).

The ICE Detention and Deportation Program has an interagency agreement with the Public Health Service for the provision of health care services to detained immigrants and aliens. These services are provided through the **Division of Immigration Health Services (DIHS)**. Under a Memo of Understanding, the ICE pays for the services of the DIHS, but the detention and deportation division has no line authority over the DIHS personnel.

Detention and deportation facilities receive immigrants and aliens from the FBP and state DOCs with deportation orders. Within 72 hours of admission to a detention facility, individuals receive an initial screening for tuberculosis and a brief physical examination. Medical emergencies are addressed immediately, and most treatment is provided at the deportation facilities. Detainees remain at deportation centers until their legal status is resolved. The DIHS has no authority to increase the length of detention for treatment purposes. Often prophylactic measures are the only treatment options possible within given time constraints (J. Glidewell, personal communication, December 1995).

On-site versus Off-site

A great deal of effort and research must go into the decision to provide health services on-site or off-site, and the type of services that must be available at the facility. Planning is the critical step in the process of designing a health care delivery system. Experts suggest creating a planning committee with a project director and representatives from the medical, custody, budgeting, information systems, and administrative divisions. The committee must have current, accurate data to determine to what extent health services are to be provided.

This setup involves many variables, not the least of which includes a health profile of the facility's current and expected population. Examples of information in a health profile include the expected inmate volume, health needs of the population, resources of the correctional system, resources available from other public agencies, staffing needs, and costs of transportation services, to name only a few.

Types of Patients

Inmates as patients present challenges for health care professionals. The goals of medicine to diagnose and cure, and corrections to punish, are sometimes in conflict. Security and personal safety are always the priority. Yet there are serious and legitimate problems that health care professionals must face when treating inmates. Recent legislation stressing more stringent sentencing restrictions ensures that inmates will stay in the correctional system longer. This and other factors will have a direct impact on the types of services and staffing required.

The inmate population overall is not well educated and enters the correctional system already in poor health. Inmates may make attempts to manipulate health staff, creating a difficult and potentially dangerous work environment. Inmates represent all age groups and a growing population of females. Age, sex, and offense can all have an effect on the delivery of health services in correctional settings.

Age

The age of the inmate population will affect the type of care, professionals, and staffing required. Younger populations are generally healthier and should require less staff. However, more juvenile offenders are entering correctional institutions in need of psychiatric and drug treatments. Older populations will have chronic conditions that require certain types of care. Inmates older than age 40 are a growing segment of the population. Geriatric issues may be faced earlier than expected in correctional settings because of related stress of incarceration and the generally poor health of inmates. Older inmates are also more likely to suffer from chronic illnesses such as hypertension, asthma, and diabetes. Conditions that are part of the aging process such as hearing and vision loss and mental confusion must also be addressed. Correctional facilities will have to be modified or built to accommodate the disabled and elderly.

Correctional facilities will also be faced with terminally ill inmates as a result of chronic diseases, especially AIDS. Terminally ill inmates have been treated in a number of ways. Some DOCs house terminally ill inmates in separate units; others offer hospice care (Bauersmith and Gent, 2002). Some facilities also allow for compassionate release or medical furlough programs when inmates are known to be terminally ill (Anno, 2001).

Sex

Gender also affects the type of health care services and professionals that must be available. Women will require access to gynecological services and obstetric and prenatal care if they are pregnant. The intake history for female inmates should include questions about menstrual cycles, pregnancy history, and gynecological problems. Female inmates need access to personal sanitary supplies, education on breast self-examinations, and annual Pap smears. When state law allows, pregnant inmates retain the right to choose abortion services.

Pregnant inmates pose a special problem for correctional facilities and should be housed together with other pregnant inmates. Their work assignments must be limited to protect their condition, and special attention should be paid to their diet.

Offense

The type of offense an inmate committed may affect the treatment received if the inmate poses a threat to security or the safety of staff. In correctional facilities, custody and security are the primary concerns, and health care is provided in a manner that does not compromise those primary concerns. Inmates are classified and confined based on the type of offense committed, and although the offense cannot be used as a reason for refusing inmates treatment, it may affect decisions to transfer inmates off-site for treatment. During periods of heightened security, such as lock-downs, health staff treat inmates in their cells.

Nature of Illness

The health status of incarcerated populations reflects and magnifies the worst trends in public health today, namely the dramatic rise in previously controlled diseases such as tuberculosis and sexually transmitted diseases, especially AIDS. This section briefly examines some of the trends health professionals working in correctional settings face today and the corresponding administrative difficulties.

Acute and Chronic Diseases

After intake examinations, many inmates are found to be in the acute stages of respiratory ailments and sexually transmitted diseases. Acute conditions may also include traumas. Although prison violence is well controlled by correctional officers and facility rules, some inmates still suffer stab wounds, blunt trauma, and other acute or urgent conditions.

Chronic conditions are on the rise in correctional institutions for several reasons, including the rise in incarceration of individuals over age 40. From 1993 to 1994, there was a 13 percent increase in the inmate population over age 55 in both state and federal facilities (ACA, 1996). Cardiovascular diseases, end-stage renal disease, and complications from AIDS are not uncommon in correctional facilities.

Communicable Diseases

Communicable diseases are commonly found in inmate populations, most notably tuberculosis and sexually transmitted diseases. The lifestyle chosen by many inmates before their incarceration includes heavy drug and alcohol use and indiscriminate sexual behavior, including prostitution. Their health is worsened by smoking cigarettes and maintaining poor nutritional habits. The treatment of chronic conditions is complicated by incarceration. Trips to on-site or off-site appointments require the use of correctional officers for escort, and use of transportation in the case of treatment that is provided outside of the facility. Basic medical information must accompany each prisoner treated. Figure 6-3 shows a health transfer summary form completed by health professionals for prisoners who are treated off-site or transferred. Educating inmates on proper administration of their medication is also difficult.

Types of Caregivers

A variety of health care professionals can be found working in a wide range of correctional settings. The extent to which services, and therefore professionals, will be available at a facility is a constant challenge for correctional administrators.

Clinical Professionals

A well-structured, adequately funded health care delivery system can employ any number of professionals. Professionals include psychiatrists, physicians, nurses (both RNs and LPNs), physician assistants, dentists, and optometrists. Other professionals

DEPARTMENT OF CORRECTIONS
Division of Program Services
DOC-3018 (Rev. 05/94)

MEDICAL HISTORY

WISCONSIN

INSTRUCTION TO OFFENDER: Complete Section II. through Signature Only, Do Not complete box below.

OFFENDER NAME				DATE OF BIRTH	DOC NUMBER
ADMISSION DATE	INSTITUTION	PULSE	RESPIRATION	BLOOD PRESSURE	TEMPERATURE

I.   Identifying Information

HEIGHT	WEIGHT	SEX	RACE	PPD	TETANUS	PREVIOUS CORRECTIONAL TIME

II. Allergies (Describe Agent and Reaction. Food, Medication, Other)

III. Language Barriers / Learning Deficits

IV. Childhood Illnesses (Indicate age of occurrence)

Measles	Mumps	Chicken Pox	Rubella	Other

V. Family Disease History (Indicate age, illness, cause of death)

	AGE	ILLNESS	CAUSE OF DEATH		AGE	ILLNESS	CAUSE OF DEATH
Mother				Sisters			
Father				Brothers			

VI. Medical Treatment (Hospitalizations and Operations, Include Psychiatric Treatment)

HOSPITAL AND LOCATION	REASON / DIAGNOSIS	DATE ADMITTED

VII. Other Information

CURRENT MEDICATIONS	

STREET DRUGS   USE OF NEEDLES ☐ Yes ☐ No

ALCOHOL USE: Type and Amount   TOBACCO USE: Type and Amount

SEXUAL HISTORY
  Homosexual Experience ☐ Y ☐ N   Number of Partners in Last Year _____
  Victim of Sexual Abuse ☐ Y ☐ N   Last Sexual Contact Date _____
  Bisexual Experience ☐ Y ☐ N   Sexually Transmitted Diseases (List)

  Contraceptive Method _____

Figure 6-3   A health assessment form and health summary completed by health professionals used when transferring health information with inmates. (Courtesy Wisconsin Department of Corrections/Bureau of Health Services.)

INSTRUCTIONS: Answer all questions. If you have any of the conditions listed below, answer YES or NO by placing an **X** in the column. If a family member has a condition listed, place an **X** in the family column.

YES	NO	FAMILY	
			1. TB or Lived with anyone who had TB
			2. Coughed up blood / Bleeding disorder
			3. Hayfever, Asthma or difficulty breathing
			4. Emphysema
			5. Sinus Problems
			6. Chronic or frequent colds
			7. Frequent nose bleeds
			8. Chest pain
			9. Heart murmur
			10. Rheumatic Fever
			11. Low or high blood pressure
			12. Stomach trouble or ulcer
			13. Frequent indigestion
			14. Hemorrhoids
			15. Frequent constipation or diarrhea
			16. Gall bladder problems
			17. Hepatitis, jaundice or liver problems
			18. Kidney Problems
			19. Blood in urine
			20. Difficulty urinating
			21. Diabetes or sugar in urine
			22. Thyroid problems
			23. Skin disease
			24. Hernia or rupture
			25. Tumor, cysts or cancer
			26. Attempted suicide
			27. Alcoholism or Drug Addictions
			28. Depression
			29. Birth defects
			30. Male genital problems
			31. Eye, ear, nose or throat trouble
			32. Vision loss or hearing loss

YES	NO	FAMILY	
			33. Glasses or contact lenses
			34. Prosthesis or other corrective device
			35. Dentures / Partials
			36. Severe tooth or gum problems
			37. Head injuries
			38. Frequent or severe headaches
			39. Loss of consciousness, dizziness or fainting
			40. Paralysis, numbness
			41. Muscle, bone or joint problem
			42. Recurrent back trouble
			43. Recurrent fever / Nightsweats
			44. Rapid weight loss
			45. Constant Fatigue
			46. Diminished appetite
			47. White spots in mouth
			48. Swollen glands
			49. Seizure Disorder

Females Only

YES	NO	FAMILY	
			50. Lumps, pain, or discharge from breast
			51. Female disorders
			52. Change in menstrual pattern
			53. Age of first period _____
			54. Last menstrual period _____
			55. Length of period _____ days
			56. Last pap smear_____
			57. A pregnancy,

57. A pregnancy,
How many pregnancies
of these:
# of live births
# of interrupted pregnancies

	YOURSELF	MOTHER

REMARKS (Explain all Yes answers checked above)

I certify that I have reviewed the foregoing information and had the opportunity to discuss it with the nurse, and that it is true and complete to the best of my knowledge.

OFFENDER SIGNATURE		DATE SIGNED

NURSE SIGNATURE	DATE COMPLETED	TIME

Nursing assessment of this data must be charted in the progress notes.

Figure 6-3 *(Continued)*

encountered may have a nonclinical role such as social workers and counselors. Sophisticated delivery systems provide case management and other support services.

Previous shortages of physicians often reflected shortages existing in the surrounding communities. Correctional facilities are often built in rural areas and many had insufficient funds to attract qualified professionals. Still other facilities refused to hire women, thus eliminating a potential source of applicants, and sometimes the working conditions discouraged clinicians from seeking employment in correctional health care (Anno, 1992).

Physicians are beginning to gain an interest in correctional health care and are less reluctant to work in correctional settings. Physicians perform the physical examinations and order medications and referrals to specialists. Some of the physician's time is spent on administrative tasks. Nurses and sometimes physician assistants are responsible for triaging patients, recording health histories and vital signs, and taking samples for laboratory analysis. Dental services must also be included in basic health services, and optometry services should be provided as well.

Ancillary Services

Pharmacy, radiology, laboratory, and dietetics are considered ancillary services. Laboratory and radiology services may or may not be performed on-site. Medications must be administered to inmates at least twice a day, 365 days a year, and some antibiotics require more frequent administration. Some correctional facilities have been successful with "keep-on-person" medication programs that allow some inmates to maintain their own small supply of medications. It is common for facilities to have a central area where inmates go to receive their daily medications (Anno, 1992).

Emergency Services

The availability of emergency services is subject to the same variables as other health services. At a minimum, however, correctional facilities must have a plan for handling medical emergencies. Facilities must designate one or more hospital emergency departments to which inmates will be transported in case of medical emergencies. The plan must also specify arrangements, including security, for emergency evacuation and identify modes of transportation to be used. Because of the remote location of many facilities, transportation can be one of the biggest problems. Some state DOCs have their own emergency medical technicians (EMTs) and/or ambulances (Anno, 2001).

Specialty Services

Depending on a facility's population, specialty health care services may include mental health, speech and rehabilitative therapies, and more extensive dental services. Some prisons must include provisions for physically handicapped inmates or those who are vision or hearing impaired. To avoid victimization of these inmates, some prisons provide separate housing (Anno, 2001).

Mental health services available at correctional facilities often come under attack for their inadequacies. Mental health screening should be part of the intake process to identify those inmates with immediate mental health needs. Aggressive mentally ill and self-mutilating inmates require careful handling and can cause extreme management problems. Many prison and jail systems now have special programs to manage aggressive mentally ill inmates (Anno, 2001).

Licensure

State licensing boards establish standards that control the number of professionals practicing in a state and determine minimum standards of competence. The licensing boards also define what activities may be legally performed under each type of license. Licensing standards do not set staffing ratios, but their requirements have staffing implications for health care facilities.

Regulatory Issues

Regulations for correctional facilities come in many forms. Those dealing with health care services and professionals are most often found in professional licensing statutes and court orders. Correctional facilities that have hospitals, satellite facilities, mental health programs, and so on must follow established legal and professional standards. Regulation of health services is usually the responsibility of the state department of health, and applicable rules can be found in state statutes.

Accreditation programs provide an opportunity for correctional institutions to evaluate their operations against national standards, identify and correct problems, and continually improve the quality of living conditions and services. Benefits most often recognized include improved management, additional defense against lawsuits, enhanced credibility, a safer environment for inmates and staff, and the establishment of objective, measurable criteria for improving the quality of programs, staff, and the physical structure of correctional facilities.

The accreditation process is initiated by completing an application with basic information about the facility. Facilities are usually encouraged to complete a self-assessment before the on-site survey. At the conclusion of the on-site survey, members of the survey team review their findings and submit a report to an accreditation committee within the accrediting organization (Anno, 1992).

The evolution of correctional standards is significant in that they enable evaluation of correctional facilities based on compliance with objective, measurable standards. Currently the **National Commission on Correctional Health Care (NCCHC)**, the **American Correctional Association (ACA)**, and the **American Public Health Association (APHA)** publish health care standards for correctional institutions. Except for the APHA, these associations offer voluntary accreditation for the administration of health care services in correctional institutions.

National Commission on Correctional Health Care

The National Commission on Correctional Health Care (NCCHC) standards were developed by a wide range of professional health care associations, including the American Health Information Management Association (AHIMA). The NCCHC used the standards of the American Medical Association (AMA) as a template and developed separate standards for jails, prisons, and juvenile detention facilities. The NCCHC standards are the most comprehensive health standards of accrediting organizations, are more measurable, and provide the most comprehensive guidance for implementation because they take into account the size and complexity of facilities and are complemented by an accreditation process. The major disadvantage to NCCHC standards is the lack of comprehensive standards addressing environmental and occupational health issues (Anno, 2001).

American Correctional Association

These standards are advantageous in that they were developed and promoted by the nation's leading professional correctional association. From a health care perspective, the ACA standards are weaker than those of the NCCHC. The focus of the ACA standards is on the administration and operation of prisons. The health services section lacks the detail found in the standards of the NCCHC and the APHA. ACA standards offer little guidance to health professionals. When health care staff are confronted with ethical issues, the ACA standards are either silent or side with security (Anno, 2001).

Joint Commission on the Accreditation of Healthcare Organizations

The ambulatory care standards are the most applicable to health services provided in correctional facilities. An advantage of the Joint Commission on the Accreditation of Healthcare Organizations (JCAHO) standards is that they reflect community standards and emphasize quality improvement. The greatest disadvantages are that the standards are not specific to corrections and do not address important concerns of the health staff. The standards also do not cover dental and mental health services (Anno, 2001).

American Public Health Association

The American Public Health Association (APHA) was not listed as an accrediting agency because it has no corresponding accreditation program for its standards. The absence of an accreditation component makes compliance with the standards difficult to verify. The APHA standards were developed by health care professionals and they are comprehensive, specific to corrections, and provide some guidance for implementation. A significant disadvantage of APHA standards is their attempt to apply to large and small institutions simultaneously, even when unwarranted or impractical (Anno, 2001).

Documentation

Published standards recognize the importance of documentation in correctional institutions, whether for health care or administrative purposes. However, reality is sometimes very different. Documentation of factual information is essential for successful management of any organization and is particularly crucial in the correctional setting. Inmates are a litigious group, and clear, precise, factual documentation is critical to a correctional facility's defense.

The Correctional Health Record

Managing correctional health information will challenge the best health information management (HIM) professional. The test of a truly successful and effective information system is its ability to adapt to the ever-changing needs of a growing inmate population.

The APHA standards require that health records be kept as a unit record. There is resistance to this method of organization from some mental health and other allied health professionals. When psychiatric and medical services operate separately, copies of psychiatric consultations and treatment reports should be provided to the health services department and kept in an envelope in the health record. This enables the physician to have access to important information, but restricts the HIM professionals from releasing the reports. The original documentation is physically maintained at another site by the counselor or psychiatrist, and any requests for copies of the information must be directed to them.

The primary purpose of the health record, regardless of the setting, is to enhance communication among health professionals providing care to patients and document the course of a patient's treatment and outcome. The secondary purpose of the health record is to serve as a legal document to protect both the facility and the patient. It also serves as an educational tool and is the basis for most quality assurance and utilization management activities (Gannon, 1988).

Format

Where facility or systemwide procedures are lacking, it is recommended that the health staff assist in establishing a standardized format for the health record. The format chosen should be based on the unique needs of the facility. HIM professionals can play an important role in educating other staff about the advantages and disadvantages of the source-oriented, problem-oriented, and integrated record formats. HIM professionals are reminded to remain flexible and open to new ideas, as must the health staff who use the record. The format should also facilitate retrieving information from the record. Abstracting is still a widely used method of accessing the wealth of information contained in health records. Neglecting to consider retrieval of information when designing the health record format and forms may hinder future efforts for automation or research.

Numbering and Filing

Inmates in state and federal prisons are assigned identification numbers upon admission to some facilities. Some large jails or detention facilities may also use ID numbers. Most state DOCs have a central office and a computer system that assigns numbers. Other methods of assigning numbers are manual and require the use of ledgers, files, and logs. Some facilities give inmates a new number if they leave and reenter the correctional system, but most assign a number that is retained for all subsequent admissions to the correctional system. The federal system also assigns inmates a computer-generated number that the inmate keeps throughout his or her confinement, even if transferred to a federal facility in another state (Gannon, 1988). In very small rural facilities, HIM professionals may be more likely to find alphabetic filing systems, whereas terminal digit filing may be used in more populated urban facilities.

Retention and Destruction

Retention and storage requirements of inactive health records are usually found in law and jurisdictional policies. In order to retain the records for the required length of time, some state prisons place records on microfilm, whereas others store older paper records off-site in a central storage facility. In the federal system, inactive records remain in the facility for one year after an inmate's release. The records are sent to a central storage facility, where they are maintained for 30 years and then destroyed. Methods of destruction vary by facility. When contracting with a vendor, the responsibilities of all parties must be clearly defined. Accurate accounts of records sent for destruction must be kept to ensure that the destruction is carried out according to the terms of the agreement.

Written policies governing retention and destruction are essential. HIM professionals must ensure that retention and destruction policies follow state laws and guidelines. The state department of archives or similar authority should know the applicable regulations for retention and destruction of correctional and health-related records. Careful thought should also be given to disaster policies, such as what should be done to protect or restore records with fire and water damage. Some companies specialize in helping facilities recover records after such disasters. Consideration should also be given to the potential for other types of natural disasters, such as tornadoes or floods.

Health records in corrections present an interesting opportunity for the energetic HIM professional. There is a great need for data analysis in the evolving field of correctional health care, and the HIM professionals should lead the way in abstracting and using the information from these records.

Transfer

Transferring inmates is a regular occurrence in correctional settings and often necessitates the transfer of health records. In some systems, a copy of pertinent information is sent with the inmate; other facilities complete a separate health summary form that may include lab results, medications, allergies, scheduled appointments, and major medical conditions such as seizure disorders. Still other facilities send the entire original record. Generally the health record will follow the inmate. The health record must be protected from physical damage, and the confidentiality of the information must be protected as well. The Wisconsin DOC uses black zippered bags that lock with "confidential" printed on the outside.

Detailed logs should be kept for tracking records that have been transferred and for copies that have been released. The records should be securely sealed by the transferring facility. The receiving facility should document the condition of the seal and record upon arrival to verify that no tampering has occurred. Correctional officers must not have access to inmates' health information, but they should be informed of a physical condition if the situation warrants.

Confidentiality

It is imperative that HIM professionals stay current on changes affecting the confidentiality of inmate health information. Current political trends often have a direct impact on the protection and release of inmate health information. Diseases such as AIDS and the mental health status of inmates may further complicate already difficult situations. HIM professionals must know under what conditions an inmate's record may be released and what constitutes a valid authorization. HIM professionals could face hostile attorneys, inmates, and other parties that may or may not be legally entitled to know the content of health records. The HIM professional must have clear, precise policies written in strict adherence to current law.

Privacy provisions of the Health Insurance Portability and Accountability Act (HIPAA) apply to correctional facilities that are deemed to be covered entities. However, there are some special provisions of HIPAA for correctional institutions. See the discussion of HIPAA in correctional health care later in this chapter.

Correctional officers and administrative personnel sometimes pose a special problem. Health and legal professionals agree that inmate health records must be maintained separately from any confinement records kept by the facility. For the protection of the inmate and institution, correctional personnel should be prohibited from accessing the record. Statutory directives require reporting medical conditions to particular authorities and agencies, and these directives must be followed.

Using inmates to supplement staffing in the health services area may create additional threats to confidentiality and the safety of some inmates. Correctional organizations have standards that detail when inmates may be used as employees. The NCCHC, ACA, and AHPA standards all prohibit inmates from providing or assisting in direct patient care, determining access of other inmates to health services, or handling medical records (Anno, 2001).

There is no substitute for careful, thorough research. Policies and procedures must be accurate, precise, and current. Consents and authorizations make up a large part of the inmate health record. HIM professionals must be well versed in informed consent statutes and current case law, which differ from state to state and between jurisdictions.

Issues surrounding inmates' right to refuse treatment and consents by juveniles arise frequently. Forms must adhere strictly to legal requirements and should not be used without approval of an attorney. Correctional settings face additional problems of handling substance abusers and mental incompetents. HIM professionals must know the legal ramifications such conditions have on individuals' ability to give consent.

Administrative Information

During litigation, considerable weight is given to administration's ability to demonstrate compliance with institutional policies and procedures and monitor staff compliance. Well-written policies and procedures imply thoughtful and well-documented organizational philosophy. For any facility, well-written policies and procedures can help reduce training time for new employees and can reduce the potential conflicts resulting from a lack of clear direction.

The first step toward a complete set of policies is to evaluate what is currently available. The policies should be read thoroughly. It is easy for busy staff members to neglect updating procedures when a modification is necessary. It is even easier for badly written procedures to be ignored. Administration must be confident that the institution's policies are consistent with current practices.

Financial Data

Accurate financial data is essential in successfully managing correctional institutions. Because of the current methods of funding (i.e., taxation), correctional facilities have difficulty receiving adequate resources to meet escalating demands for health services. Careful, accurate documentation of costs and expenditures is crucial. Once allocated, funds should be tracked and reported regularly (Anno, 2001).

Statistical Reports

Health administrators require statistical information on health care activities for budgeting, planning, and operating correctional health services. Reports should regularly reflect the number of patients served each month by each of the primary programs and information on ancillary and support services. A detailed breakdown of specific activities enhances the utility of statistical data. Statistics for off-site contracted services should be reported and monitored regularly.

Logs, Checklists, and Inspection Forms

Developing tools to monitor and measure compliance is an important contribution that HIM professionals can make. Checklists may be designed to verify compliance with other policies such as routine equipment checks. Daily operation requires tracking of patients scheduled for sick call, chronic clinics, or those with appointments outside the correctional facility. Logs are important for documenting supply use and release of information requests for health records.

Reimbursement and Funding

There is no counterpart in corrections to the reimbursement arrangements that exist in other health care settings. Funding for all corrections-related activities comes from taxes appropriated by federal and state legislatures.

The management of health care costs is often more difficult for correctional institutions than for other health care facilities. Needs frequently exceed resources, even during initial stages of budget planning, if the legislature rejects the budget and assigns less funds, or during midyear because original estimates were wrong or conditions changed unexpectedly.

There are limited options for financing correctional health services. Potential sources include additional tax revenue available from the federal or state governments, payments from inmates, and private sources including grants. Medicare and Medicaid are not generally available to state prisoners. Medicaid may be available in some states during the time when an eligible recipient becomes incarcerated, but the funds represent only a small fraction of the cost of providing care (Anno, 2001).

Correctional institutions are increasingly turning to managed care arrangements as a method of paying for care received by inmates. Decision makers view managed care systems as a way to meet inmates' increasing health care needs while containing costs. Many states have contracted with private managed care organizations (MCOs) to provide health care for incarcerated individuals. An MCO that agrees to capitation payments based on the number of inmates in the system will have more incentive to deliver care efficiently than a health care organization that is paid on a fee-for-service basis (NCJA, 1999).

Charging inmates for health care has been hotly debated over the years and continues to figure as a prominent topic of discussion at many national association meetings. Those arguing for collecting fees from inmates cite the astronomical cost of correctional health care as a burden to citizens that should rightfully belong to inmates. They also cite overutilization of health services and malingering as incentives for instituting a fee or copayment structure. Charging fees or copayments based on the facility's economy is thought to control abuse of health services. Supporters also argue that paying for their health care forces inmates to become responsible for their health and money. Inmates who spend their money to buy cigarettes rather than save it in case they become ill will continue making the same irrational choices once they are released.

Critics of this issue argue that if health care is a right, all inmates should have access to services at the continued expense of taxpayers. Another argument is that basing copayments on a facility's economy will not even begin to cover the cost of health services. Payments may constitute a high fee for some inmates, while clearly not compensating the facility for the cost of care. Critics claim copayments or fees would create a tiered system favoring "wealthy" inmates (NCCHC, 1996). Opponents of fee-for-service correctional health care argue that the use of a clinically trained "gatekeeper" would help prevent abuse of the health system by malingerers without impeding access to inmates who need health care services (Anno, 2001).

The facts of **inmate self-pay** or **copayment** are illustrated in a 1994 survey conducted by the NCCHC. At the end of 1994, the NCCHC conducted a survey of 206 jail jurisdictions. Of the 117 systems that responded, 35 percent charged inmates for health care and 15 percent were exploring it as an option. The majority of the programs required fixed payments between $2 and $10, and every jail system made provisions for providing emergency services (*Correct Care*, 1995). A National Institute of Corrections Survey in 1997 found that 33 state legislatures had authorized imposition of fees on inmates for health services (Anno, 2001).

Information Management

Careful information management is essential to providing health professionals with necessary information on which to base their treatment decisions. In principle, health information management in correctional facilities is similar to that of other health care settings.

Data and Information Flow

External data is provided to correctional facilities from government agencies such as the Federal Bureau of Investigation (FBI), local governments, quasi-governmental agencies such as the Centers for Disease Control and Prevention (CDC), and health care facilities such as hospitals and community health clinics. Internally, data is collected by various departments during the performance of daily activities, special projects, internal audits, and so forth. Most data specific to health services comes from sick call slips completed by inmates and from treatment reports provided by health staff.

One of the biggest barriers to providing inmates with adequate health care comes from a lack of access to inmate health information from hospitals and clinics. Uninformed or misinformed staff often refuse to release inmate health records to correctional facilities for the continued treatment of inmates.

In most states, release of health information is ordinarily allowed only with the prior written consent of the patient. However, information may be released without prior consent to a health professional directly involved in the care and treatment of the inmate in an emergency situation or when the inmate is unable to sign. Health information management professionals must know under what conditions inmate health information can and cannot be released. HIM professionals working in corrections should develop relationships with other professionals working in facilities with which the correctional system might contract for services. Fostering good relations will facilitate the release of information.

Coding and Classification

Coding of diseases and procedures is not routinely done in DOCs, jails, or juvenile detention centers, but the FBP does utilize ICD-9-CM coding for tracking morbidity and mortality. Classification in correctional facilities refers to the categorization of offenders according to established criteria for making housing and job assignments as well as determining security status and developing educational or rehabilitation needs. Typically the criteria include age, sex, legal status (e.g., pretrial, detention, sentenced), and inmates' physical and mental health status (Miller, 1978).

Computer Systems

A fundamental challenge to corrections is the integration of twenty-first-century information technology into nineteenth-century organizational structures. The primary purpose of current organizational structures is to maintain the integrity and hierarchy of legitimate authority positions that give bureaucratic organizations their strength. These same directives, however, tend to inhibit the flow of information within the organization (Archambeault, 1987).

Consider the general steps that must occur in an effort to automate information systems. The first step is the transformation of data, often massive amounts, into usable knowledge. The second step is collection, encoding, and storage. Indexing, cross-referencing, and retrieval comprise the third step. More complex issues involve transforming raw facts into useful operational and management knowledge. All of these steps must result in easy access and rapid retrieval for the system to be successful. Information system integrity and security are also hurdles that must be cleared, as are careful planning and training of personnel (Archambeault, 1987).

HIPAA

As the privacy provisions of HIPAA were being implemented in 2003, many correctional institutions were still unsure of their status under HIPAA. A correctional facility that provides health care services and transmits health information electronically in connection with a standard transaction would be considered an HIPAA-covered entity. However, because many correctional institutions provide self-funded health care, they do not transmit health information in electronic form and therefore would not be considered covered entities. When a correctional facility is considered a covered entity, it may designate itself as a **hybrid covered entity**, which is an organization whose activities include both covered and noncovered functions. Any correctional institution that is deemed to be a covered entity would need to appoint a privacy officer, to promulgate policies and procedures protecting the privacy of inmate health information, and generally allow inmates access to their health records (Orr and Hellerstein, 2002). Correctional institutions are granted an exception to the access rule when such access would "jeopardize the health, safety, security, custody, or rehabilitation of the individual or of other inmates, or the safety of any officer, employee, or other person at the correctional institution or responsible for transporting of the inmate" (DHHS 2000, p. 82823).

Figure 6-4 provides excerpts from the HIPAA privacy rule that pertain to correctional institutions, inmates, and health care providers that work with them. For example, a health care provider may release an inmate's health information to a correctional institution without the inmate's authorization under certain circumstances. Furthermore, health care providers do not have to account for disclosures to correctional institutions as they do for other disclosures. However, when an

---

§ 164.512 Uses and disclosures for which an authorization or opportunity to agree or object is not required....

(j) *Standard: Uses and disclosures to avert a serious threat to health or safety.*

(1) *Permitted disclosures.* A covered entity may, consistent with applicable law and standards of ethical conduct, use or disclose protected health information, if the covered entity, in good faith, believes the use or disclosure....

(ii) Is necessary for law enforcement authorities to identify or apprehend an individual....

(B) Where it appears from all the circumstances that the individual has escaped from a correctional institution or from lawful custody, as those terms are defined in § 164.501....

(k) *Standard: Uses and disclosures for specialized government functions....*

(5) *Correctional institutions and other law enforcement custodial situations.*

(i) *Permitted disclosures.* A covered entity may disclose to a correctional institution or a law enforcement official having lawful custody of an inmate or other individual protected health information about such inmate or individual, if the correctional institution or such law enforcement official represents that such protected health information is necessary for:

(A) The provision of health care to such individuals;

(B) The health and safety of such individual or other inmates;

(C) The health and safety of the officers or employees of or others at the correctional institution;

(D) The health and safety of such individuals and officers or other persons responsible for the transporting of inmates or their transfer from one institution, facility, or setting to another;

(E) Law enforcement on the premises of the correctional institution; and

---

Figure 6-4 Excerpts from HIPAA privacy regulations concerning correctional institutions and inmates (DHHS, 2000; DHHS, 2002).

inmate is released from custody, he or she regains all privacy rights (DHHS, 2000; DHHS, 2002). With regard to providing inmates with a "notice of privacy practices," correctional institutions are exempt from this requirement. They should, however, make a good-faith effort to notify former inmates who have been paroled of their privacy practices (Orr and Hellerstein, 2002). HIM professionals can play an active role in implementation and maintenance of HIPAA standards by providing expertise and guidance relating to the privacy, security, and transactions rules and regulations.

(F) The administration and maintenance of the safety, security, and good order of the correctional institution....

(iii) *No application after release.* For the purposes of this provision, an individual is no longer an inmate when released on parole, probation, supervised release, or otherwise is no longer in lawful custody.

§ 164.520 Notice of privacy practices for protected health information.

(a) *Standard: notice of privacy practices....*

(3) *Exception for inmates.* An inmate does not have a right to notice under this section, and the requirements of this section do not apply to a correctional institution that is a covered entity....

§ 164.524 Access of individuals to protected health information....

(2) *Unreviewable grounds for denial.* A covered entity may deny an individual access without providing the individual an opportunity for review, in the following circumstances....

(ii) A covered entity that is a correctional institution or a covered health care provider acting under the direction of the correctional institution may deny, in whole or in part, an inmate's request to obtain a copy of protected health information, if obtaining such copy would jeopardize the health, safety, security, custody, or rehabilitation of the individual or of other inmates, or the safety of any officer, employee, or other person at the correctional institution or responsible for the transporting of the inmate....

§ 164.528 Accounting of disclosures of protected health information.

(a) *Standard: Right to an accounting of disclosures of protected health information.*

(1) An individual has a right to receive an accounting of disclosures of protected health information made by a covered entity in the six years prior to the date on which the accounting is requested, except for disclosures....

(vii) To correctional institutions or law enforcement officials as provided in § 164.512(k)(5)

(DHHS, 2000; DHHS, 2002)

Figure 6-4   *(Continued)*

Quality Improvement and Utilization Management

Over time, different terms have been used to describe the processes of quality improvement (QI) and utilization management (UM), but the basic purposes of these processes have remained the same. The goal has always been the constant improvement of the quality of health care services and the control of costs. Today the functions of QI and UM overlap considerably and are most effective when they are coordinated with one another and with risk management programs.

Quality Improvement

QI can be defined as a process of ongoing monitoring and evaluation to assess the adequacy and appropriateness of care provided and to offer a means of initiating effective corrective action when needed.

The infrastructure of correctional facilities in large part determines health professionals' ability to deliver quality care. HIM professionals can play an important role in monitoring and improving the systems, which support the efforts of health professionals by assisting with the development of the QI program and objectives, and defining the scope and process. Critical to the success of the QI program is the ability to monitor and measure the program's effectiveness and gain the support of administrators.

Services that are provided for the correctional system by contracted professionals, organizations, or other health care facilities should also be monitored. Maintenance of statistical and other data should be forwarded to the medical director and other appropriate authorities to determine whether the terms of the agreement are being met.

Accreditation is a preferred method of external review because it provides comprehensive, objective analysis of the facility's operations with a comparison to the facility's policies and procedures. The three accrediting agencies previously cited offer self-assessment and presurvey consultation services. After an on-site survey, the survey team reviews its findings with the appropriate individuals of the correctional facility. Finally, a written report is submitted to the correctional facility and to an accreditation committee. An accreditation committee makes the final decision regarding the facility's accreditation status.

Utilization Management

Utilization management (UM) focuses on controlling the use of resources by reviewing a facility's efficiency in providing heath care services. The objective of UM is to maintain quality while ensuring appropriate utilization of services. The UM program should be a component of the organization-wide QI effort. Accurate data is crucial for a successful UM program. A facility must be able to accurately determine the costs of providing care and assess current levels of utilization. Careful monitoring of staff time and supply and equipment costs must be done initially in order to establish a baseline figure for health service costs. HIM professionals should be instrumental in the development of an effective UM program.

Risk Management and Legal Issues

Risk management (RM) and QI share similar beginnings. Both existed in other industries before emerging in health care. RM used to be distinguished from QI by its involvement with financial issues, protection of assets, and limiting professional and general liability. The legal issues faced by correctional facilities necessitate the application of RM principles and techniques.

Risk Management

The primary purpose of RM is to protect the resources of the facility and its staff. The strategies of RM and QI may sometimes overlap. Generally QI focuses on aggregate data to identify patterns and improve care; risk management focuses on individual events that may involve patients, employees, or visitors. Correctional institutions are charged with enormous responsibilities of providing a secure environment for inmates and protecting the public, both of which expose them to substantial liability that must be managed.

When the Supreme Court required correctional facilities to provide health care to inmates, it immediately exposed the facilities to additional risk. One risk management tool that has been used by correctional facilities is the inmate **grievance process**. This process is similar to the incident report process used in hospitals.

Grievances identify and document areas of potential risk exposure and allow corrective action to be taken to improve operations and reduce the incidence of litigation. The major objectives of a grievance process are to (1) improve institutional management and problem identification, (2) reduce inmate frustration and the potential for violence, (3) increase prospects for inmate rehabilitation, (4) hold down the volume of litigation, and (5) promote justice in institutional procedures (Brakel, 1983, p. 118).

Common Legal Issues

There is no limit to the number and types of lawsuits that correctional facilities may be forced to address. In the realm of correctional health care, these issues will also raise significant ethical questions.

Inmate lawsuits take up a considerable amount of time and money. Even with grievance procedures, the number of inmate lawsuits continues to rise. Lawsuits brought by inmates claiming "deliberate indifference" to their needs are common in all correctional facilities. Defining deliberate indifference is a frequently and often hotly debated legal issue. Some professional organizations are arguing for a broader definition and others for a more specific and limited definition.

Forced medications is also a frequent topic of ethical debate in corrections. In some instances of general psychiatric emergencies, state laws allow the use of psychotropic medications without the consent of the patient. Accrediting agencies have specific guidelines for the use of such medications and clearly defined rules under which they may be used. Inmates' refusal of treatment is also a topic of concern for many professionals working in correction facilities.

Perhaps the ultimate ethical issue for physicians is judging inmates' competency for execution. Physicians vow to "do no harm," but some insist this situation places them in direct conflict with that oath. The remedy offered by accreditation agencies is to use an independent expert and not a health care professional employed or under contract with the correctional facility.

Other Areas of Risk

Correctional health care delivery systems are at risk in other ways. Care delivered by contracted firms must be overseen and constantly reviewed for adequacy by the correctional facility. Reporting to the National Practitioner Data Bank and monitoring credentialing are other issues correctional facilities must address.

Role of the Health Information Management Professional

HIM professionals will find their role in correctional settings clearly defined. They will be expected to manage the inmate health records as they would manage health records in any other setting.

Correctional facilities generate and receive enormous amounts of data, but relatively little data is being converted into useful information. Even less data is shared through automated networks and databases. Statistical information is routinely requested and used by a variety of organizations and government agencies, but in too many cases the collection and retrieval of basic data must be done manually. Correctional facilities interested in surviving despite dwindling financial resources must look to technology and effective use of information.

The existing databases that collect correctional information usually reside in well-funded federal agencies such as the National Institute of Corrections and the U.S. Bureau of Justice Statistics. HIM professionals can find the greatest opportunities for improving the management of correctional data at the regional, local, and facility levels.

In 1990, the NCCHC established a certification program to elevate the level of professionalism in the field of correctional health care. The program is called the **Certified Correctional Health Professional (CCHP) Program** and is based on a two-tiered examination. Correctional health professionals begin with a self-assessment exam to earn a basic certification. Then, after three years they are eligible to sit for a proctored examination to achieve an advanced certification. Although HIM professionals have attained the CCHP credential, the majority are nurses and physicians.

Another group that offers professional development and support for correctional health care professionals is the **American Correctional Health Services Association (ACHSA)**. ACHSA provides "education, skill development and support for personnel, organizations and decision makers involved in correctional health services . . ." (ACHSA, Online).

Every setting that provides health services, without exception, can benefit from the expertise of HIM professionals. Working in correctional settings will demand the consistent application of all the principles of health information management. Ethical issues are magnified by the politically charged atmosphere. A successful HIM professional must stay current on a wide variety of legal issues and must be able to support decisions with documentation from any number of sources, including the state and federal laws, court rulings, and guidelines published by professional associations.

Opportunities for careers in corrections will continue to grow along with the industry. Mandatory sentencing, truth in sentencing, and more restrictive drug laws will continue to add to the overcrowding of correctional facilities. Opportunities for careers in corrections will continue to grow along with the industry as long as HIM professionals exhibit a high degree of excellence and maintain their professional and ethical standards. Once employed, HIM professionals should make every effort to foster relationships with educational programs and publish their experiences in professional journals.

Research is another area in which HIM professionals can excel by taking an aggressive leadership role in the proper collection and use of correctional information.

Trends

As the correctional industry continues to grow, various professions will continue to define their roles within the industry. Technology improves the quality of life and allows health care professionals to be more productive by eliminating redundant tasks. Each new application of a technology creates opportunities for new professional fields. As new technologies prove to be beneficial, increased use will lower costs. Some states have implemented the electronic health record (EHR), which automates the operations of health information management in twenty-first-century correctional facilities. Corrections has seen the introduction of technology in recent years that, as proven in private industry, has become more affordable and accessible. One technology in particular—videotelemedicine—is bringing benefits of improved access to health services and cost savings to corrections.

Videotelemedicine has been used to provide specialist consultations to inmates in some of the larger correctional institutions, for example, in Texas and Wisconsin. Primary care physicians are on-site to treat most medical problems, but specialists are sometimes needed to treat more complicated conditions. By using satellite links and computer networks, specialists are able to provide consultations to inmates while reducing the tremendous cost and risks associated with transporting inmates to off-site health care facilities. The technology also allows remote areas to have more consistent access to specialists. An additional benefit is that the primary care physicians who attend the inmates during their consultations learn how to diagnose and even treat conditions for which they were not originally trained (D. Ferguson, personal communication, July 1996).

Videotelemedicine will not eliminate the need for inpatient care, and there is a distinct disadvantage to the specialist in not being able to touch the patient, but the programs currently in operation are viewed as highly successful. Currently Georgia, Arizona, Kansas, and the Carolinas are beginning to incorporate the use of the technology in correctional health care. HIM professionals can have a tremendous impact on the way technology is introduced and applied in correctional settings.

Summary

Corrections is a rapidly growing industry, and correctional health care is growing along with it. Working in a correctional setting creates exciting and challenging opportunities for HIM professionals. Correctional health care is a relatively new industry, and the roles and responsibilities for managing the information are relatively undefined. Bright, articulate, energetic HIM professionals can achieve any measure of success they desire while creating additional opportunities for themselves and their peers as the true leaders in health information management.

Key Terms

American Correctional Association   a professional association of correctional administrators, wardens, superintendents, and other individuals and institutions that promotes improved correctional standards and studies causes of crime and juvenile delinquency and methods of crime control and prevention.

American Correctional Health Services Association (ACHSA)   a professional association of health care providers, individuals, or organizations interested in improving the quality of correctional health services.

American Public Health Association (APHA)   a professional association of health care workers, administrators, epidemiologists, planners, community and mental health specialists, and interested individuals who seek to protect and promote personal, mental, and environmental health through promulgation of standards, establishment of uniform practices and procedures, and research.

Bureau of Citizenship and Immigration Services (BCIS)   a division of the Department of Homeland Security responsible for the immigration service functions that were formerly performed by the Immigration and Naturalization Service (INS).

Bureau of Immigration and Customs Enforcement (ICE)   a division of the Department of Homeland Security responsible for the border and security functions of the former Immigration and Naturalization Service (INS).

Certified Correctional Health Professional Program (CCHP)   a certification program for health care professionals working in corrections administered by the National Commission on Correctional Health Care.

department of corrections (DOC)   a division of state government responsible for the operation of prisons.

detainee   a person held in custody awaiting trial or disposition.

Division of Immigration Health Services   the U.S. agency responsible for providing health care services to immigrants and aliens.

Federal Bureau of Prisons (FBP)   a division of the U.S. Department of Justice responsible for the administration and operation of federal correctional facilities, including penitentiaries, prison camps, and metropolitan correctional centers.

grievance process   a formal, administrative process whereby inmates may file complaints against a correctional facility for review by a panel. Institutional policy, and sometimes state statutes, determine time frames for the review process, decisions, and appeals.

health services director (HSD)   an individual responsible for the administration and operation of health services within a prison system or DOC.

hybrid covered entity   an organization whose activities include both covered and noncovered functions under HIPAA

inmate   a person confined to a correctional institution such as a prison.

inmate self-pay or **copayment**   the practice of requiring inmates to pay a (small) fee for predetermined, nonemergency medical treatments.

jail   an institution administered by local units of government (i.e., cities or counties) with the authority to detain adults for a period of 48 hours or longer and for the confinement of adults convicted of misdemeanors whose sentence does not exceed one year.

juvenile detention facility   a facility operated by a unit of government for the confinement of individuals under 18 years of age.

National Commission on Correctional Health Care (NCCHC)   a national association that offers voluntary accreditation of the health services in correctional facilities.

prisons   individual facilities operated by a unit of a state or the federal government for the confinement of adults convicted of a felony whose sentence exceeds one year.

videotelemedicine or telemedicine   the application of videoconferencing technology where a video camera and monitoring system are installed at a correctional facility and a medical facility. The monitoring systems are linked either by telephone lines, computer networks, or satellite hookups, thus allowing videoconferencing and medical images to be transmitted and received by either site.

REVIEW QUESTIONS

Knowledge-based Questions

1. List the different types of correctional facilities.

2. What Supreme Court case established a "right" to health care for inmates?

3. What are the advantages of having a health services director (HSD)?

4. How do correctional facilities become accredited and what are the benefits of receiving accreditation?

5. What is the certification that health professionals working in corrections can receive, and through which organization is the program administered?

Application-based Questions

1. Explain the different arguments for and against the use of contracted health services and privately operated correctional facilities.

2. What are the factors that will determine the type of health services that correctional facilities may need over the next ten years?

3. How are correctional institutions affected by the Health Insurance Portability and Accountability Act of 1996 (HIPAA)? In what ways are they exempt from the provisions of HIPAA according to Figure 6-4?

Web Activity

Visit the Web site of the National Commission on Correctional Health Care (NCCHC) at http://www.ncchc.org and click on their "Accreditation" link. How many institutions are currently accredited by NCCHC? What other helpful information about their accreditation program is located here? Next click on the "CCHP Certification" link. What benefits are listed for a person who obtains the Certified Correctional Health Professional (CCHP) credential?

Case Study

It is your first week as a health information supervisor of a reception facility in a prison system. During your initial interviews with staff, you hear complaints of staffing shortages and poor relationships with other facilities in the system. There are so few trained medical staff that guards and some record technicians have taken on responsibility for documenting inmate histories. The medical staff know they are performing duplicate lab tests, but the medical records are not available to verify previous tests and corroborate inmate complaints. You also learn that several inmates are filing lawsuits claiming deliberate indifference because a tuberculosis test was not performed on another inmate who infected his cellmates after being transferred from your facility. Because the medical records are stored by the discharging facility, they are not available to the reception center when inmates are readmitted. You know by law the staff must complete a health status within 24 hours and a physical exam within seven days, but most inmates are transferred after four days, which does not provide enough time to transfer records. A cursory examination of the computer system indicates a lack of relevant data on prescription drugs, dates of tests, HIV (human immunodeficiency virus) status, and allergies, and therefore cannot compensate for a lack of medical records. The staff turnover rate at the facility averages 40 percent.

1. How will you prioritize the issues you identify?
2. What recommendations would you make?

References and Suggested Readings

American Correctional Association. (1985). *Jails in America: An Overview of Issues*. College Park, MD: ACA.

American Correctional Association. (1993). *Standards for the Administration of Correctional Agencies (Central Office)*. (2nd ed.). Laurel, MD: ACA.

American Correctional Association. (1996). *Directory of Juvenile and Adult Correctional Departments, Institutions, Agencies and Paroling Authorities*. Laurel, MD: ACA.

[ACHSA] American Correctional Health Services Association [Online]. http://www.corrections.com/achsa/index.htm/

Anno, B. J. (1992). *Prison Health Care: Guidelines for the Management of an Adequate Delivery System*. Chicago, IL: NCCHC.

Anno, B. J. (2001). *Correctional Health Care: Guidelines for the Management of an Adequate Delivery System*. Chicago, IL: NCCHC.

Archambeault, W. (1987). Emerging issues in the use of microcomputers as management tools in criminal justice administration. In *Microcomputers in Criminal Justice: Current Issues and Applications*. Cincinnati, OH: Anderson Publishing Co.

Brakel, S. (1983). Ruling on prisoners' grievances. *American Bar Foundation Research Journal*, 2, 393–422.

Bauersmith, J., and Gent, R. (2002). The Broward County Jails hospice program: Hospice in the jail. *Journal of Palliative Medicine*, 5 (5), 667–670.

[BICE] Bureau of Immigration and Customs Enforcement [Online]. http://www.bice.immigration.gov/graphics/index.htm [2003, March 23].

[BCIS] Bureau of Citizenship and Immigration Services [Online]. http://www.immigration.gov/graphics/homeland.htm [2003, March 23]

Correct Care. (1995, January/February). Legal issues in correctional health care to be addressed at national conference, pp. 1, 7.

[DHHS] Department of Health and Human Services (2000). Standards for privacy of individually identifiable health information. *Federal Register, 65* (250), December 28, 82461–82829.

[DHHS] Department of Health and Human Services (2002). Standards for privacy of individually identifiable health information. *Federal Register, 67* (157), August 14, 53181–53273.

Gannon, C. (1988). *Health Records in Correctional Health Care: A Reference Manual*. Chicago, IL: NCCHC.

Klempner, J. (1981). *Juvenile Delinquency and Juvenile Justice*. New York: F. Watts.

Legal Information Institute. (2002). Law about prisons and prisoners. [Online]. http://www.law.cornell.edu [2003, March 22].

Maguire, K., and Pastore, A. L. (Eds.). (1994). *Sourcebook of Criminal Justice Statistics*. Washington, DC: U.S. Government Printing Office.

Miller, E. E. (1978). *Jail Management Problems, Programs, and Perspectives*. Lexington, MA: D. C. Heath & Co.

[NCCHC] National Commission on Correctional Health Care. (1996). *Position Statement: Charging Inmates a Fee for Health Care Services*. Chicago: NCCHC.

[NCJA] National Criminal Justice Association (1999). Managed health care. [Online]. http://www.ncja.org/managedhealthcare.html [2003, March 25].

Orr, D., and Hellerstein, D. (2002). Controversy, confusion herald HIPAA. *Correct Care, 16* (4), 1, 22. [Online]. http://www.ncchc.org/pubs/CC_archive/hipaastudy.html [2003, March 25].

Posner, M. (1992). The Estelle medical professional judgement standard: The right of those in state custody to receive high-cost medical treatment. *American Journal of Law and Medicine, 18* (4), 347–368.

[USAIS] U.S.A. Immigration Services. (2002). General naturalization requirements. [Online]. http://www.usais.org/generalnaturalizationrequirments.htm [2003, March 22].

[USDOJ] U.S. Department of Justice, Federal Bureau of Prisons. [Online]. The bureau in brief. http://www.bop.gov/ipapg/ipabib.html [2003, March 22].

World Book Encyclopedia. (1996). Chicago, IL: World Book, Inc.

Key Resources

American Correctional Association (ACA)
4380 Forbes Boulevard
Lanham, MD 20706-4322
Phone: 301-918-1800
Toll free: 800-222-5646
http://www.aca.org

American Correctional Health Services Association (ACHSA)
250 Gatsby Place
Alpharetta, GA 30022-6161
Phone: 877-918-1842
Fax: 770-650-5789
Email: achsa@mindspring.com
http://www.corrections.com/achsa

American Health Information Management Association
919 N. Michigan Avenue
Suite 1400
Chicago, IL 60611
Phone: 312-787-2672

American Medical Association
515 N. State Street
Chicago, IL 60610
Phone: 312-464-5000

American Public Health Association
1015 15th Street, NW
Washington, DC 20005
Phone: 202-789-5600

Bureau of Justice Statistics
U.S. Department of Justice
633 Indiana Avenue NW
Washington, DC 20531
Phone: 202-307-0765
http://www.ojp.usdoj.gov

Centers for Disease Control and Prevention
1600 Clifton Road, NE
Atlanta, GA 30333
Phone: 404-639-3311
http://www.cdc.gov

Division of Immigration Health Services
1220 L St., NW
Washington, DC 20005
Phone: 877-353-9834
http://www.inshealth.org

Federal Bureau of Prisons
320 First Street, NW
Washington, DC 20534
Phone: 202-307-3198
http://www.bop.gov

Legal Information Institute
Cornell Law School
Ithaca, NY 14853
E-mail: lii.law@cornell.edu
http://www.law.cornell.edu/topics/prisoners_rights.html

National Commission on Correctional Health Care
1300 W. Belmont Ave
Chicago, IL 60657
Phone: 773-880-1460
Fax: 773-880-2424
E-mail: ncchc@ncchc.org
http://www.ncchc.org

National Criminal Justice Association
444 N. Capitol St., NW
Suite 618
Washington, DC 20001
Phone: 202-624-1440
Fax: 202-508-3859
http://www.ncja.org

National Institute of Corrections (NIC), U.S. Department of Justice
Information Center
1860 Industrial Cir., Suite A
Longmont, CO 80501
Phone: (800) 877-1461 or (303) 682-0213
Email: asknicic@nicic.org
http://www.nicic.org/

Chapter 7

Mental Health: Long-Term and Acute Services

C. Harrell Weathersby, MSW, PhD

Learning Objectives

Upon successful completion of this chapter, you should be able to:

1. Describe the various settings and caregivers commonly associated with provision of mental health services.
2. Evaluate the impact of state and federal laws and regulations on the treatment of mentally ill persons.
3. Describe the components of a "typical" mental health treatment record, both inpatient and outpatient.
4. Discuss current reimbursement issues related to mental health treatment.
5. Discuss quality improvement and utilization management within mental health facilities.
6. Discuss the role of the health information manager in a mental health facility.
7. Discuss the current state and use of computer technology in managing mental health treatment information.
8. Identify the specific legal and ethical considerations associated with the confidentiality of mental health treatment records.

SETTING	DESCRIPTION	SYNONYM/EXAMPLES
Outpatient Mental Health Facility	A facility where clients receive regularly scheduled outpatient mental health treatment	Community mental health center
Group Home	Residential facility providing 24-hour supervision and daily living skills training on a time-limited basis to prepare clients for a less restrictive environment	Halfway house
Personal Care Home	A permanent living facility offering some supervision and meals, but no training, for persons who are too severely impaired to live completely independently	
Psychiatric Crisis Facility	A facility for short-term treatment of psychotic symptoms in an early stage	Acute care
Inpatient Psychiatric Hospital	A facility providing long-term inpatient treatment for persons whose symptoms do not respond sufficiently to medication to allow them to live successfully in a less restrictive environment	Institution

Introduction to Setting

The principal setting for treatment of serious mental illness is the **community mental health center (CMHC)**. CMHCs are publicly funded entities established nationally by the Mental Health Act of 1965. This congressional legislation provided the initial funding for CMHCs on a gradually decreasing scale over a period of years, with increased funding from county and state monies intended to replace the majority of the federal grants. The community mental health system was conceived as the conduit for affordable mental health services to be provided to the public in much the same way that the state departments of health were established earlier to provide a broadly based health care system to all segments of the population.

Over time, however, this service system became increasingly focused on the more chronic segment of the mentally ill population, both adults and children. The increased need for a large-scale effort to provide supportive services for this population grew out of the discovery of **psychotropic medications** in the late 1960s, which reduced the symptoms of **psychosis** and disordered thinking. Although the medications were not universally successful, the majority of persons who previously had been doomed to spend their lives in mental institutions were rendered capable of living in community settings. There followed in the 1970s and 1980s a major push to restore to the community those patients who responded well to the new medications. The process of **outpatient commitment** became feasible, making it possible for courts to place persons in need of psychiatric care in outpatient programs with stipulations regarding taking medications and so on. This mass deinstitutionalization movement resulted in the downsizing of most large mental hospitals where people had been "warehoused," as lack of any effective treatment necessitated their removal from society for their own safety as well as that of the public.

The enthusiasm with which this medical breakthrough was hailed proved, however, to be somewhat premature. The medications often had rather unpleasant and in some cases dangerous side effects. Nor did they always work as precisely as had been hoped. Additionally, many of the persons discharged into the community had lived most of their adult lives in the structured environment of the hospital. They had little idea of how to carry on daily life within society at large. Consequently, many of them experienced extremes of stress that necessitated their return to the hospital. Or worse, they skirted the mental health system and became part of the growing homeless population that burgeoned in the 1980s. Although it is difficult to get accurate statistics because of the hidden nature of the homeless persons, it is thought that approximately 20 to 25 percent of the homeless population are seriously mentally ill (Burt et al., 1999). This group consists of persons who are unwilling to receive treatment principally because of the unpleasant side effects of psychotropic medications, or who are incapable of accessing the mental health system because of their disordered thinking.

To a limited extent, some private psychiatric hospitals also provide outpatient services, but seldom on the scale and of the variety that are offered by CMHCs.

A second site for provision of mental health services is the acute care inpatient hospital. The two types of acute facilities are short-term psychiatric crisis facilities and traditional long-term care hospitals for patients who do not respond to medication.

As the effectiveness of medication continues to improve, it has become less necessary in recent years for persons with mental illness to undergo long periods of hospitalization. Often during a period of florid psychosis, they are able to access short-term acute psychiatric care that lasts on average three to four weeks. Admittance to these facilities is either voluntary or involuntary, depending on the ability of the potential patient to recognize the need for treatment. (An **involuntary commitment** is a legal process whereby individuals may be admitted to an inpatient facility even though they refuse or cannot consent to the treatment.) These inpatient facilities operate in many ways similar to long-term hospitals. Most offer the same highly structured environment, with emphasis on group therapy and recreational activities, provided in the more traditional long-term facilities. As in the case of long-term hospitals, they generally maintain capacity for restraint and isolation in case of violent behavior that poses a threat to the patient or to others. Their chief distinction is in the brevity of treatment. Patients who do not respond to this type of therapy fairly quickly are usually transferred to long-term hospitals for involuntary treatment through the usual legal commitment procedures.

Types of Clients

Although there are some similarities between services for adults and those designed for children and adolescents, there are also some differences. As one might expect, the different points within the life cycle occupied by these two groups make for some fundamental differences in status, both legal and educational, and in life tasks. In some cases, the illness also manifests itself differently within these two groups.

Adults

The two types of mental or emotional illness that adults are likely to experience are temporary emotional crisis related to traumatic event(s), or chronic, long-term mental illness. Temporary mental problems result from some traumatic event or series of events in a person's life, such as loss of a loved one, divorce, or bankruptcy. These emotional upheavals manifest most often in the form of extreme depression and/or suicidal tendencies. In these cases mental anguish and sad feelings can be clearly traced to a causal factor that has triggered the crisis and that can usually be dealt with through counseling or at times with mood-altering medication that can aid in lifting depression.

Long-term mental illness, on the other hand, cannot be traced so easily in a causal fashion. Its onset is a result of chemical changes in the brain, which we are becoming increasingly skilled, with rapidly advancing technology, at observing and describing. We are unable, however, in general to say what causes these changes to take place. This type of mental illness is chronic in nature, in that it can often be controlled with medication, but it cannot be cured. This type of mental illness receives the heaviest funding and greatest research support within the public sector, based on the concept that persons with serious, persistent mental illness are those "most in need" of the insufficient resources available for mental health treatment.

Because there are many myths about this type of mental illness, persons who have it prefer the use of terms in describing the illness that are free of the traditional connotations that arouse pity, fear, or rejection. For this reason, they particularly dislike the use of *chronic* as a descriptive term. They prefer either *long-term*, *severe*, or *serious* as descriptors of the illness, with **seriously mentally ill (SMI)** being currently the most preferred epithet. They also favor what is known as "person-first" language, that is, "a person with schizophrenia" rather than "a schizophrenic," or "persons with **manic depression**" rather than "manic-depressives." This group also has a preference in terms of how they are termed as service recipients. Since the 1970s there has been a movement toward political and social empowerment of persons with mental illness as part of the campaign against public stigmatization. Most service recipients prefer to be known as "mental health service consumers" (usually shortened to "consumers" once the context has been established). They prefer this terminology over the more traditional "client" or "patient" (except in an inpatient situation or medical relationship, as with a doctor or nurse). They feel that these latter terms connote a "one-down" relationship and imply a dependency and inability to participate in treatment planning, as opposed to the suggestion of a "customer" relationship suggested by the term *consumer*.

The most common forms of serious mental illness are schizophrenia, clinical depression, and **bipolar disorder**, which has become the favored term for what has more widely been known as manic depression. There is another large category that encompasses persons with **dual diagnoses** (two diagnoses). These persons may be dually diagnosed mentally ill with developmental disability (mental retardation) or mentally ill with alcohol and/or chemical addiction.

Schizophrenia is a type of psychosis, a state of extremely disordered thinking, manifesting as a break with reality. Persons with schizophrenia are unable to distinguish reality from **hallucinations** or **delusions** within their own minds. Hallucinations are false perceptions of the five senses (e.g., seeing images that are not present, hearing internal voices, feeling skin sensations that are not the result of external stimuli, tasting or smelling things that are not real). Delusions are false ideas that have no basis in fact (e.g., belief that the FBI is pursuing a person, that food is being poisoned, that the person has been chosen by a supreme being as the recipient of a divine message for the world). The root causes for the chemical changes in the brain that result in schizophrenic psychoses are not yet known.

Clinical depression appears as a deep feeling of melancholy and futility that is not situational in nature. It, too, results from chemical imbalances in the brain that are stress induced, but the reason for this reaction to stress in some persons and not in others remains unknown.

Bipolar disorder presents a spiral of behavior that typically begins with an episode of extreme euphoria, which in its early stages may even be highly creative, but that degenerates into hallucination and/or delusional thinking. This phase is usually followed by a very deep depression, often reaching suicidal proportions, from which only medication can lift a person.

As indicated previously, there are two types of dually diagnosed persons within the mentally ill population. Persons with developmental disabilities may become mentally ill also, in which case they will carry a diagnosis of mental illness with mental retardation. The treatment modes for this group are largely the same behavioral shaping techniques utilized for the population as a whole. The chief intervention regarding the mental illness is administration of psychotropic medication. Because of the low functioning abilities that result from the retardation, persons with this dual diagnosis often have to be followed carefully to ensure that the medication is actually being taken and in the correct dosage.

The other type of dual diagnosis occurs in persons with mental illness and an alcohol/chemical addiction, often referred to as the **MICA (mental illness with chemical addiction)** population. This group is on the rise within the mental health system. Because of the wide availability of illegal recreational drugs, many young persons in particular begin to experiment, sometimes as a way to cope with the onset of the symptoms of the mental illness. Traditionally, there has been a battle waged between substance abuse service providers and mental health professionals as to who should serve this group. Consequently, members of this group have been shuttled back and forth between the two providers, depending on which illness was most in evidence at a given time, and ill served by both. There is also a fundamental difference in treatment philosophy between the two providers, which has further reduced the likelihood of successful outcomes for the MICA population.

Substance abuse service providers typically take a confrontational approach to the addiction, with the idea that the client must face up to the addiction before help can begin. This approach often produces negative results in dually diagnosed persons because of the low self-esteem and inability to handle stress that generally accompany the mental illness. However, there has been a tendency on the part of mental health professionals to ignore the substance abuse altogether, which is equally counterproductive to a successful treatment outcome. Thus, this group has tended to have a high incidence of repeated hospitalizations: People in this group travel the cycle from achievement of sobriety in the hospital, to resumption of drug usage in the community, to onset of a psychotic episode that returns them to inpatient care, beginning the cycle all over again.

In the past several years, however, there has been a growing trend toward melding elements of both substance abuse and mental health treatment modes that are designed specifically for this population. As this cross-training occurs, it appears that an educational model is emerging. This model eschews confrontation in favor of an openness to discussion of the nature of mental illness and symptom management that incorporates material on detrimental effects of substance abuse on the efficacy of the psychotropic medications. Concomitantly the persons with mental illness are repeatedly presented with nonconfrontational invitations, in both individual and group counseling sessions, to examine the detrimental effects that the addiction has produced in their lives.

The major symptoms for these types of serious mental illness, as well as less common ones, are described in the American Psychiatric Association's ***Diagnostic and Statistical Manual of Mental Disorders-IV-Text Revision*** (DSM-IV-TR) (2000).

In the 1970s, mental health professionals and politicians began to realize that deinstitutionalization would not work without **continuity of care**, with particular emphasis on providing a smooth transition from inpatient to outpatient services. What was needed was a service system designed to maintain mentally ill persons outside the hospital. This led to the establishment of the Community Support Program (CSP) at the federal level. This initiative originated within the National Institute of Mental Health (NIMH), the federal center at that time for research around mental health issues. This branch of the institute undertook studies of what services were needed to adequately support mentally ill persons who were attempting to live independently, and how those services could best be delivered. Concurrently, the federal funding streams for mental health were diverted to this population, as the group "most in need." Disability benefits were provided in the form of **Supplemental Security Income (SSI)** for those who had not been able to establish a work history, and as **Social Security Disability Income (SSDI)** for those who had sufficient investiture in the Social Security system to be eligible. Additionally, Medicaid benefits have been tied to SSI eligibility, and Medicare benefits are also available based on age or SSDI eligibility. Because these benefits are linked to diagnosis, documentation in this area becomes an extremely important part of the person's medical history. In addition to the medical diagnoses determined through use of the DSM-IV, federal guidelines have also been set up based on criteria of physical and psychological functioning. According to these criteria:

> adults with a serious mental illness are persons age 18 and over, who currently or at any time during the past year have had a diagnosable mental, behavioral, or emotional disorder of sufficient duration to meet diagnostic criteria specified within DSM-III-R [now DSM-IV] that has resulted in functional impairment which substantially interferes with or limits one or more major life activities. (*Federal Register*, May 20, 1993)

CSP efforts to determine the best practice treatment methods for the maintenance of mentally ill persons outside the hospital gave rise to some changes in the traditional methods of aftercare following discharge from the hospital. The older concepts centered on partial hospitalization, which provided a setting in which former patients could continue during the day with nonstressful activities similar to those provided during hospitalization, such as handicrafts, group therapy, and recreational activities. Over time this emphasis on maintenance gradually changed to a focus on rehabilitation, the concept of moving the mental health consumer to a routine more nearly in keeping with that of people without the illness whose day is devoted primarily to meaningful activity. Wherever possible, the goal here is to provide actual employment, even if just part-time, because work provides to the general population one of the most powerful of all psychological connections to the society as a whole. As such, it is a major source of self esteem. More recently, the term "recovery" has become preferred over "rehabilitation" as a descriptor for the periods of time that persons with mental illness experience when the illness is brought under control. This concept, borrowed from the treatment language for persons with drug or alcohol addictions, suggests a greater potential for long periods of enfolding into routine community life similar to that experienced by addicts during successful attainment of sobriety.

This change in vision resulted in part also from a growing demand by the consumers to have an active voice in the design and purpose of mental health programming. In time the concept of **psychosocial rehabilitation** arose. This treatment modality consists of an array of support services designed to meet the changing needs of consumers based on the degree of moribundity or floridity of their symptoms at any given point in time. Because the course of the illness and the medication side effects cannot always be predicted with perfect precision, it is essential to be able to individualize treatment plans with a great deal of flexibility. The system must be designed to meet the service needs of each person as his or her needs change with regard to more structure in times of increased psychosis or sensitivity to medication and less structure as he or she becomes more stable.

Figure 7-1 provides a concept of the ideal system of support services for the mentally ill (Parrish, 1987).

The variety of services shown that are outside the mental health system per se indicates the necessity for a holistic approach to service provision to maximize the time period that a person may remain in the community without rehospitalization. Within the mental health setting, the following options are generally considered core services

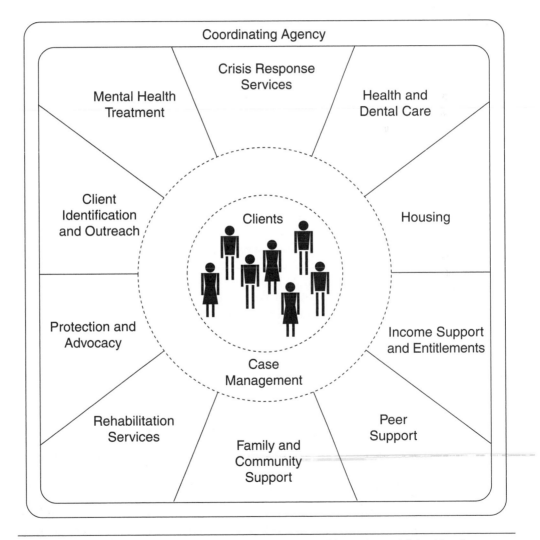

Figure 7-1   A client-centered comprehensive mental health system published by the National Institute of Mental Health. (Parrish, 1987).

likely to be needed by the majority of seriously mentally ill persons at some point in the course of their treatment (Stroul and Friedman, 1994):

- *Diagnostic evaluation and psychiatric medication management.* These services are provided by a psychiatrist, nurse practitioner, and/or nurse. If medical conditions unrelated to mental illness are present, the person is typically referred to appropriate medical personnel within the community for treatment.

- *Case management.* This service area provides linkage and brokerage to other services. Its primary function is to obtain access for the consumer to services both within and outside the mental health setting. It is thus the "glue" that provides coordination of support across the continuum and mitigates fragmentation of the service delivery system.

- *Day programming.* This area varies somewhat from system to system. The goal is to provide an opportunity for consumers to interact with both peers and professional staff. Some programs offer the more traditional partial hospitalization activities described previously. Others take a more rehabilitative approach, actively preparing and encouraging the consumer to move toward employment in the job market or volunteer work in the community and more independent functioning outside the mental health system.

- *Residential living.* This alternative is offered to consumers whose level of functioning has been impaired to the extent that they are not able upon remediation of their psychotic symptoms to maintain themselves initially in an independent setting. They are placed in group home settings (sometimes referred to as halfway houses), where they typically stay for six months to a year and practice such necessary daily living skills as cooking, money management, and personal hygiene. Acquisition of these skills will then allow them to function successfully in more independent settings such as personal care homes, where they receive some assistance with meals and medication monitoring, or in apartments or houses of their own.

- *Screening and evaluation.* Determination as to the need for short-term acute psychiatric care and/or recommendation to the courts for involuntary hospitalization is generally provided through the CMHC professional staff.

- *After-hours crisis services.* Emergency services for psychiatric crises are generally provided on a 24-hour basis through a system of on-call personnel. Where necessary, screening and evaluation for involuntary hospitalization can also be provided in this way.

Adolescents and Children

Approximately 9 to 13 percent of children ages 9 to 17 have a **serious emotional disturbance (SED)** with considerable functional impairment, and 5 to 9 percent have a serious emotional disturbance with extreme functional impairment (Friedman, 1996). A federal definition for this population has also been developed, as with mentally ill adults:

Children with a serious emotional disturbance are persons from birth to 18 who currently or at any time during the past year have had a diagnosable mental, behavioral, or emotional disorder of sufficient duration to meet diagnostic criteria specified within DSM-III-R [DSM-IV] that resulted in functional impairment which substantially interferes with or limits the child's role or functioning in family, school, or community activities. (*Federal Register,* 1993)

The first initiative to examine the extent of need for mental health services for this population was the Joint Commission on the Mental Health of Children in 1969 (Stroul and Friedman, 1994). As further studies were conducted and advocacy groups formed, Congress funded a federal initiative to address the gap in services. The National Institute of Mental Health (NIMH) established the **Child and Adolescent Service System Program (CASSP)** in 1984. As a result of the disbursement of NIMH programs in the late 1980s, this program, currently known as System of Care grants, is now under the auspices of the **Center for Mental Health Services (CMHS)** of the Substance Abuse and Mental Health Services Administration (SAMHSA), U.S. Department of Health and Human Services. The goal of the program is to assist states in creating systems of care for children and youth who have severe emotional disturbances. Since its inception in 1984, CASSP efforts to conceptualize and promulgate such a system of care across agency and service boundaries have been highly successful.

Core services needed within the mental health system itself were initially identified as follows (although "children" is used to describe the clientele, it should be understood to include adolescents unless otherwise specified) (Stroul and Friedman, 1994):

- *Early identification and intervention.* This effort necessarily crosses several service systems (e.g., health, education), but mental health has a role to play. The earlier identification of problems occurs, the better the chance for successful treatment. However, sometimes the problems or their seriousness may not become manifested clearly until latency age or adolescence. Identification of multiproblem families who seek mental health services, regardless of the age of the child, may be a first step.

- *Diagnosis and evaluation.* Again, this area may include several systems. It will usually include assessments of physical health, intelligence level, and academic achievement or potential; social and behavioral functioning; family dynamics; and environmental factors, such as degree of poverty and type of housing.

- *Outpatient treatment.* This intervention usually entails regularly scheduled appointments for individual, group, and/or family therapy, with a frequency based on need. Although there is some question as to the effectiveness of this type of treatment, some studies seem to indicate that it can be helpful (Sowder, 1979; Casey and Burman, 1985).

- *Day treatment.* This service involves an integration of educational and mental health services, whether established formally between agencies or not. Intensive treatment includes carefully integrated components of education, counseling, and family therapy and generally is provided during the school hours. Service provision may occur in a variety of settings, from regular schools, to special schools, to the mental health center. This service is much like the partial hospitalization program for adults, except for the usual inclusion and particular emphasis on the educational component.

- *Emergency services.* Crisis response is similar to that for adults, although somewhat rarer for children (Stroul and Friedman, 1994). Such services for children also may include runaway shelters and home-based services that are unique to this population.

- *Home-based services.* Other terms for this type of intervention include in-home services, family-centered services, intensive family services, and family preservation services. This category encompasses a rather wide range of actual services provided. The commonality among them all is that they are family- rather than individual-centered (Hutchinson et al., 1983), and as the term implies, the majority of the services are delivered in the home. Most of these programs have the following goals in common: "preserving the integrity of the family and preventing unnecessary out-of-home placement; linking the child and family with appropriate community agencies and individuals to create an ongoing community support system; and strengthening the family's coping skills and capacity to function effectively in the community" (Stroul and Friedman, 1994).

- *Therapeutic foster care.* This service "provides treatment for troubled children within the private homes of trained families" (Stroul and Friedman, 1994). It provides a homelike atmosphere in which treatment interventions can be applied. It looks similar to traditional foster care, but the families receive special training in how to cope with the extreme emotional disturbance that has led to removal from the family. In terms of removal from the home of origin, this setting is considered the least restrictive in the continuum of alternative placements because of its capacity to most nearly duplicate a home environment.

- *Therapeutic group home.* This type of residential setting involves congregate care somewhat similar to the adult group home. Some group homes exist primarily to serve less severely disturbed children who need care of a protective nature because of abuse or neglect. These children typically need a mental health treatment component as well as the highly structured environment typical of these programs. Generally, a therapeutic group home is defined as "a single home, located in the general community, that serves no more than eight children" (Stroul and Friedman, 1994). These entities can vary greatly in staff-to-child ratio, depending on severity of psychological impairment and intensity of treatment. Two distinct models of care are used. The teaching family model employs a married couple who live with the children in family-like arrangements, with relief help to provide time off. The other model employs shifts of workers who rotate to provide 24-hour care and supervision. Treatment approaches vary, but they generally include individual and group counseling along with a behavior modification program.

- *Inpatient hospitalization.* This setting is utilized in extreme situations. Children who demonstrate signs that they might seriously harm themselves or others are referred for hospitalization. With increasing frequency, as the home-based services become more generally available, such hospital stays are of short duration, usually a matter of days or a few weeks at most. Occasionally, however, there are situations where a child's difficulties are so severe that long-term hospitalization becomes the only option. This setting is also used for conducting comprehensive evaluations, particularly where the possible presence of neurological or other physiological complications may require extensive testing and observation over time.

As the core services have become more developed, a new concept, known as **wrap-around services**, has become the predominant method of service delivery for emotionally disturbed children and adolescents. Wrap-around services are community-based services that attempt to prevent the necessity for more restrictive levels of care. As the term "wrap-around" suggests, these are a comprehensive array of professional services that include the child's home and/or school setting. The essential features of this service approach entail individualization of services to fit the specific needs of each child and family; maximization of the strengths of the child's family and natural support systems as resources; and attention to the cultural values of the child's family and community in the way that services are developed and delivered (Furman, 1997).

As an almost necessary adjunct to wrap-around services, the notion of flexible funding has come into use. This concept allows for funding to be used for development of nontraditional services such as respite care, which allows for brief "cooling off" periods during times of high emotional crisis when the child can temporarily be cared for outside the home. Mentoring programs are another example of highly successful nontraditional services, in which successful members of the community are encouraged to volunteer as companions to troubled youths of similar culture and background, as a means of providing guidance and stability through the relationship.

Types of Caregivers

There is a wide range of professional and educational backgrounds and requirements for caregivers within the mental health system. With only a few exceptions, the types of workers providing both adults' and children's services tend to be the same. Likewise, the staff found in both the inpatient and outpatient settings tend to be the same, although their actual daily duties and responsibilities may differ in the degree of structure and control provided.

Medical Personnel

Because psychotropic medication is generally essential to the maintenance of stability in serious mental illness, the psychiatrist plays a central treatment role in performing diagnosis and evaluation and providing medication management. Many of the medications prescribed for this illness can have severe and in some cases fatal consequences if their levels are not carefully monitored at regular intervals. Dosages may also have to be adjusted from time to time because of increases or decreases in the amount of stress a person is experiencing or because of metabolic changes in the body over time. It is the role of the physician to oversee these matters. In most settings there is also a nurse to assist the physician, providing follow-up care as prescribed. These duties would typically include bloodwork and medication levels monitoring, provision of injections if the psychotropic medication is prescribed in this form, and assistance with minor side effects of the medication. Although somewhat less frequently found at present in the mental health field, there is a growing number of nurse practitioners who can, under supervision of a physician, perform some of the physician's functions, including the prescription of medication.

Therapists

This category includes a wide diversity of workers. It encompasses psychologists, master's-level and bachelor's-level social workers, and community counselors. Each of these disciplines has a certification mechanism at the national level, and most states require a state license to practice as well. Persons at the master's level or higher in social work and psychology are usually allowed to perform diagnostic and evaluation screening for mental illness. In some cases, this function is provided under supervision of a psychiatrist. In some states, psychologists have gained the authority to prescribe some drugs on a limited basis and with a physician's oversight.

Where short-term, situational emotional disturbance exists, the therapist, either bachelor's or master's level, performs a counseling function. It is generally thought that seriously mentally ill persons who are in a stable mental state do not benefit greatly from traditional talk therapy, and that in fact it may sometimes produce negative effects by increasing stress when discussion turns to unhappy events. However, one symptom of mental illness that is not always as readily apparent as the psychoses is called "poverty of thought." This symptom is characterized by an inability to generate alternative solutions to a problem. It is therefore sometimes useful to have available a person who can counsel with the consumer who is experiencing a current life crisis and cannot seem to find a viable solution. In some settings, the therapist will also conduct group therapy, especially where the traditional partial hospitalization model is used as a day care program. In the inpatient setting, group therapy is a standard form of treatment and is generally conducted by a therapist.

Case Managers

The case manager's credentials vary widely from state to state. Most possess a bachelor's degree, but there is generally great latitude as to the field of study. The chief responsibility of the case manager is to provide the consumer in the community with access to services across the spectrum of support services, as indicated in Figure 7-1. Thus the chief functions of this position are referral to needed services, coordination among service providers, and monitoring for escalation of psychotic symptoms. In general, case managers are prohibited from offering counseling and therapy, because of licensure and Medicaid restrictions. In rare cases, appropriately licensed persons are used in intensive case management programs that include a counseling component, where the target population is a small caseload (usually no more than 10) of consumers who tend to be high users of inpatient hospitalization. Persons providing the intensive home-based services to families of emotionally disturbed children would also perform many of the same functions as case managers for adults.

Aides

This group of workers goes by different appellations within the various settings where they work: direct care workers, residential living technicians, or certified nursing aides (CNAs). Their primary duties revolve around providing assistance with daily living skills to persons in the inpatient setting or in the community group homes. In each of these settings, 24-hour care and supervision are generally provided. Levels of certification vary, but generally a high school diploma or general equivalency diploma (GED) is required.

Recreation Therapists

Recreation staff is more likely to be found in the inpatient setting than in the community mental health setting, unless the program is conducting a partial hospitalization component. They are employed more often in the structured setting to provide an antidote for the lassitude that often accompanies the illness, especially in its acute state, and to provide activity and distraction, which generally ameliorate the psychotic symptoms.

Occupational Therapists

Occupational therapists typically work in the inpatient setting. They assess functioning abilities and prescribe programs designed to restore the patients' capacities to work, where feasible, and they teach daily living skills that will increase the likelihood of the patients' successful transitions to community living. They may also be found occasionally in rehabilitative roles within the community setting where the outpatient day program has an emphasis in this direction.

Regulatory Issues

The mental health centers typically receive certification from a designated state regulatory agency, usually a department or office of mental health. These agencies establish licensure standards and perform monitoring functions accordingly. As mental health consumers and their family members have become increasingly politicized in recent years, they have engaged in a steady effort to make the regulations for licensure more outcome based. The thrust is more toward measurement of quality of services than of quantity or frequency of delivery.

At the opposite end of the spectrum, the growing concern of politicians and the public regarding health care costs has motivated some states to move mental health services to a system of managed care more driven by economic concerns than quality assurance issues. The focus within a managed care system becomes the number and length of time that services are performed. This approach has been quite controversial when applied to the seriously mentally ill population because of the erratic and unpredictable nature of psychosis. The uncertainty of prognosis renders very difficult any reliable prediction as to the number and types of services a person may need over extended periods of time. Nevertheless, states have begun programs of managed care within mental health, with mixed results. Of particular concern to mental health consumers and their advocates is the tendency of managed care organizations to define narrowly the range of services that are seen as "medically necessary." This concept allows selective provision, usually limited to medication management during stable periods and hospitalization during psychotic episodes, rather than the full range of treatments and services such as case management and vocational rehabilitation options that are necessary for most persons with mental illness to maintain themselves in a community setting.

Several other regulatory entities set standards for mental health service delivery by virtue of their accrediting processes. A mental health service provider may seek accreditation by one, two, or all three of the following groups: The Joint Commission on Accreditation of Healthcare Organizations (JCAHO), the Commission on Accreditation of Rehabilitation Facilities (CARF), or the National Committee for Quality Assurance (NCQA).

JCAHO provides accreditation for both inpatient and outpatient mental health facilities. A facility licensed as a hospital is surveyed under the *Comprehensive Accreditation Manual for Hospitals (CAMH)*. If the hospital offers residential treatment, partial hospitalization, or supervised living programs, JCAHO conducts a tailored survey using selected standards from the *Comprehensive Accreditation Manual for Behavioral Health Care (CAMBHC)* in addition to the standards in the *CAMH*. Other mental health service providers that are freestanding (i.e., that are not affiliated with a hospital) are surveyed by JCAHO under the *CAMBHC* only.

CARF provides an accrediting process for mental health and psychosocial rehabilitation programs. Programs that can be accredited include case management, crisis intervention, outpatient treatment, partial hospitalization, residential treatment, community housing, inpatient treatment, community-based rehabilitation services, and so on. A mental health facility seeking accreditation from CARF would be surveyed under its *Standards Manual and Interpretive Guidelines for Behavioral Health* (Commission on Accreditation of Rehabilitation Facilities, Online)

NCQA offers an accreditation program to managed behavioral health care organizations (MBHOs). An MBHO may be a managed behavioral health care company or a behavioral health program or department within a managed care organization (MCO). At the request of an MCO or MBHO, NCQA surveys mental health services under the *Standards for the Accreditation of Managed Behavioral Healthcare Organizations* (National Committee for Quality Assurance, Online). Clinical services of MBHOs are also often accredited by URAC (formerly the Utilization Review Accreditation Commission), also known as the American Accreditation HealthCare Commission, Inc.

Another regulatory mechanism exists at the state level for both inpatient and outpatient facilities that wish to receive Medicaid. They must comply with the Medicaid guidelines set and monitored by the state agency designated as the regulatory body for this funding. Similarly, facilities that receive Medicare reimbursement must comply with the applicable *Conditions of Participation.* [Note: The "Interpretive Guidelines and Survey Procedures" for psychiatric hospitals are found in Appendix AA of the *State Operations Manual* (CMS, No date). These guidelines provide state surveyors with detailed explanations for interpreting and applying the *Conditions of Participation* during the survey of a psychiatric hospital.] Medicare and Medicaid coverage is tied to diagnosis and to a physician's prescription for the entire array of services to be provided as "medically necessary." Thus accuracy of documentation in this area is extremely important.

Documentation

There is considerable similarity among mental health case records, whether inpatient or outpatient, and other medically oriented records. Although content and arrangement vary, certain information is basic to all treatment of the mentally ill and appears in some form. These are assessment, treatment plan, progress notes, and discharge summary with plans for aftercare (Huffman, 1994).

Assessment

At the first contact between a consumer/patient and a mental health facility, an initial assessment is performed. This could occur in a telephone contact or in an emergency encounter. The initial assessment focuses on the patient's apparent needs and whether those needs can be appropriately addressed by the facility. In some instances, the result of the initial assessment is that the patient is referred elsewhere for further services. If it is determined that the patient should be admitted to the original facility, the initial assessment serves as a basis for determining which services of the facility are most appropriate.

The assessment process continues with the completion of the intake or general assessment. The mental health professional performing the intake gathers any remaining demographic information that has not yet been collected. A history of previous hospitalizations or other medical difficulties is elicited. If the consumer or patient is in a psychotic state, which renders him or her unreliable, the professional seeks this information from collateral contacts where possible. Regardless of the patient's mental status, some time should be spent gaining the consumer's perception of why he or she is present for the interview. If possible, the professional should determine the presenting problem from the point of view of the consumer/patient. It is important that the assessment be holistic in nature, so that possible physically based problems can be ruled out as contributory or ancillary to the interviewee's mental problems. For instance, diabetes can cause mania-like symptoms similar to bipolar disorder when insulin dosages are not accurate.

A complete assessment may include any or all of the following components: physical, emotional, behavioral, social, recreational, legal, vocational, or nutritional assessments (Huffman, 1994). It should also be noted that assessment is an ongoing process. It may often take several interviews for the consumer/patient to gain sufficient trust to fully state the nature of his or her problem(s). Also, these concerns may change over time, as some problems reach resolution, or in some cases, unfortunately prove to be unsolvable. Certain events or circumstances, such as the use of restraints or seclusion, a recommendation for electroconvulsive therapy, or a recommendation for a therapeutic pass, may trigger a new assessment. Most facilities have policies stating how often assessments will be routinely repeated. Comments from patients or significant others may trigger a new assessment at a date earlier than scheduled.

The *Code of Federal Regulations* outlines specific medical record requirements for psychiatric hospitals. One of these standards requires that each inpatient receive a psychiatric evaluation. The psychiatric evaluation must be completed within 60 hours of admission and must cover specific content areas such as medical history, mental status, the onset of illness, attitudes and behavior, intellectual and memory functioning, orientation, and an inventory of the patient's assets (*Conditions of Participation*, 2003).

Treatment Plan

Traditionally the assessment process has been a procedure by which the interviewer or team evaluates the consumer/patient's level of functioning. The problems have thus been defined essentially as deficits in functioning that need to be addressed in the treatment plan, with steps to mitigate or eliminate the problem outlined. As consumers have embraced the notion of empowerment, however, they have become more insistent on participation in the treatment planning process. Particularly in the outpatient setting, consumers have complained that the established method placed them in a position of inferiority in relationship to the interviewer and often resulted in a treatment plan in which they had little interest and no investiture. To expedite and encourage the consumer's participation, a strengths model of treatment planning has emerged in the community mental health sector. Using this approach, the interviewer determines from the consumer what goals he or she is interested in pursuing. The interviewer and the consumer then work out a mutual plan whereby the goal may be achieved. If the goal is a result of unrealistic thinking, the interviewer typically does not discourage the goal, but rather attempts creatively to find some facet of the goal that may be achievable. For instance, if a consumer sets as a goal the fulfillment of a lifelong dream to be a concert pianist, but has never had a piano lesson, the interviewer may suggest as a first step attendance of a music appreciation class.

In most instances, the consumer will recognize an unattainable goal, and the goal can be relinquished in favor of a more realistic one. At the same time, the professional's acquiescence to and participation in goals of interest to the consumer may open him or her to eventual consideration of goals that the professional may believe they need to work on together. If the consumer enjoys the music appreciation class, he or she may be more willing to stay on medication to avoid a relapse and the need to give up attending it. This model, and the underlying concept of client empowerment, is increasingly becoming the preferred treatment mode nationwide. A sample treatment plan form for case management using the strengths model is shown in Figure 7-2.

LIFE DOMAINS ASSESSMENT

Consumer Name: _____ Case # _____ Dx Code _____ Date _____

Admitted to Case Management: _____ Yes _____ No

Frequency of Contact: _____ High _____ Moderate _____ Low _____ Follow Along

_____   _____
              Consumer Signature   Staff Signature

LIFE DOMAINS	*CURRENT STATUS (Include Strengths and Barriers)*	*PERSONAL GOAL (What do I want?)*
LIVING ARRANGEMENTS		
Location		
Safety		
Adequacy		
LIFE SKILLS		
Home Management/Bill Paying		
ADL's		
Transportation		
Utilization of Resources		
SOCIAL SUPPORTS		
Family/Friends/Spiritual Interpersonal Relationships		
VOC/ED		
Education/Employment		
Skills		
FINANCIAL/LEGAL		
Monthly Income		
Money Management/Debts		
HEALTH/MENTAL HEALTH		
Physical symptoms/needs		
Psychological symptoms/needs		
Medication/Tx. Compliance		
Substance Abuse		
Physical/Emotional Abuse		
LEISURE/RECREATIONAL		
Exercise		
Recreation/Socialization		

CONSUMER STRENGTHS SUMMARY:

Figure 7-2   Sample treatment form for case management using the strengths model. (From the Mississippi Department of Mental Health.)

This model poses something of a challenge for health information managers, however, because it is not as easy to document progress using this model as it has been with the functional assessment approach. In using the older model, the professional typically identifies a deficit; prescribes a treatment solution and a time frame for success; and documents either a successful outcome, in which case the goal is eliminated, or a failure, in which case the goal is either dropped as unattainable or a different intervention strategy is proposed.

Although there is an increased attempt to involve the patient within an institution in treatment planning, the degree of the illness makes necessary the continued use of the functional assessment methodology to a large extent. The chief goal within the inpatient setting is virtually always stabilization to the point that the patient can be discharged into the community. Accomplishment of this aim often requires a highly structured approach to changing behaviors that are not contributory to that end. Therefore, the strengths model must be utilized in a somewhat modified form.

Progress Notes

Progress notes mark the achievement or lack thereof in the attempts of the consumer or patient to reach the goals stated in the treatment plan. Accreditation surveyors often check to see that every goal in a treatment plan has corresponding progress notes. There may be some general progress notes that do not relate to a specific treatment plan goal. However, most progress notes are tied directly to the treatment plan.

Progress notes are often also extremely important as documentation that a service was performed as a basis for reimbursement from Medicaid, Medicare, or client insurance. ("If it isn't written, it didn't happen.") As a basis for reimbursement, the timeliness of the note also becomes a central issue, as most regulatory agencies place considerable emphasis on regular intervals of review and updates of the treatment plan, which are also generally recorded in a progress note.

One of the advantages of a computer-based mental health record is that the documentation of progress notes can be electronically monitored. Some systems prompt the clinician with treatment plan goals when the clinician is writing progress notes. Some organizations prepare automated reports that indicate treatment plan goals for which no progress notes have yet been written. The same type of report can also indicate services billed that lack progress notes, or the reverse—progress notes for services performed but not billed.

For psychiatric hospitals, the *Code of Federal Regulations* specifies that physicians, nurses, social workers and others involved in active treatment of the patient must record progress notes. These standards require progress notes at least weekly for the first two months and at least once a month thereafter (*Conditions of Participation*, 2003). Because of the importance of progress notes to the care of the patient, to accreditation, and to reimbursement, there is great incentive in a psychiatric hospital to properly document progress notes.

Special Treatment Procedures

Certain procedures may be necessary in the mental health setting that may not be used in the treatment of other types of disorders. For example, a patient who is threatening injury to self or to others may be placed in restraints or in seclusion. Examples of other types of special procedures include psychosurgery and electroconvulsive therapy. When special procedures are used, proper documentation of their use is extremely important (Huffman, 1994).

The documentation regarding the use of seclusion or restraints serves as an example of the extensive documentation necessary when special procedures are used. Following a public advocacy campaign for stricter oversight of policies and procedures with regard to use of restraints and seclusion, Congress initiated an investigation of the use of these emergency safety interventions. Findings indicated an unacceptably high rate of death and injury to both staff and patients as a result of improper use or poorly planned procedures for implementation of these interventions. Accordingly, Congress called for stricter regulations governing the use of restraints and seclusion for both children and adults in facilities receiving Medicaid or Medicare funding.

As a result, the Centers for Medicare and Medicaid Services (CMS)—formerly the Health Care Finance Administration (HCFA)—promulgated the *Final Interpretive Guidelines for HCFA's Interim Final Rule, Hospital Conditions of Participation of Patients' Rights, June 2000.* These guidelines tightened considerably the rules for conditions under which these interventions could be used, as well as the procedures to be followed during use. Accordingly, documentation surrounding the entire event of the use of such emergency safety interventions—from the decision-making process through implementation of the procedure and including follow-up evaluative measures—must be very carefully done.

Restraints are defined as being of two types: physical and chemical. **Physical restraint** is described as:

> mechanical or personal restriction that immobilizes or reduces the ability of an individual to move his or her arms, legs, or head freely, not including devices . . . for the purpose of conducting routine physical examinations or tests or to protect the resident from falling out of bed or to permit the resident to participate in activities without the risk of physical harm to the resident. . . ." (P. L. 106-310, 2000, pp. 1195–1196).

Chemical restraint is defined as use of a drug or medication that is not part of a person's usual medical regimen that is administered to control behavior or restrict freedom of movement (P. L. 106-310, 2000).

The rules for applying restraint or seclusion require an order from a board-certified psychiatrist or a physician with specialized training and experience in diagnosis and treatment of mental disorders. Assessment of the need for such procedures must include consideration of all possible alternatives and rationale for the chosen intervention. At bottom the issue must be the safety of the patient. Such intervention must also be the least restrictive possible in order to achieve the desired outcome. Within one hour of initiation of such an emergency safety intervention, there must be a face-to-face assessment of the psychological and physical well-being of the patient conducted by a physician or registered nurse qualified by special training in the use of emergency safety interventions (*Federal Register*, 2001).

The new regulations emphasize in particular the issue of training for all staff who are involved in any way in the process of emergency safety intervention. Such training must be conducted upon hire and updated semiannually. Documentation of the type of training developed and staff in attendance at each session is required. Time limits for the physician's order for the procedure have also been changed: no more than four hours for patients ages 18 to 21, two hours for patients ages 9 to 17, and one hour for residents under age 9. Distinction is also made between time-out, which by definition implies that the patient is not physically restrained from leaving the area, and the more restrictive nature of emergency safety interventions, although staff is also required to monitor persons placed in time-out. In the case of minors, parents or guardians must also be notified of the intervention as soon as possible, and notification must be documented. During restraint, trained staff must be physically present and continually monitoring the physical and psychological well-being of the patient and the safety of the restraining device. Use of seclusion requires trained staff either physically present or just outside the seclusion room, continually monitoring and assessing the patient's physical and psychological well-being. Staff administering the procedure must document its use in the patient's record by the end of the shift in which the intervention has taken place. A physician or appropriately trained registered nurse must conduct an evaluation of the patient's well-being immediately after cessation of restraint or seclusion. Within 24 hours after the use of an emergency safety intervention, involved staff and the patient must have a face-to-face discussion. Within the same time frame, a second debriefing is to occur with all involved staff and appropriate supervisory and administrative staff. A chief topic in both meetings is to see how such an intervention might be avoided in the future. Staff must document both of these meetings. If a patient is seriously injured or dies during or possibly because of use of restraint or seclusion, the facility must report the incident to both the state Medicaid agency and the state-designated Protection and Advocacy agency by no later than close of business the next business day (*Federal Register*, 2001).

Additionally, Congress enacted the Children's Health Act of 2000. This legislation applied specific restrictions to utilization of emergency safety interventions with children and youth, particularly those residing in nonmedical community-based residential facilities receiving Medicaid. Most notably, use of mechanical restraints with children was altogether prohibited in these facilities. Also defined is the concept of "physical escort," which is contrasted with "physical restraint." Whereas physical restraint is defined as a restriction that immobilizes an individual or severely limits his or her ability to move arms, legs, or head freely, as defined previously, "physical escort" is defined otherwise and is permitted. The latter is defined as "temporary touching or holding of the hand, wrist, arm, shoulder, or back for the purpose of inducing a resident who is acting out to walk to a safe location" (P. L. 106-310, 2000, p. 1196). Distinction is also made between time-out and restraint. Time-out is described as a separation of a resident from his or her peers for the purpose of calming; most important, the separation is within an unlocked setting, so that no physical limitation is imposed.

A two-sided form, such as the one depicted in Figures 7-3 and 7-4, may be used to help meet these special documentation requirements.

Discharge Summary and Aftercare Plans

The discharge summary contains the reason for discharge, noting whether the person left in a timely manner or against program advice, and if the person is living in the community. Hospital discharge includes the doctor's orders certifying that the person is no longer a danger to self or others, and therefore ready for discharge. Although some hospitals have begun to make the determination of readiness for discharge a decision of an interdisciplinary team, the treating physician has ultimate responsibility for discharge. Documentation related to discharge summarizes what the goals of the treatment plan have been and the progress made. It includes linkages with other programs, including mental health, to which the person has been referred, any appointments that have been made, and a prognosis statement as to future expectations for the person's physical health and mental health. Other details documented in the discharge summary in a psychiatric hospital include the final diagnoses, medications and instructions, disabilities (if any), dietary instructions, and with whom the patient was discharged.

Although discharge summary documentation is important in both institutional and community settings, it is especially important to have it completed in a timely manner in the inpatient setting. Community programs often have policies that prohibit recent patients from participating in their programming until they have received the discharge summary from the hospital. There are several reasons for this policy. First, it is more difficult to assist with a treatment plan if the worker does not know where the potential candidate for the program fits on the scale of recovery. Also, the program workers are made aware of any special conditions or needs that were discovered in the hospital, particularly related to physical health needs. It is also vital to identify linkages for funding, such as supplemental security income (SSI) or food stamp eligibility, or to enter the community mental health system via an appointment set up before discharge. These continuity of care issues are of absolute importance in preventing immediate relapse and return to the hospital. How quickly and how well the former patient is reoriented to community living is a key factor in successful transition from the institution. The discharge summary, with its delineation of aftercare plans, provides community mental health professionals with invaluable information with which to assist in that process.

MISSISSIPPI STATE HOSPITAL
SECLUSION/RESTRAINT/PROTECTIVE DEVICE
OBSERVATION REPORT

Addressograph

DATE:	TIME STARTED:	BUILDING:	Explanation of initiation and goal for discontinuation of seclusion/restraint given to patient/significant other: Time: _____ Nurse's Signature: _____

TYPE OF BEHAVIOR WARRANTING SECLUSION/RESTRAINT/PROTECTIVE DEVICE:
☐ Agitated/Combative   ☐ Self Destructive   ☐ Invasion of Other's Personal Space   ☐ Other: _____
☐ Confusion   ☐ Threatening

CRITERIA FOR DISCONTINUATION: ☐ Maintains relaxed, non-threatening posture   ☐ Ceases verbal threats
☐ Can discuss alternative behavior   ☐ Agrees to follow plan for safety (Contracts)   ☐ Other: _____

PRIOR INTERVENTION:
☐ Time Out   ☐ Visual Contact   ☐ I:I Observation   ☐ Behavior Management   ☐ Medication
☐ Limit Setting   ☐ Family Participation   ☐ Supervised Physical Activity   ☐ Reduced Stimulation   ☐ Redirection
☐ Frequent Reorientation   ☐ Peer Isolation   ☐ Other: _____

TYPE OF INTERVENTION:
☐ Seclusion
☐ Restraint
☐ Protective Device
☐ Behavior Management Program

TYPE OF DEVICE:
☐ Restraint Bed   ☐ Helmet   ☐ Sleeved Jacket/Vest
☐ Wrist Restraint   ☐ Mittens   ☐ Papoose Board
☐ Ankle Restraint   ☐ Pelvic Holder   ☐ Restraint Chair
☐ Lap Belt   ☐ Jump Suit   ☐ Other: _____

CODE - OBSERVATION (More than one may be used)
1. Yelling or Screaming
2. Attempting Self Harm
3. Kicking
4. Threatening Violence
5. Mumbling Incoherently
6. Talking Coherently
7. Biting
8. Restless
9. Requesting Release
10. Sleeping
11. Quiet/Calm/Resting
12. Attempting Removal of Restraint
13. Other: _____
14. Other: _____

CODE - INTERVENTIONS (More than one may be used)
A. Offered Fluids **(q 1 hour)**
B. Offered Bathroom **(q 2 hours)**
C. Circulation/Skin Checks **(q 2 hours)**
D. "A, B, C"
E. Refused Fluids
F. Refused Bathroom
G. Released from Seclusion
H. Released from Restraints
I. Released from Protective Device
J. Restraints Reapplied
K. Did not meet criteria for d/c, renew restraints up to 4 hrs.
L. Other: _____
M. Other: _____

BEHAVIORAL CARE ONLY: Observation documentation required Q 15 minutes.....Reassessment for release/renew documentation Q 4 hours

	Initials	O	I		Initials	O	I		Initials	O	I
7:00 am				3:00 pm				11:00 pm			
7:15 am				3:15 pm				11:15 pm			
7:30 am				3:30 pm				11:30 pm			
7:45 am				3:45 pm				11:45 pm			
8:00 am				4:00 pm				12:00 am			
8:15 am				4:15 pm				12:15 am			
8:30 am				4:30 pm				12:30 am			
8:45 am				4:45 pm				12:45 am			
9:00 am				5:00 pm				1:00 am			
9:15 am				5:15 pm				1:15 am			
9:30 am				5:30 pm				1:30 am			
9:45 am				5:45 pm				1:45 am			
10:00 am				6:00 pm				2:00 am			
10:15 am				6:15 pm				2:15 am			
10:30 am				6:30 pm				2:30 am			
10:45 am				6:45 pm				2:45 am			
11:00 am				7:00 pm				3:00 am			
11:15 am				7:15 pm				3:15 am			
11:30 am				7:30 pm				3:30 am			
11:45 am.				7:45 pm				3:45 am			
12:00 pm				8:00 pm				4:00 am			
12:15 pm				8:15 pm				4:15 am			
12:30 pm				8:30 pm				4:30 am			
12:45 pm				8:45 pm				4:45 am			
1:00 pm				9:00 pm				5:00 am			
1:15 pm				9:15 pm				5:15 am			
1:30 pm				9:30 pm				5:30 am			
1:45 pm				9:45 pm				5:45 am			
2:00 pm				10:00 pm				6:00 am			
2:15 pm				10:15 pm				6:15 am			
2:30 pm				10:30 pm				6:30 am			
2:45 pm				10:45 pm				6:45 am			

MSH-31B

Figure 7-3   Front of Seclusion/Restraint/Protective Device Observation Report.
(Courtesy of Mississippi State Hospital.)

Pre-Seclusion/Restraint Search and Removal Of Items:

Items Removed	Description	Disposition	Initials
☐ Clothes			
☐ Belt			
☐ Shoes			
☐ Smoking Materials			
☐ Money			
☐ Other			

Patient Wishes Family/Correspondent to be Notified?
☐ Yes
☐ No

Date/Time of Notification:
Notified By: _____ _____ at _____ AM/PM
                    Signature/Title   Date   Time

Date/Time Released:
Date: _____   Time: _____ AM/PM

Debriefing:
What could you have done differently to have prevented/avoided seclusion/restraint? _____
_____

Do you feel like hurting yourself?
☐ Yes   Explain: _____
☐ No

Do you feel like hurting anyone else?
☐ Yes   Explain: _____
☐ No

Debriefed By: _____ _____ at _____ AM/PM
                    Signature/Title   Date   Time

Trauma Experienced?
☐ Yes   Explain: _____
☐ No

Treatment Plan Modification Needed and documentation of need placed on Accountability?
☐ Yes   Explain: _____
☐ No

First Name	Last Name	Title	Initials	First Name	Last Name	Title	Initials

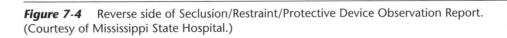

Figure 7-4   Reverse side of Seclusion/Restraint/Protective Device Observation Report. (Courtesy of Mississippi State Hospital.)

Reimbursement and Funding

The principal sources of funding for CMHCs are client fees, Medicaid, Medicare, and block grant funding for special projects. Client fees are calculated on a sliding scale based on income and account for a small percentage of the overall budget. The majority of the income for community mental health comes from Medicaid and Medicare reimbursement. Some funding comes from federal block grants, which is typically distributed through the state mental health agency to support special initiatives. CMHCs also receive a prescribed millage from the counties they serve. The great variety of funding streams makes for a complex billing and accounting system that could well become a specialized area into which health information managers might wish to venture.

The larger inpatient institutions have traditionally been supported for the most part by state funds, with a small percentage coming from patient fees. The trend in recent years, however, has been toward becoming accredited through the JCAHO. This credentialing leads to eligibility for the institutions for payment through Medicaid funding.

In 2003, CMS published a proposed rule to create an inpatient psychiatric facility prospective payment system (IPF PPS) for Medicare payments to both freestanding psychiatric hospitals and psychiatric units in acute care hospitals. Under the proposed rule, inpatient psychiatric facilities (IPFs) would receive per diem payments that are adjusted up or down by patient factors, such as the diagnosis related group (DRG), the patient's age, and additional comorbidity factors for certain nonpsychiatric diagnoses. In addition, the facility would receive higher per diem payments for the first eight days of the patient's stay. The proposed rule also included a Case Mix Assessment Tool (CMAT), a form designed to capture additional information about the patient's psychiatric symptoms, level of cognitive functioning, and ability to perform activities of daily living, along with limited information on services or treatments provided and diagnostic studies performed. Although the CMAT does not affect payment under the initial proposal, CMS plans to use this instrument to collect data for future refinements of the IPF PPS (Medicare program, 2003).

Managed care is becoming more prevalent as a payer. States have begun to contract with MCOs to provide mental health services for their Medicaid programs. Such a program may be capitated, meaning that payment is made based on the number of program participants in their service area. In other types of managed care arrangements, the MCO may authorize the number of services that will be paid during a certain period. This period could be six months or a year, or it could be defined as an **episode of care**. An episode of care involves a variety of services (inpatient and/or outpatient) provided by an organization to an individual during a given episode of illness.

Information Management

Beginning in 1975 there was a movement toward creation of a uniform, integrated statistical reporting system for mental health at the national level. In 1975, the Division of Biometry and Epidemiology (DBE) proposed the undertaking to create such a system

(Patton and Leginski, 1983). As a result, the **Mental Health Statistics Improvement Program (MHSIP)** within the National Institute of Mental Health (NIMH) suggested that the state mental health authorities work cooperatively with NIMH to create a broad-based data collection spearheaded by the state efforts. The goals were to be as follows:

> (a) Enhance state, local, and national mental health agencies' capacity to respond to local, state, and national needs for mental health program management data; (b) train sufficient systems and statistical personnel to collect, process, and analyze the data generated by these systems; (c) provide an ongoing cost sharing mechanism for the production of data required by the Federal system. (Patton and Leginski, 1983)

An ad hoc advisory group made up of personnel from local, state, and federal programs undertook the early work of establishing data sets that were widely accepted as appropriate and useful. Following the reorganization of NIMH, this initiative was placed with the Center for Mental Health Services (CMHS) branch of the Substance Abuse and Mental Health Services Administration (SAMHSA).

In 1984, the initiative received a second strong impetus with a mandate from Congress to create a system for data collection regarding mental health and substance abuse. Unlike the substance abuse system, where the move toward uniformity was translated into a set of federally mandated standards for data collection, the mental health system chose to promote guidelines rather than specific standards. Thus, participation in the initiative continued to be voluntary. The congressional directive led NIMH to publish the next year the *Data Standards for Mental Health Decision Support Systems* **("FN 10")**. This manual became the basis for all subsequent work in the effort to create a compatible data reporting system. It produced a significant impact on the direction and scope of the current thinking about mental health data, as it made a strong case for including more than just client service data. The case was made for expanding the data collection into such areas as finances and human resources as "auxiliaries" to the direct service arena (Leginski et al., 1989). The MHSIP/FN-10 initiative has since entered a second phase, termed Decision Support 2000+. Planning for this version includes incorporation of the Health Insurance Portability and Accountability Act of 1996 (HIPAA) regulations regarding confidentiality as well as other more recent developments in the field.

In order to encourage and assist the effort to establish the data system, the federal government provided approximately 30 three-year grants on a competitive basis. These were conceived as the first in a series of three such three-year initiatives. Hence, the project was envisioned as a nine-year effort. Decreased funding greatly stymied this progress, however, and the number of grants given each year decreased accordingly. Much of the early work that was accomplished was done through creation of task forces made up of a mixture of state and federal personnel working voluntarily. This means the project has remained alive and has made some progress, although not at the rate that was anticipated at the beginning.

A second grant initiative was begun in 2001, with awarding of Data Infrastructure Grants (DIGs). The first series of these grants was awarded noncompetitively in 2001. The goal of this initiative is to have all state mental health authorities enabled to report on tables of data—12 "basic" and 7 "developmental"—in their mental health block grant applications. This entire process is currently in transition, with the new terminology for the block grants being Performance Partnership Grants (PPGs). The guiding intention is that state mental health agencies and SAMHSA will collaborate on setting goals and reporting data that indicates where the state is using the PPG process.

Several other factors have also affected the move toward a uniform data system. In recent years, the cry for increased democratization of the mental health service delivery system has broadened to include the ways in which those services are measured and quantified. This movement has occurred within the societal context of the growing popularity of consumer service orientation in management. Such an information system would arise from an entirely different paradigm from the traditional collection and analysis of data, shifting MHSIP's present focus "from persons *served within* individual specialty mental health *organizations* toward *persons with significant needs* for mental health services and supports, *regardless of* the number or type of *organizations* that may or may not serve them" (Campbell and Frey, 1993). The emphasis would become one of identifying need across systems and organizations in a much broader context than just the mental health system. Obviously, such a system, where highly individualized data is being sought and shared in a variety of settings, raises special concern around issues of confidentiality (see "Confidentiality," later). Yet it can be done. South Carolina is currently the only state that has achieved creation of an information system for mental health consumers that reaches across agencies in this way.

The other, and quite antithetical, influence on current discussions of data standards and information systems development springs from the managed care system. Here, of course, the driving force is economic considerations. The emphases on fiscal responsibility and cost/benefit considerations of this model of service delivery place paramount value on the very type of data supporting organizational accountability that the proponents of "person-centered" information systems find unsatisfactory. The debate within the managed care camp has focused on use of outcome measures versus performance indicators. Outcome measures are more suitable to situations where an illness has a usual duration and generally ends in cure. Obviously, there is a measurable outcome in such cases. Because of the chronic nature of mental illness, it is difficult to measure outcome with accuracy. So many factors enter into the possibility of relapse that we are hard-pressed to say what particular factors prevent or produce recidivism. Nor can we always predict duration of a psychotic episode and its aftermath, much less the long-term prognosis of the illness. For these reasons there is a strong belief among mental health professionals that a much more accurate way of measuring success is by using performance indicators. Such indicators focus on consumer satisfaction with services delivered, rather than treatment outcomes. To some extent this approach also bows in the direction of consumer empowerment, as it provides a vehicle by which the consumer can register his or her satisfaction or unhappiness with the mental health system.

Data and Information Flow

Intake procedures vary within the community mental health system. Because of staff constraints, few CMHCs are able to take walk-ins except those in emergency situations, usually defined as persons in need of inpatient commitment as a danger to self or others. Typically, applications are received and screened as to the seriousness of the case, and appointments are established, including an appointment with a psychiatrist if it is clear from the application that one is needed for medication issues. Priority is generally given to persons who have been discharged from inpatient care; these appointments are generally set up by the social worker at the institution before the person's discharge.

A file for recording service delivery, billing data, and other pertinent information is usually established just before the intake interview. Intake provides an opportunity to gather additional demographic information not included or unclear on the application form. Assessment is conducted and an initial plan of treatment is agreed on by consumer and therapist, with the understanding that it can be modified as needed as the treatment progresses. If necessary, an appointment is made to see a psychiatrist for possible medication. If appropriate, other services are offered, such as participation in the case management program; attendance at a day program; either psychosocial rehabilitation aimed at vocational opportunity or partial hospitalization; and/or placement in a group home designed to increase daily living skills for a more independent living arrangement in the future. In most cases, these services will be paid for by Medicaid and/or Medicare, so the psychiatrist will need to certify under signature that they are "needed services." From this point, the course of treatment becomes individualized, based on the consumer's needs and preferences as to the services available.

There is no universal standard for content or order of arrangement of information in the consumer's file. (See Figure 7-5 for sample items from a large psychiatric hospital.) If the services are offered in a satellite office, the essential, most up-to-date information will, quite naturally, be contained in the record on that site. Some CMHCs have a central file for all clients in their main office, with copies of material sent periodically from the satellite file for inclusion in the central record. Others have only the one record at the satellite office. Billing information, in particular reporting of units of service (15-minute increments in the case of Medicaid) provided, is contained in the record. Surveyors and auditors are thus able to match billing information with documentation of service delivery in the progress notes section of the record.

Voluntary admission to the hospital, which has become a rare phenomenon in recent years, would follow much the same process as that for admission for treatment in the community. The documentation process for involuntary admission to the inpatient facility begins, of course, with the information assembled during the commitment proceedings, from screening and evaluation through the legal order of commitment. This data usually arrives with the patient. It typically becomes the responsibility of the institutional social worker to assemble and augment the information received by performing a social history, including contact with family members whenever possible. In most inpatient settings the patient's treatment plan is developed by an interdisciplinary team that usually includes at least a psychiatrist, a nurse, a psychologist, and

Identification and Personal Data
  Demographic Data
  Legal Status (commitment vs. voluntary
    admission)

Physician's Orders

Treatment Plan and Behavioral Documentation
  Treatment Plan
  Treatment Plan Update/Review Note
  Anger Management Assessment
  Psychiatric Intervention History
  Patient/Family Education Record
  Individual Patient Schedule
  Behavior Modification Plan

Progress Notes, including…
  Initial Integrated Summary
  Admission Note
  Transfer Notes
  Elopement Notes
  Diagnostic Summary or Addendum to
    Diagnostic Summary
  Audiology Alert Sheet
  Discharge Summary

Nurses' Notes, including…
  Nursing Assessment
  Child/Adolescent Addendum
  Abnormal Involuntary Movements
  Fall Assessment
  Nursing Discharge Summary

Medication Records
  Monthly Medication Administration Records
    (MARs)
  Monthly PRN medications
  Medication Information Documentation
    Form
  Specialized medication records (for example,
    for patients with diabetes mellitus)

Other Health Records
  Vital Signs Record
  Menstrual Record
  Intake/Output
  Fluid Accountability Record

Other Health Records *(continued)*
  Seizure Record
  Immunization and TB Record
  Summary of Ambulatory Visits
  Outpatient Procedure Report

Ancillary Services
  Lab Reports
  X-ray Reports
  EKG

Consultations
  Medical
  CT Scans
  EEG
  Outpatient Unscheduled Visit

Physical Exam

Alcohol and Drug Abuse Needs
  Assessment/Aftercare Plan

Psychology
  Psychology General Assessment
  Psychology Progress Notes
  Psychological Evaluation

Social Service
  Social Service Assessment/Plan
  Social Service Clinical Progress Notes
  Spiritual Assessment
  Social History

Dietary
  Nutritional Assessment
  Dietary Clinical Progress Notes

Pharmacy Medication Review

Activities
  Therapeutic Recreation Assessment
  Rehab Clinical Progress Notes
  Leisure Assessment

Rehabilitation
  Rehabilitation Services Screening Assessment
  Rehabilitation Clinical Progress Notes

Figure 7-5   Examples of items that may be found in the records of a large psychiatric hospital. (Excerpted and adapted from procedures of Mississippi State Hospital, Whitfield, MS. Used with permission.)

Rehabilitation *(continued)*
  Restorative Therapy Note
  Physical Therapy Evaluation Report
  Kinesiotherapy Evaluation Report
  Occupational Therapy Evaluation
  Feeding Evaluation
  Upper Extremity Evaluation
  Splint Information
  Speech, Language, Pathology Assessment
  Dysphagia Assessment

Education
  Education Clinical Progress Notes
  Patient Education Progress Report
  Psychosocial Education Program
  Functional Needs Assessment
  Psychosocial Education Program
  Art Assessment
  Music Evaluation
  Hearing and Vision Screening Results

Dental
  Dental Record
  Dental Treatment Plan

Residential Living
  Patient Care Flow Sheet
  Patient Observation Reports

Legal
  Advance Directives
  Admission Checklist
  Patient's Rights Statement

Legal *(continued)*
  Smoking Policy
  Ethics Fact Sheet
  Notice of Privacy Practices
  Consent Forms
  Contraband Search, Seizure, Disposition
  Admission Papers (Commitment orders)
  Legal Guardianship
  Legal Correspondence

Miscellaneous
  Visitors' Permits
  Patient Transfer Form
  Transfer and Referral Form
  Patient's Valuable Form
  Missing Patient Reports
  Hearing Reports
  Patient's Pass/Discharge Record
  Pass Evaluation Checklist
  Vocational Rehab
  Sheltered Workshop forms
  Work Opportunity forms
  Transitional Living Forms and Progress
    Reports

Electroconvulsive Therapy (ECT)
  ECT Checklist
  Progress Report
  Anesthesia Record
  Electroconvulsive Nursing Care Plans
  Consent for ECT
  Referral for ECT

Figure 7-5   *(Continued)*

a social worker. The patient is encouraged to participate in the planning to whatever extent possible. An attempt is made to provide a highly structured atmosphere, as activity often alleviates the psychotic symptoms and the debilitating side effects of some of the medications. Progress notes are entered into the case file by the various disciplines in the same way that persons are followed in the outpatient setting. The team meets periodically and decides whether the patient's condition indicates long-term hospitalization or whether progress is being made toward release. The social worker usually begins to develop a tentative discharge plan very early in treatment so that the necessary steps are in place when the time comes to put them into action. As the actual time of discharge nears, the social worker takes steps to ensure continuity of care beyond the hospital. These steps include at a minimum assurance of housing, establishment of monetary benefits if the patient is eligible, and contact with the community mental health system to set up an initial appointment.

Coding and Classification

Behavioral health organizations use a variety of coding systems. The system used will depend on the purpose of coding and other factors. Psychiatric diagnoses are commonly coded using the *Diagnostic and Statistical Manual of Mental Disorders, Fourth Edition (DSM-IV)*, published by the American Psychiatric Association. DSM-IV provides not only a classification system but also diagnostic criteria to assist clinicians in making psychiatric diagnoses. The latest revision of *DSM-IV* is the *Diagnostic and Statistical Manual of Mental Disorders, Fourth Edition, Text Revision (DSM-IV-TR)*. *DSM-IV-TR* provided mostly textual changes and did not significantly alter the system of codes. More information on the structure and utilization of *DSM-IV* may be found in Chapter 8.

For billing purposes, behavioral health organizations submitting electronic bills must use the HIPAA standard code sets, which do not include *DSM-IV*. Therefore *ICD-9-CM* and *CPT/HCPCS* codes are used as appropriate.

Data Sets

Although considerable work has been done at the federal level of the mental health system to develop standardized data collection procedures, there is currently no strong legal mandate for their use. Use of the DIG tables is currently considered voluntary. Language in the PPG indicates that the concept of penalties traditionally used in the block grants (10 percent of funding to be withheld for failure to meet plan objectives) may be removed. The emphasis has been on producing guidelines for the development of relevant data standards, rather than promulgation of a uniform system of data fields and collection procedures. In part the reluctance to mandate uniformity has stemmed from the enormous impact of the consumer empowerment movement, which changed not only the programming for service delivery but also the perception of what constitutes success in the rendering of those services.

The absence of such a uniform data system has encouraged the development within the private sector of numerous software vendors who specifically target the CMHCs for marketing of programs designed to capture data related to mental health service delivery. There is also some targeting of inpatient hospitals, but the software tends to be considerably more expensive for these institutions, so that the inpatient market consists more of private hospitals for whom information management is linked to profit, making such expenditures more immediately justifiable.

An innovation of interest in information management is relational database technology. This method of data storage and retrieval, based on set theory, allows for tremendous expansion of the number of fields that can be stored. For example, the consumer's file may allow storage of only two diagnoses. If there is a third diagnosis, in the past there has been no way of including this data. The relational database system allows for the storage of a table of diagnoses that can be linked to fields in the consumer's individual file. In this way, the amount of data that can be retrieved is greatly increased. Another innovation is relational and object-oriented technology, which links graphics, video segments, or portions of taped interviews to the service recipient's file, using the same methodology described previously. In this way, information other than what is written can be retrieved by virtue of the identifier that is attached to the file containing the audio/visual or other media, without having to be stored within the consumer's file.

As previously mentioned, the data elements of the FN-10 have served as the foundation for standardized data collection efforts for mental health since their publication in 1989. As a part of the Decision Support 2000+ initiative, the FN-11 workgroup began revising the FN-10 in 1997. The data elements included in the draft of the FN-11 data set are summarized in Figure 7-6 (MHSIP, 1998).

Type of Data Element	Number of Data Elements
Client Master Data	9
Client Eligibility Data	5
Client Periodic Data	23
Encounter Data	16
Provider/Organization Data	4
Provider/Organization Periodic Data	3
Human Resources Data	15
Financial Data	16

Figure 7-6　Types of elements included in the September 3, 1998 draft of the FN-11 data set (MHSIP, 1998).

Quality Improvement and Utilization Management

The mental health field has been at least as susceptible as other segments of our society to the current focus on total quality management (TQM), or its more recent manifestation as **continuous quality improvement (CQI)**. The focus that both of these management techniques place on customer satisfaction and sharing of decision-making power between administrative and line staff make a natural fit with the mental health consumer movement toward empowerment. These concepts have been for the most part well accepted by now and in general incorporated into both the outpatient and the inpatient systems of care. Client-centered approaches permeate the mental health system, affecting all aspects of service delivery, from programming that encourages self-determination, emphasizing consumer strengths rather than functional deficits, to data collection that focuses on client satisfaction and feedback mechanisms. The Joint Commission on Accreditation of Healthcare Organizations (JCAHO) has added an impetus to the incorporation of CQI into the management structure of inpatient facilities by adopting its principles as one of the standards by which it provides accreditation. Because this accreditation is generally accepted by major funding sources such as Medicare and Medicaid, it is frequently sought after by the inpatient facilities.

Utilization management has led over the years to the downsizing of large public mental institutions. The move to deinstitutionalization, while resulting in part from the improvement in stabilization through medication, has also been driven in part by economic considerations. It has proved much less expensive, generally speaking, to maintain consumers in the community with a variety of support services than to keep them in the hospital, with its more costly medical orientation. Because the funding from the hospitals did not always follow the consumer to the community, however, some would argue that the consumers have received uneven and often inadequate support outside the hospital. Thus, the lowered cost of community services may in part be a reflection of the inadequate funding that may deprive its customers of a decent quality of life, and in this sense be somewhat deceptive as to what the actual costs ought to be.

In both the outpatient and inpatient settings, steps have been taken to further reduce costs. Many CMHCs have created a staff position that serves as the "single point of entry" (SPOE) for emergency hospitalization in either the acute care psychiatric units or the long-term institution. Data is sometimes gathered regarding high users of inpatient services, with an eye to providing more or different supports to those who fall into this category. Bed allocation is a further device, particularly within institutions, to encourage utilization of community resources to the fullest before resorting to hospitalization. This method assigns beds on a regional basis using formulas that take into account such factors as total population and past usage of the facility. Then a certain amount of "borrowing" of beds among regions is allowed to take care of emergencies.

Risk Management and Legal Issues

Risk management as an organized program exists more frequently in the inpatient than in the outpatient treatment sector. The function of this program is to predict and thereby reduce or eliminate sources of likely injury and accident or of other potential financial loss to the institution. Such responsibility obviously includes avoidance of litigation, which leads to involvement in treatment issues that carry a high risk of violation of patients' rights, such as use of restraints, informed consent regarding administration of medications, and timely discharge when stabilization has occurred. Additionally, protection of confidentiality is of particular importance, especially since implementation of the Health Information and Portability Act (HIPAA) regulations in April 2003. (See Chapter 1, "Introduction," for details regarding HIPAA.) This concern has direct impact on the duties of the health information manager, who has ultimate responsibility for protection of such information.

Confidentiality

Patient information in mental health settings has always been highly confidential. It was more restricted than other types of medical information until passage of HIPAA, which tightened restrictions on all types of medical information and brought confidentiality more in line with practices already largely in place within mental health. For example, before HIPAA, in settings outside mental health, information such as patient name and dates of service was considered nonconfidential and could be disclosed in the absence of a specific request by the patient to prohibit disclosure (Huffman, 1994). However, in mental health facilities, such information has traditionally been legally protected; even acknowledging that a patient has been treated at a facility has been considered a breach of confidentiality. Mental health facilities have always placed great emphasis on strictest confidentiality, and long before HIPAA have generally required all employees and vendors to sign confidentiality agreements prohibiting staff and vendors alike from disclosing any information regarding patients who have been treated at the facility.

HIPAA provides a greater degree of protection to psychotherapy notes than to other types of protected health information. The use or disclosure of psychotherapy notes requires a valid authorization, even for treatment, payment, or health care operations, with the following exceptions: (1) the originator of the notes may use them for continuing treatment; (2) students, trainees, or practitioners may use psychotherapy notes in supervised mental health training programs; (3) the covered entity may use the notes when necessary to defend itself in a legal action brought by the individual; and (4) notes may be used as needed for health oversight activities or other activities as required by law (Standards for privacy of individually identifiable health information, 2002).

As a general rule, the mental health consumer's right to strictest confidentiality regarding matters of illness and treatment is carefully guarded. Legal protections of this right have been enacted legislatively in every state as well as at the federal level. Traditionally the relationship of mental health professionals to the consumer/patient has been considered privileged in the same way as that of lawyer to client or priest to confessing parishioner. The only way in which such information could be released has been through a formal, documented procedure whereby the consumer, patient, or patient's guardian provided written consent. Even where consent has been granted, constraints have been placed on the specific type of information to be released, the exact recipient of the information, and a stated limit on the duration of time for such release of information.

Although these strictures continue to hold true in general, certain court decisions in recent years have somewhat eroded the concept of near absolute confidentiality. Perhaps the most profound impact on the traditional notion of the inviolability of the therapist/client relationship has been the emergence of the concept of **"duty to warn."** This idea stems from a 1976 court decision *(Tarasoff v. Regents of the University of California)*, which held that a therapist has an obligation to warn persons against whom their clients make threatening statements, regardless of the fact that such threats are made within a privileged context. The theory behind the decision appears to be that safety from violent assault outweighs the breach of confidentiality and the risk of erroneous warnings. Since this court decision, there has been a trend to legislate "duty to warn" clauses into the states' laws regarding confidentiality.

There are other instances where case information may be required, such as in determining client eligibility for benefits, but these vary somewhat from state to state. Frequently the courts will accept release of a summary of the case record along with specific sections that pertain directly to the legal questions of the case. In cases where specific designation of information to be released is not provided by the court, responsibility for such summaries and/or selections of pertinent material will most often fall to the information manager, with possible collaboration with risk management and/or legal counsel staff.

Technological advances have also complicated the maintenance of confidentiality. Organizations must take an aggressive approach to security to protect information stored on computers from mischievous or malicious "hackers." Widespread use of facsimile (fax) machines has likewise created a potential source of information leakage, through human error of misdialing the correct fax machine number or through machine malfunction, in either case resulting in transmission of confidential information to unintended recipients. In a study undertaken at the request of the National Library of Medicine, the National Research Council recommended that efforts to protect patient privacy focus on the potential of computer-based patient records to improve the security of health information. However, health care organizations must adopt strong security practices if computer-based records are to become as secure or more secure than paper-based records. The National Research Council's report recommended specific policies, practices, and procedures to improve the security of computer-based patient information (Dowell and Frawley, 1997). Public concern over these issues was a major factor in passage of the HIPAA legislation, which now mandates many of the policies and procedures that were previously left to the discretion of the mental health system.

Court-Ordered Treatment

One of the most tragic aspects of serious mental illness is that persons who are in the grips of psychosis are victims of disordered thinking, which prevents their recognition of the fact that they are indeed ill. They are often unable to make decisions that are in their best interest, such as recognizing their need for psychotropic medication, and may be led by their delusions to acts that are dangerous to themselves or to others. In such cases, the mentally ill person may be in need of court-ordered treatment.

Treatment under court order is generally predicated by a procedure that is similar throughout the nation, with slight variations from state to state, and in some states, even from county to county. Generally, there is an examination of the person deemed in need of treatment by a physician and/or mental health professional (at least master's-level psychologist or social worker). The usual criterion for court-ordered commitment to an inpatient institution is the professional's certification that the person is "a danger to self and/or others." In recent years there has been an effort to broaden the rationale for commitment to include "person in need of care." Such a concept provides greater latitude for the court's decision as to whether institutionalization would be a means of improving a person's quality of life even if that person does not pose a direct threat to anyone. It takes into account the ill person's quality of life around such issues as homelessness resulting from the inability to access resources because of disordered thinking, or the degree of mental misery inflicted by paranoia and delusional thinking, which might be remediated by medication. While family members and the general public support this concept, particularly as a means of dealing with the homeless population, some consumer groups are opposed. They fear that such latitude can be misused and would return us to the era of widespread abuse of the commitment laws as a means of removing undesirables from the community who were not actually mentally ill, resulting in the "snake pit" conditions of mental institutions widely publicized by the media in the 1930s and 1940s.

Yet another solution to the dilemma of recognizing persons who are in need of supervision but who do not pose a threat to anyone is the outpatient commitment, which consists of a court order that outlines guidelines for behavior (e.g., regularly taking prescribed medication, refraining from abusing nonprescribed drugs or alcohol, reporting for mental health appointments), and may include commitment to a particular residence located in the community (e.g., a group home, a family residence). Failure to abide by the prescribed conditions may result in a new court appearance and the likelihood of inpatient commitment if the person's condition has deteriorated.

Role of the Health Information Management Professional

Increased interest in technological advances in data management is expanding the potential role of health information managers in the field of mental health as in other areas of health care. The traditional role function of the profession has been in the institutional sector of mental health services, where the recording, storing, and monitoring of patient information have been the chief responsibilities. Increasingly, however, the community mental health centers are finding that decision making around management information systems is growing increasingly complex and requires an expertise of its own. This area would seem a logical extension of the present health information manager in the era of computer technology.

Outside the domain of client data collection, another major potential for the expansion of the traditional role of the health information manager within CMHCs is in the area of billing. Because of the multiple and disparate nature of the sources of funding for community mental health services, this is a complex arena for information storage and management (refer back to "Reimbursement and Funding" for further details).

Health information managers may also assume roles in quality improvement and risk management or they may work as consultants to mental health facilities. A health information management (HIM) consultant could advise a mental health facility on issues related to accreditation, information management, or automation of patient information. A consultant assisting with the automation of patient information could have responsibilities ranging from helping to write requests for proposals for new information systems to assisting with the actual implementation of a new system.

Trends

One of the continuing major efforts in the area of mental health information management is the attempt to create nationally standardized data sets along with a universal system of data collection. Several mutually antagonistic factors have somewhat impeded this movement, although some progress has been made. The thrust toward managed care has created interest in data that in essence justifies an organization's decision making in service delivery based on cost/benefit issues. On the other hand, the interest in "client-centered" information systems that focus largely on client satisfaction rather than on treatment efficacy per se, predicates moving in another direction in the development of data collection and analysis. The emphasis at the national level has therefore been more on quality of the standards for data management than on uniformity.

Even without standardization, the movement toward use of computer technology has increased tremendously in the past decades, particularly in the community mental health sector. Beyond this statement, however, it becomes very difficult to generalize. The level of sophistication of the technology varies widely from locale to locale, as does the capacity for linkages, whether interagency or to statewide systems. The almost universal dependence on this form of technology has implications, however, for health information managers. As the level of complexity of these systems continues to climb, there will be a call for increased sophistication and specialization in their utilization as a tool for data collection. Decisions about a multitude of data-related questions will need to be addressed, from which computer system best suits the needs of the particular agency to which programs will best capture the information needed by a particular service provider. Such questions are clearly within the purview of the HIM profession.

In terms of treatment innovations, there have also been several developments in recent years. There has been an emphasis placed on client strengths, rather than on functional deficits. This change in focus results in a shift in the type of data collected, with increasing emphasis on satisfaction with services, as opposed to specific goals accomplished or failed. As a part of this trend, the concept of "recovery" has been borrowed from substance abuse to contrast with the older mental health concept of "stabilization," which means a reduction of symptomology, but does not imply return to the level of functioning before the illness. To capture progress in this type of program emphasis is rather difficult and calls for creative and innovative approaches to data collection and analysis.

These are some of the challenges facing health information managers in the area of developing client data systems. There are also other areas opening for exploration in the profession. Collection of other types of data besides the client service information is also a possible area of expansion of the profession. As mentioned earlier, the billing process in the outpatient facilities is a complicated weave of funding sources that also require a knowledge of computer-based information storage and retrieval.

Additionally, there is the possibility of entrepreneurial enterprise in developing and marketing software designed to meet the growing and changing data collection needs of the mental health system. Consultation around data system development targeted at specific program needs is also a possible avenue for the skills of health information managers.

Summary

As in other areas of health care, treatment of mental health service consumers has shifted from the inpatient to the outpatient setting because of advances in treatment methodologies and other factors. Mental health services consumers may also be called *clients* or *patients*. Among adults, the most common forms of serious mental illness are schizophrenia, clinical depression, and bipolar disorder. Adolescents and children may also suffer from mental disorders, and specific services have been identified to benefit these categories of mental health services consumers. A variety of caregivers, including medical personnel, therapists, case managers, aides, recreation therapists, and occupational therapists provide services to clients.

Mental health service providers are licensed by the state. Voluntary accreditation is available from the Joint Commission on Accreditation of Healthcare Organizations for both inpatient and outpatient providers. The Commission on Accreditation of Rehabilitation Facilities offers accreditation for programs that offer rehabilitation services. Medicare and Medicaid guidelines apply to facilities that receive payment from these sources.

Documentation is very important in mental health services. Various assessments help determine the patient's treatment plan. To demonstrate that every goal in the treatment plan is being addressed, there must be progress notes documenting services provided and the patient's progress toward achieving the treatment goals. Discharge summaries and aftercare plans are also important in the continuing care of the patient.

Several forces have helped mental health service providers improve the quality of data and information. The National Institute of Mental Health, now Center for Mental Health Services, has worked with state agencies to improve, broaden, and standardize data collection activities. The increase in managed care in the mental health arena has also caused providers to pursue high-quality data and information. High-quality information in the individual patient's record is also important to the patient and to the provider. Mental health information is extremely confidential, and the health information manager must ensure that appropriate HIPAA-compliant policies and procedures are in place to safeguard it. The health information manager can find opportunities in mental health hospitals and community mental health centers in a traditional information management role or in risk management, quality assurance, reimbursement, or information services. The increasing use of aggregate data for mental health services also presents opportunities for health information managers as data analysts in a variety of agencies.

Key Terms

bipolar disorder a form of serious mental illness in which a person alternates between states of ecstatic mania and severe depression. Also known as manic depression.

Center for Mental Health Services (CMHS) the federal agency that oversees administration of demonstration and research grants and other initiatives at the federal level related to mental health issues. This entity and its parent organization, the Substance Abuse and Mental Health Services Administration (SAMHSA), were created within the U.S. Department of Health and Human Services as a part of the reorganization of the National Institute of Mental Health (NIMH), which formerly carried these responsibilities.

chemical restraint the use of a drug or medication that is not part of a person's usual medical regimen that is administered to control behavior or restrict freedom of movement (P. L. 106-310, 2000).

Child and Adolescent Service System Program (CASSP) an initiative begun by the National Institute of Mental Health to create a comprehensive network of services for emotionally disturbed children and adolescents through a series of demonstration grants. The program is now overseen by the Substance Abuse and Mental Health Services Administration (SAMHSA) within the U.S. Department of Health and Human Services.

clinical depression a serious mental illness appearing as a deep feeling of melancholy and futility that is not situational in nature.

community mental health centers (CMHC) publicly funded mental health organizations established in communities throughout the United States by the Mental Health Act of 1965.

continuity of care a concept that refers to creation of a comprehensive system of care for persons with serious mental illness, with particular emphasis on smooth transition from inpatient to outpatient services.

continuous quality improvement a management concept that focuses on customer involvement in planning services and obtaining feedback as to satisfaction with service delivery. This concept has been an important feature of the mental health consumer empowerment movement. Also known as total quality management (TQM).

Data Standards for Mental Health Decision Support Systems a major reference source for creation of a national mental health services database. Also referred to by its series number, "FN-10."

delusion a form of disordered thinking in which a person holds unrealistic beliefs (e.g., that they are receiving communications from aliens in outer space or that their food is being poisoned). See **psychosis**.

Diagnostic and Statistical Manual of Mental Disorders, fourth edition (DSM-IV) a classification system and nomenclature of mental disorders developed by the American Psychiatric Association with a stated purpose of providing "clear descriptions of diagnostic categories in order to enable clinicians and investigators to diagnose, communicate about, study, and treat people with various mental disorders" (APA, 1994, p. xxiii). It is also used as a coding system for mental disorders.

dually diagnosed persons persons who have two diagnoses. Most commonly refers to persons with mental illness and chemical or alcohol addiction, but may also refer to persons who are diagnosed as developmentally disabled and seriously mentally ill.

"duty to warn" a legal concept that holds that it is the duty of a mental health professional to warn a person whom a mentally ill client has threatened to harm, despite the usual protections of confidentiality in the client/professional relationship.

episode of care a period during which a variety of services (inpatient and/or outpatient) are provided to an individual for a given episode of illness.

"FN-10" see *Data Standards for Mental Health Decision Support Systems*.

hallucination a form of disordered thinking in which a person reports sensory experience that is not valid, such as seeing, hearing, smelling, or feeling things that are not real. See **psychosis**.

involuntary commitment a legal process by which individuals who are deemed to be a danger to themselves or to others may be admitted to an inpatient facility even though they refuse or cannot consent to the treatment.

manic depression see **bipolar disorder**.

Mental Health Statistics Improvement Program (MHSIP) an initiative begun by National Institute of Mental Health and continued by Substance Abuse and Mental Health Services Administration to create a uniform data system nationwide for reporting of mental health statistics. The work has largely been done by a voluntary ad hoc group made up of local, state, and federal personnel and has thus far focused more on assuring standards of high quality for collection of information than on creation of a specific database. Decision Support 2000+, the second phase of this initiative, includes planning for inclusion of regulations from the Health Insurance Portability and Accountability Act (HIPAA).

MICA common acronym for persons or programs for persons dually diagnosed with mental illness and chemical/alcohol addiction. Also sometimes written as MIDA or MICAA.

outpatient commitment judicial diversion, from inpatient to outpatient care, of a person who has been certified as in need of psychiatric care, with stipulations regarding behaviors such as taking medications, remaining sober, and maintaining residence in a designated place. Failure to abide by the stipulations generally results in involuntary commitment to an inpatient facility.

physical restraint "mechanical or personal restriction that immobilizes or reduces the ability of an individual to move his or her arms, legs, or head freely, not including devices . . . for the purpose of conducting routine physical examinations or tests or to protect the resident from falling out of bed or to permit the resident to participate in activities without the risk of physical harm to the resident . . . ." (P. L. 106-310, 2000, pp. 1195-1196).

psychosis state of extreme disordered thinking in which a person demonstrates such symptoms of serious mental illness as hallucinations and delusions. See **hallucination** and **delusion**.

psychosocial rehabilitation mode of treatment for serious mental illness that focuses on provision of an array of community support services (e.g., development of job skills, if needed) for persons with mental illness sufficient to allow them to live in the least restrictive environment possible outside an institution.

psychotropic medication a variety of medications designed to reduce psychotic symptoms by altering the chemical processes within the brain. Also sometimes referred to as "neuroleptics."

schizophrenia a psychosis represented by a state of extremely disordered thinking, manifesting as a break with reality.

serious emotional disturbance (SED) a condition in which a young person (from birth to age 18) has a diagnosable mental, behavioral, or emotional disorder resulting in functional impairment that substantially interferes with or limits the child's role or functioning in family, school, or community activities.

serious mental illness (SMI) a condition in which a person has a diagnosable mental, behavioral, or emotional disorder resulting in functional impairment that substantially interferes with or limits one or more major life activities.

Social Security Disability Income (SSDI) federal benefits paid to persons with disability who have worked a sufficient length of time to qualify to receive Social Security benefits. A frequent source of income for persons with serious mental illness who are not able to work.

Supplemental Security Income (SSI) federal benefits paid to persons with disability who have not worked a sufficient length of time to qualify for Social Security benefits. A common, and often only, source of income for the seriously mentally ill who are unable to work.

wrap-around services predominant method of mental health service delivery to emotionally disturbed children, adolescents, and their families. The concept consists of a comprehensive array of professional services that may include home and/or school settings and that are tailored to meet the specific needs of the child and his/her family.

REVIEW QUESTIONS

Knowledge-based Questions

1. Explain the difference between situational emotional disturbance and serious mental illness.

2. Name the three most prevalent types of serious mental illness.

3. What are two categories of dual diagnoses?

4. Give the term by which persons with mental illness who are living in the community prefer to be called.

5. Name the two commonalities that all children's home-based services share.

6. Define outpatient commitment.

7. Name the main components of the mental health consumer case record.

8. What is the relationship between the treatment plan and progress notes, and why is it important?

9. How did the "duty to warn" originate, and how does it affect confidentiality of mental health information?

10. What are the FN-10 and the FN-11?

Application-based Questions

1. Explain how the mental health consumer empowerment movement has affected development of mental health data collection systems.

2. Discuss some of the areas in mental health services into which health information managers may expand their roles.

Web Activity

1. Visit the Substance Abuse and Mental Health Services Administration (SAMHSA) National Mental Health Information Center web site at http://www.mentalhealth.org. Find a feature or article that interests you and write a brief summary.

2. Visit the "Medicare Payment Systems" page at the CMS web site at http://www.cms.hhs.gov/paymentsystems. Review this page and follow appropriate links to determine whether or how the inpatient psychiatric facility prospective payment system (IPF PPS) has been implemented.

Case Study

As a health information manager, you have been hired as a consultant to design a data collection system for a short-term acute care facility in the planning stages. The facility is connected to a mental health center and is expected to draw most of its funding from Medicaid-eligible patients who will remain hospitalized an average of 21 days. It is likely that most of the persons discharged from the unit will be engaged in the ongoing services of the CMHC, such as case management and partial hospitalization. Formulate a recommendation as to whether the CMHC should use a data system that is client centered, which is the type it is using for its ongoing services, or whether the CMHC should investigate use of a system more oriented to managed care. Develop a list of reasons for and against adoption of each system and provide a final recommendation with a rationale for your choice.

References and Suggested Readings

American Medical Record Association. (1990). *Professional Practice Standards for Mental Health*. Chicago, IL: American Medical Record Association (now the American Health Information Management Association).

American Psychiatric Association. (2000). *Diagnostic and Statistical Manual of Mental Disorders-IV-Text Revision*. Washington, DC: American Psychiatric Association.

Buckley, S. (1993). Moving MHSIP toward a person-centered paradigm. Unpublished concept paper submitted to CMHS and the MHSIP Ad Hoc Advisory Group.

Burt, M., Aron, L., Douglas, T., Valente, J., Lee, E., & Iwen, B. (1999). *Homelessness: Programs and the People They Serve*. Washington, DC: Interagency Council on the Homeless.

Calvert, C. L., and Lee, F. W. (1993). The health information manager in a residential treatment facility: An innovator, a change agent, an educator. *Journal of the American Health Information Management Association, 64* (10), 48–50.

Campbell, J., and Frey, E. (1993). Humanizing decision support systems. Unpublished position paper.

Casey, R., and Berman, J. (1985). The outcome of psychotherapy with children. *Psychological Bulletin, 98*, 388–400.

Center for Mental Health Services. (1996). *MHSIP Consumer-Oriented Mental Health Report Card: The Final Report of the Mental Health Statistics Improvement Program (MHSIP) Task Force on a Consumer-Oriented Mental Health Report Card*. Washington, DC: Center for Mental Health Services.

[CMS] Centers for Medicare and Medicaid Services. (No date). Appendix AA: Psychiatric hospitals—Interpretive Guidelines and Survey Procedures. State Operations Manual [Online]. http://www.cms.hhs.gov/manuals/pub07pdf/AP-a.pdf [2003, July 10].

Commission on Accreditation of Rehabilitation Facilities. (1997). *Standards Manual and Interpretive Guidelines for Behavioral Health*. Tucson, AZ: Commission on Accreditation of Rehabilitation Facilities.

Commission on Accreditation of Rehabilitation Facilities. [Online]. Behavioral health documents. http://www.carf.org.

Conditions of Participation for Hospitals, *Code of Federal Regulations*, Title 42, Pt. 482, Subpart E—Requirements for Specialty Hospitals, 2003 ed.

Dowell, S. P., and Frawley, K. A. (1997, July–August). National research council report provides clear direction to industry. *In Confidence, 4*, 4–5.

Federal Register. (1993, May 20). Definitions of adults with a serious mental illness and children with a serious emotional disturbance, pp. 29422–29425.

Federal Register. (2001, January 22). Psychiatric residential treatment facilities providing psychiatric services to individuals under age 21; use of restraint and seclusion, pp. 7147–7164.

Friedman, R., Katz-Leary, J., Manderscheid, R., and Sondheimer, D. (1996). Prevalence of serious emotional disturbance in children and adolescents. In R. Manderscheid and M. Sonnenschein (Eds.), *Mental Health: United States* (pp. 71–98). Washington, DC: U.S. Government Printing Office, DHHS Publication Number (SMA) 96-3098.

Furman, R. (1997). Wrap-around services: A comprehensive approach to adolescent mental health services. *Advocates Forum, 4* (1), 8–9.

Huffman, E. (1994). *Health Information Management* (10th ed.). Berwyn, IL: Physicians' Record Company.

Hutchinson, J., Lloyd, J., Landsman, M., Nelson, K., and Bryce, M. (1983). *Family-Centered Social Services: A Model for Child Welfare Agencies.* Iowa City, IA: The University of Iowa School of Social Work, National Resource Center on Family Based Services.

Joint Commission on Accreditation of Healthcare Organizations. (1997). *1997–1998 Comprehensive Accreditation Manual for Behavioral Health Care.* Oakbrook Terrace, IL. Joint Commission on Accreditation of Healthcare Organizations.

Joint Commission on Accreditation of Healthcare Organizations. (1997). *Comprehensive Accreditation Manual for Hospitals.* Oakbrook, Terrace, IL. Joint Commission on Accreditation of Healthcare Organizations.

Leginski, W., Croze, C., Driggers, J., Dumpman, S., Geertsen, D., Kamis-Gould, E., Namerow, M., Patton, R., Wilson, N., and Wurster, C. (1989). *Data Standards for Mental Health Decision Support Systems. Series FN No. 10.* Rockville, MD: U.S. Department of Health and Human Services.

Medicare program: Prospective payment system for inpatient psychiatric facilities; proposed rule. (2003, November 28) *Federal Register,* pp. 66919–66978.

[MSHIP] Mental Health Statistics Improvement Program. (1998). Summary List. *FN-11 Tables* [Online]. http://www.mhsip.org/fn11/summary.htm [2003, July 11].

National Committee for Quality Assurance. (2004). *Standards and Guidelines for the Accreditation of Managed Behavioral Healthcare Organizations (MBHOs).* Washington, DC: National Committee for Quality Assurance.

National Committee for Quality Assurance. [Online]. Frequently Asked Questions http://www.ncqa.org/Programs/faq/index.asp [2003, July 11].

P. L. 106-310. (2000). Children's Health Act of 2000 [Online]. http://www.access.gpo.gov/nara/publaw/106publ.html [2003, July 11].

Parrish, J. (1987). *Ideal Community-Based Mental Health Service System for Adults with Long-Term, Disabling Mental Illness.* Washington, DC: Substance Abuse and Mental Health Services Administration.

Patton, R., and Leginski, W. (1983). *The Design and Content of a National Mental Health Statistics System. DHHS Publication (ADM) 83-1095.* Rockville, MD: U.S. Department of Health and Human Services.

Sowder, B. (1979). *Issues Related to Psychiatric Services for Children and Youth: A Review of Selected Literature from 1970–1979.* Bethesda, MD: Burt Associates.

Standards for privacy of individually identifiable health information; final rule. (2002, August 14). *Federal Register,* pp. 53181–53273.

Stroul, B. (1986). *Models of Community Support Services* (1986). Boston, MA: Center for Psychiatric Rehabilitation.

Stroul, B., and Friedman, R. (1994). *A System of Care for Children and Youth with Severe Emotional Disturbances.* Washington, DC: Georgetown University Child Development Center.

Tarasoff v. Regents of the University of California, 17 Cal 3d 425, 131 Cal Rptr 14, 551 P 2d 334 (1976).

Key Resources

Commission on Accreditation of Rehabilitation Facilities (CARF)
(See Chapter 1 for contact information.)

Joint Commission on Accreditation of Healthcare Organizations
(See Chapter 1 for contact information.)

National Alliance for the Mentally Ill
200 North Glebe Road, Suite 1015
Arlington, Virginia 22203-3754
Helpline phone: 800-950-NAMI (6264)
Office phone: 703-524-7600
Fax: 703-524-9094
http://www.nami.org

National Committee for Quality Assurance (NCQA)
2000 L Street NW, Suite 500
Washington, DC 20036
Phone: 202-955-3500
http://www.ncqa.org

National Institute of Mental Health (NIMH)
Office of Communications
6001 Executive Boulevard, Room 8184, MSC 9663
Bethesda, MD 20892-9663
Phone: 1-866-615-NIMH (6464)
http://www.nimh.nih.gov

URAC
1220 L Street, NW
Suite 400
Washington, D.C. 20005
Phone: 202-216-9010
Fax: 202-216-9006
http://www.urac.org

U.S. Department of Health and Human Services
Substance Abuse and Mental Health Services Administration
Center for Mental Health Services
National Mental Health Services Knowledge Exchange Network
P.O. Box 42557
Washington, DC 20015
Phone: 800-789-2647
http://www.mentalhealth.org

Chapter *8*

Substance Abuse

Frances Wickham Lee, MBA, RHIA
Kimberly D. Taylor, RHIA
Melissa King, RHIA

Learning Objectives

Upon successful completion of this chapter, you should be able to:

1. Describe the various settings and caregivers commonly associated with substance abuse treatment.
2. Evaluate the impact of state and federal laws and regulations on the treatment of substance abuse clients.
3. Describe the role of CARF and JCAHO in setting substance abuse treatment standards.
4. Describe the components of a "typical" substance abuse client record, both inpatient and outpatient.
5. Discuss current reimbursement issues related to substance abuse treatment.
6. Compare DSM-IV and ICD-9-CM as they relate to coding of substance abuse client records.
7. Discuss quality improvement and utilization management within substance abuse facilities.
8. Discuss the role of the health information manager in a substance abuse facility.
9. Discuss the use of computer technology in managing substance abuse client information.
10. Identify the specific legal and ethical considerations associated with the confidentiality of substance abuse client records.

SETTING	DESCRIPTION	SYNONYMS/EXAMPLES
Outpatient Substance Abuse Facility	A facility where clients receive regularly scheduled outpatient substance abuse treatment	Substance abuse treatment program or center
Intensive Outpatient Substance Abuse Facility	A facility where clients spend at least nine hours per week in substance abuse treatment, but do not stay overnight	Partial hospitalization Day treatment IOP (Intensive Outpatient Program)
Residential Inpatient Substance Abuse Treatment Setting	A setting where clients are treated for substance abuse in a nonmedical residential setting	Rehabilitation 28-day program Residential treatment program Chemical dependency unit
Medically Managed Intensive Inpatient Substance Abuse Treatment Setting	A setting where clients are treated for substance abuse under the direction of a physician, and that includes all services of an acute care hospital	Acute inpatient treatment Inpatient detoxification
Substance Abuse Education and Prevention Program	A program designed to prevent substance abuse problems in individuals or families	Early intervention School intervention programs Children of addicted families programs Alcohol and other drug prevention programs
Self-help Recovery Groups	Support groups established to assist individuals in maintaining sobriety and a drug-free lifestyle	Alcoholics Anonymous Narcotics Anonymous 12-step programs Rational Recovery
Aftercare	Usually follows intensive in/outpatient treatment. Weekly individual and group sessions. Lasts up to two years.	Continuing Care Program Relapse Prevention Program

Introduction to Setting

In the American Psychiatric Association's ***Diagnostic and Statistical Manual of Mental Disorders, fourth edition (DSM-IV)***, various substance use disorders (e.g., alcohol use disorder, cocaine use disorder) are generally divided into the broad categories of substance abuse and substance dependence, depending on the severity of the condition and the presence of withdrawal and other symptoms of addiction. General synonyms for substance abuse include alcohol and other drug abuse and psychoactive substance abuse. Alternate terms that are commonly used in place of substance dependence include *alcohol and other drug dependence*, *psychoactive substance dependence*, *drug addiction*, *alcoholism*, or *chemical dependency*. These terms may be substituted where appropriate for *substance abuse* throughout the various care settings discussed in this chapter. It is also important to note that individuals seen in substance abuse treatment settings are often referred to as clients, rather than patients, because the term *patient* implies a more medically oriented model of care.

Substance abuse is a major health problem in the United States. Many different types of treatment settings are available to substance abuse clients seeking assistance, including public and private facilities that provide a full range of services, from educational programs to medically managed intensive inpatient care. In excess of $3 billion a year is spent for substance abuse treatment and prevention (American Psychiatric Association). The public sector has traditionally assumed a major responsibility for the operation of substance abuse treatment centers, particularly outpatient treatment centers. According to the *National Survey of Substance Abuse Treatment Services (N-SSATS): 2000*, 55 percent of all clients in treatment were in private nonprofit facilities. Private for-profit facilities accounted for 24 percent of substance abuse clients (SAMHSA, 2002). Publicly owned treatment centers generally receive their funds from state, city, and county governments, federal grants and contracts, and some client fees and third-party reimbursement. Private substance abuse treatment facilities, on the other hand, rely primarily on direct client payments and third-party reimbursement for their funds. Figure 8-1 shows the primary focus of facilities according to ownership.

The evolution of modern substance abuse treatment in the United States began in the 1950s with the development of freestanding residential programs for the treatment of alcohol dependency and with the continued growth and recognition of **Alcoholics Anonymous** and its 12-step recovery philosophy. Early alcohol treatment programs were not considered by the medical community to be truly part of the health care system and were often staffed and run by nonprofessionals, some of whom were recovering alcoholics themselves. Treatment for drug addiction was even more removed from mainstream health care, and clients were often referred to drug treatment centers by the

PERCENT DISTRIBUTION ACCORDING TO FACILITY OWNERSHIP

Primary Focus	Total	Private nonprofit	Private for-profit	Local govt	State govt	Federal govt	Tribal govt
Substance Abuse Treatment Services	66.8	67.1	74.6	56.0	67.5	43.3	73.5
Mental Health Services	5.5	6.0	4.8	5.9	5.8	2.7	—
General Health Care	3.2	2.3	0.4	1.5	1.6	37.9	5.2
Both Substance Abuse and Mental Health	22.6	22.6	18.3	34.5	24.4	14.6	21.1
Other	1.9	1.9	1.9	2.2	0.7	1.5	0.2

SOURCE: Office of Applied Studies, Substance Abuse and Mental Health Services Administration, National Survey of Substance Abuse Treatment Services (N-SSATS).

Figure 8-1   Substance abuse treatment clients by facility ownership, according to facility ownership and primary focus of facility, October 1, 2000.

criminal justice system. Although the American Medical Association classified alcoholism as a disease in 1956, it was not until the 1970s that the public began to recognize alcoholism as a disease and third-party payers began to offer some reimbursement for inpatient treatment. Outpatient treatment became more prevalent in the 1980s and 1990s as providers and third-party payers realized that substance abuse clients needed a full range of treatment options (American Society of Addiction Medicine, 1991). Outpatient rehabilitation was the most widely available type of care, with non–intensive and intensive rehabilitation offered by 78 percent and 46 percent of all facilities, respectively. Residential rehabilitation was offered by 26 percent of all facilities, while hospital inpatient rehabilitation was offered by 5 percent of facilities. Sixteen percent of all facilities provided partial hospitalization programs. Outpatient detoxification was available at 13 percent of facilities, while residential detoxification and hospital inpatient detoxification were each provided by 8 percent of all facilities (SAMHSA, 2002).

Care Settings

The following list represents some of the more common settings for substance abuse treatment and services; however, it should not be considered an exhaustive list. For simplicity, the programs discussed in this chapter have been grouped by care setting under the following general headings:

1. Outpatient treatment
2. Intensive outpatient or partial hospitalization treatment
3. Inpatient treatment
4. Aftercare/Continuing Care
5. Educational programs
6. Self-help recovery groups

Within the substance abuse treatment community, however, similar programs can sometimes be found in an inpatient, outpatient, or community setting. For example, the Alcoholics Anonymous (AA) 12-step philosophy and program originated as a part of a self-help recovery network, but over the years, this philosophy has also been incorporated into programs at both inpatient and outpatient treatment facilities.

The discussion of the first three care settings in this section is based on the levels of care as defined in *American Society of Addiction Medicine Patient Placement Criteria, Second Edition Revised (ASAM PPC-2R)* (ASAM, 2001). The levels of care are:

- Level 0.5, Early Intervention
- Level I, Outpatient Treatment
- Level II, Intensive Outpatient/Partial Hospitalization
- Level III, Residential/Inpatient Treatment
- Level IV, Medically Managed Intensive Inpatient Treatment

Within these broad levels of service is a range of specific levels of care. As a general rule, clients should be treated at the lowest or least intensive level of care that will accomplish their treatment goals. The levels are discussed in this chapter as discrete entities, but in reality they represent the continuum of substance abuse treatment services available to clients in most areas of the country.

Outpatient Treatment

ASAM describes Level I **outpatient treatment** as follows:

> Level I encompasses organized services that may be delivered in a wide variety of settings. Addiction or mental health treatment personnel provide professionally directed evaluation, treatment and recovery service. Such services are provided in regularly scheduled sessions and follow a defined set of policies and procedures or medical protocols.
>
> Level I outpatient services are designed to treat the individual's level of clinical severity and to help the individual achieve permanent changes in his or her alcohol- and drug-using behavior and mental functioning. To accomplish this, services must address major lifestyle, attitudinal and behavioral issues that have the potential to undermine the goals of treatment or inhibit the individual's ability to cope with major life tasks without the non-medical use of alcohol or other drugs (ASAM, 2001, p. 2).

Outpatient providers, such as mental health centers, hospital-based outpatient centers, and freestanding drug and alcohol treatment centers, currently treat substance abuse clients through a variety of treatment modalities, such as individual, group, and family therapy. Individual therapy is currently the most common form of outpatient treatment, accounting for 78 percent of all treatment sessions (Wheeler et al., 1992). Specialized outpatient programs are also found throughout the substance abuse treatment system. Some examples of specialized outpatient treatment programs are methadone maintenance programs for heroin addicts, organized school intervention programs for adolescents, court-related programs for individuals convicted of substance abuse–related offenses, and employee assistance programs that contract with companies within the community to provide care to their employees. The "Types of Clients" section in this chapter provides more information on these and other specific client populations. Outpatient therapy is typically a long-term commitment for a client, lasting up to a year or more.

Intensive Outpatient or Partial Hospitalization Treatment

ASAM defines **intensive outpatient or partial hospitalization treatments** as follows:

> Level II is an organized outpatient service that delivers treatment services during the day, before or after work or school, in the evening or on weekends. For appropriately selected patients, such programs provide essential education

and treatment components while allowing patients to apply their newly acquired skills within "real world" environments. Programs have the capacity to arrange for medical and psychiatric consultation, psychopharmacological consultation, medication management, and 24-hour crisis services (ASAM, 2001, p. 3)

Intensive outpatient treatment requires a minimum of nine hours of weekly attendance, usually in increments of three to eight hours a day for five to seven days a week. This treatment is often recommended for patients in the early stages of treatment or those transitioning from residential or hospital settings. This environment is suitable for patients who do not need full-time supervision and have some available supports but need more structure than is usually available in less intensive outpatient settings. This treatment encompasses day treatment programs that may offer a full range of services, including outpatient detoxification. The frequency and length of session is usually tapered as patients demonstrate progress, less risk of relapse, and a stronger reliance on drug-free community supports. An evening program can provide clients with an alternative to inpatient treatment that would necessitate an extended leave from work or school. Intensive outpatient treatment programs allow adult clients to continue working and adolescent clients to continue schooling, while providing a structured treatment environment. Partial hospitalization programs are generally day treatment programs that provide a greater number of treatment hours for clients with a more severe level of illness. Clients spend all day in the treatment program, but return home each evening (ASAM, 1991; APA, 1995).

Inpatient Treatment

Under certain circumstances a substance abuse client may require an inpatient stay at a hospital or residential treatment facility. These clients may be in need of medically managed detoxification, have substance abuse–related medical problems, or come from environments that make outpatient treatment ineffective. ASAM recognizes two levels of inpatient treatment: **residential/inpatient treatment** and **medically managed intensive inpatient treatment**. Both levels require a planned regimen of 24-hour professionally directed evaluation, care and treatment.

Residential/Inpatient Treatment

Residential/inpatient treatment is directed at clients with subacute medical, behavioral, or emotional problems. Residential treatment provides a live-in facility with 24-hour supervision. This type of treatment is better than outpatient treatment for consumers with an overwhelming substance abuse problem. The consumers in this program typically are without the motivation or social supports to abstain from abusing. The length of stay in these facilities ranges from short term to long term. There are programs that offer less restrictive types of treatment, such as halfway and quarter-way houses, to help the consumer's transition back into the community (APA, 1995).

Medically Managed Intensive Inpatient Treatment

In a medically managed environment, the clients' problems are acute, and a full range of medical and support services that can be found in a general hospital should be available to them. The treatment settings for medically managed intensive inpatient treatment include acute care general hospitals, acute psychiatric hospitals or units, and chemical dependency specialty hospitals that have the appropriate medical and nursing services available (ASAM, 2001). According to the APA, this level of inpatient hospitalization includes around-the-clock treatment and supervision by a multidisciplinary staff that emphasizes medical management of detoxification or other psychiatric crisis. The length of stay at this level of care is usually short term (APA, 1995).

Educational Programs/Early Intervention

Society places a significant emphasis on awareness and prevention of substance abuse problems. Substance abuse facilities, particularly those in the public sector, are frequently involved in providing structured prevention, education, and awareness programs. The clients served by these programs differ from those who receive substance abuse treatment; these clients do not necessarily have substance abuse or dependence diagnoses, but are considered to be at risk for problems in the future. Many participants in educational programs are children or adolescents who have been identified by the schools, social service agencies, or legal system as having the potential to develop substance abuse problems or who have family members with existing substance abuse problems. A program that targets children of addicted families is one example of a service that might be offered by a substance treatment facility to help children who are affected by substance abuse within their families. Drug Abuse Resistance Education (D.A.R.E.) is a school-based prevention program. Researchers found that students participating in a revised DARE curriculum scored 6 percent higher on decision-making skills and 5 percent higher on drug-refusal skills than students in a control group (Study: Revamped D.A.R.E. curriculum shows promise, 2002).

Self-Help Recovery Groups

It can be argued that it is not appropriate to include the self-help recovery groups in a list of substance abuse care settings, because they are designed to be voluntary and to provide support rather than treatment for the recovering addict. However, these groups provide lifelong assistance to many individuals with substance abuse problems and are considered a significant factor in many successful recoveries. The most widely recognized self-help organization is Alcoholics Anonymous, a program in which members follow a 12-step program that leads to recovery. AA was founded in 1935 and had reached national prominence by the 1950s (Alcoholics Anonymous World Services, Inc., 1957). Since that time, AA has spawned other self-help groups, such as Narcotics Anonymous (NA), that adhere to a similar 12-step philosophy. No records are kept by 12-step support groups, since anonymity is a key element in the recovery programs.

However, 12-step programs have reached such prominence in the substance abuse treatment community that many providers actually integrate the philosophy into their treatment services, and this will be reflected in client records.

AA is the most widely accepted network of substance abuse self-help groups, but it is not without critics. Some individuals with substance abuse problems and some care providers have questioned the religious underpinning of 12-step programs, leading to the formation of alternatives. For example, Rational Recovery (RR) is a self-help system for individuals with alcohol or drug addiction problems that has a cognitive orientation in contrast to AA's spiritual one (Galanter et al., 1993).

Types of Clients

Within the various types of substance abuse settings and programs, the clients served may range in age from infants to the elderly, and come from all socioeconomic backgrounds. In addition to identifying broad categories of clients, such as inpatients and outpatients, facilities will often further identify segments of their client populations by factors such as age, sex, type of referral, or legal status. This categorization facilitates program planning and administration. In many cases, educational and treatment programs can be tailored to meet the needs of particular client groups. Some examples of client groups served by specific programs or protocols because of their special needs are adolescents, women, clients referred to employee assistance programs, clients who have been dually diagnosed with a mental disorder and a substance abuse disorder, and clients who have been court referred. Many other special programs are offered in substance abuse treatment centers throughout the United States, but examining this sample will provide an overview of the scope of clients served.

Adolescents

In addition to potentially causing problems with family, friends, and schoolwork, use of alcohol and other drugs by adolescents can lead to dangerous patterns of lifelong abuse. Statistics indicate that more than 88 percent of all seniors have tried alcohol (Drug Enforcement Administration, Online). Health care providers, teachers, and parents now recognize that an adolescent can develop serious abuse and addiction problems as a result of this early experimentation. A 1990 government study found that approximately 115,000 adolescents are treated each year in the United States for substance abuse problems, and the majority of these clients are treated in a clinical setting that is specifically structured for treating adolescents (Marshall and Marshall, 1993). Treating an adolescent substance abuse problem is quite different from treating an adult problem. The youthful client's unique emotional, social, and educational needs must be incorporated into his or her treatment plan. To highlight the need to use care in selecting a treatment program for adolescents, the American Academy of Pediatrics (AAP) has developed a list of program selection criteria that addresses, among other concerns, such issues as:

- Knowledge of the clinicians about adolescent behavior and development, in addition to chemical dependency treatment
- Low staff-to-patient ratio
- Separation of the adolescent unit from an adult unit
- Availability of academic and vocational activities (Muramoto and Leshan, 1993)

The treatment settings for adolescents span all levels of care and include in-school intervention programs, outpatient therapy, intensive outpatient programs, short-stay inpatient treatment, and extended-stay inpatient treatment.

Women

There is growing awareness within the substance abuse treatment community that women, particularly pregnant women and women who are parents of young children, have special care and support needs, as do their children. In 1999, 4 percent of women of childbearing age who entered publicly funded substance abuse treatment were pregnant when admitted (SAMHSA, 2003). Treatment of pregnant women should be made a priority, because the welfare of both the mother and the unborn baby are at stake. Fetal alcohol syndrome and cocaine addiction in newborns can lead to serious health and developmental problems for children. Pregnant women with substance abuse problems need prenatal care along with substance abuse treatment, and their children need monitoring for potential medical and emotional problems. Programs developed for pregnant women might include child care that incorporates therapeutic activities to assist the children in learning to deal with issues related to living with an addicted parent and easy access to intensive prenatal care and case management services. The levels of service provided in women's substance abuse programs include outpatient, intensive outpatient, and inpatient treatment, depending on the severity of the substance abuse and the individual's treatment plan.

EAP Clients

Many substance abuse agencies and treatment facilities have established **employee assistance programs (EAPs)** to serve working adults and their employers. Businesses contract with local substance abuse organizations to provide services to their employees. Employers have come to recognize that substance abuse problems will have a negative impact on job performance, and that it is in their best interest and that of their employees to encourage treatment of these problems. The actual scope of the substance abuse services provided by the EAP is specified in a contract negotiated between the business and the provider. The contract generally includes at least an assessment, at little or no out-of-pocket cost for the employee, and, if needed, referral to one of the education or treatment options available through the provider's existing programs. Employees can be referred to the EAP by their employers, or in some cases, the employees will seek out the EAP services for themselves. As in other substance abuse treatment programs, the strict confidentiality of EAP client information is maintained, regardless of the referral source.

Dually Diagnosed Clients

A portion of the substance abuse client population is **dually diagnosed** with both a substance abuse or dependency disorder and a chronic mental illness. These clients typically have difficulty succeeding in traditional alcohol and drug treatment programs and self-help groups, which has led to the development of programs designed to meet their special care needs. In some states, and in some private facilities, substance abuse and mental health services are offered in the same location or by a single organizational unit, allowing dually diagnosed clients access to treatment for both their substance abuse and their mental health disorders. However, states do not have to provide mental health and substance abuse services through one agency in order to develop programs for dually diagnosed clients. For example, the New Hampshire Division of Mental Health and Developmental Services, in collaboration with the state's Office of Alcohol and Drug Abuse, has been offering integrated treatment services for dually diagnosed clients since 1987 (Drake et al., 1991).

Court-Referred Clients

Individuals who are arrested and convicted of alcohol- and other drug-related offenses are frequently referred to substance abuse treatment programs for drug and alcohol awareness education, a substance abuse assessment, or substance abuse treatment. For additional information on court-ordered treatment, refer to the "Risk Management and Legal Issues" section. When an individual is convicted of driving while intoxicated (DWI) or driving under the influence (DUI) of alcohol or drugs, the court may, for example, order that individual to enroll in an awareness program and to obtain a substance abuse assessment to determine whether treatment would be required. In some states, the assessment or education program may actually be required by law, creating a situation in which law enforcement, the court system, and the substance abuse treatment center must work closely together. DUI clients are not the only court-related clients seen by substance abuse facilities; persons arrested and convicted of other alcohol- or drug-related offenses may also be referred or ordered to obtain assessment and treatment.

Types of Caregivers

The types of caregivers who work with substance abuse clients are quite varied. They include individuals who possess a wide range of educational and professional backgrounds, from residential aids to psychiatrists and other physicians. Each of these caregivers is an important member of the substance abuse treatment team, bringing unique experience and expertise to the overall treatment process. The following discussion is a representation of direct caregivers who work with substance abuse clients; however, there may be several others who are involved in the clients' care. Clients treated in an acute inpatient setting are cared for by the various ancillary departments and other medical and allied health specialists found in the hospital. It is not unusual to see professionals such as occupational therapists, recreation therapists, and dietitians working in substance abuse programs.

Physicians

Some physicians specialize in the treatment of chemically dependent patients. However, there are also psychiatrists, family practitioners, or other physicians with a general practice orientation involved in substance abuse treatment. Any treatment plan that requires a medical intervention, such as prescription medications or detoxification services, is monitored, if not managed, by a physician. Depending on the level of care and the treatment setting, for example, public or private, inpatient or outpatient, medical services may be provided by full-time staff physicians or by part-time contract physicians.

Physician Assistants and Nurse Practitioners

As in other segments of health care, the role of physician extenders—physician assistants (PAs) and nurse practitioners (NPs)—varies from state to state and from facility to facility. As a general rule, these professionals treat clients under the supervision of a physician; however, some states allow more independent practice.

Nurses

Clients in inpatient substance abuse facilities have nursing care needs, in addition to medical care needs and substance abuse treatment. The extent of nursing service provided by a facility depends on the level of care offered by the facility. An acute care hospital setting provides 24-hour nursing care to its substance abuse patients, just as it does to other patients.

Counselors

Substance abuse counselors are professionals, such as social workers and psychologists, with special training and experience in the treatment of clients with substance abuse problems. The educational background of these individuals varies and may depend in part on the state's facility licensure, practitioner licensure, and Medicaid regulations. The counselor provides individual, group, and/or family therapy to the client and the client's family according to the treatment plan. Frequently, the counselor is recognized as the client's primary therapist, particularly in an outpatient setting. The primary therapist is the caregiver responsible for coordinating the treatment of the client, including ensuring that all documentation requirements are met.

Case Managers

As with substance abuse counselors, substance abuse case managers come from a variety of professional and educational backgrounds. They may be nurses, social workers, or educational specialists. The role of the case manager in substance abuse treatment depends on the level of care and the particular care setting. In an inpatient setting, the case manager may focus primarily on reimbursement issues and organizing follow-up care. The case manager in an outpatient setting assists the client with these and other nontreatment activities, such as obtaining adequate housing, securing financial assistance, keeping medical and counseling appointments, and so on. A case manager differs from a counselor in his or her relationship with the client; the case manager provides assistance with obtaining and coordinating services for clients rather than actual therapy.

Recreational Therapists

Long-term inpatient and other residential treatment programs often employ recreational therapists to work with clients. Recreational therapists design therapeutic recreational activities for residents while they are undergoing treatment. For example, a residential treatment program for adolescents might incorporate a challenge course or other outdoor activities designed to build trust and self-esteem.

Regulatory Issues

Several public and private agencies regulate or set standards for substance abuse treatment facilities and programs. One important set of federal regulations, *42 CFR, Part 2, Confidentiality of Drug and Alcohol Abuse Records*, mandates that strict confidentiality guidelines and legal procedures be adhered to by any federally assisted substance abuse treatment program. Substance abuse treatment records are the only category of health-related record, except those created in government-operated health care facilities, such as veterans affairs and Indian health service hospitals, whose security and confidentiality are specifically protected by a comprehensive federal law. A detailed discussion of 42 CFR, Part 2, is in the "Risk Management and Legal Issues" section of this chapter. As discussed in an earlier chapter, HIPAA provides guidelines for confidentiality of protected health information (PHI). With HIPAA, the awareness of confidentiality has been raised. The federal law that protects substance abuse programs and their information is more comprehensive than the HIPAA requirements in many ways. Therefore, the substance abuse programs have not fundamentally changed their approach to maintaining confidentiality. The other regulatory agencies that are discussed in this section set standards for substance abuse treatment facilities along with other health care facilities with the intent of promoting high-quality care. There are two major private, not-for-profit, voluntary accrediting agencies that set standards for substance abuse facilities: the Joint Commission on Accreditation of

Health Care Organizations (JCAHO) and the Commission on Accreditation of Rehabilitation Facilities (CARF). The government standards that are most frequently applied to substance abuse treatment programs are state Medicaid guidelines. Facilities treating Medicare clients also have to comply with the applicable *Conditions of Participation*.

As the best-known voluntary health care accreditation agency in the United States, JCAHO's original focus was on improving the quality of hospital-based patient care. Over the years, however, JCAHO has developed distinct accreditation programs for nonhospital settings, such as outpatient mental health and substance abuse treatment, ambulatory care, long-term care, and others. Although JCAHO accreditation is voluntary, in some states substance abuse treatment facilities, particularly inpatient facilities and hospital-based programs, that are accredited do not have to undergo additional surveys for licensure and certification. Inpatient substance abuse facilities, as well as hospital-based ambulatory, residential, or partial hospitalization substance abuse programs, follow the standards outlined in JCAHO's *Comprehensive Accreditation Manual for Hospitals* (CAMH). This is the same manual that is used by acute care hospitals, but specific standards within the CAMH address services to behavioral health patients, including substance abuse clients. Community-based outpatient substance abuse programs follow the standards outlined in a separate JCAHO accreditation program manual, the *Comprehensive Accreditation Manual for Behavioral Health Care (CAMBHC)*. This manual and its corresponding accreditation program are designed to meet the needs of nonhospital programs serving mental health, substance abuse, and developmentally delayed clients. Hospital-based and inpatient substance abuse programs are more likely to seek JCAHO accreditation, often as a part of an organization-wide effort, than are community outpatient programs. Although there are definite advantages for substance abuse treatment programs to seek JCAHO accreditation, it can be a costly process, and many publicly funded outpatient programs often choose not to participate.

The mission of the **Commission on Accreditation of Rehabilitation Facilities (CARF)** is "to promote the quality, value, and optimal outcomes of services through a consultative accreditation process that centers on enhancing the lives of the persons served" (CARF, Online). CARF's core values emphasize the rights of the individuals served by rehabilitation facilities. These values address the importance of treating individuals with respect and empowering them to make their own informed choices. Substance abuse programs can be accredited under several of CARF's core programs, including detoxification, drug court treatment, employee assistance, outpatient treatment, partial hospitalization, prevention, or residential treatment, to name a few. Two CARF standards manuals are relevant to substance abuse programs: the *Behavioral Health Standards Manual* and the *Opioid Treatment Program Standards Manual* (CARF, Online).

Another major category of regulators of substance abuse treatment is the various state agencies that are responsible for state Medicaid programs. Medicaid is a federally mandated program that provides medical assistance to low-income individuals, as authorized by Title XIX of the Social Security Act of 1965. However, the actual Medicaid costs are shared by the federal government and the states. The percentages for this cost sharing and the actual dollar amount spent for Medicaid vary significantly from state to state. State Medicaid agencies are granted a fair amount of independence in determining the levels of coverage and the payment mechanisms they will employ, provided the basic services as required by the federal regulations are covered. Consequently, the majority of the standards governing Medicaid providers are developed at the state level and also vary from one state to another. One basic tenet of Medicaid is that it provides for reimbursement of care that is "medically necessary." For substance abuse treatment programs, this translates into the need for physician involvement and clear documentation of the medical necessity of the prescribed substance abuse treatment for Medicaid clients.

Documentation

As in other health care settings, substance abuse facilities require clear and consistent documentation. Good-quality documentation of care, whether it is done manually or electronically, is essential. The primary purpose for maintaining client records is to support client treatment. Other purposes for the records include to improve communication among care providers, to serve as legal records of care provided, to support reimbursement claims, to monitor the quality of care, and to provide data for research and education. The types of documents, computer systems, files, and forms vary considerably from organization to organization. However, each facility should develop and maintain standards, policies, and procedures governing its specific documentation requirements. The following list represents typical information that might be found within a substance abuse client's record, divided into two general groups: legal/administrative documentation and clinical documentation (SCDAO-DAS, 1995*b*).

Legal/Administrative Documentation

The legal/administrative portion of the client record typically includes essential nonclinical information such as demographic and identifying information, along with any required legal documentation. Some examples include:

- Admission information
- Commitment papers
- Fee agreement and financial assessment
- Insurance authorization
- Special-program enrollment forms
- Program or agency rules
- Consents to treatment
- Consents to release of information
- Client rights information

Clinical Documentation

The clinical portion of the client's record documents the direct care provided and might include such items as:

- Clinical assessment
- Medical assessment, if necessary
- Individualized treatment plan
- Clinical service notes or progress notes (They may be daily or weekly summary notes depending on the type of program and applicable standards.)
- Discharge summary
- Follow-up information
- List of medications

Two key documents in the substance abuse record are the **clinical assessment** and the **individualized treatment plan**. (See Figures 8-2 and 8-3.) Each client should receive a thorough clinical assessment before the development of his or her individualized treatment plan. This assessment typically includes documentation of:

- Identifying information
- Presenting problem
- Health, medical, and/or developmental history
- Family and social history
- History of psychoactive substance use
- History of psychological factors impacting the client's condition
- Educational/vocational history
- Client abilities, strengths, needs, and preferences
- Preliminary diagnoses
- Admission to program information, including specific reasons when admission is denied
- Initial problem list
- Clinical assessment summary

The severity and unique treatment considerations of substance abuse problems vary significantly from one client to another, so an individualized plan of treatment must be established for every case, even if the clients' diagnoses are the same. For example, one client with a diagnosis of cocaine abuse might require both an inpatient stay and outpatient therapy, whereas another client might only need outpatient therapy. The individualized treatment plan (ITP) is the document in the client's record that is intended to guide the clinician and the client through the treatment process, and

Clinical Assessment Outline

Client Name (Last, First, MI)	ID#

Presenting Problem: Include reason for entry, source of referral, legal involvement, self-identified problems and recent stressors.

_____

_____

_____

_____

_____

_____

_____

_____

_____

_____

_____

_____

_____

_____

_____

Health/Medical History: Describe general health, nutrition, medical problems, medications, hospitalizations, disabilities, tuberculosis screening and HIV-risk behaviors.

_____

_____

_____

_____

_____

_____

_____

_____

_____

_____

_____

_____

_____

_____

_____

_____

_____

Page 1 of 4

Figure 8-2   Clinical assessment forms. (Courtesy of South Carolina Department of Alcohol and Other Drug Abuse Services.)

Family/Social Interaction: In chronological order, describe family of origin and present family, including relationships with all family members. Include family history of substance use/abuse and current family use. Describe other intimate and social relationships. Include peer group functioning. Include cultural, ethnic and spiritual factors and expectations. Include any physical and/or sexual abuse history.

_____
_____
_____
_____
_____
_____
_____
_____
_____
_____
_____
_____
_____
_____
_____
_____
_____
_____
_____
_____
_____
_____
_____
_____
_____
_____
_____
_____
_____

Figure 8-2   (*Continued*)

Client Name (Last, First, MI) | **ID#**

Psychoactive Substance Use History

Drug	Age at First Use	Frequency (last 6 months)	Quantity (specify time frame)	Last Use	How Used
Alcohol					
Amphetamine					
Caffeine					
Cannabis					
Cocaine					
Hallucinogen					
Inhalant					
Nicotine					
Opioid					
PCP					
Sedative Hypnotic					

Psychoactive Substance Use: Include other relevant substance use factors such as loss of control, tolerance, treatment history, patterns of use and problems related to use. Include data to differentiate between use, abuse and dependence.

Figure 8-2　(Continued)

Psychological: Include mental status, activities of daily living, communication skills/abilities, present emotional state, management of emotions, violence, suicide attempts/thoughts and psychiatric history (to include history of eating disorder behaviors).

_____
_____
_____
_____
_____
_____
_____
_____
_____
_____

Educational/Vocational: Include years of education, military service, job history, financial status and leisure activities.

_____
_____
_____
_____
_____

Strengths and Needs: Describe client and clinician perceptions and unique factors affecting the course of treatment.

_____
_____
_____
_____
_____

Sources of information other than client:

Name _____   Relationship _____

Name _____   Relationship _____

Assessment Interview Information		
Assessment Date	Client Time	Clinician Signature and Title
_____	_____	_____
_____	_____	_____
_____	_____	_____

Figure 8-2   *(Continued)*

Clinical Assessment Summary

Client Name (Last, First, MI)	ID#

Identifying Information

DOB _____ Age _____ Sex _____ Ethnic Group _____

Marital Status _____ Occupation _____ Education _____

Multiaxial Diagnosis

	Code #	Description
Axis I:	_____	_____
	_____	_____
	_____	_____
Axis II:	_____	_____
Axis III:		_____

Axis IV: Psychosocial Stressors: _____

Severity: _____

Axis V: GAF = _____ (current)

Master Problem List: In concise statements, list the most immediate problems the client is presenting. Indicate whether each problem will be addressed on the Treatment Plan (T); whether it will be referred (R) for services elsewhere; or whether it will be monitored (M). Place the letter that corresponds to the appropriate disposition in the space provided to the left of each problem statement.

_____ 1)_____

_____ 2)_____

_____ 3)_____

_____ 4)_____

_____ 5)_____

_____ 6)_____

_____ 7)_____

_____ 8)_____

Admitted to services _____ yes _____ no   Reason for non-admission _____

_____

Figure 8-2   (*Continued*)

Interpretive Summary: Include an integration and interpretation of all pertinent assessment information; the client's perception of his/her needs, strengths, limitations or problems; clinical judgments regarding the course of treatment; recommended treatments; and anticipated level and length of care.

Clinician Signature and Title	Date

Figure 8-2 (*Continued*)

Six Month Individualized Treatment Plan

1. Client Name (Last, First, MI)			ID#	

2. Diagnosis and Justification for Treatment or Continuation of Treatment

3. Proposed Treatment Process

a. Date Service Ordered	b. Type Service	c. Estimated Frequency	d. Goals	e. Expected Achievement Date

4. Client Signature	Date
5. Clinician Signature and Title	Date

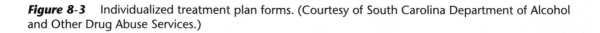

Figure 8-3   Individualized treatment plan forms. (Courtesy of South Carolina Department of Alcohol and Other Drug Abuse Services.)

6. Summary of FIRST 90 Day Progress
   (Address progress on goals, appropriateness of service being provided, and need for continued treatment.)

7. Clinician Signature and Title	Date

8. Summary of SECOND 90 Day Progress
   (Address progress on goals, appropriateness of service being provided, and need for continued treatment.)

9. Clinician Signature and Title	Date

Figure 8-3 (*Continued*)

it must be based on the client's comprehensive clinical assessment. An ITP typically includes:

- Identifying information
- DSM-IV diagnoses
- Justification or reason for treatment
- Proposed treatment process including type of service and frequency
- Treatment goals and objectives that are measurable, with target achievement dates

The ITP is updated periodically to reflect changes in the client's condition and revised treatment goals. The ITP should be a flexible document designed to meet the treatment needs of the individual client. Both CARF and JCAHO have developed standards for the ITP.

Reimbursement and Funding

The reimbursement issues facing inpatient substance abuse facilities are essentially the same as those for other types of inpatient mental health services. However, the funding stream for outpatient substance abuse treatment is complex, involving several government agencies at both the state and federal levels, as well as private insurance companies and client fees.

In a community (outpatient or residential) substance abuse treatment center, for example, revenues may come from any combination of the following sources:

- *Client Fees.* In the public sector client fees do not account for a major portion of revenue, but they are collected, generally on a sliding-scale basis (i.e., clients' out-of-pocket fees are set according to their ability to pay). Both family size and income are taken into consideration in determining the clients' copayments.

- *Private Insurance.* Individual insurance policies may cover substance abuse services at the inpatient or outpatient level. In public facilities, the insurance company is generally billed first, before any federal insurance is billed or any applicable sliding-scale copayment is determined.

- *Medicaid.* Medicaid program costs are shared by the federal and state governments. Therefore, eligibility, reimbursement rates, and payment mechanisms (fee-for-service, capitation, etc.) for substance abuse treatment vary from state to state. Most publicly supported substance abuse facilities rely heavily on Medicaid as a source of revenue.

- *Medicare.* Medicare covers a limited amount of substance abuse treatment for eligible clients. Services such as inpatient treatment, outpatient treatment, and detoxification are covered for a preset number of days or visits.

- *Other Government Funding Sources.* Several federal agencies administer a variety of block grants and contracts to support substance abuse treatment or prevention.

The agency that administers the federal substance abuse prevention and treatment (SAPT) grants is the Substance Abuse and Mental Health Services Administration (SAMHSA). These grants, and others, are generally awarded to individual states, which in turn distribute the money to eligible community agencies. In some of these agencies, federal funding may account for up to 75 percent or more of total revenue. Certain community-based treatment programs, such as school-based intervention programs, may actually be funded up to 100 percent by specific grants or contracts.

Information Management

Many of the information management issues facing substance abuse facilities are shared by other types of health care settings, which makes sense, because the purpose of maintaining client information in substance abuse facilities is basically the same as in other facilities: to facilitate the documentation of care and services provided, to support quality review activities, to optimize financial reimbursement, to meet all legal requirements, and to meet a variety of administrative, research, and educational needs. There are, however, a few issues that are either unique to substance abuse or are more commonly found in this setting. The following sections describe some of these issues related to the areas of data and information flow, coding and classification, data sets for substance abuse, and computerization of client information.

Data and Information Flow

Each substance abuse facility has its own distinct flow of client information, from the time of admission through discharge and follow-up care. This information flow may or may not include computer-based information, but it should reflect the course of treatment provided to the clients. Figure 8-4 represents a typical flow of information in an outpatient substance abuse center. Once a client enters the system, whether as a court-ordered admission or as a voluntary admission, the intake process is the first step in collecting client information and determining the appropriate treatment. During intake, clerical personnel gather all necessary demographic and financial information, as well as the necessary consent to treatment and release-of-information forms. After the intake, designated clinical staff conduct a complete substance abuse assessment to determine the level of care and program that is most appropriate for the client. The client's program-specific individualized treatment plan is then developed by his or her treatment team. This treatment plan lists, among other things, the client's individualized treatment goals and objectives and serves as a "blueprint" to his or her care. While the client is involved in active treatment, all other documentation is tied to the treatment plan and should reflect progress toward the treatment goals. Most substance abuse programs have aftercare

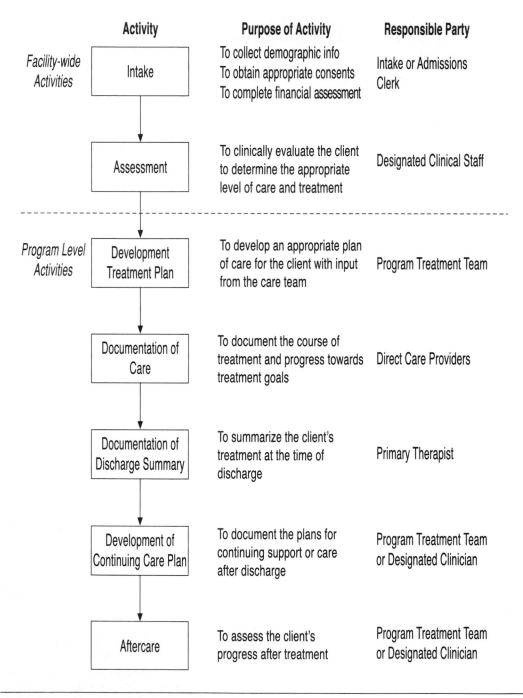

Activity	Purpose of Activity	Responsible Party

Facility-wide Activities

Intake — To collect demographic info / To obtain appropriate consents / To complete financial assessment — Intake or Admissions Clerk

Assessment — To clinically evaluate the client to determine the appropriate level of care and treatment — Designated Clinical Staff

Program Level Activities

Development Treatment Plan — To develop an appropriate plan of care for the client with input from the care team — Program Treatment Team

Documentation of Care — To document the course of treatment and progress towards treatment goals — Direct Care Providers

Documentation of Discharge Summary — To summarize the client's treatment at the time of discharge — Primary Therapist

Development of Continuing Care Plan — To document the plans for continuing support or care after discharge — Program Treatment Team or Designated Clinician

Aftercare — To assess the client's progress after treatment — Program Treatment Team or Designated Clinician

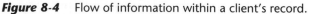

Figure 8-4   Flow of information within a client's record.

staff, who follow up on their discharged clients to evaluate their continued progress once active treatment has been completed.

Coding and Classification

The selection of a coding or classification system for a substance abuse treatment facility depends on the level of care provided by that facility and the type of funding that is used to support its programs. In general, when ICD-9-CM and CPT codes are required for reimbursement purposes they are assigned to substance abuse client diagnoses following the same rules that apply to other inpatient and outpatient settings. The one significant difference in substance abuse coding is the availability of the *Diagnostic and Statistical Manual of Mental Disorders, fourth edition, text revision* (DSM-IV-TR). DSM-IV-TR is a classification system and nomenclature of mental disorders that was developed by the American Psychiatric Association with a stated purpose of providing "clear descriptions of diagnostic categories in order to enable clinicians and investigators to diagnose, communicate about, study, and treat people with various mental disorders" (American Psychiatric Association, 2000, p. xxxvii). The term *mental disorders* in DSM-IV-TR includes conditions related to substance abuse and dependence. In addition to providing diagnostic criteria sets for clinicians to use in assigning mental health diagnoses, DSM-IV includes a five-character coding system that is based on ICD-9-CM. Although there is a high degree of compatibility between the codes found in DSM-IV and those found in ICD-9-CM, there are some significant differences.

Another interesting feature of DSM-IV is that it offers clinicians the option of assessing clients and recording their findings in a multiaxial format. According to the American Psychiatric Association, a multiaxial system is one that "involves an assessment on several axes, each of which refers to a different domain of information that may help the clinician plan treatment and predict outcome" (APA, 2000, p. 27). The first three axes in DSM-IV are generally thought of as the basic components of the multiaxial reporting system. They are described in the following table (Lee, 1995).

Axis	Title	Used for reporting . . .
Axis I	Clinical Disorders Other Conditions That May Be a Focus of Clinical Attention	All the disorders or conditions found within DSM-IV (including substance abuse and dependence diagnoses), except Personality Disorders and Mental Retardation
Axis II	Personality Disorders Mental Retardation	Personality Disorders and Mental Retardation
Axis III	General Medical Conditions	General medical conditions that impact the treatment of the client. ICD-9-CM codes are used for reporting diagnostic codes on Axis III.

The remaining axes, Axes IV and V, are less frequently used in assessing clients:

Axis	Title	Used for reporting . . .
Axis IV	Psychosocial and Environmental Problems	Psychosocial and environmental problems that may affect the treatment of the client, such as unemployment, victim of child neglect, etc.
Axis V	Global Assessment of Functioning	The client's overall level of functioning. Clinicians may report this using the Global Assessment of Functioning (GAF) scale contained within the DSM-IV or another appropriate functioning scale. The GAF scale is reported as number between 0 and 100, with 100 representing the highest level of functioning.

The advantage of using DSM-IV in a substance abuse treatment setting is that it represents the latest research findings and acceptable diagnostic terms associated with mental health and substance abuse disorders. The disadvantage is that most third-party payers do not accept DSM-IV codes in lieu of ICD-9-CM codes. To offset this disadvantage, the American Health Information Management Association (AHIMA) published the *DSM-IV Crosswalk: Guidelines for Coding Mental Health Information*, which provides an easy-to-use tool for translating DSM-IV codes to the equivalent ICD-9-CM codes (Albaum-Feinstein, 1999).

Data Sets

In 1988, Congress passed Public Law 100-690, which required the collection of data on the national incidence and prevalence of both mental illness and substance abuse. The message that Congress sent by passing this law was that states had to be able to substantiate the need for federal block grant money. The National Institute of Drug Abuse (NIDA) and the National Institute of Alcohol Abuse and Alcoholism (NIAAA) were the federal agencies charged at that time with the administration of a national database of substance abuse client information to meet the substance abuse reporting component of the law. In 1995, this function was taken over by the Substance Abuse and Mental Health Services Administration, which has attempted to integrate the two existing substance abuse data sets, the Treatment Episode Data Set (TEDS) and the National Survey of Substance Abuse Treatment Services (N-SSATS), formerly known as the Uniform Facility Data Set (UFDS), with a third data set, the National Facility Register (NFR). TEDS, which was previously called the Client Data System, was developed to collect uniform data from states that was client specific, but not client identifiable. Facility-specific information is collected through N-SSATS (Brooks, 1990). The goal of this integration process is to establish one data system that provides national and state-level data on substance abuse clients and on the facilities that receive federal grants or contracts to provide substance abuse treatment.

Computer Systems

It is difficult to generalize about computer information systems that exist within the substance abuse treatment community today, because they vary greatly from facility to facility. There are treatment programs in the United States that have sophisticated electronic client information systems, and there are programs where one computer is shared among an entire staff. Some of this variability comes from the differences in levels of care and funding sources. A substance abuse treatment unit within a progressive acute care hospital, for example, will benefit from the hospital-wide information systems that are in place. On the other hand, a public community treatment program with limited funds may not have much in the way of computer development. One generalization that can be made, however, is that as the health care industry moves toward more integrated delivery systems and computer-based patient records, client information systems within the substance abuse treatment community will take on new importance. Substance abuse treatment facilities will be competing with other health care entities for scarce health care dollars, and the government and other payers are demanding outcomes-oriented data to support continued direct funding or reimbursement. This increased need for timely, accurate data should lead to increased development of computer-based substance abuse client information systems.

Quality Improvement and Utilization Management

Quality improvement (QI) and utilization management (UM) are two additional areas within substance abuse facilities about which it is difficult to make general statements. Substance abuse treatment organizations do include the QI and UM functions, but the level of sophistication of the QI and UM processes depends on the level of care provided by that facility and its primary funding source.

Quality Improvement

Providers of substance abuse treatment must ensure that they offer quality care and service. The type of QI or quality assurance activities found within substance abuse treatment facilities is often related to the level of care provided and whether the facility seeks JCAHO or CARF accreditation. Some states have specific Medicaid standards that also address the need for an organized quality improvement or quality assurance process. A substance abuse treatment unit in a JCAHO-accredited hospital would participate in the hospital-wide quality improvement program, which would include activities such as continuous quality improvement (CQI) and outcomes assessment using critical pathways. Public outpatient facilities, on the other hand, may rely on periodic chart review to meet their quality objectives.

Utilization Management

Providers of substance abuse treatment, just as other health care providers, must demonstrate fiscal responsibility and solid clinical decision making that is based on the individual needs of the client. It is important that facilities ensure that each client receives the level of care appropriate to his or her severity of illness. As a general rule, clients should be served at the least intensive level that will meet their treatment objectives, such as outpatient therapy, and should move on to a more intensive level, such as residential treatment, only when it is justified by their specific treatment needs.

Severity indexes and other treatment review instruments have also been developed for evaluating treatment and the utilization of services within the substance abuse treatment community. As discussed earlier, the American Society of Addiction Medicine (ASAM) publishes a placement criteria manual that defines levels of care and the specific criteria that should be used in placing both adolescent and adult clients in the appropriate treatment setting. The "Care Settings" section of this chapter describes these levels of care. Managed care organizations have endeavored to use these or similar levels of care to place patients in the most cost-effective settings, yet still achieve the desired treatment results (Kosanke et al., 2002). Another instrument that is used in utilization management and to facilitate client care is the **Addiction Severity Index (ASI)**, which was developed in 1979. ASI is designed to be administered through an interview process by a trained technician to measure seven substance abuse–related problem areas: medical condition, drug use, alcohol use, employment, illegal activity, social relations, and psychological findings. The data from the client interview is tabulated and results in a severity "score" for the client. The score can be stated as a 10-point severity rating for clinical use or as a mathematically weighted score for use as an outcomes measure in research studies (Grissom, 1991).

Risk Management and Legal Issues

Risk management is defined as "a four step process designed to identify, evaluate and resolve the actual and possible sources of loss. The four steps are risk identification, risk evaluation, risk handling, and risk monitoring." (Roach and Aspen Health Law and Compliance Center, 1998, p. 333). Organized risk management programs are found in inpatient substance abuse treatment settings more often than they are found in the outpatient settings, because Medicare, Medicaid, and many state regulations actually require hospitals to have adequate risk management in place (Roach and Aspen Health Law Center, 1994). There are, however, a variety of other important legal issues, such as confidentiality and release of information, court-ordered treatment, and commitments, that are commonly associated with all levels of substance abuse treatment.

Confidentiality and Release of Information

Confidentiality of client information is extremely important in substance abuse treatment facilities. Clients seeking alcohol and drug abuse prevention and treatment services must be assured of the greatest possible privacy, because of the stigma attached to "alcoholic" and "addict" labels and because use of illicit drugs and use of alcohol by underage minors constitute crimes. Clients must feel that they will be not be subject to a law enforcement investigation if they seek treatment. In the early 1970s, the federal government enacted two laws that were written to guarantee this strict level of confidentiality: the Comprehensive Alcohol Abuse and Alcohol Prevention, Treatment and Rehabilitation Act of 1970 and the Drug Abuse and Treatment Act of 1972 (Legal Action Center, 1991). The federal regulations, known as 42 CFR *(Code of Federal Regulations)*, Part 2, *Confidentiality of Alcohol and Drug Abuse Patient Records*, which implemented these confidentiality statutes, were issued in 1975 and revised in 1987 and 1995.

The regulations in 42 CFR, Part 2, are more restrictive than the privacy provisions of the Health Insurance Portability and Accountability Act (HIPAA). Except under certain specified conditions, disclosure of information concerning any client who is seen in a federally assisted alcohol or drug abuse program is strictly prohibited. A program is defined as "any person or organization that, in whole or in part, provides alcohol or drug abuse diagnosis, treatment or referral for treatment" (42 CFR, Part 2). There are a few exceptions to this general prohibition written into the regulations. Disclosure can be made:

- With the written consent of the patient
- For internal communications on a need-to-know basis
- When there is no patient-identifying information
- In a bona fide medical emergency
- With a court order (with special procedures)
- When a crime is committed at the treatment program or against program personnel
- For research and audits
- In child and vulnerable adult abuse reporting, under the provisions of the applicable state law
- Under the provisions of a qualified service organization agreement (QSOA), through which an organization, such as a commercial laboratory or a private occupational therapy group, has a written agreement to provide services to the clients within the substance abuse program

No information about a substance abuse client should be disclosed unless the facility can state how these exceptions permit disclosure. However, it is very rare to release information based on exceptions. Confidential substance abuse information can be released with a written authorization from the patient (Legal Action Center, 2003), but this authorization must contain specific items to be considered valid. Figure 8-5 outlines the required elements for an authorization to release drug and alcohol treatment information. Other elements, such as the signature of a witness, may be added to the authorization form at the discretion of the facility. When the information is released, it must be accompanied by a written statement notifying the

The name or general designation of the program(s) making the disclosure

The name of the individual or organization that will receive the disclosure

The name of the patient who is the subject of the disclosure

The purpose or need for the disclosure

How much and what kind of information will be disclosed

A statement that the patient may revoke the consent at any time, except to the extent that the program has already acted in reliance on it

The date, event, or condition upon which the consent expires if not previously revoked

The signature of the patient (and/or other authorized person)

The date on which the authorization is signed

Figure 8-5   Required elements for an authorization to release information from an alcohol or drug program, from 42 CFR, Part 2, *Confidentiality of Alcohol and Drug Abuse Patient Records.*

recipient that the information is "protected by Federal confidentiality rules" and that the recipient may not redisclose the records to a third party (42 CFR, Part 2).

Court-Ordered Treatment

A portion of the substance abuse client population enters treatment as a result of a court order. The court order may come from a conviction for driving under the influence of alcohol or drugs (DUI). In some states, substance abuse assessment is mandated by law for all persons with a DUI conviction, and if the assessment indicates that the individual needs further treatment, this treatment is also mandated. Typically, if the DUI client fails to fulfill an established court-ordered assessment and treatment protocol, he or she will not be reissued a driver's license. Thus, it is necessary to establish a good working relationship between the substance abuse treatment centers and the legal system. One community substance abuse center in North Carolina, for example, met this challenge through the development of an active partnership with the municipal court system. A treatment center employee was assigned to be present in court during the DUI hearings to facilitate the enrollment of these court-ordered clients. All necessary consents and authorizations to release information back to the court were signed and appropriate fees were collected before the client ever left the courthouse.

DUI convictions are not the only court procedures that lead to court-ordered substance abuse treatment. Examples of situations that might result in a court order for treatment are child abuse, possession of illegal drugs, sexual assault, underage alcohol consumption, burglary, or assault, when the court feels that the perpetrator's substance abuse was a factor. Typically the judge will order the client to seek substance abuse treatment as a stipulation in a suspended or reduced sentence or probation. On occasion the court might actually order an incarcerated individual to obtain appropriate substance abuse treatment, if it is available through the correction facility.

Involuntary Commitments

Involuntary commitment is a legal process by which individuals who are deemed to be a danger to themselves or to others may be admitted to a treatment program even though they refuse or cannot consent to the treatment. Involuntary commitment is governed by state statutes, and the criteria and procedures vary from state to state. All states require that the person being committed have a mental illness or mental disorder; however, many states do not define the terms *mental illness* or *mental condition*, or define them very broadly. Several states, such as North Carolina, Louisiana, and Hawaii, specifically cite substance abuse as a mental disorder or as a potential cause for involuntary commitment (Beis, 1984).

In states where involuntary commitment for substance abuse treatment is permitted, the actual procedure varies depending on the state laws, but the following steps represent a typical series of events in the overall process:

- A petitioner, law enforcement officer, or other responsible person files a petition that states that the client meets the criteria for involuntary admission (i.e., he or she is a danger to himself or herself or to others).
- The client is detained for an evaluation by a physician or other qualified clinician for a period of time that may vary from state to state.
- The clinician certifies that the client meets the standard for involuntary commitment.
- The petition and the certificate are filed with the court and a hearing date is set.
- The court determines whether or not the client meets the standard for involuntary admission.
- The court will require that the client be admitted if the client meets the standard (this admission may be to an inpatient or outpatient program, depending on the needs of the client and the state guidelines) (Beis, 1984).

See Figure 8-6 for an example of a form used to evaluate individuals in a commitment recommendation screening process.

Role of the Health Information Management Professional

The role of the health information manager is becoming increasingly important in substance abuse treatment settings. The changing health care environment is increasing the need for substance abuse facilities to collect, analyze, and maintain timely and reliable client information. Managed care organizations and other payers, including the

---

DEPARTMENT OF MENTAL HEALTH
Community Counseling Services
Pre-evaluation Screening Form
DMH/013   5/02

Name: _____

Case #: _____

IN THE _____ COURT OF _____ COUNTY   RE: _____
          (Type of Court)   *(Name of County)*

CASE NO. _____ SERVICE CODE _____ UNITS OF SERVICE _____ DATE _____

Respondent having been evaluated and pre-screened for commitment pursuant to M.C.A. Section 41-21-67, Region _____
Mental Health Center Offers the following:

Legal Charges Pending: Yes ☐   No ☐

PERSONAL DATA INFORMATION

NAME: _____ SOCIAL SECURITY NO: _____ DOB: _____

RACE: _____   MARITAL STATUS: ☐Single   ☐Married   ☐Divorced   ☐Widowed   SEX: ☐Male   ☐Female

ADDRESS: _____

_____

_____

NAME OF SPOUSE/NEXT OF KIN: _____ COUNTY OF RESIDENCE: _____

MEDICAID# _____ MEDICARE # _____

EDUCATION *(Circle Highest Grade Completed)* 1 2 3 4 5 6 7 8 9 10 11 12 13 14 15 16 17 18 GED

OCCUPATION: _____ PRESENTLY EMPLOYED: ☐ Yes   ☐ No

EMPLOYER: _____ LENGTH OF EMPLOYMENT: _____ years ____ months

HOUSEHOLD COMPOSITION *(Mark All That Apply)*

☐ Lives Alone   ☐ With Siblings   ☐ With Parents   ☐ With One Parent   ☐ With Children
☐ With Spouse   ☐ With Relatives   ☐ With Legal Guardian   ☐ With Others   ☐ Others

NUMBER OF DEPENDENT(S): _____

NAME OF AFFIANT *(Person Filing Papers)*

Name: _____ Relationship: _____ Phone: (H) _____ (W) _____

Address: _____ City _____ State _____ Zip Code _____

FAMILY CONTACT

Name: _____ Relationship: _____ Phone: (H) _____ (W) _____

Address: _____ City _____ State _____ Zip Code _____

PERSON WITH <u>LEGAL CUSTODY</u>, GUARDIANSHIP, and /or Conservatorship

Name: _____ Relationship: _____ Phone: (H) _____ (W) _____

Address: _____ City _____ State _____ Zip Code _____

Figure 8-6   Pre-commitment evaluation screening form. (Courtesy of Community Counseling Services, Starkville, Mississippi.)

MEDICAL HISTORY INFORMATION

PREVIOUS MENTAL HEALTH HOSPITALIZATION, SERVICE, A&D TREATMENT (*List Where & When*)_____

_____

_____

_____

_____

CURRENT MEDICATIONS (*List Names and Dosage*)

Name	*Dosage*
_____	_____
_____	_____
_____	_____
_____	_____
_____	_____
_____	_____

COMPLAINT WITH MEDICATIONS: ❑ Yes ❑ No ❑ Unknown

ALLERGIES: ❑ Yes ❑ No If Yes, Explain _____

PREVIOUS SURGERY: ❑ Yes ❑ No If Yes, Explain _____

CONCURRENT PHYSICAL CONDITIONS (*Mark all that apply*)

❑ Diabetes ❑ Emphysema/Cold ❑ Heart Condition ❑ Seizures
❑ Hypertension ❑ S.T.D. ❑ TB ❑ Cancer
❑ Contagious Disease ❑ Other Chronic Illness ❑ (Please State) _____
❑ Hepatitis
Elaborate on acute medical conditions of conditions marked (if needed) _____

FAMILY PHYSICIAN: _____

BEHAVIORS EXHIBITED BY RESPONDENT
Also consider information from affiant and/or affidavit.
(*Mark appropriate answer and/or write in additional pertinent descriptions.*)

History or Present Danger to Self ❑ Yes ❑ No *(If Yes, Mark Appropriate Statements Below)*

❑ Thoughts of suicide ❑ Threats of suicide ❑ Plan for suicide ❑ Pre-occupation with death
❑ Suicide gesture ❑ Suicide attempts ❑ Family history of suicide ❑ Self-mutilation
❑ Inability to care for self ❑ High risk behavior ❑ Provoking harm to self from others
❑ Other _____

Describe: _____

History or Present Danger to Others ❑ Yes ❑ No *(If Yes, Mark Appropriate Statements Below)*

❑ Thoughts to harm others ❑ Threats to harm others ❑ Plans to harm others
❑ Attempts to harm others ❑ Stalking ❑ Has harmed others
❑ Felt like killing someone ❑ Inability or unwillingness to care for dependents
❑ Other _____

Describe: _____

Figure 8-6 (*Continued*)

Pre-evaluation Screening Form *(page three)*   Name:_____   Case#:_____

Failure to Care for Self   ❏ Yes   ❏ No   (If Yes, Mark Appropriate Statements Below)

Failure or inability to provide necessary: ❏ Food   ❏ Clothing   ❏ Shelter   ❏ Safety   ❏ Medical care for self

❏ Other _____

Antisocial/Criminal Behavior   ❏ Yes   ❏No   (If Yes, Mark Appropriate Statement Below)

❏ Frequent lying   ❏ Stealing   ❏ Running away from home   ❏ Excessive fighting
❏ Destroys property   ❏ Fire setting   ❏ Cruelty to other   ❏ Cruelty to animals
❏ Arrests   ❏ Gang membership   ❏ Brandishing weapons   ❏ Convictions
❏ Imprisoned   ❏ Promiscuity   ❏ Exhibitionism   ❏ Family desertion
❏ Uses assumed name   ❏ Identify any legal charges which may be pending

❏ Other _____

Describe: _____

Drug Use/Abuse   ❏ Yes   ❏No   (If Yes, Mark Appropriate Statement Below)

❏ Has abused   ❏ Is abusing   ❏ Narcotics   ❏ Amphetamines ❏ Barbiturates   ❏ Hallucinogens
❏ Cocaine   ❏ Marijuana   ❏ Absenteeism ❏ Job loss   ❏ Arrests
❏ Has required hospitalization   ❏ Family problems due to drug use   ❏ Currently under the influence of drugs

❏ Other _____

Describe: _____

Alcohol Use/Abuse   ❏ Yes   ❏No   (If Yes, Mark Appropriate Statement Below)

❏ Drinking problem suspected   ❏ Intoxicated Now   ❏ Has required hospitalization
❏ D.T. s   ❏ Black-outs   ❏ Absenteeism
❏ Job loss   ❏ Arrests/DUI   ❏ Family problems due to drinking
❏ Currently under the influence of alcohol (BAL, if available)
❏ High-risk behavior occurs primarily when under the influence of alcoholic beverages, including beer.

❏ Other _____

Describe: _____

Depressive-Like Behaviors   ❏ Yes   ❏No   (If Yes, Mark Appropriate Statement Below)

❏ Sadness   ❏ Fatigue   ❏ Low Energy   ❏ Loss of interest   ❏ Extreme Withdrawal
❏ Crying   ❏ Poor Concentration   ❏ Weight loss or gain   ❏ Guilt feelings
❏ Feelings of worthlessness   ❏ Hopelessness about the future   ❏ Hypoactive
❏ Thoughts/threats of suicide   ❏ Sudden drop in grades or change in friends (especially in adolescents)

❏Other _____

Describe: _____

Manic-Like Behavior   ❏ Yes   ❏No   (If Yes, Mark Appropriate Statement Below)

❏ Euphoria   ❏ Hyperactivity   ❏ Grandiosity   ❏ Over talkativeness and/or pressured speech
❏ Irritability   ❏ Sexual promiscuity   ❏ Sleep disturbance ❏ Extravagance with money

❏ Other _____

Describe: _____

Dementia-Like Characteristics   ❏ Yes   ❏No   (If Yes, Mark Appropriate Statement Below)

❏ Confusion   ❏ Wanders Off   ❏ Disorientation   ❏ Impaired Judgement
❏ Absent-mindedness ❏Getting Lost   ❏ Confusion   ❏ Significant short-and/or long term memory
❏ Decline in activities of daily living (Consider age of respondent)   ❏Impaired Abstract Thinking

❏ Other _____

Describe: _____

Figure 8-6   (*Continued*)

Psychotic-Like Behavior   ❑ Yes   ❑No   *(If Yes, Mark Appropriate Statement Below)*

❑ Poor personal hygiene ❑ Loose Association   ❑ Suspiciousness   ❑ Bizarre or obscene acts
❑ Withdrawn   ❑ Incoherence   ❑ Unmanageable   ❑ Flat or inappropriate affect
❑ Talks often   ❑ Wanders off   ❑ Illusions   ❑ Disorientation time, place, people)
❑ Delusions   ❑ Confusion   ❑ Forgetfulness   ❑ Poor judgment
❑ Doesn't make sense   ❑ Irritability   ❑ Hallucinations
❑ Emotional turmoil   ❑ Disorganized speech or behavior

❑ Other _____

Describe: _____

ADDITIONAL INFORMATION

Child/Adolescent Conduct Disturbance   ❑ Yes   ❑ No   *(If Yes, Mark Appropriate Statement Below)*
(Current Behavior or During Childhood)

❑ Theft   ❑ Fire-setting   ❑ Cruelty to people   ❑ Cruelty to animals   ❑ Destruction of property
❑ Aggression   ❑ Arrest/detainment   ❑ Sexual Misconduct   ❑ Combativeness/aggression
❑ Refusal to attend school   ❑ Running away   ❑ Defiance of authority and rules
❑ Possession/Use of weapons
❑ Other _____

Mental Retardation   ❑ Yes   ❑No   *(If Yes, Mark Appropriate Statement Below)*

❑ History of special education placement   ❑ Documented IQ below a70
❑ Inability to care for self or activities of daily living   ❑Significantly sub-average intellectual functioning before age 18
❑ Substantial limitations in adaptive skills *(communication, self-care, home living, social skills, community use, self-direction health and safety, leisure and work)*
❑ Other _____

Other   ❑ Yes   ❑No   *(If Yes, Mark Appropriate Statement Below)*

❑ Anxiety   ❑ Panic   ❑Eating disorders   ❑Sexual disorders   ❑ Impulsive disorders
❑ Obsessive disorders ❑ Other _____

RECOMMENDATIONS

Examination for Commitment: ❑ Yes   ❑ No

If yes, is outpatient commitment currently an option for the respondent?   ❑ Yes   ❑No   Explain:

_____
_____
_____

If no, explain why outpatient commitment is not an option for the
        respondent:_____
_____
_____

SPECIFIC RECOMMENDATIONS
(Include Treatment Options)

_____
_____
_____

_____   _____   _____
Screener/Credentials   Date   Print Name

Figure 8-6   *(Continued)*

federal government, want "proof" that their enrollees are receiving quality services at the lowest possible cost.

Opportunities for the health information manager within substance abuse facilities are found in the areas of traditional client record management, electronic client record systems, risk management, utilization management, quality improvement, release-of-information services, and client rights coordination. One of the most challenging aspects for the health information manager working in substance abuse treatment is to be an advocate for client confidentiality. Most health information managers in substance abuse facilities fill the role of the confidentiality "expert" and must be thoroughly familiar with the federal regulations governing alcohol and drug abuse treatment records. Health information managers can assist in developing policies to meet the requirements of existing and newly developed regulations.

Trends

The trends in substance abuse treatment can be divided into treatment trends and economic or funding trends. The currents trends in treatment include many innovative approaches, some of which are discussed in this chapter. Examples of current treatment trends include the growth of programs for women, adolescent prevention programs, and treatment for the dually diagnosed. Substance abuse treatment centers are involved with an increasing number of Employee Assistance Programs (EAPs) and are also becoming more active in identifying needs of inmates in city or local jails. The economic trends are related to the changing health care environment and to the government's continuing struggle to spend taxpayers' dollars wisely.

Because government support is an essential source of revenue to many substance abuse treatment facilities, the changing political and economic climate will affect the future of the delivery of substance abuse services. Substance abuse education, prevention, and treatment have been important social issues in the United States for several decades. Congress, in partnership with state governments, has directed a substantial amount of government funds toward increasing awareness of substance abuse issues, as well as toward increasing the availability of treatment services across the socioeconomic spectrum. The national political and economic climate, however, has changed considerably since the 1970s, as taxpayers are asking for validation that their tax dollars are spent appropriately and are questioning the high cost of health care.

One of the most significant trends to affect health information management within the substance abuse treatment community is the government's increased emphasis on the need for data to substantiate the effectiveness of government-funded programs. Programs are being held accountable for the government dollars that they are awarded, and this accountability means providing supporting data back to the funding agency. In many cases, the information systems within substance abuse facilities are inadequate to provide this type of outcome-oriented data in a timely and accurate manner. To thrive in the current climate, substance abuse facilities will need improved information systems.

Another political and economic factor that is impacting substance abuse treatment services, along with the other segments of the health care delivery system, is the increase in the role of managed care organizations (MCOs). Not only are private MCOs increasing their services across the United States, but many states are opting to develop managed care models for Medicaid. Dealing with MCOs will necessitate *significant* changes in the way substance abuse facilities have traditionally operated. The need for more sophisticated information systems that can provide financial and client outcomes data will be an important part of this change.

Along with changes in government funding procedures and the increase in the number of MCOs, substance abuse facilities will also be affected by the trend of multiple health care organizations building alliances and partnerships to develop integrated health delivery systems. Hopefully, substance abuse treatment will be valued as an important component of any comprehensive health delivery system. However, this raises important issues related to integrated client information systems, access to this information, and client confidentiality that will need to be addressed. This is an era of significant change in health care delivery systems, of which substance abuse treatment services are an important element.

Summary

Modern substance abuse treatment emerged in the 1950s as residential facilities for the treatment of alcohol dependency began to develop across the United States. Since that time, the number of different treatment settings for clients with alcohol and other drug problems has grown to include outpatient treatment, intensive outpatient and partial hospitalization treatment, residential/inpatient treatment, and medically managed intensive inpatient treatment settings. The number of programs within the treatment settings has also grown to include special programs for women, adolescents, court-referred clients, children of addicted families, and many others. Substance abuse treatment settings can be either publicly funded or privately funded. Substance abuse treatment and prevention has been a national issue for several decades, with the government granting significant amounts of money to states that are specifically targeted for substance abuse treatment and prevention programs. Public substance abuse treatment settings have traditionally assumed a major responsibility for providing substance abuse treatment services to the community, and they receive the majority of their funds from the federal and state governments. However, reimbursement from private insurance companies and client fees account for a portion of their revenue.

Health information managers working in substance abuse treatment facilities not only provide the traditional services associated with health information management, but they must gain expertise in several other areas, as well. For example, substance abuse treatment is regulated by federal and state governments and by voluntary accreditation organizations, such as JCAHO and CARF. Many state regulations, and the CARF and JCAHO standards, address quality of care and information management issues. Health information managers working in substance abuse treatment facilities need to be aware of all relevant regulations and standards, as they are often seen as the information management and quality assurance experts within the facilities. Another very important aspect of managing substance abuse client information is maintaining strict client confidentiality. The federal regulations, 42 CFR, Part 2, *Confidentiality of Alcohol and Drug Abuse Records*, mandate that all federally assisted substance abuse programs follow certain procedures before releasing client information. The health information manager often oversees compliance with 42 CFR, Part 2.

The national trends in health care, such as cutting government spending on health care, the growth of managed care, and the development of integrated delivery systems, have had an impact on substance abuse treatment facilities. Centers that had few financial worries when government substance abuse grants were plentiful are now faced with competing for scarce dollars with other segments of the health delivery system. One potentially positive development to result from this changing environment may well be growth in the use of computer technology to develop and maintain integrated client information systems that provide data that are timely, accurate, complete, legible, and accessible.

Key Terms

42 CFR, Part 2, Confidentiality of Drug and Alcohol Abuse Records   federal regulations that mandate strict confidentiality of drug and alcohol patient information in federally assisted substance abuse treatment programs.

Addiction Severity Index (ASI)   a rating scale that was developed to be used by clinicians to measure the severity of a client's substance abuse problems. The ASI measures seven substance abuse–related problem areas: medical condition, drug use, alcohol use, employment, illegal activity, social relations, and psychological findings.

Alcoholics Anonymous (AA)   a worldwide organization of self-help recovery groups that support individuals in maintaining sobriety. AA is based on a 12-step recovery process, and AA and other programs that follow the 12-step recovery process are sometimes referred to as 12-step programs.

clinical assessment   a clinical assessment is conducted by a clinician for every client that enters a substance abuse treatment program. The clinical assessment is used as a basis for the client's diagnosis and individualized treatment plan.

Commission on Accreditation of Rehabilitation Facilities (CARF)   a voluntary accreditation agency that sets standards that promote "the delivery of quality services to people with disabilities" (CARF, 1994). CARF standards include a section devoted to alcohol and other drug treatment programs.

Diagnostic and Statistical Manual of Mental Disorders, fourth edition **(DSM-IV)**   a classification system and nomenclature of mental disorders developed by the American Psychiatric Association with a stated purpose of providing "clear descriptions of diagnostic categories in order to enable clinicians and investigators to diagnose, communicate about, study, and treat people with various mental disorders" (APA, 1994, p. xxiii). It is also used as a coding system for mental health disorders. Each diagnosis is assigned a unique code number that is based on ICD-9-CM.

dually diagnosed clients   clients with both a substance abuse disorder and a chronic mental illness. These clients typically have special treatment needs.

employee assistance programs (EAPs)   substance abuse assessment and treatment programs established through a contractual arrangement between an organization and a substance abuse treatment facility to serve the employees within the organization.

individualized treatment plan (ITP)   a written plan developed by the client's treatment team that is used to identify the type and frequency of services needed by the client. It includes measurable goals and objectives that address the problems identified in the clinical assessment and should be updated periodically (usually every six months) as the client's treatment needs change.

intensive outpatient or partial hospitalization treatment   "an organized outpatient service that delivers treatment services during the day, before or after work or school, in the evening or on weekends" (ASAM, 2001, p. 3).

involuntary commitment   a legal process by which individuals who are deemed to be a danger to themselves or to others may be admitted to a substance abuse (or mental health) treatment program even though they refuse or cannot consent to the treatment.

medically managed intensive inpatient treatment   substance abuse treatment programs that "provide a planned regimen of 24-hour medically directed evaluation, care and treatment of mental and substance related disorders in an acute care inpatient setting. They are staffed by designated addiction-credentialed physicians, including psychiatrists, as well as other mental health- and addiction-credentialed clinicians" (ASAM, 2001, p. 4).

residential/inpatient treatment   substance abuse treatment "services staffed by designated addiction treatment and mental health personnel who provide a planned regimen of care in a 24-hour live-in setting. . . . They are housed in, or affiliated with, permanent facilities where patients can reside safely. They are staffed 24 hours a day. Mutual and self-help group meetings generally are available on site" (ASAM, 2001, p. 3).

outpatient treatment   "professionally directed evaluation, treatment and recovery services . . . provided in regularly scheduled sessions" (ASAM, 2001, p. 2).

REVIEW QUESTIONS

Knowledge-based Questions

1. Describe three different settings in which substance abuse treatment can take place.

2. Define the role of a case manager versus the role of a counselor in substance abuse treatment settings.

3. What is Alcoholics Anonymous? How does it relate to substance abuse treatment?

4. List the key elements that should be included in an individualized treatment plan.

5. Name two voluntary accreditation organizations that set standards for substance abuse treatment facilities. What standards are used for outpatient centers? inpatient programs?

6. Define involuntary commitment. What are the basic steps to obtain an involuntary commitment?

Application-based Questions

1. Why is it important for a health information manager to be familiar with the ASAM *Patient Placement Criteria Manual*? What is the purpose of this manual?

2. The role of the health information manager in a substance abuse treatment facility often involves serving as the confidentiality expert. Why is confidentiality of special concern in a substance abuse treatment program?

3. Briefly discuss current trends in the overall health care delivery system that you believe will impact substance abuse treatment services.

Web Activity

1. Go to the *Code of Federal Regulations* at http://www.gpoaccess.gov/cfr/index.html to search for a sample consent form in 42 CFR, Part 2, "Confidentiality of Alcohol and Drug Abuse Patient Records." Upon arriving at the site, locate the hyperlink, "Retrieve by CFR citation" located on the left side of the screen. Follow this link to the next screen, then enter "42" as the Title, "2" as the Part, leave the section number blank, then enter "C" as the subpart. You may select either "TEXT" or "PDF" as the file type. Then click the "Go" button. Find the sample consent form in Subpart C and use it to begin developing a consent form for the fictitious facility, Seven Acres Substance Abuse Treatment Services. Find the notice of prohibition of redisclosure in the same subpart and use it in developing a form to accompany information released from the Seven Acres facility.

2. Visit the Web site of the Legal Action Center at http://www.lac.org to look at the sample forms available there. Upon arriving at the site, select "Publications and Videos." Then click on the "Free Publications" hyperlink. Scroll down to find the sample forms. Select the "Sample Consent Form," which is a consent for the release of confidential information. How does this form compare to the form you developed in Activity 1?

Case Study

Sarah Johnson is the health information manager for the Columbus County Alcohol and Drug Treatment Center, a CARF-accredited, publicly funded treatment facility. As a member of the quality improvement (QI) committee, Sarah has been reviewing client records, focusing on written clinical assessments and treatment plans. The QI committee is interested in evaluating how consistently the clinicians document appropriate treatment goals, based on the information found in the clinical assessment. One of the records that Sarah reviewed is an outpatient record for Ann Wilson, a 24-year-old female client enrolled in the center's womens' program. Based on the following summaries of Ms. Wilson's clinical assessment and treatment plan, what specific feedback should Sarah give to the committee? Do the treatment goals and objectives relate to the person's goals? Are they written in measurable terms? Do they specify treatment interventions and their frequency?

Clinical Assessment

Presenting Problem: The 24-year-old, white female with a history of alcohol and cannabis abuse was referred by the county inpatient alcohol and drug treatment program. She is in need of continuing treatment for her longstanding problem with alcohol and drugs.

Health/Medical History: No current health problems. Client has two children, aged 2 years and 4 years. Other than childbirth and her recent substance abuse treatment, this client has not had any previous hospitalizations.

Family/Social Interaction: Client was raised in a physically abusive environment by her mother and alcoholic stepfather. Natural father was killed in a nightclub when the client was 10 years old. Client indicates that her natural father was also an alcoholic. She is currently living in public housing with her two children. She has little family or other emotional support. Her boyfriend of several years (father of her 2-year-old child) recently moved in with another woman.

Psychoactive Substance Use History

Drug	Age at First Use	Frequency (last 6 mo)	Quantity	Last Use	How Used
Alcohol	11	Daily	Pint of bourbon per day	One month ago	Oral
Cocaine	18	Once in the last year	Unknown	6 months ago	Smoked
Cannabis	15	Weekly	Two per week	One month ago	Smoked

DSM-IV Diagnoses

Axis I	Alcohol Dependence
	Cannabis Abuse
	Cocaine Use
Axis II	Diagnosis deferred
Axis III	None currently

Clinical Impression: This client recently completed a 28-day inpatient rehabilitation program. Client realizes she has a problem and is ready to seek treatment on a voluntary basis. Client feels relapse risks are high due to her lack of support. She will be admitted to the womens' program so her children can benefit from the day care services and she can benefit from the support network. Anticipated level of care is weekly individual counseling sessions, as well as participating in group therapy twice a week.

Individualized Treatment Plan

Justification for Treatment: Referred by inpatient program.

Goals: Date Service Ordered: 8/20/XX   Expected Achievement Date: 2/22/XX

1. Client will improve her knowledge of addiction by:
   a. Read chapters 2 and 3 from the book on addiction behavior and list 10 addictive behaviors.
   b. Remember a drug is a drug.
   c. Acknowledge problems related to alcohol use.
2. Improving self-esteem
   a. Client shall report three personal strengths about herself.
   b. Client will use at least three "I statements" per day.

References and Suggested Readings

[42 CFR, Part 2] Confidentiality of alcohol and drug abuse patient records, *Code of Federal Regulations*, Title 42, Pt. 2, 2002 ed.

Albaum-Feinstein, A. L. (1999). *DSM-IV Crosswalk: Guidelines for Coding Mental Health Information*. Chicago, IL: American Health Information Management Association.

Alcoholics Anonymous World Services, Inc. (1957). *Alcoholics Anonymous Comes of Age: A Brief History of A.A.* New York: Author.

American Psychiatric Association. (2000). *Diagnostic and Statistical Manual of Mental Disorders: DSM-IV-TR* (4th ed. text revision). Washington, DC: Author.

[ASAM] American Society of Addiction Medicine. (2001). *American Society of Addiction Medicine Patient Placement Criteria, Second Edition Revised (ASAM PPC-2R)*. Chevy Chase, MD: Author.

American Society of Addiction Medicine. (1997). *Patient Placement Criteria for the Treatment of Substance Related Disorders* (2nd ed.). Chevy Chase, MD: Author.

Beis, E. B. (1984). *Mental Health and the Law.* Rockville, MD: Aspen.

Brooks, S. R. (1990). Establishment of national datasets for mental health and substance abuse treatment services. *Journal of the American Medical Record Association, 61* (6), 33–36.

Commission on Accreditation of Rehabilitation Facilities. (1997). *Standards Manual and Interpretive Guidelines for Behavior Health.* Tuscon, AZ: Author.

[CARF] Commission on Accreditation of Rehabilitation Facilities. [Online.] http://www.carf.org [2003, December 4].

Dayhoff, D. A., Pope, G. C., and Huber, J. H. (1994). State variations in public and private alcoholism treatment at specialty substance abuse treatment facilities. *Journal of Studies on Alcohol, 55* (5), 549–560.

Drake, R. E., Antosca, L. A., Noordsy, D. L., Bartels, S. J., and Osher, F. C. (1991). New Hampshire's specialized services for the dually diagnosed. *New Directions for Mental Health Services, 50,* 57–67.

Drug Enforcement Administration, U.S. Department of Justice. [Online.] TEAM UP: A Drug Prevention Manual for High School Athletic Coaches. http://www.usdoj.gov/dea/demand/team-up.htm [2003, April 10].

Galanter, M., Egelko, S., and Edwards, H. (1993). Rational recovery: Alternative to AA for addiction? *American Journal of Drug and Alcohol Abuse, 19* (4), 499–510.

Grissom, G. R. (1991). Addiction severity index: Experience in the field. *International Journal of the Addictions, 26* (1), 55–64.

Joint Commission on Accreditation of Healthcare Organizations. (1997). *1997–1998 Comprehensive Accreditation Manual for Behavioral Health Care.* Oakbrook Terrace, IL: Author.

Joint Commission on Accreditation of Healthcare Organizations. (1995). *1996 Comprehensive Accreditation Manual for Hospitals.* Chicago, IL: Author.

Kosanke, N., Magura, S., Staines, G., Foote, J., and DeLuca, A. (2002). Feasibility of matching alcohol patients to ASAM levels of care. *The American Journal on Addictions, 11,* 124–134.

Lee, F. Wickham (1995). *Using the DSM-IV to ICD-9-CM Crosswalk.* Chicago, IL: American Health Information Management Association.

Legal Action Center. (2003). *Confidentiality and Communication: A Guide to the Federal Alcohol & Drug Confidentiality Law and HIPAA, 2003 Revised Edition.* New York: Author.

Marshall, M. J., and Marshall, S. (1993). Homogeneous versus heterogeneous age group treatment of adolescent substance abusers. *American Journal of Drug and Alcohol Abuse, 19* (2), 199–207.

Muramoto, M. L., and Leshan, L. (1993). Adolescent substance abuse. Recognition and early intervention. *Primary Care: Clinics in Office Practice, 20* (1), 141–154.

Of Substance. Bimonthly newsletter of the Legal Action Center. New York.

Roach, W. H., and the Aspen Health Law and Compliance Center (1998). *Medical Records and the Law.* (3rd ed.) Gaithersburg, MD: Aspen.

South Carolina Department of Alcohol and Other Drug Abuse Services [SCDAODAS]. (1995a). *FY95 Standard Operating Procedures for Act 301 Medicaid Providers.* Columbia, SC: Author.

SCDAODAS. (1995*b*). *Uniform Clinical Records*. Columbia, SC: Author.

Study: Revamped D.A.R.E. curriculum shows promise. 2002. *Alcoholism & Drug Abuse Weekly, 14* (43), 4, 6.

[SAMHSA] Substance Abuse and Mental Health Services Administration, Office of Applied Studies. (2002). *National Survey of Substance Abuse Treatment Services (N-SSATS): 2000. Data on Substance Abuse Treatment Facilities.* DASIS Series: S-16, DHHS Publication No. (SMA) 02-3668, Rockville, MD: Author. http://wwwdasis.samhsa.gov/00nssats/nssats2000report.pdf [2003, April 10].

[SAMHSA] Substance Abuse and Mental Health Services Administration, Office of Applied Studies. (2003). *Pregnant Women in Substance Abuse Treatment.* Available http://www.samhsa.gov/oas/2k2/pregTX/pregTX.cfm [2004, January 4].

Wheeler, J. R. C., Fadel, H., and D'Aunno, T. A. (1992). Ownership and performance of outpatient substance abuse treatment centers. *American Journal of Public Health, 82* (5), 711–718.

Key Resources

Alcoholics Anonymous
General Service Office
475 Riverside Drive
Box 459, Grand Central Station
New York, NY 10163
Phone: 212-870-3400
http://www.aa.org

American Psychiatric Association
1000 Wilson Boulevard, Suite 1825
Arlington, VA 22209-3901
Phone: 703-907-7300
http://www.psych.org

American Society of Addiction Medicine
4601 North Park Avenue
Arcade Suite 101
Chevy Chase, MD 20815,
Phone: 301-656-3920
Fax: 301-656-3815
E-mail: Email@asam.org
http://www.asam.org

Center for Substance Abuse Prevention
5600 Fishers Lane
Rockville, MD 20857
Phone: 301-443-0365 or 301-443-8956
E-mail: info@samhsa.gov

Commission on Accreditation of Rehabilitation Facilities (CARF)
(See Chapter 1 for contact information.)

Drug Enforcement Administration
Mailstop: AXS
2401 Jefferson Davis Highway
Alexandria, VA 22301
Phone: 202-307-1000
http://www.usdoj.gov/dea/index.htm

Joint Commission on Accreditation of Healthcare Organizations
(See Chapter 1 for contact information.)

Legal Action Center
153 Waverly Place
New York, NY 10014
Phone: 212-243-1313
Fax: 212-675-0286
http://www.lac.org

Narcotics Anonymous
World Service Office
P.O. Box 9999
Van Nuys, CA 91409
Phone: 818-773-9999
Fax: 818-700-0700
http://www.wsoinc.com

National Clearinghouse for Alcohol and Drug Information (NCADI)
11426 Rockville Pike
Rockville, MD 20852
Phone: 800-729-6686
Fax: 301-468-6433
http://www.health.org or http://ncadi.samhsa.gov

National Institute on Alcohol Abuse and Alcoholism (NIAAA)
Willco Building
6000 Executive Boulevard
Bethesda, MD 20892-7003
Phone: 301-443-3860
http://www.niaaa.nih.gov

National Institute on Drug Abuse
National Institutes of Health
6001 Executive Boulevard, Room 5213
Bethesda, MD 20892-9561
Phone: 301-443-1124
http://www.nida.nih.gov

Substance Abuse & Mental Health Services Administration
Parklawn Building
Room 16-105
5600 Fishers Lane
Rockville, Maryland 20857
http://www.samhsa.gov

Chapter 9

Facilities for Individuals with Mental Retardation or Developmental Disabilities

Elaine C. Jouette, MA, RHIA
Judy S. Westerfield, MEd

Learning Objectives

Upon successful completion of this chapter, you should be able to:

1. Identify the major differences in services provided to an individual living in an ICF/MR as compared to other settings.
2. Explain various methods of record keeping and the natural separation of information into sections or divisions for long-term care in an ICF/MR setting.
3. Explain the need for utilizing various coding systems, all of which are designed to provide for the care of the individual.
4. Explain the need for utilizing various coding systems to study and research the causes of mental retardation and developmental disabilities in order to help prevent their occurrence.
5. Discuss the process involved in risk management in the tracking of all accident/incident reports.
6. Apply the technical features of this chapter to assist with health information management in practical work settings.

SETTING	DESCRIPTION	SYNONYMS/EXAMPLES
ICF/MR	Intermediate care facilities for mentally retarded and developmentally disabled individuals May be operated as private, religious, or governmental	Persons classified with autism, cerebral palsy, dual diagnosis, special education; parameters set for services based on age, functioning level, and condition

Introduction to Setting

Federal regulations classify an organization providing specialized services for persons with mental retardation as an **intermediate care facility for the mentally retarded (ICF/MR)**. In addition to routine medical and nursing care, these facilities must be responsive to the unique needs of this population and provide individualized training in such areas as sensorimotor, cognitive, emotional, communicative, vocational, and social development. An organization licensed as an ICF/MR is eligible to receive payment for its services from Medicaid (Title XIX). These facilities may be called "schools," "training centers," "development centers," or some other similar name.

Individuals who live on the premises of an ICF/MR may have a wide range of needs, so a particular ICF/MR may provide a wide range of living arrangements. A typical center may have a campus with several homes or dormitories in which persons live. Such a center may provide one building that resembles a small nursing home with 24-hour nursing care for individuals with severe physical and mental disabilities. The same center may house persons with less severe disabilities in a group home setting where direct care staff with no nursing background provide supervision. Federal regulations encourage the grouping of individuals by age and developmental level, but prohibit segregating them solely on the basis of physical disability. For example, persons who are deaf or blind must be integrated with others of comparable social and intellectual development (*Conditions of Participation*, 1996).

Typically, each building or home houses a small number of individuals—in the range of 3 to 24. A common standard is six persons per group home. However, the total number of individuals on a campus can be quite large, ranging from less than 100 to more than 1,000. It should be noted that between 1996–2000, the number of individuals residing in public or private institutional facilities for 16 or more persons declined by 15 percent (Braddock et al., 2002).

The ICFs/MR differ from other settings in that individuals are on a 24-hour training schedule. Tasks that can be easily accomplished by the "normal" population, such as tying one's shoes, may take months and even years to master by these special needs individuals, and the ICF/MR is required to include such **training objectives** in its plans for each person. ICFs/MR are committed to helping individuals reach their fullest potential. These facilities strive for the best quality of life for persons by providing care, treatment, training, and a safe environment for those for whom they are responsible.

Types of Individuals Served

Persons receiving services from an ICF/MR are affected by **mental retardation**, which is "a disability characterized by significant limitations both in intellectual functioning and in adaptive behavior as expressed in conceptual, social, and practical adaptive skills. This disability originates before age 18" (AAMR, 2002, p. 13). The term "**developmental disability**" is used almost interchangeably with the term "mental retardation," although it has been defined slightly differently. A *developmental disability* is caused by either a mental or physical impairment that begins before age 22 (AAMR, 1992).

The admission of these persons may be voluntary, court committed, or the result of an emergency situation. The state and/or regional departments usually make the referrals of the individual to the ICF/MR facility.

The facility conducts a preliminary examination (preadmission screening) of the referred individual. This evaluation can be conducted by an admission committee that focuses on two major areas: (1) do the facility's services meet the needs of the individual? and (2) is this the least restrictive environment for the individual?

The individual admitted to an ICF/MR facility must be in need of receiving **active treatment** services. Therefore, the facility's primary responsibility is to provide for the health care, training, and habilitative services for individuals with mental retardation or developmental disabilities under the supervision of qualified professionals.

These individuals over time have been referred to as patients, students, residents, clients, or customers. The synonyms have changed over the years for these individuals as there has been a move away from the medical model toward the person-centered approach. The medical model leans toward institutions, "patients," care/basic needs, doctors, and restoration to health with the emphasis on good care. The developmental model stresses deinstitutionalization. Services strive for skill development/behavior change using the **interdisciplinary team** approach for establishing services for development/growth in the active treatment process. The individual supports model is more community based with the individual/consumer obtaining support services based on self-determination that is outcome oriented. Also, facilities may be under different departments and services and the synonyms tend to favor the service the department renders. For instance, individuals with cerebral palsy may come under the Department of Special Education; therefore, *students* may be the preferred term. However, co-authors Amy Hewitt and Susan O'Nell (1998) in addressing labels for persons with mental retardation or developmental disabilities remind us that "it's the person, not the service, that matters. It's a sign of respect" (p. 5).

Types of Caregivers

Personnel vary from facility to facility depending on the size and scope of the services the facility provides. However, all ICFs/MR must focus on activities that build or strengthen the person's skills (Janicki, 1992). To this end, an interdisciplinary team identifies and addresses each person's needs. The members of an individual's interdisciplinary team should represent the professions, disciplines, or service areas that are relevant to the person's needs (*Conditions of Participation*, 2002). Any of the following may serve on an interdisciplinary team: physician, psychologist, social worker, registered nurse, pharmacist, dietitian, physical therapist, occupational therapist, speech-language pathologist, audiologist, dentist, recreational staff member, vocational staff member, education staff member, or resident services staff member. The individual also participates as a member of the team, as well as family members and friends or advocates invited by the individual.

In the traditional planning approach established in the *Conditions of Participation*, the interdisciplinary team reviews and discusses the past progress and current status of the individual. From this review, a program is developed based on individual **assessments** and identification of needs by the interdisciplinary team exclusively for the individual. A summary of essential assessment information that facilitates the identification of needs and provides necessary information to staff members who are responsible for working with the person is developed along with the goals, objectives, and a service plan for meeting the individual's prioritized needs. This document becomes the product of the interdisciplinary team process, which is a review and revision of services provided. Although federal regulations governing this process have not changed, the expectation for including the expressed needs and desires of the individual receiving services is critical. Several self-advocacy models can be incorporated into the team process that allow persons and their families to make choices and have a major role in the development of the program plan. This shift in the planning process toward more personal choice is based on the belief that every person has the right to plan a life that is meaningful and satisfying.

A **qualified mental retardation professional (QMRP)** is responsible for coordinating and monitoring each person's active treatment program. A QMRP has "at least one year of experience working directly with persons with mental retardation or other developmental disabilities" and is a physician, an RN, or a person with a bachelor's degree in a relevant profession (*Conditions of Participation*, 2002, p. 550).

Health Care Staff

These individuals are responsible for providing and administering proper health care in order to maintain the physical and mental well-being of the person receiving services. These caregivers include, but are not limited to, the following:

- Physicians
- Dentists

- Podiatrists
- Nursing service
- Health information staff
- Laboratory technicians
- X-ray technicians
- Respiratory therapists
- EEG technicians
- EKG technicians
- Occupational therapists
- Physical therapy
- Dietary staff
- Pharmacists
- Central supply staff

Habilitative Staff

The facilities utilize the habilitative method. This is a process by which a person is assisted to acquire and maintain life skills that enable him or her to cope more effectively with personal and environmental demands and to raise the level of physical, mental, and social efficiency. **Habilitation** includes, but is not limited to, programs of structured education and training. The operative force in the habilitation process is often accomplished by the "person first" philosophy. Employees are involved in creating an environment for individuals that encourages continuous improvement. The person-centered approach has been instrumental in improving the services rendered as the least restrictive program alternative, meaning the available program is the least confining for the person's condition, service, and treatment, which is provided in the least intrusive manner reasonably and humanely appropriate to the individual's needs and preferences. These staff members include, but are not limited to, the following:

- Qualified mental retardation professional (QMRP)
- Social service workers
- Psychologists
- Speech-language pathologists
- Audiologists
- Special education staff
- Vocational/life skills coaches
- Recreational therapists
- Music therapists
- Direct care staff

Administrative Staff

These individuals work within the guidelines of the ICF/MR federal regulations to produce positive outcomes regarding individuals. They manage funds in order to provide quality care. They are responsible for the smooth operation of the facility in order to maintain the health, safety, and quality of life for the individuals being served. Administrative staff members include, but are not limited to, the following:

- Administrator
- Finance officer
- Personnel staff
- Health information services staff
- Home life directors/managers/supervisors
- Housekeeping staff

Types of Settings

Facilities for individuals with mental retardation or developmental disabilities may be operated by a variety of groups, such as the government, religious groups, private interests, and everything in between. Also, the facilities may be designated by the type of services rendered. Some facilities may provide services based on age limits for the persons they serve, such as from the age of 3 to 22. Some may provide services only to individuals with a specific diagnosis, such as those with cerebral palsy, autism, and dual diagnoses.

In general, no admission should be considered permanent. The facility provides the individual with the training and guidance necessary to develop and acquire the skills needed to function in a less restrictive setting. This normalization training model has been a major force for individuals with developmental disabilities.

Once these goals have been reached, the discharge planning objectives are obtained by referring the person to the appropriate setting, such as group homes, supervised living, or supported living where the person chooses where and with whom he or she will live with assistance as needed.

Regulatory Issues

The majority of the ICF/MR facilities are funded by Title XIX (Medicaid) and must therefore meet the standards in the *Conditions of Participation* for ICFs/MR. In order to obtain a state license, the facilities must go through this survey process in order to be funded at the level of service assigned to the facility. Because funding is tied into the survey process, it is the goal of all facilities to meet regulatory requirements the first time around. However, if deficiencies are noted that may endanger the safety of the client, the facility can be fined several hundreds to thousands of dollars per day, depending on the infraction, until the deficiency has been rectified.

Voluntary accreditation is also available to facilities serving persons with mental retardation or developmental disabilities. The Joint Commission on Accreditation of Healthcare Organizations (JCAHO) offers accreditation for organizations serving persons with mental retardation or developmental disabilities through its behavioral health care division. The standards that are used to survey these organizations are found in the *Comprehensive Accreditation Manual for Behavioral Health Care*.

Another accrediting body, The Council on Quality and Leadership in Supports for People with Disabilities (formerly the Accreditation Council on Services for People with Developmental Disabilities), has also set standards for facilities serving persons with mental retardation or developmental disabilities. There are currently around 200 organizations accredited by the Council. The Council is sponsored by the following organizations and service providers: American Association on Mental Retardation, American Network of Community Options and Resources, American Occupational Therapy Association, American Psychological Association, The Arc (formerly Association for Retarded Citizens of the United States), Association for Behavior Analysis, Autism Society of America, Epilepsy Foundation of America, National Easter Seal Society, and United Cerebral Palsy Associations, Inc. The Council's accreditation standards are found in its publication, *Personal Outcome Measures* (Council on Quality and Leadership in Supports for People with Disabilities, 2000).

Generally, voluntary accreditation surveys performed by the Council or the JCAHO are more stringent than the states' ICF/MR surveying processes. Usually when accreditation is obtained, the facility is considered to be performing above and beyond the state licensing requirements. Although the majority of ICFs/MR may not undergo voluntary accreditation by the Council or JCAHO, they sometimes use the publications of these organizations to improve the quality of the services they offer.

Documentation

Individual records are the official files on each person at an ICF/MR facility. Although in theory they should consist of only one chart, these records are often divided into administrative, health, and habilitation/training sections. All sections must be kept confidential in secure areas when not in use.

The major difference between individual records in an ICF/MR and other long-term settings relates to the fact that some type of training is occurring on a 24-hour basis. For example, persons may practice toileting or grooming skills in their living areas. Thus, it is important that these records are housed in the living units or homes. This also makes the records more user-friendly for the authorized chart handlers who follow the 24-hour schedules for daily observation and documentation of training factors for their monthly statistics. These statistics are gathered for **annual staffings**, or meetings of the interdisciplinary team. They are needed to demonstrate the accomplishment or failure of goals set forth for each person.

Likewise, the health section of the record documents the health/medical needs of the person, and the data meets with the standards of practice for the caregivers. Table 9-1 is a generic tabular listing of data that may be maintained on an individual in an ICF/MR facility. The tabular arrangement is based on what meets the needs of the facility and the user of the various sections of the document. Often forms are designed to meet several types of charting needs, such as two-sided copies, multipart forms for distribution purposes, and forms that can meet the needs of two or more departments/services. For example, a weight chart could meet both dietary and nursing requirements. Forms should be designed to keep the bulk of the chart down while meeting the appropriate documentation standards.

Reimbursement and Funding

Medicaid is the primary source of funding for most ICFs/MR. A facility that meets the federal *Conditions of Participation* is certified to receive payment from Medicaid for persons who have been determined to need its services. A state's mental health or mental retardation authority determines whether a particular individual needs "a continuous specialized services program, which is analogous to active treatment" (Preadmission Screening and Annual Review of Mentally Ill and Mentally Retarded Individuals, 1996). When the person has been determined to need active treatment in a facility setting, then the ICF/MR receives a per diem payment for each day of care provided to that individual. Other sources of funding include state offices of family services, Veterans Affairs, railroad retirement funds, and so on. Some persons qualify for services covered by Medicare, as well.

In some states, the level of care needed by each person determines the amount of the per diem payment received by the facility. Individuals with more medical complications, behavior problems, and disabilities would be funded at higher levels because they need more specialized treatment and service modalities provided by a variety of professionals and caregivers. Various methods for determining the level of care needed are used in different states. Several standardized assessment tools that can be used for diagnostic and planning purposes can also be used to determine the level of services needed. Some states have begun using these assessment instruments to establish case-mix reimbursement systems. Under such a system, the provider typically receives a case-mix-adjusted per diem payment for each individual receiving services. For example, the **Inventory for Client and Agency Planning (ICAP)** is an assessment instrument used by some states that provides service scores that can be used to adjust payments to providers.

Managed care proposals have been offered as a mechanism for paying for services for persons with mental retardation or developmental disabilities. Managed Care proposals should consider some of the differences between care for this

Table 9-1   Generic Listing of Individual Data in a ICF/MR Facility

---

Administrative Data

Personal Account
Personal Funds Ledger
Savings Accounts
Long-Term-Care Certification
Medicare/Medicaid
Insurance
   Funeral Home Preference/Verification
Financial Agreements
Admission Agreements
Legal Data
Guardianships
Interdictions
Court Commissions
Authorizations
   Authorizations for Release of Information
   Authorizations for Administration of Long-
   Term Estrogen Substances
Consents
   Consents for Disclosure of Information
   Consent to Medical Treatment–Therapy–
   Surgery Procedures
   Consent Regarding Emergency Medical
   Treatment
   Consents for Off-Campus Visits/Activities with
   Authorized Individuals

Consent for Seizure Medications
Consent to Photograph or Record
Consent for Behavior Program Using
   Restricted Procedures
Consent for Psychotropic Medications and
   Treatment Plan
Consent for Religious Activities
Consent for Off-Campus Activities
Correspondence
   Letters, Memos, Forms
Resident's Rights
   Bill of Rights
   Explanation of Rights of Individuals Served
   Review/Approval by Behavior Management
   Committee
   Human Rights Committee Review or Approval
   Data
   Abridgement of Rights
Office of Family Services Notifications
Pre-Admission Data
Birth Certificate
Discharge and Follow-up
Discharge Summary

Training Data

Individual Habilitative Program (IHP) Addenda
Psychological (Comprehensive/Annual) Behavior
Treatment Plans
Individual Education Plan (IEP)
Special Education Assessments
   Education Correspondence
Activity Schedule (24 hours)
Training Assessments
   Core Team Notes
   QMRP Monthly Reviews
   Monthly Core Team Progress Notes
   Social Service Assessments

Vocational (Life Skills) Assessment/Evaluations
Speech and Language Updates
   Comprehensive Evaluations
Audiology Evaluations and Screenings
Occupational Therapy Evaluations and
Updates
   Wheelchair Evaluations
   Adaptive Equipment Evaluations
Physical Therapy Evaluations and Updates
Recreation Therapy Evaluations and Updates
Music Therapy Evaluations and Updates

Table 9-1   *(Continued)*

Health Care Data (Medical and Nursing)

Medical	*Nursing*
Major and Minor Problem Lists	Height/Weight/Head Circumference
Physician Orders	Nursing Assessments
Health Care Progress Notes	Quarterly
Consultations	Initial
Neurology/EEGs	Medication Administration Records
Occupational	Medication History
Ophthalmology	Pharmacy Medication/Drug Reviews
Orthopedic	Medication Destruction Records
Physical Therapy	Medication on Leave of Absence Form (Visits)
Psychiatry	Seizure Records
Physical Exams	Restraint and Checklist
Referrals	Accident/Incident Report Forms
Off-Campus Clinics/Health Care Facilities	Graphic Data
Laboratory	Female Health Care Records (Copies of
Hematology	Consents for Oral Contraceptives and
Chemistry	Estrogen Usage)
Medication Levels	Diabetic Record
Urinalysis	Immunization Record
Microbiology	Dietary Data
Serology	Nutritional Evaluations
Parasitology	Dietary Notes
Miscellaneous	Tube Feedings
X-Ray	Growth Graph (under 18 years of age)
X-rays	Death Certificate
EKGs	Autopsy Reports
Dental	Death Summary
Progress and Treatment Received	

population and the other types of care that are usually provided in a managed care program. For example, people with developmental disabilities need more than just health care—they need training and other types of supports. States considering managed care proposals may find it difficult to determine an appropriate capitation rate because of these differences. Advocates for persons with mental retardation or developmental disabilities are urging attention to the special needs of these individuals in any managed care programs developed for them (The Arc, 2003).

Information Management
Data and Information Flow

Chronologically, data tends to flow as follows:

Admission of the Individual
↓
Comprehensive Diagnostics
↓
Interdisciplinary Team Assessments/Updates
↓
Receipt of Treatment/Services
Documentation of these in the individual record
↓
Discharge/Death of the Indvidual
↓
Follow-up Documentation

The physical flow of the record varies from facility to facility. However, Figure 9-1 depicts a typical flow of information in a paper-based system from decentralized storage on the person's living unit to centralized storage in the health information department.

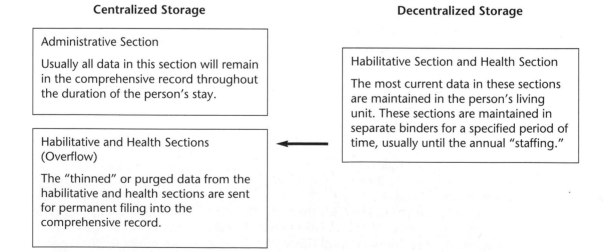

Centralized Storage

Administrative Section

Usually all data in this section will remain in the comprehensive record throughout the duration of the person's stay.

Habilitative and Health Sections (Overflow)

The "thinned" or purged data from the habilitative and health sections are sent for permanent filing into the comprehensive record.

Decentralized Storage

Habilitative Section and Health Section

The most current data in these sections are maintained in the person's living unit. These sections are maintained in separate binders for a specified period of time, usually until the annual "staffing."

Figure 9-1   Tabulated centralized comprehensive record located in health information department.

In a paper-based system, data is filed in the centralized comprehensive record as it is received from the living units and other sources. For ease of reference, the centralized record is usually maintained in sections, such as the administrative section, the habilitative or training section, and the health section. Because the active records can be voluminous, some facilities commit portions of the paper record to microfilm while the individual is still being served by the facility. Other facilities may use optical imaging for storage of active records.

At the death or discharge of the individual, the active record is closed and retained for the duration of the statute of limitations. If a facility utilizes a microfilming program for active records, the remaining portions of the closed records are often microfilmed at the death or discharge of the person. However, some facilities prefer to avoid the additional cost of microfilming the entire record and microfilm only selected portions for research or administrative purposes. The remainder of the paper record in these facilities is destroyed upon reaching the statute of limitations or other legal retention period.

Coding and Classification

In the ICF/MR facilities, employees may need to become familiar with three types of coding systems, depending on established policies and procedures.

ICD-9-CM

International Classification of Diseases, 9th Revision, Clinical Modification is the more widely used coding system. Codes may be assigned on an accumulative basis or based on individual "infirmary," "sick call," or "acute care" stays or visits. Often this tool may be selected when a survey is in process so that individual records containing specific diagnoses or conditions can be obtained for tracking during the actual survey. Traditionally, this type of coding often appears in the summary sheet, which encompasses the screening of the infirmary, sick call, or acute care stays whenever these services are rendered in the ICF/MR facility. Facilities often prefer to use an accumulative type of diagnoses/procedures sheet that is chronological in nature and is an inclusive listing of the individual's conditions and procedures coded for reference purposes. However, diagnoses and procedures information may also be required on identification sheets for quick reference and may be used as well on the order sheets since condition for medication is also required. Whatever format is utilized, it should be developed in conjunction with facility services and references needs in mind. A sample of this format, which would be used in the infirmary section, is as follows:

Mental Retardation [mild, moderate, severe, profound]
Etiology: Due to _____

Additional diagnosis and conditions are then listed.

DSM-IV (1994)

The *Diagnostic and Statistical Manual of Mental Disorders, Fourth Edition, (DSM-IV)* or the revised edition (DSM-IV-TR) is mainly used by psychologists and psychiatrists in their evaluations and consultations. (For more information on DSM-IV, see Chapter 8.) Mental Retardation is coded in Axis II of DSM-IV. DSM-IV recognizes four degrees of severity of mental retardation: mild, moderate, severe, and profound. IQ test results are used to determine the degree of severity. (American Psychiatric Association, 1994). This information may be recorded on the consultation, evaluation, or data sheet for retrieval purposes, or in the computer system for networking needs.

Manual on Terminology and Classification in Mental Retardation, 1983 Edition

This manual was published by the American Association on Mental Retardation (AAMR) in 1983 and is still cited as the source of definitions of mental retardation in the *Code of Federal Regulations* (Preadmission Screening and Annual Review of Mentally Ill and Mentally Retarded Individuals, 1996). The AAMR has replaced this reference with a publication called *Mental Retardation: Definition, Classification, and Systems of Supports*. However, the older publication is still used for classification purposes in many ICFs/MR.

This manual attempts to provide a definitive classification system for use in the mental retardation field. Classifications may be simply a scientific procedure for systematic arrangement of individuals, units, or events into groups with one or more common denominators. They may be useful for administrative purposes and for preliminary planning for groups identified by the system. Classifications can lead to benefits that arise when funds are allocated and personnel trained to provide special services. Once an individual is classified as mentally retarded, it is imperative to periodically reassess the diagnosis and classification and service needs.

The manual includes ten major categories and seven secondary categories, both with sublistings, as well as tertiary categories. Coding is usually done at the time of admission to encompass the necessary information for the care and treatment of individuals for establishing the comprehensive plan of care required of the facility. An example of this type of coding would be as follows:

Primary

Secondary

Tertiary
  Genetic
  Cranial anomaly
  Sensory impairment
  Perception
  Convulsive disorder
  Psychological impairment

The major and minor categories of this classification system are designed to include a variety of helpful levels concerning both the behavioral and medical classifications to standardize the data needed for statistical reporting. The major medical divisions in this manual follow those listed in the ICD-9-CM and the DSM coding systems.

Mental Retardation: Definition, Classification, and Systems of Supports, Tenth Edition

Mental Retardation: Definition, Classification, and Systems of Supports is the latest publication on classification from the American Association on Mental Retardation. This publication uses four dimensions for defining and classifying mental retardation: Dimension I, Intellectual functioning and adaptive skills; Dimension II, Psychological/emotional considerations; Dimension III, Physical/health/etiology considerations; and Dimension IV, Environmental considerations (AAMR, 2002). This publication provides a framework for assessing the individual and identifying needed supports. It also includes a table, which can be used as a coding system to describe the etiology of mental retardation.

Computer Systems

Computer systems may vary from facility to facility and/or within the facility. Acute health care settings are, in general, more advanced than the long-term care facilities, but with additional requirements of various licensing and accreditation agencies, the use of computers is becoming more prevalent.

Some ICF/MR facilities use purchased programs, but the majority have individually designed programs to meet the needs and types of persons served. The current trend is to utilize personal computers with interchangeable software programs.

Private ICF/MR facilities are considered to be businesses. The acceptance of the various functions and features needed to accomplish the business aspects of the overall facility operation are seen as vital to the business's survival. The need to control the "paper tiger" has grown to encompass a variety of other areas including, but not limited to, the individual record.

When a facility becomes committed to computerization, it takes an average of three years for it to begin to reap the benefits of the various computerized features. These benefits may range from financial reports to program planning, or from time keeping to rapidly producing all information requested during a survey. The first priority in many facilities is to begin to integrate the various systems that have been developed over time to address specific needs. As various departmental systems begin to interface with each other or with a central system, a partially computerized record can be useful. Attempting to go to a paperless record by implementing an optical imaging system in a mental retardation facility would probably not be cost-effective in most facilities at present. More benefits are likely to be achieved by developing databases to help manage individual data and information. A completely computerized record is not possible until computers or workstations are available on all units and in all services.

It is imperative that the health information director become an active participant in the establishment of standardized forms and reports. With the ease of formatting and designing forms on computers, every department or service will tend to develop a desirable form or record. Some type of facility-wide forms control is vital to the success of the computerized record.

Data Sets

As stated earlier in this section, it may take several years to experience the fruits of the facility's computerized program(s). For discussion and illustration purposes of the data sets, a conservative selection of forms and specific features has been made to hopefully share some of the positive outcomes and information tools vital to the operation of a 24-hour ICF/MR.

This listing is not inclusive. Many variables can affect the choice of forms and the management of their use, such as variations of state laws, survey requirements, types of facilities, and even the choice of computer hardware and software. The selected forms serve a twofold purpose. One purpose is to meet requirements, and these forms have a filing designation on them to ensure that they are filed in the correct sequence and tab heading. Other selected forms are simply tools that may not become part of the permanent file, but can be shredded once they have met their service needs.

Administrative and Assessment Data

Assessment of the individual is a requirement in most states to determine eligibility for services. Assessment processes vary from state to state and may include psychological, psychiatric, and medical evaluations. To assist in determining services that the individual may need, many states use standardized assessment instruments. For example, adaptive and maladaptive behavior can be assessed with a variety of instruments, such as the Scales of Independent Behavior—Revised (SIB-R), the Vineland Adaptive Behavior Scales, the AAMR Adaptive Behavior Scales (ABS), and the Inventory for Client and Agency Planing (ICAP). The use of such instruments can assist both with diagnosis and program planning. Some states use this type of instrument to provide data for case-mix reimbursement systems as well.

Authorizations/Consent Forms

Based on individual computerized data, a variety of consents and authorizations can be generated, such as psychotropic drug use and birth control pills.

Individual Information Release Record

This record is maintained for the control and authorized release of requested information in the individual records, thus providing an audit tool of this task area.

Ongoing Inventory of Individual Belongings

This inventory is one of the most useful computer-generated forms, making it easy to update inventories by the touch of a key to add, delete, and/or change the information. Although there is still manual labor involved in the inventory process, just keeping up with each person's clothes is a monumental task in itself. Clothing is listed by long sleeves, short sleeves, and a variety of identifying items to be accounted for in a specific area of the form.

Training Data

This section of the individual record is unique to an ICF/MR. The following specific forms are described as examples of training data forms.

The Updating Worksheet

This worksheet is a computerized tool used by the interdisciplinary team at the full team staffings for updating the person's record in specific service areas. This tool not only addresses the services rendered and the responsible staff member providing the service, but readily adapts to immediately making these changes into the person's individual programming plans.

The Draft Referral to Staffing

This form is used throughout the year to provide updates to the current individual program plan. It eventually becomes a part of the permanent record as an addendum to the current staffing, which illustrates that program updates have been initiated and approved by appropriate staff members.

The Individual Program Plan

The **individual program plan (IPP)** is a composite summary of the goals and the objectives that the staff will assist the individual to attain during the coming year. This individualized program plan is used in the overall care of the person and outlines how the program will guide the resident toward achieving the set goals. The program includes brief summaries of all services rendered for the past year and the establishment of goals for the coming year. Figure 9-2 is an excerpt from an individual program plan, illustrating the portion of the plan that summarizes the person's current status and progress. Figure 9-3 is an excerpt that demonstrates how goals and plans to accomplish these goals may be documented in the individual program plan.

Core Team Summary Sheet

The core team summary sheet (Figure 9-4) is a tracking form used to implement the individual program plan. As needs are identified by the staff, they are added to the core team summary sheet. Because this is a working tool used by the staff, there is no problem if there are write-overs and strikeouts to indicate when goals have been met or when new information is added. A new summary sheet for review purposes is

PECAN GROVE TRAINING CENTER

INDIVIDUAL PROGRAM PLAN

April 24, XXXX

NAME: TYPE OF ADMISSION: Family

PGTC: # A-Unit   LEGAL STATUS: Noninterdicted Major

DATE OF ADMISSION: 7-22-XX   HOME OF RECORD: Anywhere, LA

RELIGION: Catholic

BIRTHDATE: 11-23-XX

AGE: 25 years and 6 months

CURRENT STATUS AND PROGRESS:

MEDICAL: _____ is currently monitored through a Medical Care Plan. Her condition is considered to be chronic stable due to her convulsive disorder. _____ remains in optimal physical health. She has had no serious illnesses or injuries during the past year. _____ had one chronic medication change, when Surfak was discontinued. _____'s bowel movements are monitored and she is given a suppository for relief of constipation as needed. _____ has quarterly head circumferences taken, as she has a shunt, and there has been no change. _____ is seen by her podiatrist for routine care. Because of her lack of cooperation, she required sedation before her visit. _____ has a prescriptive behavioral program, and she required manual restraint thirty-one times since her last review as part of her prescriptive behavioral program, to promote relaxation when positive and less restrictive measures failed to control behavior endangering self and others.

DENTAL: _____'s recent dental examination revealed her oral hygiene is at its highest level. She is void of any carious lesions, and her periodental support tissues are healthy. No other dental treatment is indicated for her at this time. _____ is scheduled for fluoride treatment next month. She receives dental treatment as needed at Dr. Doe's office in the community.

Figure 9-2   Individual program plan (excerpt).

printed on or before a 90-day interval with the recommended revisions. Because care is rendered on a 24-hour basis, the summary sheets are also used in developing the 24-hour active treatment schedules, described as follows.

The 24-Hour Active Treatment Schedule

The 24-Hour Active Treatment Schedule works in conjunction with the individualized program plan and the summaries (see Figure 9-5). It specifically sets into time frames the who, what, why, when, and where of the individual's treatment program.

RECREATION:

1. Promote effective use of leisure time and improve socialization skills.	1. Continue to organize small-group activities and encourage participation through 4-30-XX.
2. Maintain high level of participation in community-based activities.	2. Continue to provide outings into community through 4-30-XX.
3. Expand range of interests and activities.	3. Provide a variety of activities for a broader recreational program through 4-30-XX.

DIETARY:

1. Maintain adequate nutritional status. Gain weight of approximately 2 pounds to help reach her ideal weight range of 137–147.	1. Provide present diet as ordered by physician: regular high-fiber diet, with no seconds and low-fat milk.
2. Increase intake of fiber.	2. Provide foods high in fiber at meals.

Figure 9-3   Individual program plan (excerpt).

Although the IPP and the 24-hour schedules are developed for a period of one year, periodic revisions/summaries/assessments are done at a minimum of 90-day intervals and more frequently if warranted by the service and treatment modalities of the IPP and schedule change. Often surveyors use this form to ensure that a service or activity is being followed by the **direct care staff**. If the facility is not adhering to the individualized program based on the time frame set forth, it can be cited for a deficiency in that particular area of care or service.

Annual Assessments

When the full team conducts its annual assessments, forms such as nutritional assessment, recreational assessment, and vocational assessment are used to summarize and address the services rendered by these specialty areas.

Identification Data

Generally, identification sheets illustrate a variety of information/features vital to the care and management of the individual's records. The design of the form provides for a view of the individual's information at a glance. This form is usually reviewed and updated as required, at least yearly at the **annual staffing**.

CORE TEAM REVIEW SUMMARY FOR X

(Based Upon Client & Staff Interviews and 20–25% Random Sampling of Daily Documentation)

COVERING THE REVIEW PERIOD 02/02/XX THROUGH 04/19/XX

RTA MEMO: SEIZURES: Monitor closely and report to Nursing. Wash hair every Wednesday. Apply activator daily. Encourage her to carry purse.

1. Praise good behavior and give extra attention when good. Give attention to dress and appearance.

2. Offer (when patting stomach) to take X to bathroom often (each half hour).

3. Direct her to bathroom and offer shower when highly upset.

4. Remove from loud areas when upset.

5. When agitated and aggressive, contact supervisor.

6. Call for help as needed.

7. Do not "back off" from X; this increases problems.

8. Monitor closely when around Y (May bite when upset).

Time:	Location:	Code:	Current Training Objective:					Flags:	Recommendations
08:15 AM	DAYROOM/GYM	BC61L -005AAAD	**BASIC COMMANDS**/ Also scheduled: 04:45 PM						
			Will remain dressed in same outfit for half						
			hour (RTA to reward with edible)						
			does this on verbal command 1 Out of 3 trials						
			to be completed by 08/30/XX						DATE
			PERIOD ENDING:	09/01/XX	11/17/XX	02/02/XX	04/19/XX		
			PROGRESS:	82.30 %	79.76 %	80.00 %	78.90 %		DECLINE
			OBJECTIVE:	BC53G	BC53G	BC53G	BC53G		
			LEVEL:	005 D	005 D	004 D	004 D		

Figure 9-4 Core team summary sheets (excerpt).

08:30 AM BEDROOM HK125N-005 D

HOUSEKEEPING/ Also scheduled: 04:30 PM
Will carry two items of dirty clothing
to dirty clothes bucket in bathroom
does this on verbal command
to be completed by 09/30/XX

PERIOD ENDING:	09/01/XX	11/17/XX	02/02/XX	04/19/XX	
PROGRESS:	0.00 %	0.00 %	85.19 %	86.14 %	
OBJECTIVE:			HK79B	HK79C	RECENT OBJECTIVE CHANGE
LEVEL:			011AAAD	011 D	RECENT LEVEL CHANGE

08:30 AM BATHROOM [At Workshop]
BATHROOM TO15f-005AMAS

TOILETING/ Also scheduled: 10:00 AM 12:15 PM
Will wash hands after toileting for
30 seconds (RTA to monitor closely)
does this on verbal command to be trained throughout day
to be completed by 10/31/XX

PERIOD ENDING:	09/01/XX	11/17/XX	02/02/XX	04/19/XX	
PROGRESS:	81.15 %	94.23 %	83.03 %	76.67 %	DECLINE
OBJECTIVE:	TO19G	TO19G	TO3B	TO3B	
LEVEL:	011 D	011 D	005AMAD	005AMAS	RECENT LEVEL CHANGE

Figure 9-4   (*Continued*)

	Weekday Client Active Treatment Schedule	
	12:00 A.M.—11:45 P.M.	
TIME:	**LOCATION:**	**SCHEDULED TRAINING:**
06:00 AM	BEDROOM/BR	Rise; Personal Hygiene Care
06:15 AM	BEDROOM/GYM	TOILETING SKILL Formal Training
07:00 AM	BEDROOM	GROOMING Formal Training
07:30 AM	DINING ROOM	Scheduled Mealtime
08:15 AM	BATHROOM	ORAL HYGIENE Formal Training
08:30 AM	BEDROOM/GYM	TOILETING SKILL Formal Training
09:00 AM	GYM/CR 7	STIMULATION Formal Training
09:15 AM	GYM/CR 7	READING Formal Training
09:30 AM	CLASSROOM 6	KITCHEN MANAGEMENT Formal Training
09:45 AM	BEDROOM/GYM	TOILETING SKILL Formal Training
10:00 AM	CANTEEN	Snack/allowance on Thursdays
10:15 AM	GYM/CR 7	DISCRIMINATION Formal Training
10:30 AM	GYM/CR 7	TIME KNOWLEDGE Formal Training
10:45 AM	BATHROOM	BATHING Formal Training
11:00 AM	BEDROOM	Leisure time until 11:30 AM
11:30 AM	BEDROOM	PERSONAL INFORMATION Formal Training
12:00 PM	BEDROOM/GYM	TOILETING SKILLS Formal Training
12:15 PM	BATHROOM	GROOMING Formal Training
12:30 PM	DINING ROOM	Scheduled Mealtime
01:15 PM	BATHROOM	ORAL HYGIENE Formal Training

A.M. Medication Times: None

P.M. Medication Times: None

PGTC #:   CLIENT:

Figure 9-5   24-hour schedule—weekday/weekend.

The second form is a baseline information sheet applicable at the time of admission and maintains the same information throughout the person's stay. It is very important for the completion of vital records such as death certificates.

The third form is used at the time of death/discharge and provides necessary information for tracking and follow-up and basically is used to officially close out the individual's record.

Physician Data

Standing orders are individualized forms listing medications, contraindications, allergies, use of restraints, and so forth (see Figure 9-6).

Orders sheets list every medication the person is taking and list a diagnosis. For example, if the person is a diabetic, there must be proof of diagnosis in order for medication to be provided for the control of this condition.

Physician progress notes may be hand-written or may be generated from a computer program.

Because most ICF/MR facilities do not maintain full-time medical staff members but must utilize available community medical services, the use of the transfer and referral record is vital not only for the individual's care but for the communication of the care rendered. This is especially true in emergency transfer situations. The front of the form deals with information that the facility furnishes when the person is transferred, and the reverse side of the form provides for communication of the treatment, evaluation, and consultation rendered.

Specialty services such as X-rays and laboratory work are often provided by outside sources. When they are requested and the facility documentation of the service rendered is recorded on this form, it is also used for accounting purposes.

The transportation request form is used when the individual must obtain health care services in the community. This is not only a request but is required for accounting purposes.

The physical exam form is used at the time of annual staffing. As noted, the primary and additional diagnoses, as well as personal information, are furnished to the physician. This data enables the physician to screen more methodically. For example, if the individual has a heart problem, it would be in the diagnosis section, and the physician could address the status of the heart with a cardiovascular entry.

Nursing assessments are performed throughout the year and with the physical exam provide the data needed to annually summarize the overall medical and nursing care rendered.

Nursing Data

The chronological drug regimen review is a form used on a monthly basis by the consultant pharmacist, who conducts a review of not only the medication and administration of drugs but also specific protocols required of the staff to follow in the use of the medications prescribed for the individual.

HUDSPETH REGIONAL CENTER
PHYSICIAN'S STANDING ORDERS

1. PASSES: To include therapeutic leaves: Individualized activities, school and programming; off campus consultations, appointments and follow-up visits with physicians in clinic, and other diagnostic studies done off campus and other purposes.

2. ROUTINE TREATMENT FOR WOUND CARE AND INJURIES:
    1. Superficial wounds: Clean with saline twice a day and apply antibiotic ointment (Neosporin or Bacitracin) until healed.
    2. Ice pack as needed.
    3. For sutures: Clean with saline twice a day and apply antibiotic ointment and remove sutures in 7 days, unless otherwise ordered.

3. FEVER/PAIN:
    For fever greater than 100.5^0 F. rectally (99.5^0 oral, 98.5^0 axillary), or above, and/or for pain give:
    1. Tylenol 10 mg. per kg up to 650 mg. q. 4 hours as needed or
    2. Tylenol Suppository 325 mg. per rectum for clients weighing less than 45 pounds and 650 mg. per rectum for clients weighing more than 45 pounds q. 4 hours as needed.

    For fever not relieved by Tylenol within 1 hour:
    May give Ibuprofen 10 mg. per kg. up to 800 mg. q. 6 hrs. PRN.

    For temperature of 103^0 rectally (102^0 oral, 101^0 axillary) or above:
    3. Use a cooling blanket.
    4. Give tepid sponge bath and Tylenol/Ibuprofen as noted above.
    5. CBC with differential on A shift closest to occurrence of fever
    6. Check complete set of vital signs and Notify M.D.

4. HYPOTHERMIA: (temp less than 96^0 rectal, 95^0 oral, 94^0 axillary)
    1. Put socks and cap on client.
    2. Wrap client up with a regular blanket.
    3. If temperature does not respond, put on heating blanket.

5. NAUSEA AND VOMITING: (New Onset)
    1. Check for fecal impaction
    2. If positive, follow orders for impaction. If negative, and after vomiting 2 times, give Phenergan Suppository 25 mg., 1 whole one for clients over 45 pounds, ½ for clients under 45 pounds.

NAME:_____CASE NUMBER:_____

Figure 9-6   Physician's standing orders. (Courtesy Hudspeth Regional Center, Whitfield, MS. Used with permission.)

6.   DIARRHEA: (New Onset)
       1.   Hold any laxatives or prune juice for 48 hrs.
       2.   Immodium 2 mg. P.O. after 3rd loose stool. May repeat once within an hour.

7.   SEIZURES:
       After 2nd Grand Mal seizure:
       1.   Check for impaction.
       2.   Give Ativan 2 mg. IM for clients weighing greater than 50 pounds or 1 mg. IM for clients weighing less than 50 pounds.
       3.   Check complete set of vitals and notify MD if seizures not resolved.
       4.   If impaction was positive, follow orders for impaction.

8.   IMPACTION:
       1.   Give one Dulcolax or Bisacodyl Suppository per rectum.
       2.   May manually disimpact as needed.

9.   CONSTIPATION:
       1.   Give MOM 30 cc by mouth or PEG.

10.   MOUTH INJURIES:
       1.   Glyoxide application 3 times a day for 5 days.
       2.   Refer to the physician or dentist as needed.

11.   RUNNY NOSE: Nalex-A:
                               1.   Age greater than 12, give 1 tablet or 2 teaspoons 3 times a day X 5 days, or
                               2.   Age less than 12, give 1 teaspoon or ½ tablet 3 times a day X 5 days with first and last dose being at least 12 hours apart and middle dose being at least 4 hours from first and last. (Ex. 7am,4pm, 8pm, or 8am, 12am, 8pm)

                       OR

                       Rondec:
                               1.   Age greater that 6, give 1 tablet or 1 tsp three times a day X 5 days, or
                               2.   Age less that 6, give ½ tsp. of the liquid three times a day X 5 days with first and last dose being at least 12 hours apart and middle dose being at least 4 hours from first and last. (Ex. 7am,4pm, 8pm, or 8am, 12am, 8pm)

NAME:_____CASE NUMBER:_____

Figure 9-6   *(Continued)*

12.   FOR RED EYES WITH DRAINAGE/CONJUNCTIVITIS: Bacitracin or Neosporin Ophthalmologic Ointment 3 times a day for 5 days with first and last dose being at least 12 hours apart.

13.   DIAPER RASH: A & D Ointment as needed and with every diaper change.

14.   PURULENT EAR DRAINAGE: Cortisporin Otic Suspension or Cortaine-B, 4 drops in affected ear 4 times a day for 7 days. Do not use if there is a known tympanic membrane perforation or PE Tubes.

15.   COUGH:
  1.   For clients 12 and above, give Robitussin DM 3 teaspoons 4 times a day for 7 days.
  2.   For clients 12 and under, give 2 teaspoons of Robitussin DM 4 times a day for 7 days.

16.   EAR WAX REMOVAL: (Do not use if there is a known tympanic membrane perforation or PE Tubes.)
  1.   Cerumenex 3 or 4 drops in effected ear at 8 PM and repeat again at 8 AM the next morning. OR
  2.   For more stubborn cerumen: Cerumenex 3 to 4 drops in affected ear 3 times a day for 5 days
  3.   Then irrigate with warm water after the Cerumenex treatment.

17.   FINGER STICK GLUCOSE: Do a finger stick glucose for signs and symptoms of hypoglycemia or hyperglycemia (nausea, diaphoresis, shakiness, decreased level of consciousness).

  1.   If glucose is less than 70, give juice and sugar or Instaglucose and recheck in 15 minutes. If still less than 70, continue with juice and sugar and/or Instaglucose, check complete set of vitals and notify MD.
  2.   If glucose is greater than 400, check complete set of vitals and notify MD.

18.   ROUTINE MEDICATION ORDERS THAN RUN OUT ON THE WEEKENDS OR HOLIDAYS: Continue same medications and dosages until the next working day.

19.   For any acute illness or change in status, check a complete set of vitals (Blood Pressure, Temperature, Pulse, Respirations) and notify MD.

DO NOT GIVE ANY OF THE ABOVE MEDICATIONS IF ALLERGIC. ANY SPECIFIC ORDERS ON ANY CLIENT SUPERCEDES THESE STANDING ORDERS.

| Physician | Date | Nurse | Date |

NAME:_____CASE NUMBER:_____

Figure 9-6   (*Continued*)

The medication administration record (MAR) is a tool used by the nursing staff to initial for the medication administered during their shift. The reverse side of the form is used to explain why medications were not administered, for example, the person was out on pass, NPO (nothing by mouth) prior to surgery, or the person refused medication.

The director of nursing and the pharmacist use this form in their medication reviews to check for problem areas, for incidents in medication administration, and in guidelines when in-service training or more severe corrective measures are required in reference to the issues noted in the review.

The individual medication and chart audit review summary is used on a monthly basis to audit services provided to the person such as medications and behavior monitoring activities. This form is used primarily by the director of nursing in medication reviews for checking problem areas, such as incidents in medication administration, and in guidelines when in-service training or more severe corrective measures/actions are required. This information could be noted on the medication administration record or individual medication and chart audit review summary. Some facilities and nursing staffs may elect to conduct their medication review and chart audit on a separate form.

The medication worksheet is a computerized summary used by the nursing staff to assist in the review and audit of medication administrations and may be used in conjunction with the process covered in this section.

Self-administration of medication progress forms is valuable for recording persons' skills in their self-medication administration.

The medication destruction record is used when the medication becomes outdated or unused quantities of medications must be destroyed.

The discharge from facility release of responsibility and medication form is vital when individuals leave the facility and medication is being administered. Often medication issues can be addressed and staff alerted to possible medication problems by the use of this form. The medication count can reveal if the individual was overdosed, underdosed, or the medication was not given correctly.

The seizure chart provides documentation on individuals with convulsive disorder. This form provides staff with the frequency, time of day, and kinds of seizures, and can assist the staff in the medication adjustments for the control of seizures.

Behavior modification is often a major problem in an ICF/MR. In order to meet the legal and medical needs set forth, forms such as restraint documentation are required in the tracking of restraint use and become valuable in addressing such issues on a timely basis, such as in quarterly summary reviews.

Graphic records, such as weight, are important to various services. For example, the dietary department must provide menus based on the individual's diagnosis and nutritional needs. Nursing may need to check the weight records for the administration of medications, especially for children. Monitoring of vital signs and menstrual information is also done.

The influenza vaccine authorization and administration record serves a dual purpose. The form is sent to the family to obtain permission and/or refusal for the flu vaccine. In the event that the response is affirmative, the second portion of the form is used to document the administration of the vaccine.

Quality Improvement and Utilization Management

To continue providing excellent care and supports to individuals, every area of a facility must be involved in continuous quality improvement. To make sure that individuals are in the right setting, utilization management is essential.

Quality Improvement

The quality improvement (QI) function includes each department and service in order to accomplish the mission correctly. This task is ultimately a facility-wide endeavor. Quality must be incorporated into all of the services provided and measured according to acceptable standards. These standards are usually developed as guidelines in meeting licensing and accrediting requirements.

QI can involve studies conducted by the Infection Control Committee; comparisons of the frequency of accidents/incidents, medication errors, or seizure frequency; and review of yearly required training in universal precautions and cardiopulmonary resuscitation. Review of the various drills for fire, weather conditions, and toxic spills can be included in the QI function. Audits of documentation requirements on a monthly, quarterly, and yearly basis are other examples of QI in action.

Utilization Management

Utilization management (UM) relates to caring for each individual in the most appropriate setting and also to the efficient use of resources. The interdisciplinary team reviews the person's progress at regular intervals and places the individual in the most appropriate care setting. UM is also part of the work of various standing committees. For example, the formulary committee attempts to obtain the medications recommended by the medical and dental staff at the most reasonable price. Department heads and supervisors can also practice UM techniques in their daily activities as they strive to provide efficient, quality services.

Risk Management and Legal Issues

Risk management includes, but is not limited to, reviewing deaths, studying incidents and accidents, correcting errors, changing records properly, and using new technology correctly. Legal issues that must be considered are confidentiality, production of records, policies and procedures for health information, and record retention.

Risk Management

Depending on the organization of the ICF/MR, the governing body along with its legal counsel oversees the legal issues and sets the parameters under which it must operate. The records maintained by the facility can be risk management's best friend or worst enemy depending on the documentation contained within the record. The following are some of the areas in which risk management may be involved in the ICF/MR.

Deaths

Usually every death is automatically reviewed in-depth, no matter if the death occurred in-house or in another health care facility. The risk management committee leaves no stone unturned in verifying that all necessary steps were taken to prevent the death from occurring. This investigation is very important in deaths that have occurred unexpectedly and without previous disease process.

Incidents and Accidents

Risk management may study every incident and accident report to see if the situation could possibly have been avoided. Often computer programs are designed to study the incident/accident and the time of day, by shift and hour, place, cause of incident, most effective interaction, and the injury sustained. This information is placed on a grid. From the computer printout, the staff may ascertain something as simple as a hole in a shower curtain allowing puddles of water to accumulate. With this information, the staff can correct the situation and prevent individuals from being placed in an unsafe environment.

Method of Correcting Errors

In order to eliminate any suspicion of fraudulent documentation, staff must use the proper method to correct documentation errors. A single line through the incorrect entry without completely obliterating the erroneous entry is the correct method for changing an entry. The person making the correction should also date and initial the correction.

Editing Documentation in Records

Addenda should be used when information in a person's record is incorrect. By retaining the original form and including the addendum, legal questions to a change should be reduced. The addendum should include the date, time, reason for the change, and the signature of the person entering the addendum followed by professional credentials, such as MD, RN, or other.

New Technology

The risk management staff may want to investigate the possible legal issues in the use of computers and the various features they have, such as electronic signatures and faxing of information. The facility's policies and procedures should address the elements in the use of new technology. Watching for changes in the laws governing the high-tech equipment of the present and future is definitely a major function of risk management.

Legal Issues

Confidentiality

Confidentiality issues are a major concern in an ICF/MR. Medical professionals and other professional staff generally receive training in the safeguarding of confidential information during their formal educational programs. As records are made more user-friendly and placed in the areas where individuals live, direct care workers must be provided with in-depth in-service training in protecting confidential information. All chart handlers should sign statements agreeing to protect the confidentiality of individual information, and a breach of this responsibility would make the employee subject to severe action, up to and including dismissal.

The confidentiality statement should be obtained from all authorized record handlers before their first handling of any records. All data contained within the record may not be discussed with anyone who has not obtained the appropriate clearance for use of the record. As a rule of thumb, no person should be allowed to review an individual's record who does not have a job-related need to do so.

With the ease of copy machines and computer printers, often unnecessary copies of records are made. All data produced by the facility (originals) should become a part of the person's permanent record. Copies of information from other health services and copies of data retained for reference and/or proof of work completed should be stamped with a "copy" indicator, which would signal to the staff that this information is to be retained as a permanent record. All unnecessary data should be destroyed by shredding.

The Health Insurance Portability and Accountability Act (HIPAA) intensified the need for scrutiny in maintaining confidentiality of protected information in ICF/MR facilities. Facilities have taken steps to ensure compliance with both the privacy and security standards of HIPAA. In taking the protection of confidentiality to a higher level, facilities have typically appointed privacy and security officers and enhanced staff training programs. Policies involving actions such as release of records to third parties, use of photos on bulletin boards, persistence in obtaining parental permissions, and labeling personal articles have been reviewed and brought into compliance. Training procedures have been put into place for business associate activities that require identification of individuals. Maintenance of these higher standards will require that facilities make compliance with the federal law everyone's responsibility through continued staff training and advocacy for individual rights. Health information managers have a vital role in this process.

Production of Records

Individual records are the property of the facility and as such should be protected from loss, damage, tampering, or use by unauthorized individuals. Records may be removed from the facility's jurisdiction and safekeeping only in accordance with court order, subpoena, or statute.

Written Policies and Procedures

There should be written policies and procedures governing access to, publication of, and dissemination of information from individuals' records. Some points to consider in the management of information are as follows.

The policy sections of the manual should be inclusive and applicable on a facility-wide basis. Training sessions should also be implemented to provide in-service for new employees and serve as a reminder and reference to tenured employees. Procedures can be department/service specific and are not necessarily on the facility-wide level.

Policies and procedures may vary in the ICF/MR setting depending on the type of facility and the services rendered, but there must be established guidelines. Some infractions in the day-to-day handling (mishandling) of an individual's records could lead not only to dismissal of the employee for not performing his or her job according to policy/procedure but also fines, imprisonment, and even the loss of license, certification, or accreditation, depending on the severity of the offense.

Record Retention

Laws vary from state to state; therefore, the retention schedule should be consistent with the state statute of limitations.

For historical and research purposes, it would be highly recommended that if the individual's records are not retained in their entire original format after the retention period, that at least a "skeleton" of the most vital data be considered for retention for archival purposes.

Health information managers should work with administration, legal staff, or state research (genetic) centers to determine what may be the most useful information in the individual's records to retain to enhance specialty study areas and general population data requirements.

On average, an ICF/MR may receive from five to ten requests annually for information about a family member who was in the facility. Today the public is much better informed, and many individuals want to know firsthand if they are at risk of having a child who could be mentally and/or physically challenged.

In working with genetic specialists, they often find that the cause of disability was simply a "fluke," but if this is not the case, the person(s) in turn can make a very informed decision as to the risks of producing a child with inheritable conditions.

The "overretention" of beneficial information in essence becomes a judgment call. The cost of maintaining the data in the original, microfilmed, or electronic format is an important decision factor. It has to be weighed against an individual's need to know this helpful information.

Role of the Health Information Management Professional

The role of the HIM professional may be either as a regular employee or as a consultant to the facility. The health information manager serving as a regular employee performs duties and responsibilities covering all levels of management, but in a functional format. When issues and problems in the management of the records arise, the expertise of this professional is sought facility-wide. This is doubly true because the most active portion of the individual's record is not housed in the HIM department, but rather on the living unit. Development of policies and procedures in the handling of records must consider activities more far-reaching than the processes occurring in the centralized department of health information services.

Major duties and responsibilities fall into the following categories:

Management

Risk management/legal aspects

Supervision

Implementation and maintenance of health information systems

Designing health care records to address the health needs of the facility and the client it serves

Retrieval and storage of health information

Maintenance of various statistical data

Coding and indexing of records

Quality improvement

Completion of all phases of the record including:
    Active
    Overflow
    Closed records
    Maintenance and storage of microfilmed records

Data analysis

The health information manager consultant assists administration to establish policies and procedures to address the maintenance, preservation, completion, and confidentiality of records and release of information. In order to accomplish facility objectives for this service, the consultant supervises and trains personnel assigned to record-keeping services, including on-the-job training and in-service education methods.

The major function of the consultant involves quality management in the review and auditing of the facility records. This task includes all facility-wide records—administrative, habilitative, and health records.

Trends

The provision of services for individuals with mental retardation or developmental disabilities is a health industry in a state of constant change. As mentioned in the introduction of this chapter, the number of persons receiving services in large public or private facilities is decreasing: "Since the 1970s many states have vigorously reduced their reliance on institutional facilities and developed community residential settings including group homes, foster care, and supported living options" (Braddock et al., 2002, p. 1). Reasons for the expansion of community services are varied. The number of persons needing services is increasing partly because of the aging of our society and the increased longevity of persons with developmental disabilities. Many individuals and their families are becoming vocal in expressing their needs and desires and want more choices in the types of supports made available: "The enactment of the **Home and Community Based Services (HCBS) Waiver** in 1981 enabled states to expand federal Medicaid support for community services. . . . In 2000, federal HCBS Waiver reimbursement totaled $5.5 billion and supported 293,713 participants" (Braddock et al., 2002, pp. 15, 17). Services provided by the waiver such as respite care, home health aides, supported employment, transportation, and various health therapies can delay or prevent placement in a facility.

Litigation is another factor influencing the growth of community-based programs: "On June 22, 1999, the United States Supreme Court held in Olmstead vs. L.C. that the unnecessary segregation of individuals with disabilities in institutions may constitute discrimination based on disability. The court ruled that the American with Disabilities Act may require states to provide community-based services rather than institutional placements for individuals with disabilities" (National Association of Protection and Advocacy Systems, Inc., 2001). As of March 2002, nine Olmstead lawsuits had been filed. Other class action suits have been filed to force states to expand services to persons on waiting lists and for those persons who have been found to be eligible for Medicaid services but did not receive them (Braddock et al., 2002). As states often struggle with a weak economy and limited funds to initiate new desired services, the likelihood of additional lawsuits is great. Care in an institutional setting is one option in the array of services utilized by individuals with mental retardation or developmental disabilities; however, future growth is most likely to occur in the provision of supports that enable individuals to remain in their home communities.

Summary

This chapter has reviewed the technical aspects of the ICF/MR services and how they apply to the practical daily work environment. With the guidelines, suggestions, and recommendations furnished in this chapter, the health information manager has at his or her fingertips basic information that should serve as a quick reference in the management of individual records.

This chapter should provide health information managers, as members of an interdisciplinary team, with a solid foundation from which to build their skills, talents, and knowledge to best meet the needs, objectives, and goals of individuals receiving services in an ICF/MR.

Key Terms

active treatment   each individual must receive a continuous active treatment program that includes aggressive, consistent implementation of specialized and generic training, treatment, health services, and related services.

annual staffing   informal term for the annual meeting of the interdisciplinary team during which the individual program plan is reviewed and revised for the coming year; not to exceed 365 days from the previous annual or initial staffing.

assessment   the process of identifying an individual's functional level, strengths, needs, causes of disabilities, and conditions hindering development.

developmental disability   a disability "attributable to a mental or physical impairment that begins before age 22 and is likely to continue indefinitely and that results in substantial functional limitation in three or more areas of major life activity" (AAMR, 1992).

direct care staff   personnel whose daily responsibility is to manage, supervise, and provide direct care to individuals in their residential living unit.

habilitation   the process by which a person is assisted to acquire and maintain life skills that enable the person to cope more effectively with personal and environmental demands and to raise the level of his or her physical, mental, and social efficiency. Habilitation includes, but is not limited to, programs of structured education and training.

Home and Community Based Services (HCBS) Waiver   a federal program that allows states to use Medicaid funding to serve persons in their own homes and communities, not just in institutional settings.

individual habilitative or individual program plan (IHP or IPP)   a comprehensive individualized assessment that serves as the major tool in the care and services rendered to the individual.

interdisciplinary (ID) team   a group that develops an integrated habilitation or program plan that provides individualized services to the individual.

intermediate care facility for the mentally retarded (ICF/MR)   a facility that provides care and training for persons with mental retardation in order to increase their adaptive skills, such as self-care skills, language skills, social skills, vocational skills, and so on.

Inventory for Client and Agency Planning (ICAP)   a standardized assessment instrument that can be used for program planning and is also used in several states as a data collection tool for case mix reimbursement to ICF/MR organizations.

mental retardation   low intelligence with significant disabilities in two or more adaptive skill areas with age of onset before age 18. Mental retardation may be classified in terms of etiology or causal factors including conditions caused by infection, intoxication, brain injury, disorders of metabolism and neoplasms.

qualified mental retardation professional (QMRP)   a person assigned to monitor and coordinate all activities related to development and implementation of the individual program plan.

training objective   single outcome expected to be achieved by the individual within one year, as a result of training. Measurable outcome, criteria for measuring progress, and projected completion date should be specified relative to strengths, needs, and established goals.

REVIEW QUESTIONS

Knowledge-based Questions

1. What types of coding may be utilized in an ICF/MR?

2. Name the sections into which the individual's charts may be divided.

3. Is an admission to an ICF/MR facility permanent? Why or why not?

4. Who performs regular surveys of an ICF/MR facility?

5. Why is it important to establish the legal guardianship for individuals in an ICF/MR over 18 years of age?

Application-based Questions

1. What would you consider to be one of the major issues in an ICF/MR facility? Why?

2. The HIM professional employed on a regular basis and the HIM consultant would have different job roles. How would their jobs be different?

3. Describe how the services rendered to an individual in an ICF/MR are different from those in other settings.

4. Explain why accident and incident situations are important to study.

Web Activity

Visit the Centers for Medicare and Medicaid Services *Conditions of Participation/Conditions for Coverage* Web site at the following URL: http://www.cms.hhs.gov/cop/1.asp.

Scroll down to find the listing Intermediate Care Facilities for Persons with Mental Retardation and click on the links to reach the current *Conditions*. What term is used to refer to individuals receiving services from an ICF/MR?

Case Study

The interdisciplinary team in the XYZ facility was experiencing problems with the habilitative portion of the individuals' records in that changes in the program were not being addressed by the direct care staff. Recommendations were being made on the quarterly team reviews but were not getting into the program records to be instituted by the direct care staff as required for the continuity of care.

Jean Deaux, a health information management professional, was contacted about this discrepancy in the program. She noted the recommended changes and the problem of the program not being carried out, and the lack of some documentation to tie these two together.

After studying the problem and the frequency with which it was occurring, she made the following recommendation: The suggested changes were to be covered in an addendum format, so that any time throughout the year when a major change in the individual's program was instituted, the change would be reflected in the 24-hour schedule, thus alerting the direct care staff of the addition, deletion, and/or change in the program.

In order to better track the documentation requirements, Ms. Deaux elected to monitor whether program changes were being documented appropriately in her monthly audit of the records and to submit any variance in the program to the assigned QMRP.

1. Could this problem be averted if the facility records were computerized?

2. Even if the records were computerized, would there still be a need to utilize some sort of tracking mechanism?

3. What steps would you have taken to solve the problem?

References and Suggested Readings

American Association on Mental Retardation. (1983). *Manual on Terminology and Classification in Mental Retardation* (1983 ed.). Washington, DC: Author.

American Association on Mental Retardation. (2002). *Mental Retardation: Definition, Classification, and Systems of Supports* (10th ed.). Washington, DC: Author.

American Psychiatric Association. (1994). *Diagnostic and Statistical Manual of Mental Disorders* (4th ed.). Washington, DC: Author.

Braddock, D., Hemp, R., Rizzolo, M. C., Parish, S., and Pomeranz, A. Coleman Institute for Cognitive Disabilities and Department of Psychiatry, The University of Colorado. (2002, June). *The State of the States in Developmental Disabilities: 2002 Study Summary* [Online]. http://www.cu.edu/ColemanInstitute/stateofthestates/summary_2002.pdf [2003, June 3].

Centers for Medicare and Medicaid Services. *Interpretive Guidelines—Intermediate Care Facilities for the Mentally Retarded*.

Conditions of participation for intermediate care facilities for the mentally retarded. *Code of Federal Regulations*, Title 42, Pt. 483, Subpart I, 2002 ed.

Council on Quality and Leadership in Supports for People with Disabilities. (1997). *Personal Outcome Measures*. Towson, MD: Author.

Council on Quality and Leadership in Supports for People with Disabilities. (Online) Accredited Organizations. http://www.thecouncil.org.

Hewitt, A., and O'Nell, S. (1998, August). Preface. *I Am Who I Am* [Online]. Y. Bestgen (Ed.). http://www.ncor.org/AuthorsBK4.html [2003, June 3].

Janicki, M. P. (1992). Lifelong disability and aging. In Rowitz, L. (Ed.), *Mental Retardation in the Year 2000*. New York: Springer-Verlag.

Joint Commission on Accreditation of Healthcare Organizations. (1997). *1997–1998 Comprehensive Accreditation Manual for Behavioral Health Care*. Oakbrook Terrace, IL. JCAHO.

Louisiana Code. Chapter 4. *Mental Retardation Law*. R.S. 28-380 to 28-452

National Association of Protection and Advocacy Systems, Inc. (2001, January). *Olmstead vs L. C.* [Online]. http://www.protectionandadvocacy.com/lcolmste.html [2003, June 3].

Preadmission screening and annual review of mentally ill and mentally retarded individuals. *Code of Federal Regulations*, Title 42, Pt. 483, Subpart C, 1996 ed.

Rowitz, L. (ed.) (1992). *Mental Retardation in the Year 2000*. New York: Springer-Verlag.

The Arc & UCP Public Policy Collaboration: 2003 Legislative Goals in Cooperation with AAMR (2003, March 8) [Online]. http://www.aamr.org/Policies/LegGoals03Web.pdf [2003, June 3].

Key Resources

American Association on Mental Retardation
444 North Capitol Street, NW
Suite 846
Washington, DC 20001-1512
Phone: 800-424-3688
http://www.aamr.org

The Arc of the United States
1010 Wayne Avenue
Suite 650
Silver City, MD 20910
Phone: 301-565-3842
Fax: 301-565-3843 or 301-565-5342
http://TheArc.org

Council on Quality and Leadership in Supports for People with Disabilities
(formerly Accreditation Council on Services for People with Developmental Disabilities)
100 West Road, Suite 406
Towson, MD 21204
Phone: 410-583-0060
Fax: 410-583-0063
http://www.thecouncil.org

Joint Commission on Accreditation of Healthcare Organizations
(See Chapter 1 for contact information.)

Chapter 10

Long-Term Care

Kris King, MS, RHIA, CPHQ
Barbara A. Gorenflo, RHIA

Learning Objectives

Upon successful completion of this chapter, you should be able to:

1. Describe the type of care typically associated with long-term care facilities.
2. Discuss the stringent impact of federal regulation on the long-term care industry and the relationship that this has on information management documentation content.
3. Identify the significance of state and **federal surveys** to long-term care facilities.
4. Describe the types of reimbursement and payer relationships within a long-term care facility.
5. Describe the purpose of the Minimum Data Set 2.0 and its use in the federal survey process and in case-mix payment systems.
6. Identify the priorities for health information management in the long-term care setting.

SETTING	DESCRIPTION	SYNONYM/EXAMPLES
Freestanding Nursing Facility	A facility or a portion of a facility licensed by the state as a nursing facility where the majority of patients are regarded as permanent residents for long-term nursing care	Nursing home Long-term care facility Intermediate care facility
Freestanding Skilled Nursing Facility	A facility or a portion of a facility licensed by the state as a skilled nursing facility and certified, either wholly or in part, as a Medicare Part A skilled nursing facility provider	Skilled nursing facility Skilled nursing unit Distinct part Medicare SNF unit
Acute Care Hospital	A designated area, attached wing, or a separate structure on the hospital campus that is licensed for skilled nursing care	Skilled nursing facility Skilled nursing unit SNF unit
Long-Term Acute Hospital	A facility providing specialized acute care for patients averaging a length of stay of 25 days or more	Long-term care hospital LTAC, LTCH, or LTACH

Introduction to Setting

Long-term care typically describes care of the frail, institutionalized elderly or those who are permanent residents of a nursing facility. For purposes of this chapter, long-term care does not include boarding care, assisted living, residential care, long-term care for the mentally ill, mentally retarded, or developmentally disabled (ICF/MR), or other types of institutionalized care that are not subject to the federal long-term care regulations or the state licensure regulations for **nursing facilities (NFs)**, or **skilled nursing facilities (SNFs)**, or long-term acute care hospitals (LTCH). With the exception of ICF/MR facilities, which are discussed in Chapter 9, these other components of the care continuum are less regulated and do not have the broad range of caregivers as found in the typical long-term care facility. With regard to federal regulations, the term "nursing facility" is a facility that is qualified for reimbursement under the Medicaid program. A "skilled nursing facility" meets the requirements for reimbursement under Medicare (CMS, 2002e).

Most of the discussion of the long-term care setting in this chapter relates to nursing facilities and skilled nursing facilities. However, there is another type of long-term care facility—the **long-term acute care hospital** (abbreviated **LTAC, LTACH,** or **LTCH**). Although both nursing facilities and LTCHs are considered "long-term care," LTCHs and skilled nursing facilities represent two distinctly different levels of care, with different licensing and different payment systems. LTCH facilities are licensed as hospitals and have their own prospective payment system (PPS) under Medicare. An LTCH can be a freestanding facility or it can be a "hospital within a hospital." In the 1980s, the Medicare program defined the characteristics of LTCH facilities and exempted them from the original hospital inpatient PPS (ALTHA, No date). By the year 1997, there were 195 LTCHs in the United States. In the year 2002, a specialized PPS for LTCHs was implemented (CMS, 2002f). The LTCH PPS will be discussed later in this chapter.

As the percentage of our population age 65 and older continues to grow, there will likely be several different care settings that will fall under the global term of *long-term care*; however, this chapter addresses long-term care as it applies to the settings and care descriptions identified.

Types of Patients

In the long-term care setting, *patient* is often replaced with *resident* because the person receiving care is not only a recipient of nursing care but in most cases is also permanently residing in the facility. The nursing facility becomes the home or place of residence, and as such, the facility is responsible for providing quality of care as well as high quality of life under the long-term care regulations. Within the broad category of *long-term care*, more specific distinctions can be drawn to describe the types of residents and the care they receive. As specialization of services increases within the long-term care industry, facilities find the need to categorize levels of care, and often physically separate types of care to distinct units or floors within the same facility. Therefore, residents can be placed in areas with other residents of similar care needs.

Permanent Residents Receiving Nonskilled Care

These residents are distinguished by their need for general oversight and supervision in performing **activities of daily living (ADL)** (e.g., bathing, eating, dressing); however, their needs can be generally met without the direct care or services of a licensed professional on a 24-hour basis. While a licensed practical nurse or registered nurse supervises their general care under the direction of the attending physician, their immediate care needs do not involve direct skilled treatment on a daily basis such as injections, intravenous therapy, parenteral feeding, or skilled wound care. From a level of care perspective, these residents require a higher level of care than those in a residential, boarding, or assisted living environment, either due to cognitive impairment or as a result of physical incapacity. For example, these residents could not, either due to physical or cognitive impairment, negotiate their way to safety in the event of an emergency. However, their daily care needs do not require continual intervention by a licensed nurse or other skilled health care professional.

Permanent Residents, Special Care

Special care units (SCUs) are often found as a distinct part within a long-term care facility. For example, some of these units are designed to specifically care for the Alzheimer's residents who benefit from a physical environment that is quiet, home-like, and adapted to their specific cognitive impairment. The physical separation of the unit assures that these residents are afforded the opportunity to move throughout the area without fear of wandering off the property. In addition, the staff assigned to these units generally receive special training in the care of Alzheimer's residents because their needs are typically more behavior oriented than medically oriented. Other special care units may be designed for patients using ventilators or other residents with special needs.

Permanent Residents, Skilled Care

In contrast to the permanent residents who do not receive daily skilled care, these residents receive services from one or more licensed professionals on a frequent and often daily basis. Typically these residents have received as much benefit from rehabilitation services as can be reasonably expected and their improvement or progression has plateaued. As a result, their potential to be discharged is not good. Types of care would include the need for continuous tube feeding, long-term ventilator care, complex wound care, and/or an aggregate combination of nursing and restorative professionals to meet the daily care needs of feeding, performing ADLs, and maintaining the highest functional level for as long as possible. Often the term *heavy care* is used to describe these residents because of the intensity of their dependence on the staff for mobility, toileting, bathing, eating, and performing all ADLs. Their care can be described as more custodial in nature.

Short-Term Patients (less than 100 days)

A short-term patient in a long-term care facility would generally be considered one who has a length of stay of less than 100 days and in the traditional health care sense would be regarded as a *patient* because the intent is to ultimately discharge the patient to a more independent level of care. In some long-term care facilities, this distinct unit is categorized as a subacute unit where patients are provided with a higher level of care than that associated with the traditional skilled nursing setting. Care in these distinct units is skilled care for treatment of a specific condition, and often placement is temporary because the goal of treatment is rehabilitation to discharge the patient home or to a lower level of care. In some situations, discharge from this unit may correlate with an internal transfer to a long-term care bed within the same facility.

Long-Term Acute Care Hospital Patients

Patients admitted to a long-term care hospital (LTCH) are generally more acutely ill than patients in other long-term care settings. In fact, patients are often admitted to the LTCH directly from a short-stay hospital intensive care unit (ALTHA, No date). Their medical conditions are complex (e.g., respiratory conditions with ventilator dependence), and they require more acute type services such as cancer treatment, head trauma treatment, and pain management. Comprehensive rehabilitation is also a common service provided to LTCH patients. As opposed to a short-stay acute care hospital, the average length of stay in an LTCH is 25 days or more. (Liu et al., 2001).

Respite Care

Respite care is a short stay for the purpose of providing relief or "respite" to the primary caregivers of the frail elderly who cannot live in an independent environment and do not require the intensity of services and supervision required of the traditional long-term care facility. The period of respite care may range anywhere from overnight to several weeks, depending on the caregiver's needs. For the respite care admission, a long-term care facility is providing meals and general supervision to assure that necessary medications are administered and is providing a safe environment for the respite resident with opportunities for socialization, with there being no need for active care intervention.

Types of Caregivers

Licensed Physicians

Doctors of medicine and osteopathy are responsible for the overall medical supervision in the long-term care facility; however, their physical presence in the nursing facility is generally limited. Frequency of visits to a long-term care resident can range from once a month to once a year depending on the level of care required of the resident. In some instances, the physician does not actually visit the nursing facility but requires that the resident be transported to his or her office for necessary medical examinations. Therefore, the majority of communication with the physician is done through the nursing staff via telephone as opposed to physical contact with the physician. In the skilled nursing facility (SNF) or subacute units of long-term care facilities, frequency of physician involvement is generally greater and can range to several visits a week, with monthly visits being the outside range depending on the level of acuity of the SNF/subacute unit. The minimum visit requirement for physician visits in the SNF and subacute units is once every 30 days for the first 90 days and then every 60 days thereafter.

The physician visit pattern in LTCHs is different from that found in long-term care nursing facilities. In the long-term hospital setting, daily physician visits are more common (ALTHA, No date).

Physician Extenders

Nurse practitioners, clinical nurse specialists, and physician assistants are used by physicians to assist in caring for their patients who reside in long-term care facilities. Particularly in rural settings, the addition of these personnel to the physician office practice affords greater contact with the resident than may occur if only the physician were making visits to the nursing facility.

Registered Nurses

Registered nurses are the primary coordinators of daily care within the long-term care facility. Because there is limited physical contact with the physicians in most long-term care settings, care is nursing driven. The director of nursing in most regulatory environments is required to be a licensed, registered nurse. Depending on the number of beds, the facility will employ additional registered nurses for supervisory positions, or as charge nurses on specific nursing units.

Licensed Practical Nurses

Licensed practical nurses are the most predominant caregivers among the licensed professionals in the long-term care nursing facility setting. Their responsibilities range from administering medications, tube feedings, and treatments to charging a nursing division and serving in a supervisory capacity within the nursing department.

Nursing Assistants

Nursing assistants comprise the bulk of the nursing department in a long-term care nursing facility. They are nonlicensed staff members who have completed a basic training course for providing daily care needs to the geriatric patient, including basic skills in bathing, transfer training, lifting, range of motion, and related supportive services that would be provided under the general supervision of a licensed nurse.

In some facilities, a distinction is made for nursing assistants who strictly provide restorative therapy, called a restorative aide or rehabilitation aide. With additional training from the licensed therapists, the restorative or rehabilitation aides are given responsibility for providing maintenance services to residents after skilled rehabilitation has been discontinued. At this point in the resident's care, a plateau has been reached and no active improvement is expected from continued skilled therapy. The restorative therapy is intended to maintain the level of functioning that has been achieved from skilled therapy and/or to prevent further functional decline.

Certified Medication Technicians

In some states, a certified medication technician (CMT) is a distinct type of caregiver in the long-term care setting, provided for in the state long-term care regulations. Requirements for this position are generally a minimum of nursing assistant training with an additional course in medication administration, the scope of competency requirements varying with the individual state regulations. The purpose of this caregiver category is to recognize a lower-cost health care position with limited responsibilities that can lessen the workload of the licensed nursing professionals.

Social Services

Provision of the medically related social services of residents is assigned to the department that is typically described as *social services* in the long-term care setting. Depending on the size of the facility, this department may or may not be staffed with a credentialed social worker (BSW or MSW). Federal long-term care regulations require that a facility with more than 120 beds employ a full-time social worker or a person with qualifications outlined in the federal requirements.

These requirements describe a qualified social worker as an individual with a bachelor's degree in social work or a bachelor's degree in a human services field including but not limited to sociology, special education, rehabilitation counseling, and psychology and with one year of supervised social work experience in a health care setting working directly with individuals.

In the long-term care setting, the social services staff takes on many responsibilities that impact on the care and well-being of the resident such as making arrangements for adaptive equipment, clothing, and financial assistance; coordinating discharge planning; coordinating and initiating referrals and appointments with outside services; providing counseling to residents, family members, and facility staff as it relates to the care needs of individual residents; and providing any other services that promote the psychosocial well-being of the resident. Social services staff are advocates for many residents who are no longer able to realize or protect their rights to decision making, fair treatment, dignity, respect, and so on.

Activities/Therapeutic Recreation

Although therapeutic recreation is not a direct care service as one considers administration of a treatment or a medication, providing stimulating activities or therapeutic recreation services is extremely important in the long-term care setting. In most long-term care facilities, the activity program is not necessarily directed by a licensed or credentialed individual. Licensing of activity professionals other than recreational therapists is not universal in each state, and federal regulations provide several alternative options as qualifications for an activity professional including two years of direct experience in a patient activities program in a health care setting and/or completion of a training program approved by the state agency.

The activities staff is responsible for assessing the therapeutic recreational needs and preferences of each resident and developing an individualized program that responds to those needs. This includes providing sufficient group and individual activity and recreational programs to respond to the needs of the various levels of care within the facility. The types of activity programs that fall within the scope of the typical long-term care facility include planning and providing for outings such as shopping and recreational activities off the premises of the facility; planning and providing supplies and materials for independent, in-room activities; establishing small group programs for the cognitively impaired such as reminiscent therapy; conducting in-room, one-on-one activities for the roombound and unresponsive resident such as music therapy and tactile stimulation; and planning and conducting facility-wide social events for residents and their families.

If a facility population consists of mostly alert and oriented residents with limited physical impairments, the recreational program will be far different than that for the population that consists of semicomatose residents or residents with severe dementia. As a result, the therapeutic activities program must be responsive to the varying needs of the resident population.

Independent Contractors

In the long-term care facility, most of the ancillary services and many of the professional services are provided through independent contracts with outside resources, including laboratory, radiology, pharmaceutical, and rehabilitation services such as physical, occupational, speech, and respiratory therapy services. As independent contractors, these providers are not employees of the facility and are generally not physically present within the facility on a full-time basis.

Laboratory and Radiology

Laboratory and radiology services may be necessary to further evaluate or treat chronic or acute medical conditions, and these services are performed in accordance with physician orders. Laboratory and radiology services are evaluated in terms of their timeliness of response to stat and routine calls and for the additional services they provide for enhancing the overall quality of health information. For example, laboratory services generally provide the facility with a monthly computerized report outlining the types of tests performed in the previous month, patterns and trends with respect to nosocomial infections, use of antimicrobial agents, and related infection control issues.

Rehabilitation Services

Rehabilitation services (PT, OT, speech, and RT) are most often provided through independently contracted arrangements because the volume of rehabilitation cases in the typical long-term care facility does not warrant full-time employees in any of the respective rehabilitation disciplines. Registered physical and occupational therapists visit the facility based on the volume of skilled therapy services required by the resident population. Often services are supplemented with physical therapy and occupational therapy assistants, who provide the daily therapy under the general supervision of the registered therapist. Speech therapists provide daily skilled therapy for dysphagia and dysphasia, primarily in postacute care of patients suffering from a cerebrovascular accident.

Respiratory Therapists

Respiratory therapists are more prevalent in facilities with long-term ventilator patients or facilities with a high number of residents requiring daily suctioning and respiratory therapy treatments.

Registered Dietitians

Federal regulations and many licensure regulations require the services of a registered dietitian on either a full-time or consulting basis. In the larger long-term care facilities of more than 150 beds, a registered dietitian may be a full-time employee of the long-term care facility, particularly if the resident population is predominantly skilled care with more complex nutritional care needs. If a registered dietitian is not employed in the facility on a full-time basis, the day-to-day management of the dietary service is the responsibility of a food services manager while the dietitian approves menus for therapeutic diets and provides individual clinical assessments for those residents with high risk or clinically complex nutritional needs during regularly scheduled consultation visits. Diet technicians may also be utilized to assist with nutritional care under the supervision of a registered dietitian.

Registered Pharmacists

With rare exception, pharmaceutical services are not available directly within a long-term care facility and are provided by a supplier that is remote to the facility. The services of a pharmacist are also required by the long-term care federal regulations, either on a full-time or on a part-time or consulting basis. The consulting pharmacist role may or may not be provided by the same entity that services the facility as the pharmaceutical supplier. The provider of drugs and biologicals or the actual pharmaceutical service is responsible for ensuring that medications are dispensed to the facility in a timely and appropriate manner. The responsibilities of the facility pharmacy consultant are somewhat different in that consultation extends to all aspects of the provision of pharmacy services within the facility to include performing a monthly drug regimen review for each resident in the facility to evaluate potential irregularities in medication administration. This includes monitoring for unnecessary drugs, evaluating proper dosages and indications for psychotropic medications, and evaluating internal storage and administration procedures within the facility. This review is required in the federal regulations and can be accessed by long-term care surveyors in the event of a question regarding the medication profile of a particular resident.

Regulatory Issues

The long-term care industry is one of the most, if not *the* most, highly regulated industries in the United States. In addition to federal regulations for long-term care facilities participating in Medicare and Medicaid, each state has separate licensure laws for long-term care facilities, and in the case of overlapping or conflicting laws, the facility is obligated to abide by the more stringent of the two. **Standard surveys** are unannounced and conducted at least every 15 months. The two general survey outcomes are termed *substantial compliance* and *substandard quality of care*. **Substantial compliance** means that any deficiencies found by the surveyors were deemed to be of minimal potential for harm to the residents. **Substandard quality of care** means that surveyors found one or more deficiencies that constitute either immediate jeopardy to resident health or safety; a pattern of widespread actual harm that is not immediate jeopardy; or a widespread potential for more than minimal harm, but less than immediate jeopardy, with no actual harm (CMS, 2002a). Results of all surveys are accessible to the public, with federal regulations requiring that the most recent survey be posted in a public area of the facility for easy access by residents, family members, and inquiries from the general public. In addition to the certification and **licensure surveys**, long-term care facilities are subject to surveys conducted in response to complaint investigations, which result from calls to the state agency concerning care concerns and potential regulatory violations. These survey findings are also subject to public access and can affect the facility license in the event of substantial noncompliance. Table 10-1 provides examples of several surveys unique to long-term care.

Effective July 1, 1995, federal enforcement regulations were implemented by the Health Care Financing Administration (now CMS) that outline remedies, including **civil money penalties** of up to $10,000 per day, for findings of substantial noncompliance and

Table 10-1   Types of Surveys Unique to a Long-Term Care Facility

Surveying Agency/Entity	Purpose and Frequency	Potential Impact and Outcome
State licensing agency	Annual licensure renewal and interim review depending on state law (unannounced)	Written deficiencies requiring a plan of correction and revisit Monetary fines Ban on admissions and other penalties and restrictions depending on state law
State licensing agency	Complaint investigation in response to state hotline calls concerning abuse and/or neglect (unannounced)	Written deficiencies requiring a plan of correction and revisit Monetary fines Ban on admissions and other penalties and restrictions depending on state law Full survey in response to findings of substantial noncompliance
Centers for Medicare and Medicaid Services (CMS)	Annual certification for participation in Title XVIII or XIX federal programs (unannounced)	Written deficiencies requiring a plan of correction and letter of credible allegation stating date corrections will be implemented Revisit may or may not be conducted to determine facility compliance Federal agency may conduct follow-up survey to validate findings of state agency Civil money penalties, temporary ban on admissions and denial of payment for Medicare/Medicaid admissions or current residents depending on scope and severity of noncompliance
Joint Commission on Accreditation of Healthcare Organizations (JCAHO)	Optional survey for long-term care facilities and special care and subacute units within long-term care facilities (announced every three years for fully accredited facility)	Full accreditation with commendation Provisional accreditation

substandard quality of care. In addition to federal enforcement regulations, individual states may pass legislation that also gives the state agency authority for fines and civil money penalties. Therefore, findings of substandard quality during a facility survey can result in civil money penalties from both the federal and the state licensing agency. Furthermore, federal enforcement regulations also provide for mandated temporary management of a facility, termination from the Medicare/Medicaid program, denial of Medicare/Medicaid payment for new admissions and/or for all current nursing facility residents in addition to the civil money penalties. As a result, the regulatory environment and impact of state and federal regulation on the long-term care facility is without comparison in other sectors of the health care industry.

State Licensure

If a long-term care facility does not participate in the Medicare or Medicaid program, federal regulations do not apply, and the facility is subject only to the state licensure requirements. These requirements are passed by the respective state legislative bodies, and consequently, there is great variability among the 50 states with regard to the scope of issues promulgated in their long-term care requirements.

JCAHO Accreditation

Although the number of long-term care facilities seeking Joint Commission on Accreditation of Healthcare Organizations (JCAHO) accreditation is increasing, the number is still relatively insignificant as a total percentage of licensed long-term care facilities. There is no clear advantage for a long-term care facility to seek JCAHO accreditation, unless it is required as part of an overall hospital accreditation for hospital-owned and -operated long-term care facilities. JCAHO has sought deemed status from the Centers for Medicare and Medicaid Services that would present long-term care facilities with the option of choosing between the current survey system by state and federal agencies or applying for JCAHO long-term care accreditation. However, at this writing this option is not available for long-term care.

Documentation

Documentation in the resident's record has tremendous significance to the nursing facility. Documentation is vital in the evaluation of how a facility has contributed to and/or affected the quality of care and quality of life of individual residents, strongly linking documentation with regulatory compliance. In addition, accuracy and appropriateness of documentation affects facility reimbursement by Medicare, Medicaid, and commercial insurance. Finally, as litigation involving negligence for poor care outcomes becomes more pervasive in the long-term care industry, proper documentation can be crucial in defending a provider against a wrongful claim for failure to provide quality care and services.

Although documentation of key information is important when a resident is transferred or discharged, the primary emphasis on routine documentation monitoring should be concurrent for detecting significant omissions in individual records as well as in identifying key training issues for ongoing staff education and quality improvement.

Federal Requirements

The quality of documentation is highly significant in the federal survey process in that the resident record is used as a means of validating positive and negative care outcomes both in the annual survey and in complaint investigations. Survey procedures for the federal long-term care survey process include two separate tasks in which the record is used for evaluating compliance with care issues, Task 5C—Resident Review, Part F—Closed Record Review, and Part I—Record Review (CMS, 2002a).

The **comprehensive resident assessment** is the primary vehicle for evaluating care outcomes in the federal long-term care survey process. Comprehensive resident assessment refers not only to the actual resident assessment document but also to the federally mandated **resident assessment instrument (RAI)** process. The RAI consists of three basic components: the **minimum data set (MDS), resident assessment protocols (RAPs)**, and utilization guidelines specified in the *State Operations Manual (SOM) Transmittal #272*. As a process, each of the three basic components flows into the next. The MDS is a core set of screening, clinical, and functional status elements that constitutes a standardized means of assessing all residents in Medicare and/or Medicaid certified facilities (CMS, 2002e).

The Omnibus Budget Reconciliation Act (OBRA) "regulations have defined a schedule of assessments that will be performed for a nursing facility resident at admission, quarterly, and annually, whenever the resident experiences a significant change in status, and whenever the facility identifies a significant error in a prior assessment. These are known as 'OBRA assessments.' MDS assessments are also required for Medicare payment purposes. . . . When the OBRA and Medicare assessment time frames coincide, one assessment may be used to satisfy both requirements. When combining OBRA and Medicare assessments, the most stringent requirement for MDS completion must be met. It is important for facility staff to fully understand the requirements for both types of assessments in order to avoid unnecessary duplication of effort" (CMS, 2002h, p. 2-1).

The RAPs are a structured process for assessing social, medical, and psychological problems by providing a systematic method of reviewing key components of the MDS and directing caregivers to evaluate causes, interrelationships, and particular strengths that affect the development of the **care plan** (CMS, 2002e). As of this writing there are 18 RAPs:

1. Delirium
2. Cognitive loss
3. Visual function
4. Communication

5. ADL functional/rehabilitation potential
6. Urinary incontinence and indwelling catheter
7. Psychosocial well-being
8. Mood state
9. Behavioral symptoms
10. Activities
11. Falls
12. Nutritional status
13. Feeding tubes
14. Dehydration/fluid maintenance
15. Dental care
16. Pressure ulcers
17. Psychotropic drug use
18. Physical restraints

Based on the resident data entered on the MDS, resident assessment protocols may or may not be triggered, indicating a need for further evaluation of the RAP utilization guidelines. If a RAP is triggered, the interdisciplinary team must document the outcome of their assessment process for that particular RAP and their decision regarding care planning for a particular problem or need. The location of this assessment information is documented on the **RAP summary** form, and this information is used by surveyors to evaluate whether nursing facility staff have properly utilized MDS information to assess and plan care for avoidable negative outcomes and to recognize resident strengths in the development of a comprehensive care plan.

According to federal regulations, a comprehensive assessment must be completed for each resident admitted to a certified bed within 14 days of admission or after any significant change in condition and on at least an annual basis thereafter. Between comprehensive assessments, staff must complete a quarterly review of specific assessment categories of physical, mental, and psychosocial information.

Although the comprehensive assessment (MDS form) and the quarterly reviews are actual data sets, they are regarded as a permanent part of the long-term care resident record. Therefore, these documents are not only valuable in providing aggregate care information concerning intensity of services and ongoing care outcomes, but they are also used to track individual resident care outcomes in the long-term care survey process. As changes occur with regard to assessed categories on the MDS, there should be explicit documentation in the resident record to explain and individualize these changes in condition, particularly if negative outcomes such as unplanned significant weight loss or acquired pressure ulcers are reflected in the course of care.

The data from the MDS has a variety of uses in the long-term care industry. Depending on the state, the MDS data may be used as the basis for Medicaid reimbursement for the nursing facility. In many states MDS data is required to be submitted to the state agency on a monthly basis, either in paper or electronic form. The state agency uses the data to evaluate care trends and may use the information as a presurvey evaluation tool for targeting potential care concerns before a formal survey. For example, MDS data can be used to track the number of residents with facility-acquired pressure sores, urinary tract infections, increased use of indwelling catheters, decline in functional ability, increased use of antipsychotic medications, increased use of physical restraints, and number of residents receiving rehabilitation and restorative services. Consequently, the data is valuable not only to the state agencies and surveyors but also to the individual provider. As a result, accurate and focused documentation is extremely important in its relationship to the comprehensive assessment. Documentation must support the assessment information in the MDS and should explain and describe how this information affects the individual resident.

The record review portion of the long-term care federal survey procedures instructs surveyors to evaluate the care and outcome of care provided to residents as portrayed through direct observation of staff and through assessed improvement/decline as noted on the MDS. In this phase of the survey, the record is used as a source of information to determine if the assessment process is accurate and consistent with what is actually observed with the residents and to evaluate if the staff are properly planning and implementing care goals and interventions to avoid decline and/or facilitate improvement in physical or psychosocial well-being *(CMS Guidance to Surveyors—Long Term Care Facilities)*. If there is an identified negative care outcome with a particular resident, documentation of the RAP process and other elements of the resident record would be used as a means of validating whether the negative outcome was facility related as compared to clinically unavoidable.

Care Plan

The care plan content and use is linked to the comprehensive assessment in the federal long-term care survey process. Depending on the individual state licensure regulations, additional emphasis may be placed on care plan documentation; however, this varies from state to state. In some states, care plans are not specifically required for residents who are not in Medicare or Medicaid certified beds.

In the federal long-term care regulations, the care plan is a subcategory of the comprehensive assessment regulation [483.20(d)]. These requirements specify content as well as timeliness guidelines. The care plan must be completed within seven days of the comprehensive assessment and should be an interdisciplinary process that involves not only the professional disciplines involved in the care of the resident but also the attending physician and the resident or resident's legal representative.

Specific documentation guidelines for the comprehensive care plan include the following items:

- Measurable objectives and timetables to meet medical, nursing, and mental and psychosocial needs that are identified in the comprehensive assessment
- Description of the services that are to be furnished to attain or maintain the resident's highest practicable physical, mental, and psychosocial well-being
- Description of the services that would otherwise be required but are not provided due to the resident's exercise of rights including the right to refuse treatment *(CMS Guidance to Surveyors—Long Term Care Facilities)*

Because the care plan is an inherent part of federal regulatory compliance, it is not only viewed as a tool for direct caregivers but it also has far-reaching implications from a legal point of view. If the content of the care plan does not support that appropriate and individualized care was provided to a resident, the facility has increased vulnerability to claims of poor and/or inappropriate care if there are avoidable negative care outcomes (Sullivan, 1996). Furthermore, if the facility has a survey record of noncompliance with care plan requirements that can be correlated with **quality of care** deficiencies, the legal vulnerability of the facility is heightened.

The care plan is viewed as the focal point for communicating significant care findings and goals for the individual long-term care resident. For that reason, a well-documented care plan should reflect an individualized view of the resident such that it introduces the resident to each caregiver on the interdisciplinary team from the nursing assistant on each tour of duty to the licensed therapists and physicians who care for the resident on a less frequent basis. Consequently, standardized or computerized care plans that do not reflect individualization of care routines based on specific resident strengths and care priorities are not regarded as individualized or resident specific. Individualization of care information is the single most important content characteristic of a care plan in the long-term care setting from the perspective of a long-term care survey.

Discharge/Transfer

In the closed record review, documentation is evaluated in reference to the circumstances surrounding the transfer and/or discharge of the resident from the facility. Particular emphasis is placed on whether federal regulations were followed concerning involuntary transfer or discharge of a resident to another health care facility. Federal regulations outline specific circumstances in which a facility may transfer or discharge a resident involuntarily, and proper documentation is critical in demonstrating compliance with these requirements:

(1) The transfer or discharge is necessary for the resident's welfare and the resident's needs cannot be met in the facility;
(2) The transfer or discharge is appropriate because the resident's health has improved sufficiently so the resident no longer needs the services provided by the facility;

(3) The safety of individuals in the facility is endangered;

(4) The health of individuals in the facility would otherwise be endangered;

(5) The resident has failed, after reasonable and appropriate notice, to pay for (or to have paid under Medicare or Medicaid) a stay at the facility. For a resident who becomes eligible for Medicaid after admission to a nursing facility, the nursing facility may charge a resident only allowable charges under Medicaid.

When the facility transfers or discharges a resident under any of the circumstances specified in paragraphs (a) (2) (i) through (v) of this section, the resident's clinical record must be documented. The documentation must be made by:

(i) The resident's physician when transfer or discharge is necessary under paragraph (a)(2)(i) of this section; and

(ii) A physician when transfer or discharge is necessary under paragraph (a)(2)(iv) of this section. *(CMS Guidance to Surveyors—Long Term Care Facilities)*

In addition, circumstances leading to the transfer, discharge, or death are evaluated to identify if any specific avoidable negative care outcomes or lapses in care contributed to the final status of the resident. Consequently, discharge and transfer documentation is crucial in determining key quality of care and **quality of life** compliance issues.

Resident Rights

Resident rights represent a major focus in the long-term care setting, and often documentation becomes crucial in the evaluation of potential resident rights issues and whether a facility has properly acknowledged and recognized the rights of residents in the provision of care and services. Documentation affects the evaluation of compliance with resident rights requirements in a variety of ways. In addition to providing each resident or resident's legal representative with a written explanation of his or her basic rights under state and federal law, ongoing documentation of care preferences and explanations for various care outcomes becomes essential in determining compliance with resident rights requirements.

For example, if a resident has a particular diet order (such as an order for a diabetic diet) but the resident is not compliant with that diet and is frequently eating candy and other items that are restricted on that diet, documentation becomes essential as a resource for determining whether staff members are aware of this dietary compliance concern and how they manage the situation and balance clinical priorities with observance of residents' rights. Ideally, documentation would reflect that staff had advised the resident of the adverse complications associated with dietary noncompliance. If the resident knowingly chooses to continue with a behavior that has potentially negative consequences, documentation should reflect ongoing attempts to educate and reverse the behavior as well as the ongoing assessment of the resident's ability to understand and participate in this decision-making process. Although the need to recognize the rights of residents to participate in their own care and care planning is significant, there is an equally important need for the facility to demonstrate that staff acted appropriately and responsibly to supervise the care needs of the resident and to inform appropriate individuals of the consequences of their actions or inactions. Often these types of situations are portrayed differently depending on the perspective, that is, resident or caregiver. Therefore, documentation plays a crucial role in the balance between observing resident rights and providing necessary care and services for the well-being of the resident.

In addition to ongoing documentation by caregivers, various consents are necessary in order to document that permission has been obtained for specific activities that are specified in the federal regulations, and additional resident rights issues may also be included in state-specific requirements. These include but are not limited to permission to open mail, designation of attending physician and pharmacy service, permission to be photographed, handling of funds deposited with the facility, and informed consent for use of physical and chemical restraints. New resident rights under the Health Insurance Portability and Accountability Act (HIPAA) include the residents' right to know what information is obtained about them, and how it is used and disclosed. Residents have the right to review and amend their information and have an accounting of all disclosures.

State Licensure Requirements

As stated earlier in this chapter, the scope and intensity of state long-term care licensure requirements varies. In some states, the need for specific documentation above and beyond the content of the federal regulations may be extensive, whereas in other states the focus may be less stringent. From a health information management standpoint, it is essential that the long-term care facility evaluate documentation needs from the perspective of both state and federal requirements. If a facility is not certified for Medicare or Medicaid, state licensure requirements provide the regulatory structure for documentation standards. If, however, a facility is certified for Medicare or Medicaid, both the federal and the state requirements must be met. In some cases, the state requirements may require more stringent documentation than the federal requirements. For example, in the state of Missouri, the state licensure requirements specify that telephone orders must be signed within seven days. There is no federal requirement specifying a time frame for signature of telephone orders; however, long-term care facilities in Missouri would be obligated to both understand and comply with this separate licensure requirement during a state licensure survey.

JCAHO Long-Term Care Accreditation Requirements

The emphasis on comprehensive assessments and care plans is reflected equally in the long-term care accreditation requirements of JCAHO. In many respects, JCAHO long-term care requirements are a mirror image of the federal long-term care requirements, although there are not specific RAPs in the JCAHO accreditation standards. The standards do, however, refer to the need for the facility to establish and follow specific care protocols depending on the scope and intensity of services provided in a particular facility or unit.

In addition to long-term care accreditation standards, JCAHO also has standards for special care units that specialize in the care of the Alzheimer's type dementia residents and for subacute units. Therefore, if a facility is seeking accreditation for all three types of care, all three standards must be utilized in determining documentation and accreditation compliance. (Note: Beginning in 2004, JCAHO planned to integrate the standards in its subacute protocol into its overall long-term care standards.) From the facility perspective, compliance with multiple JCAHO standards and federal and state long-term care standards presents a significant challenge to all clinical disciplines.

Reimbursement and Funding

Reimbursement ranges from the very simple to the extremely complex in the long-term care setting because of the various sources of payment, the type and level of care provided by the facility, and whether a facility participates in Medicare and/or Medicaid. Within the industry as a whole, Medicaid reimbursement methodology varies from state to state. Moreover, depending on the type of long-term care facility, care and services may be billed to Medicare Part A and B, Medicaid, managed care, commercial insurance, and private pay, depending on the licensure and certification of the facility and the type and scope of services provided. A general overview of the various payment categories that are typically found in a long-term care facility is provided in Table 10-2. Depending on the degree to which a long-term care facility participates in each of these types of payer options, the complexity of documentation and information systems increases proportionately. The most simplistic environment is the strictly private pay facility in which all care and services are billed to the resident or resident's guarantor on a monthly basis. The most complex setting is one in which the facility participates in both Medicare Part A and Medicaid, has managed contracts for **subacute care**, bills directly for Medicare Part B services, and has residents with commercial insurance policies that pay on a fee-for-service basis for daily care.

Medicaid per Diem Based on Overall Facility Costs

The Medicaid program is an indigent program for the institutionalized elderly that is promulgated by individual state legislation. Therefore, depending on the type of reimbursement methodology adopted by the state agency, the type of coverage and system for determining reimbursement rates will vary. A common methodology is to calculate an overall facility per diem rate based on basic facility cost reporting. In these types of systems, there is no level of care distinction and all residents are reimbursed at a flat daily rate based on facility-specific cost data using a reimbursement formula developed by the state agency.

Medicare Part A Skilled Nursing Facility Benefit

Medicare Part A coverage is limited in that a resident must first be eligible for Medicare Part A coverage and qualify with a 3-day hospital stay within the previous 30 days of admission to a Medicare-certified bed and require the services of a skilled professional

Table 10-2 Basic Reimbursement Categories and Pay Sources

ITEM	Medicaid	Medicare Part A	Medicare Part B	Managed Care	Commercial Insurance	Private Pay
Daily room and board	If all other financial resources have been exhausted and resident meets state criteria, basic care services are reimbursed at a daily rate.	If residents meets eligibility and level of service criteria, pays up to 100 days per spell of illness.	Does not apply.	For rehabilitation and subacute patients, individual and/or provider contracts are negotiated for room and board and other services.	Depending on the policy, daily care is reimbursed at the skilled level or at a daily cap outlined in the individual policy.	Paid by patient or family funds.
Durable medical equipment	Coverage varies from state to state; most equipment is expected to be provided by the facility as a part of the daily rate. Medicaid will pay as a secondary payor for care/ services billed and paid under Medicare Part B.	Daily Medicare Part A rate is all inclusive for the period of certification. Use and cost of supplies and equipment is tracked for cost-reporting purposes.	Ancillary services such as physician visits, use of rehabilitation services outside of a Part A bed, some durable medical equipment, injections.	Reimbursement for durable medical equipment may be a part of the daily negotiated rate or negotiated and reimbursed separately by the managed care payer.	Coverage of durable medical equipment varies with individual policy.	Billing for use of special equipment and services over and above room and board varies from facility to facility.
Drugs	Specific coverage of drugs in the Medicaid program varies from state to state.	Cost of pharmaceuticals during care under Medicare Part A is included in the daily rate.	Coverage of medication is limited to that reimbursed under Part B.	Reimbursement for medications and treatments may be a part of the daily negotiated rate or negotiated and billed separately to the managed care payer.	Coverage for medications varies with individual policy.	Generally the supplier bills the facility who in turn bills the resident or guarantor on a monthly basis.

on a daily basis. If these criteria are met, the duration of the SNF coverage is limited to the need for daily skilled care up to a maximum of 100 days per spell of illness. Therefore, not every admission to a nursing facility will qualify for Part A benefits, and not every long-term care facility chooses to participate in the Medicare Part A program. Consequently, if a resident chooses to utilize the Medicare SNF benefit following discharge from an acute care facility, he or she must select a facility/provider that is certified to participate in the Medicare program unless the resident is covered under a Medicare risk contract with a health maintenance organization.

Beginning in 1998, Medicare payments to SNFs changed from a cost-based reimbursement to a prospective payment system (PPS). Medicare Part A payment rates now utilize a case-mix adjusted per diem rate. The per diem payments for each qualified admission are based on **Resource Utilization Groups III (RUGs)**, a case-mix methodology driven from the MDS. One of the 44 groups is assigned, and that payment is reimbursed to the facility for a specific period of time or until the next MDS is completed according to the defined schedule.

The SNF PPS also assigns billing responsibility for the entire package of care that residents receive during a stay to the SNF. This concept is called **consolidated billing**. For example, physical therapy services are billed by the SNF (not by the physical therapy provider) as part of the package of care. The physical therapy provider, in turn, receives payment from the SNF. There are some exceptions to the consolidated billing requirement. For example, Medicare does make separate payments for physicians' professional services, certain dialysis-related services, and other items (CMS, No date).

From a health information management perspective, the case-mix reimbursement greatly affects documentation and accurate submission of MDS data. Therefore, the quality and accuracy of documentation has a direct relationship with the financial viability of a facility heavily dependent on Medicare reimbursement.

Medicaid per Diem Based on Level of Care

In some states, a Medicaid per diem or daily rate is established based on a level of care distinction for intermediate or skilled care or on a case-mix methodology developed by the state agency. In some states, the MDS is used as a resource document for calculating the level of care and extent of resources utilized for individual residents and for the facility as a whole. Depending on the state methodology, additional reimbursement may be recognized for intensity of services, such as may be the case with care of AIDS, or for specific quality of care outcomes such as would apply for improvement in functional independence as a result of rehabilitation and restorative services.

Resource Utilization Groups III in Medicaid Reimbursement

Resource utilization groups (RUGS) III reimbursement methodology is a specific case-mix payment system used in a growing number of states for long-term care Medicaid reimbursement. Using the MDS as the foundation for the data collection, states categorize reimbursement for individual residents based on their characteristics and service needs. From a very general perspective, the methodology is based on the premise that if a resident has special or heavy care needs, the facility will be reimbursed at a higher rate than that for a resident who is more independent in care and requires less skilled or clinically complex services. In addition to a direct care rate, the facility is also reimbursed a nondirect rate that includes cost of administrative services, capital costs, and other financial categories that are not directly related to the provision of individual care and services. As with the Medicare SNF PPS, attention to documentation and the accuracy of MDS data is crucial when RUGs form the basis of a large portion of a provider's reimbursement.

Commercial Insurance

Commercial insurance coverage for long-term care services is growing and is projected to increase with the aging of our population. There is great variability, however, in terms of the type and duration of services that are covered as there is no standard definition of long-term care coverage as there is, to some degree, with *major medical* in relation to acute hospitalizations. In some instances, coverage mirrors the Medicare Part A SNF benefit and will reimburse the beneficiary only for a maximum of 100 days or for the period of time that daily skilled care is needed. In other instances, room and board expenses are reimbursed for a predetermined period of time regardless of level of care. Often the commercial insurance carrier will request copies of the resident medical record on a monthly basis to verify services rendered and to substantiate the level of care required of the beneficiary. Depending on the specific policy coverage, documentation of the level of care and scope/intensity of services is essential for assuring reimbursement from the third-party payer.

Managed Care Payers

Although the penetration of managed care into the long-term care industry is likely to increase over time, the predominant influence at this time is in the Medicare SNF and subacute sector of the long-term care industry. Managed care payers have entered into Medicare **risk contracts** (a contract between an HMO and CMS to provide services to Medicare beneficiaries under which the health plan receives a fixed monthly payment for enrolled Medicare members) and therefore assume responsibility for the SNF benefit for their enrollees. In addition, an increasing number of managed care payers are contracting with long-term care facilities for the care of non-Medicare enrollees who require the intensive postacute rehabilitation and nursing services provided by SNF and subacute units. In order to control cost of care, managed care payers are seeking affiliations with long-term care facilities that can provide the same or higher-quality outcomes at a lesser cost per care episode than the acute care setting. Consequently, managed care reimbursement is projected to increase in the long-term care setting for the low-cost, high-quality providers.

Managed care reimbursement can occur as a result of a variety of affiliations with a long-term care facility. For those facilities that are a part of a large, multifacility chain, managed care payers and health maintenance organizations (HMOs) may enter into national agreements on an exclusive basis. Facilities that are a part of an integrated delivery system may be involved in a managed care payment situation for an entire episode of care for enrollees. An example might be a worker's compensation claim in which the global care episode is reimbursed at a designated rate that includes acute care, postacute care, and related physician or other outpatient services. On an individual facility basis, negotiation with a managed care payer is done on both an individual or patient-to-patient basis and on a capitated basis based on predetermined levels of care and reimbursement. These negotiated rates may or may not include separate charges for pharmaceuticals, durable medical equipment, and/or rehabilitation services beyond a designated minimum number of units per day. As the term *negotiation* implies, there is a certain degree of bargaining on both sides in that the managed care payer is looking for the lowest price and the provider is looking for the highest price for the same outcome. For this reason, information becomes essential to the successful managed care negotiator. If a provider has insufficient or inaccurate information from which to understand where specific care costs can be controlled, profits maximized, and losses minimized, a capitated rate can be financially devastating if care needs exceed reimbursement.

Private Pay

Private pay in the long-term care setting denotes payment by the individual without any third-party payer. In some facilities, a global daily rate is billed to the resident on a monthly basis, including all meals, treatments, and supplies with no additional line item charges other than medications supplied by the pharmacy. In other facilities, a basic daily rate includes only room, board, and a nominal list of supplies/services with additional services being charged for restorative services, incontinent care, specialized therapeutic activity programs, feeding assistance, and other services that are regarded as "nonroutine" by the facility. The degree to which additional services are charged over and above routine services varies from provider to provider.

Long-Term Care Hospital Prospective Payment System (LTCH PPS)

Since October 1, 2002, Medicare payments to long-term care hospitals (not nursing facilities) have been determined by a diagnosis related group (DRG)–based prospective payment system (PPS). Although the numbers and titles of most of the long-term care diagnosis related groups (LTC-DRGs) are similar to those of inpatient DRGs, the LTC-DRGs differ from inpatient DRGs in relative weights and in their associated lengths of stay. LTC-DRGs are also similar to inpatient DRGs in that they are based on the patient's principal diagnosis, additional diagnoses, procedures performed during the stay, age, sex, and discharge status. The LTCH PPS calculates a per-discharge payment to the facility based on the product of the LTC-DRG relative weight multiplied times a federally determined payment rate. Other factors beyond the scope of this discussion may also affect Medicare payment to the LTCH (CMS, 2002c).

Information Management

Management of information is an area of growing significance in the long-term care setting not only from a reimbursement perspective but also from a regulatory compliance and risk management perspective. This need is seen more dramatically in facilities participating in Medicare and Medicaid because of the information emphasis in the survey process and successful management of information-based reimbursement.

Coding and Classification

Although coding has a place in tracking various types of care, reimbursement is not dictated by codes in the residential long-term care setting. As a general rule, ICD-9 codes have limited value in describing the level of care or intensity of services required for a long-term, chronically ill institutionalized resident. Consequently, while coding is used for billing of services and tracking clinical information in NFs and SNFs, its role is somewhat diminished when compared to the acute care environment.

ICD-9

International Classification of Diseases, 9th Revision, Clinical Modification (ICD-9) diagnosis codes must be used for submitting Medicaid, Medicare Part A SNF, and Medicare Part B claims; however, their role is not significant in dictating the level of reimbursement the facility receives for an individual resident. Although inaccurate or incomplete codes may affect the timely processing of claims or increase the chances of a claim being isolated for medical review, reimbursement decisions are not solely linked to ICD-9 codes. ICD-9 codes may be used by the individual facility to track reasons for admission and hospitalization and to monitor clinical care issues such as incidence of acquired pressure ulcers, urinary tract infections, fractures, and other care outcomes that would be relevant to the overall monitoring and surveillance of quality. The use of ICD-9 codes for tracking of clinical information beyond basic admission and discharge data varies from provider to provider.

ICD-9 codes are also a part of the diagnosis reporting information included in the minimum data set (Section I). In this section, diagnoses are to be recorded in relation to current ADL status, cognitive status, mood and behavior status, medical treatments, nursing monitoring, or risk of death. A minimum amount of space is provided for recording actual ICD-9 codes because the majority of diagnosis information is entered by checking the relevant box on the form. If a diagnosis code provides more specific information relative to intensity of care or level of skilled services, then a code should be entered in preference over the checked box. For example, if a resident has insulin-dependent diabetes mellitus or uncontrolled diabetes, there is a greater degree of skilled supervision and monitoring required than with a resident whose diabetes is diet controlled. Consequently, an ICD-9 code would provide greater information concerning that resident's level of care than would the simple description "diabetes mellitus." However, diagnoses and/or diagnosis codes are not adequate to describe the level and intensity of care required by the long-term care resident. Therefore, there is less intensity on use and value of ICD-9 codes in the long-term care setting in terms of having a direct impact on facility reimbursement and monitoring of quality of care.

Current Procedural Terminology Codes

Current Procedural Terminology (CPT) codes are used for billing Medicare Part B services for rehabilitation (PT, OT, speech) and for physician visits to residents in a nursing facility. For the rehabilitation services, CPT codes indicate the type of therapy provided. For physician visits, the CPT codes describe the level of service provided, which thereby dictates the reimbursement for the visit performed. In a retrospective review of claims by the Medicare carrier, physician documentation must support that the level of service billed was actually performed and was medically justified. Therefore, if a CPT code is used that correlates with a more intensive visit, documentation should support that a greater amount of time was involved than a routine physician visit.

Often billing for Part B physician services is not done directly by the nursing facility because these services are billed through the private practice. Therefore, nursing facility staff have much less familiarity with CPT codes as compared to ICD-9 codes.

Data and Information Flow

Management of data and use of automation for data management has increased dramatically in the long-term care industry in the 1990s. In large part this has been due to the efforts of the Centers for Medicare and Medicaid Services to mandate automation of the MDS for all facilities participating in the Medicare and/or Medicaid programs. Although this effort has not been fully realized as of this writing, individual state agencies are increasing their own requirements for electronic submission of MDS data on a monthly basis. Consequently, discussion of data and flow of information is relevant not only from the internal facility viewpoint but also from the perspective of reporting information to external agencies.

Data and Information Flow within the Facility

MDS Data

In the Medicare- and/or Medicaid-certified facility, data and information flow centers around the MDS, which is not only a vehicle for a clinical assessment process but is also a mandated data set linked to regulatory compliance. Therefore, timeliness and accuracy of assessment information must be coordinated between the various disciplines and is a significant activity within the facility. From a data management perspective, the facility must ensure that systems are in place to monitor timeliness of completion of the MDS and accuracy of reported items (see Table 10-3). Furthermore, a system must be in place to ensure that significant changes in condition are properly

Table 10-3   Monitoring Assessment Timeliness and Content

Time	Content of Information
Within 14 days of admission	MDS information is consistent with interdisciplinary assessment information recorded in the resident record.
Within 14 days of significant change in condition	Care plan content reflects appropriate use of triggered RAPs for development of goals and interdisciplinary interventions.
At least annually	Documentation explains the clinical reason(s) for not completing a new comprehensive assessment if some significant change criteria are met based on a quarterly review and/or at any time between scheduled assessment or review intervals.
Review of specific data elements quarterly	

identified, assessed, and communicated to the appropriate individuals as this represents an area of federal regulatory compliance.

Once the MDS is completed, information is used to establish which RAPs are triggered, either through an automated RAI process or through manual review of the MDS trigger legend. Therefore, coordination of completion among the various disciplines is an ongoing process within the nursing facility. In addition, information regarding changes in resident condition must be monitored continually to determine if specific criteria are met, which indicate a possible need for a new comprehensive assessment. The criteria for determining if a resident has experienced a significant change in condition, either through improvement or decline, are included in the federal long-term care regulations, and as such are a significant part of evaluating compliance with the resident assessment regulations. Consequently, concurrent information regarding resident condition must be communicated and evaluated on an ongoing basis.

Federal regulations define a "significant change" as a major change in the resident's status that is:

1. Not self-limiting
2. Impacts on more than one area of the resident's health status
3. Requires interdisciplinary review and/or revision of the care plans *(CMS Guidance to Surveyors—Long Term Care Facilities)*

According to this definition, a significant change reassessment would be indicated if decline or improvement is consistently noted in two or more areas of decline or two or more areas of improvement. Following are examples that *could* indicate a significant change:

Decline

- Any decline in ADL functioning where a resident is newly coded as 3, 4, or 8 (extensive assistance, total dependency, activity did not occur);
- Increase in the number of areas where behavioral symptoms are coded as "not easily altered";
- Resident's decision-making changes from 0 to 1, 2 or 3;
- Resident's incontinence pattern changes from 0 or 1 to 2, 3 or 4, or placement of an indwelling catheter;
- Emergence of sad or anxious mood as a problem that is not easily altered;
- Emergence of an unplanned weight loss problem (5% in 30 days or 10% in 180 days);
- Begin to use trunk restraint or a chair that prevents rising for a resident when it was not used before;
- Emergence of a condition/disease in which a resident is judged to be unstable;
- Emergence of a pressure ulcer at Stage II or higher, when no ulcers were previously present at Stage II or higher;
- Overall deterioration of resident's condition; received more support (e.g., in ADLs or decision making).

Improvement

- Any improvement in ADL physical functioning where a resident is newly coded as 0, 1, or 2 when previously scored as a 3, 4, or 8;
- Decrease in the number of areas where Behavioral Symptoms or Sad or Anxious Mood are coded as "not easily altered";
- Resident's decision-making changes from 2, 3, or 4 to 0 or 1; or
- Overall improvement of resident's condition; resident receives fewer supports. *(CMS Guidance to Surveyors—Long Term Care Facilities)*

Level of Care Evaluation

There are different reasons for residents requiring permanent care in a long-term care facility. Some require a higher level of skilled intervention on a daily basis, whereas others may need less intensive care. Depending on their diagnoses and overall condition, residents may decline rapidly and require more intensive services. For this reason, facilities develop methods for defining individual resident acuity and care needs and will attempt to place residents with similar needs in the same physical area or unit of the facility. As residents' conditions change, their care needs change, and relocation to more appropriate areas within the facility may be required. Generally the type of information that would be utilized for this assessment would depend on the care issues outlined in Figure 10-1.

Skilled Nursing Requirements	**Dependence on Staff for Activities of Daily Living**
• Enteral feedings	• Supervised feeding or totally fed by staff
• Wound care	• Number of staff required for transfer and/or mobility
• Ostomy care	• Number and extent of staff assistance required for dressing and personal hygiene
• Acute, unstable condition requiring skilled monitoring	

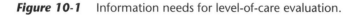

Figure 10-1   Information needs for level-of-care evaluation.

Utilization of Supplies and Services

Regardless of the pay source of the resident, information regarding utilization of central supply items and special services must be maintained for cost-accounting purposes. Some facilities manage supply information with the use of scanners where charge information is automatically captured at the point of use. In other instances, supply utilization is managed totally by a manual tracking system. Improper management of this key area of the facility operations can result in tremendous amounts of lost revenue to the long-term care facility.

For those facilities participating in managed care contracts with capitated payments, concurrent monitoring of supply utilization is essential to the successful provider. If the facility is paid a negotiated rate of a certain amount per day, it is important that the facility have a system in place that ensures effective monitoring of actual facility cost versus what the managed care payer will reimburse. This also applies to use of pharmaceuticals and durable medical equipment.

External Data Reporting

Facilities participating in the Medicare and/or Medicaid programs are required to submit MDS data to the state agency. Depending on the individual state requirements, facilities may be required to submit individual resident MDS data to the state agency electronically. Both the state and federal agencies utilize individual resident and aggregate facility data to monitor quality by individual provider and to evaluate trends in care throughout various regions of the country. In some states, MDS data is also used to establish the facility Medicaid reimbursement.

Computer Systems

With the advent of mandated computerization of MDS data in certain states, the long-term care industry has seen a growing number of computer vendors specializing in long-term care software. However, the degree to which facilities are able to totally computerize clinical and financial data is still dependent on the financial constraints of the average long-term care provider. As a result, there are wide ranges of utilization of computer systems within the industry from stand-alone systems used strictly for processing MDS data to systems that successfully integrate all financial and clinical information within the facility.

Some of the more common applications of computer software are as follows:

- Computerized physician orders, medication and treatment records either within the facility or provided by the pharmacy service off-site
- Computerization of financial information (census, payroll, billing, cost-reporting data)
- Computerization of MDS, RAP triggering system, and care plans

Often these systems are not integrated and/or are not designed such that the facility has full advantage of the data in a repository. As the impact of concurrent information management grows within the long-term care industry, there will be an increasing demand for effective and affordable automated systems.

CMS provides free software, called RAVEN, for entering and transmitting MDS assessment data. The RAVEN software "imports and exports data in standard MDS record format, maintains facility, resident, and employee information, enforces data integrity via rigorous edit checks, and provides comprehensive on-line help. It includes a data dictionary, RUGs and RAPs calculators . . ." (CMS, 2002g, p. 1). Facilities may also choose to submit MDS data using software purchased commercially through a vendor, provided that the software meets the CMS standards.

Data Sets

MDS has become the universal data set for the long-term care industry. Although some states have made additional data submission requirements to accommodate their Medicaid reimbursement systems, effective January 1, 1996, the MDS 2.0 became the universal basic reporting instrument for all 50 states. The initial goal of CMS in establishing MDS was to combine the benefits of a standardized clinical assessment tool with a universal data set for monitoring key information within the long-term care industry.

Now that the MDS also supplies information important to reimbursement, CMS is concerned with the potential for fraudulent reporting of MDS data. Effective September 2000, a formal statement certifying accuracy of information was developed for all MDS forms. Each staff member completing a portion of the MDS document must certify the accuracy of that portion by signing an attestation statement, which includes verbiage regarding Medicare fraud and penalties that may apply. Figure 10-2 includes an example of the attestation statement as incorporated into the MDS tracking form.

A shortened version of the MDS data set is also now available. The Medicare PPS Assessment Form (MPAF) provides facilities with the option of answering only the areas on the MDS that affect reimbursement and will also calculate a RUG III category. The MPAF is only for use with PPS. The OBRA assessment requirements supercede the use of the abbreviated form. Figure 10-3 is the first page of the four-page MPAF.

Numeric Identifier_____

MINIMUM DATA SET (MDS) — *VERSION 2.0*
FOR NURSING HOME RESIDENT ASSESSMENT AND CARE SCREENING

BASIC ASSESSMENT TRACKING FORM

SECTION AA. IDENTIFICATION INFORMATION

1.	RESIDENT NAME⊚	a. (First)	b. (Middle Initial)	c. (Last)	d. (Jr/Sr)

2.	GENDER⊚	1. Male	2. Female

3. BIRTHDATE⊚
Month — Day — Year

4. RACE/⊚ ETHNICITY
1. American Indian/Alaskan Native
2. Asian/Pacific Islander
3. Black, not of Hispanic origin
4. Hispanic
5. White, not of Hispanic origin

5. SOCIAL SECURITY⊚ AND MEDICARE NUMBERS⊚ [C in 1st box if non med. no.]
a. Social Security Number
b. Medicare number (or comparable railroad insurance number)

6. FACILITY PROVIDER NO.⊚
a. State No.
b. Federal No.

7. MEDICAID NO. ["+" if pending, "N" if not a Medicaid recipient] ⊚

8. REASONS FOR ASSESS-MENT
[Note—Other codes do not apply to this form]
a. Primary reason for assessment
1. Admission assessment (required by day 14)
2. Annual assessment
3. Significant change in status assessment
4. Significant correction of prior full assessment
5. Quarterly review assessment
10. Significant correction of prior quarterly assessment
0. *NONE OF ABOVE*

b. *Codes for assessments required for Medicare PPS or the State*
1. *Medicare 5 day assessment*
2. *Medicare 30 day assessment*
3. *Medicare 60 day assessment*
4. *Medicare 90 day assessment*
5. *Medicare readmission/return assessment*
6. *Other state required assessment*
7. *Medicare 14 day assessment*
8. *Other Medicare required assessment*

9. Signatures of Persons who Completed a Portion of the Accompanying Assessment or Tracking Form

I certify that the accompanying information accurately reflects resident assessment or tracking information for this resident and that I collected or coordinated collection of this information on the dates specified. To the best of my knowledge, this information was collected in accordance with applicable Medicare and Medicaid requirements. I understand that this information is used as a basis for ensuring that residents receive appropriate and quality care, and as a basis for payment from federal funds. I further understand that payment of such federal funds and continued participation in the government-funded health care programs is conditioned on the accuracy and truthfulness of this information, and that I may be personally subject to or may subject my organization to substantial criminal, civil, and/or administrative penalties for submitting false information. I also certify that I am authorized to submit this information by this facility on its behalf.

Signature and Title	Sections	Date
a.		
b.		
c.		
d.		
e.		
f.		
g.		
h.		
i.		
j.		
k.		
l.		

GENERAL INSTRUCTIONS

Complete this information for submission with all full and quarterly assessments (Admission, Annual, Significant Change, State or Medicare required assessments, or Quarterly Reviews, etc.)

⊚ = Key items for computerized resident tracking

☐ = When box blank, must enter number or letter   [a.] = When letter in box, check if condition applies

MDS 2.0 September, 2000

Figure 10-2 MDS tracking form and attestation.

MDS MEDICARE PPS ASSESSMENT FORM
(VERSION JULY 2002)

Numeric Identifier _____

AB5.	**RESIDENTIAL HISTORY 5 YEARS PRIOR TO ENTRY**	*(Check all settings resident lived in during 5 years prior to date of entry.)* a. Prior stay at this nursing home b. Stay in other nursing home c. Other residential facility—board and care home, assisted living, group home d. MH/psychiatric setting e. MR/DD setting f. NONE OF ABOVE
A1.	**RESIDENT NAME**	a. (First) b. (Middle Initial) c. (Last) d. (Jr/Sr)
A2.	**ROOM NUMBER**	
A3.	**ASSESSMENT REFERENCE DATE**	a. Last day of MDS observation period Month — Day — Year
A4a	**DATE OF REENTRY**	Date of reentry from most recent temporary discharge to a hospital in last 90 days (or since last assessment or admission if less than 90 days) Month — Day — Year
A5.	**MARITAL STATUS**	1. Never married 3. Widowed 5. Divorced 2. Married 4. Separated
A6.	**MEDICAL RECORD NO.**	
A10.	**ADVANCED DIRECTIVES**	*(For those items with supporting documentation in the medical record, check all that apply)* b. Do not resuscitate c. Do not hospitalize
B1.	**COMATOSE**	*(Persistent vegetative state/no discernible consciousness)* 0. No 1. Yes *(If Yes, skip to Section G)*
B2.	**MEMORY**	*(Recall of what was learned or known)* a. Short-term memory OK—seems/appears to recall after 5 minutes 0. Memory OK 1. Memory problem b. Long-term memory OK—seems/appears to recall long past 0. Memory OK 1. Memory problem
B3.	**MEMORY/ RECALL ABILITY**	*(Check all that resident was normally able to recall during last 7 days)* a. Current season b. Location of own room c. Staff names/faces d. That he/she is in a nursing home e. NONE OF ABOVE are recalled
B4.	**COGNITIVE SKILLS FOR DAILY DECISION-MAKING**	*(Made decisions regarding tasks of daily life)* 0. INDEPENDENT—decisions consistent/reasonable 1. MODIFIED INDEPENDENCE—some difficulty in new situations only 2. MODERATELY IMPAIRED—decisions poor; cues/supervision required 3. SEVERELY IMPAIRED—never/rarely made decisions
B5.	**INDICATORS OF DELIRIUM— PERIODIC DISORDERED THINKING/ AWARENESS**	*(Code for behavior in the last 7 days.)* **[Note: Accurate assessment requires conversations with staff and family who have direct knowledge of resident's behavior over this time].** 0. Behavior not present 1. Behavior present, not of recent onset 2. Behavior present, over last 7 days appears different from resident's usual functioning (e.g., new onset or worsening) a. EASILY DISTRACTED—(e.g., difficulty paying attention; gets sidetracked) b. PERIODS OF ALTERED PERCEPTION OR AWARENESS OF SURROUNDINGS—(e.g., moves lips or talks to someone not present; believes he/she is somewhere else; confuses night and day) c. EPISODES OF DISORGANIZED SPEECH—(e.g., speech is incoherent, nonsensical, irrelevant, or rambling from subject to subject; loses train of thought) d. PERIODS OF RESTLESSNESS—(e.g., fidgeting or picking at skin, clothing, napkins, etc; frequent position changes; repetitive physical movements or calling out) e. PERIODS OF LETHARGY—(e.g., sluggishness; staring into space; difficult to arouse; little body movement) f. MENTAL FUNCTION VARIES OVER THE COURSE OF THE DAY—(e.g., sometimes better, sometimes worse; behaviors sometimes present, sometimes not)

C4.	**MAKING SELF UNDERSTOOD**	*(Expressing information content—however able)* 0. UNDERSTOOD 1. USUALLY UNDERSTOOD—difficulty finding words or finishing thoughts 2. SOMETIMES UNDERSTOOD—ability is limited to making concrete requests 3. RARELY/NEVER UNDERSTOOD
C6.	**ABILITY TO UNDERSTAND OTHERS**	*(Understanding verbal information content—however able)* 0. UNDERSTANDS 1. USUALLY UNDERSTANDS—may miss some part/intent of message 2. SOMETIMES UNDERSTANDS—responds adequately to simple, direct communication 3. RARELY/NEVER UNDERSTANDS
D1.	**VISION**	*(Ability to see in adequate light and with glasses if used)* 0. ADEQUATE—sees fine detail, including regular print in newspapers/books 1. IMPAIRED—sees large print, but not regular print in newspapers/books 2. MODERATELY IMPAIRED—limited vision; not able to see newspaper headlines, but can identify objects 3. HIGHLY IMPAIRED—object identification in question, but eyes appear to follow objects 4. SEVERELY IMPAIRED—no vision or sees only light, colors, or shapes; eyes do not appear to follow objects
E1.	**INDICATORS OF DEPRESSION, ANXIETY, SAD MOOD**	*(Code for indicators observed in last 30 days, irrespective of the assumed cause)* 0. Indicator not exhibited in last 30 days 1. Indicator of this type exhibited up to five days a week 2. Indicator of this type exhibited daily or almost daily (6, 7 days a week)

VERBAL EXPRESSIONS OF DISTRESS
a. Resident made negative statements—e.g., "Nothing matters; Would rather be dead; What's the use; Regrets having lived so long; Let me die"
b. Repetitive questions—e.g., "Where do I go; What do I do?"
c. Repetitive verbalizations—e.g., calling out for help, ("God help me")
d. Persistent anger with self or others—e.g., easily annoyed, anger at placement in nursing home; anger at care received
e. Self deprecation—e.g., "I am nothing; I am of no use to anyone"
f. Expressions of what appear to be unrealistic fears—e.g., fear of being abandoned, left alone, being with others
g. Recurrent statements that something terrible is about to happen—e.g., believes he or she is about to die, have a heart attack

h. Repetitive health complaints—e.g., persistently seeks medical attention, obsessive concern with body functions
i. Repetitive anxious complaints/concerns (non-health related) e.g., persistently seeks attention/reassurance regarding schedules, meals, laundry, clothing, relationship issues

SLEEP-CYCLE ISSUES
j. Unpleasant mood in morning
k. Insomnia/change in usual sleep pattern

SAD, APATHETIC, ANXIOUS APPEARANCE
l. Sad, pained, worried facial expressions—e.g., furrowed brows
m. Crying, tearfulness
n. Repetitive physical movements—e.g., pacing, hand wringing, restlessness, fidgeting, picking

LOSS OF INTEREST
o. Withdrawal from activities of interest—e.g., no interest in long standing activities or being with family/friends
p. Reduced social interaction

E2.	**MOOD PERSISTENCE**	One or more indicators of depressed, sad or anxious mood were not easily altered by attempts to "cheer up", console, or reassure the resident over last 7 days 0. No mood indicators 1. Indicators present, easily altered 2. Indicators present, not easily altered

MDS 2.0 PPS July 2002

Figure 10-3   Excerpt from the Medicare PPS Assessment Form (MPAF).

Quality Improvement and Utilization Management

Quality Improvement

MDS-derived quality indicators have been developed by Dr. David Zimmerman at the University of Wisconsin. These indicators can be utilized to monitor quality, both in process and outcome, through the automated use of MDS data. Figure 10-4 is a summary of the quality indicators developed as a result of this project. From a facility perspective, many of these indicators also correlate directly with compliance monitoring for key federal quality of care and quality of life regulations as noted in Figure 10-4.

CMS has contracted to implement an ongoing system of verifying and improving the accuracy of the MDS. Data Assessment and Verification (DAVE) is an audit system that is being phased in. Although the beta-testing phase included only a few selected states, DAVE will ultimately be rolled out nationwide. Data analysis will identify patterns that may signify potential data accuracy issues, focusing on whether the MDS is accurate and supported by the record and whether coverage criteria were met and payment was accurate. It is expected that automated provider feedback reports will be available through the MDS submission system and will give providers access to results of data analyses, possible patterns identified, and tools that can be used in reviewing their own data for accuracy as part of the internal QA/QI process. CMS also plans to include home health OASIS data (discussed in Chapter 12) in the DAVE project (CMS, 2003a).

As part of the CMS Nursing Home Quality Initiative, CMS hosts a "Nursing Home Compare" Web site that provides information about nursing homes in the form of quality measures. This information is posted for nursing homes in all states effective October 2002 with the intent of assisting potential residents and their families in making an informed selection if they need to consider nursing home placement. Quality measures are derived from the MDS, with some being adjusted per facility profile. Providers can utilize the information to compare themselves to similar nursing homes in a QI process. CMS started with six quality measures for chronic care residents and four for short stay residents. Some of these include pain, pressure sores, physical restraints, infections, delirium, worsening function in activities of daily living, and improvements in walking. CMS plans to change and expand the measures over time (CMS, 2003b).

Utilization Management

In the long-term care setting, utilization management applies to the Medicaid, Medicare Part A, and managed care residents who may be in an SNF or subacute unit of the facility. Each state has individual requirements for qualifying for Medicaid nursing home payments, and the manner in which this process is monitored varies from state to state. In some instances, qualification is monitored through the MDS data in conjunction with additional state-specific information submission. In other instances, a separate review process is adopted by the state agency to determine initial and continuing Medicaid eligibility.

Quality Indicator	Quality of Care and Quality of Life Requirement (F-tag)
Accidents	F323, F324—The facility must ensure that (1) the resident environment remains as free of accident hazards as is possible; and (2) each resident receives adequate supervision and assistance devices to prevent accidents.
Behavioral and emotional patterns	F319, F320—Based on the comprehensive assessment of a resident, the facility must ensure that (1) a resident who displays mental or psychosocial adjustment difficulty, receives appropriate treatment and services to correct the assessed problem; and (2) a resident whose assessment did not reveal a mental or psychosocial adjustment difficulty does not display a pattern of decreased social interaction and/or increased withdrawn, angry, or depressive behaviors, unless the resident's clinical condition demonstrates that such a pattern is unavoidable.
Infection control/ prevalence of UTIs	F316—A resident who is incontinent of bladder receives appropriate treatment and services to prevent urinary tract infections and to restore as much normal bladder function as possible.
Prevalence of weight loss	F325—Based on a resident's comprehensive assessment, the facility must ensure that a resident maintains acceptable parameters of nutritional status, such as body weight and protein levels, unless the resident's clinical condition demonstrates that this is not possible.
Prevalence of tube feeding	F321, F322—Based on the comprehensive assessment of a resident, the facility must ensure that (1) a resident who has been able to eat enough alone or with assistance is not fed by nasogastric tube unless the resident's clinical condition demonstrates that use of a nasogastric tube was unavoidable; (2) a resident who is fed by a nasogastric or gastrostomy tube receives the appropriate treatment and services to prevent aspiration, pneumonia, diarrhea, vomiting, dehydration, metabolic abnormalities, and nasal-pharyngeal ulcers and to restore, if possible, normal eating skills.
Prevalence of dehydration	F327—The facility must provide each resident with sufficient fluid intake to maintain proper hydration and health.
Incidence of decline in late loss ADLs	F310—A resident's abilities in activities of daily living do not diminish unless circumstances of the individual's clinical condition demonstrate that diminution was unavoidable. This includes the resident's ability to (1) bathe, dress, and groom; (2) transfer and ambulate; (3) toilet; (4) eat; and (5) use speech, language, or other functional communication systems.

(continues)

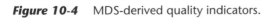

Figure 10-4 MDS-derived quality indicators.

Incidence of contractures	F317, F318—Based on the comprehensive assessment of a resident, the facility must ensure that (1) a resident who enters the facility without a limited range of motion does not experience reduction in range of motion unless the resident's clinical condition demonstrates that a reduction in range of motion is unavoidable; and (2) a resident with a limited range of motion receives appropriate treatment and services to increase range of motion and/or to prevent further decrease in range of motion.
Psychotropic drug use	F328—Each resident's drug regimen must be free from unnecessary drugs. F330—Based on a comprehensive assessment of a resident, the facility must ensure that residents who have not used antipsychotic drugs are not given these drugs unless antipsychotic drug therapy is necessary to treat a specific condition as diagnosed and documented in the clinical record and F331—Residents who use antipsychotic drugs receive gradual dose reductions, and behavioral interventions, unless clinically contraindicated, in an effort to discontinue these drugs.
Quality of life: prevalence of daily physical restraints	F221—The resident has the right to be free from any physical or chemical restraints imposed for purposes of discipline or convenience, and not required to treat the resident's medical symptoms.
Prevalence of stage 1–4 pressure ulcers	F314—Based on the comprehensive assessment of a resident, the facility must ensure that (1) a resident who enters the facility without pressure sores does not develop pressure sores unless the individual's clinical condition demonstrates that they were unavoidable.

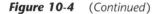

Figure 10-4   *(Continued)*

For the Medicare Part A SNF benefit, utilization must be monitored to ensure that the condition of the resident meets ongoing criteria for daily skilled care. In addition, the facility must be aware of SNF days that the resident may have used before being admitted to the SNF unit to ensure that the stay does not exceed the maximum benefit of 100 days per spell of illness. If the level of care of the resident changes such that the facility feels that care no longer meets Medicare skilled criteria, an internal denial letter must be issued to the beneficiary (or the beneficiary's representative). In addition, the beneficiary must be advised of the right to submit a demand billing to the intermediary if the denial decision is questioned or challenged.

Utilization management for managed care residents, typically those in an SNF or subacute bed, is a dynamic process that requires frequent monitoring by the facility case manager to ensure that care needs and progress are communicated to the managed care case manager on an ongoing basis. The facility must be in a position to communicate changes in resident status and discharge plans to the managed care payor. If care needs increase such that additional services must be ordered or are recommended by the attending physician, this must be communicated and generally approved through the managed care case manager. Most often this monitoring and communication process is the responsibility of the facility RN case manager who serves as the primary communicator of care progress with the managed care payor.

Role of the Health Information Management Professional

Credentialed health information managers (i.e., RHIT, RHIA) are not required in the federal long-term-care regulations but may be required on either a part-time or consulting basis in some of the state long-term care licensure laws. The trend toward automation and use of health information in long-term care reimbursement has increased the importance of the credentialed health information manager in the long-term care setting. As a result, independent facilities and long-term care management corporations are increasing their use of full-time registered health information technicians (RHITs) and registered health information administrators (RHIAs).

Auditing

One role of the health information manager in long-term care is to design and implement auditing systems. Of significant importance to the long-term care facility is the content, completion, accuracy, and timeliness of medical record documentation. Documentation affects the quality of care provided. Assessment and ongoing care planning are determined in part by what is written in the medical record. Documentation is also an important factor in outcomes for reimbursement systems, survey compliance, and in the event of legal action. The medical record serves as a tool in QI studies and is used in facility planning.

Health information managers or other trained staff can be a valuable asset to the long-term care organization by conducting routine documentation audits against established criteria. Results of such audits can be used to help ensure quality care, survey readiness, and proper reimbursement. Additionally, audit outcomes can be utilized as measures in training health care staff and for system evaluation and improvement.

Audits can be quantitative or qualitative in nature. Quantitative audits include review of whether medical record forms are complete, timely, and signed by the author of the form. Qualitative audits generally require more training because they are a more in-depth look at the actual content of the medical record as compared to regulations and standards of practice.

Typical intervals for auditing records in long-term care are when admission assessments are complete, concurrently at regularly scheduled intervals throughout the resident/patient stay (such as quarterly), and upon discharge. The purpose of regular ongoing monitoring is to identify any problems or trends in documentation while correction is possible or when changes can be made. In many cases, because of the extended length of stay and volume of the record, delaying review of documentation until discharge is not as effective as an ongoing review system. Incomplete documentation often cannot legally be completed at a time well after the event and most likely would not be to anyone's benefit.

Utilizing a defined set of criteria for auditing or use of a review form promotes consistency and objectivity. Audit forms can be created by giving consideration to regulatory requirements and what the facility defines as useful information to collect. Some typical items on a long-term care audit form might include the following:

- Timeliness of MDS assessments
- Physician orders signed
- Advance directives addressed
- Allergies identified
- Assessments completed by each discipline
- Medication orders are consistent with medication records
- Physician progress notes coincide with required visit schedule
- Laboratory results are in the record for all lab testing ordered

The auditor can review several items in a sample of records or focus on one issue in a larger sample of records. In order to be effective, it is important in any type of auditing to accurately report the results in a timely manner. Problems or trends should be identified, a plan of correction developed, and further monitoring done to measure improvement.

External Consultant versus Full-Time Employee

Services of the health information management (HIM) professional were deleted from the federal long-term care regulations in 1990; however, some state licensure regulations still include a requirement for a facility to utilize the services of an RHIT or RHIA on a consulting basis.

As a consultant, the HIM professional conducts periodic visits ranging from monthly to quarterly, to monitor documentation trends within the facility, particularly as this relates to potential regulatory compliance concerns. The HIM professional brings expertise in terms of resident confidentiality and release of confidential information, and also serves as an ongoing resource for development of forms and documentation systems and procedures that facilitate compliance and promote proper reimbursement. With the increase in automation, the HIM consultant also is a useful resource in selection of computerized systems that are suited to the needs of the facility while also meeting specific state and federal requirements pertaining to automation of resident information. From that perspective, the HIM professional offers expertise in terms of evaluating the adequacy of existing, traditional paper systems and provides valuable insight as to the necessary steps for streamlining and preparing manual systems for the gradual transition to a computerized resident record.

Because of the resident's length of stay and the scrutiny that nursing home documentation receives, HIM staff must ensure that the medical record, whether automated or paper, is safeguarded throughout the resident's stay as well as thereafter. HIM staff members must be diligent in protecting privacy and confidentiality by adhering to proper release of information standards.

Whether as a full-time employee or as an independent consultant to the long-term care facility, the HIM professional is often the key resource for monitoring federal regulatory compliance and alerting the facility to potential survey compliance concerns. Monitoring of key quality of care concerns is often detected through the current documentation in residents' records. As a result, the HIM professional can serve as an ongoing compliance monitor for the facility.

In some long-term care facilities, the documentation of assessments and progress notes by social services, activities, and dietary staff is the responsibility of noncredentialed personnel who have limited training for their jobs. As a result, the HIM professional is a valued resource for training these personnel in the proper methods and procedures for charting and for emphasizing the importance of their documentation as a part of the permanent medical record.

Training and education of long-term care facility staff is ongoing with respect to the various documentation requirements affecting long-term care reimbursement and regulatory compliance. This need is seen in all of the departments of the nursing facility as new graduates in nursing enter the long-term care setting and as more personnel from the acute care setting are moving into the long-term care and subacute care facilities. The HIM professional is a valuable resource for ongoing in-service with all disciplines and for providing initial training as to the role of the MDS and the proper procedures to follow in the RAI and care planning processes.

The expertise of the HIM professional offers numerous opportunities in the long-term care environment, particularly as information management becomes more crucial to monitoring regulatory compliance and ensuring proper reimbursement from Medicare, Medicaid, and managed care payers. Skills in streamlining work flow, management of information for QI initiatives, and data collection and analysis for critical pathways are growing areas in the SNF and subacute care settings in which the HIM professional can offer tremendous value.

Summary

As the population continues to age, the demand for long-term care facilities will continue to grow. Often referred to as one of the most regulated industries in the country, long-term care has unique information system needs and documentation requirements. Consequently, health information managers have valuable skills to offer this growing segment of the health care industry. Prior federal regulations required the services of a credentialed health record practitioner as either an employee or a consultant of long-term care facilities participating in the Medicare or Medicaid programs.

Although this regulation was deleted in the early 1990s, there has been a growing trend for long-term care facilities to employ credentialed health information managers as a result of the increasing demand for efficient and effective documentation and information systems.

Key Terms

activities of daily living (ADL)   for purposes of the federal long-term care regulations, activities of daily living include the resident's ability to (1) bathe, dress, and groom; (2) transfer and ambulate; (3) toilet; (4) eat; and (5) use speech, language, or other functional communication systems *(CMS Guidance to Surveyors—Long Term Care Facilities)*. Federal regulations include ADL as a component part of the quality of care requirements, and information concerning individual resident ADL capability is a significant portion of the monitoring information in the minimum data set.

care plan   a documented plan developed by an interdisciplinary team that includes measurable objectives and timetables to meet a resident's medical, nursing, and mental and psychosocial needs that are identified in the comprehensive assessment. A care plan must describe (1) the services that are to be furnished to attain or maintain the resident's highest practicable physical, mental, and psychosocial well-being; and (2) any services that would otherwise be required but are not provided because of the resident's exercise of rights including the right to refuse treatment *(CMS Guidance to Surveyors—Long Term Care Facilities)*.

case-mix reimbursement   a long-term care reimbursement methodology designed to provide a mechanism for facilities to be paid in a manner that reflects the types of residents served and the types of services provided. The system is also designed to provide greater access to nursing facility beds for heavier care residents and to improve the quality of care for all nursing facility residents. Payment is based on a specific methodology that considers direct care costs, care-related costs, administrative and operating costs, and property.

civil money penalties   penalties or fines levied by the federal government against providers who are found to be in substantial noncompliance with federal regulations. These penalties may be as much as $10,000 per day.

comprehensive resident assessment   as defined by the long-term care federal regulations, a comprehensive resident assessment describes the resident's ability to perform daily life functions and significant impairments in functional capacity. Specifically, it includes at least the following information: (1) medically defined conditions and prior medical history; (2) medical status measurement; (3) physical and mental functional status; (4) sensory and physical impairments; (5) nutritional status and requirements; (6) special treatments or procedures; (7) mental and psychosocial status; (8) discharge potential; (9) dental condition; (10) activities potential; (11) rehabilitation potential; (12) cognitive status; and (13) drug therapy *(CMS Guidance to Surveyors—Long Term Care Facilities)*.

consolidated billing   under Medicare a skilled nursing facility is responsible for billing the entire package of care that residents receive during a stay with certain specified exceptions, such as physicians' professional services.

federal survey   a survey based on the federal long-term care requirements using the federal long-term care survey procedures required for long-term care facility participation in the Medicare and/or Medicaid programs.

federal surveyor   a surveyor from one of the 10 regional or the central health care financing office. Federal surveyors may conduct surveys in long-term care facilities to determine the accuracy and validity of surveys by state agencies and may also participate in on-site evaluations of state surveyors during their survey of a long-term care facility.

licensure survey   a survey conducted by the state agency to determine long-term care facility compliance with state licensure laws.

long-term acute care hospital (LTAC, LTACH, or LTCH)   a facility providing specialized acute care for patients averaging a length of stay of 25 days or more.

minimum data set   a core set of screening and assessment elements, including common definitions and coding categories, that forms the foundation of the comprehensive resident assessment for all residents of long-term care facilities certified to participate in Medicare or Medicaid. The items in the MDS standardize communication about resident problems and conditions within facilities, between facilities, and between facilities and outside agencies *(CMS State Operations Manual)*.

nursing facility   an institution or a distinct part of an institution that provides skilled nursing care, rehabilitation services, or health-related care to individuals who because of their condition require services above the level of room and board. Either a registered nurse or a licensed practical nurse is on active duty at all times. If properly licensed and certified, a nursing facility may receive reimbursement under the Medicaid program.

quality of care federal requirements   a broad category of the long-term care federal regulations that requires a facility to provide the necessary care and services to attain or maintain the highest practicable physical, mental, and psychosocial well-being, in accordance with the comprehensive assessment and plan of care. Substantial noncompliance with quality of care requirements subjects a facility to potential civil money penalties and other punitive measures in the federal enforcement regulations.

quality of life federal requirements   a broad category of the long-term care federal regulations that requires a facility to care for its residents in a manner and in an environment that promotes maintenance or enhancement of each resident's quality of life. Substantial noncompliance with quality of life requirements subjects a facility to potential civil money penalties and other punitive measures in the federal enforcement regulations.

RAP summary   the CMS-required document that identifies which RAPs have been triggered from the MDS, where the assessment information is located in the resident record, and if the RAP assessment resulted in care planning for a specific condition, concern of care, or resident issue.

resident assessment instrument (RAI) an instrument that requires for completion the performance of a standardized assessment system, comprised of the MDS and utilization guidelines (including the RAPs and triggers). This assessment system provides a comprehensive, accurate, standardized, reproducible assessment of each long-term care facility resident's functional capabilities and identifies medical problems *(CMS State Operations Manual)*.

resident assessment protocols (RAPs) a component of the utilization guidelines, the RAPs are structured, problem-oriented frameworks for organizing MDS information and additional clinically relevant information about an individual that identifies medical problems and forms the basis for individual care planning *(CMS State Operations Manual)*.

Resource Utilization Groups (RUGS) a case-mix methodology based on data submitted on the MDS. RUGs are used to adjust per diem payments to SNFs under the Medicare PPS and to NFs under some state Medicaid programs.

risk contract also known as a Medicare risk contract. A contract between an HMO and CMS to provide services to Medicare beneficiaries under which the health plan receives a fixed monthly payment for enrolled Medicare members, and then must provide all services on an at-risk basis (Kongstvedt, 1993).

skilled nursing facility an institution or a distinct part of an institution that provides skilled nursing care or rehabilitation services. Either a registered nurse or a licensed practical nurse is on active duty at all times. If properly licensed and certified, a skilled nursing facility may obtain a Medicare provider agreement and be reimbursed under the Medicare program.

standard survey a periodic, resident-centered inspection that gathers information about the quality of service furnished in a facility to determine compliance with the requirements of participation in the federal Medicare and Medicaid programs *(CMS State Operations Manual)*.

subacute care a transitional type of care that represents a level of service that is less intensive than traditional acute care but more goal oriented and resource intensive than what is generally regarded as skilled nursing care.

substandard quality of care one or more deficiencies related to participation requirements under 42 CFR 483.13, resident behavior and facility practices, 42 CFR 483.15, quality of life, or 42 CFR 483.25, quality of care, that constitute either immediate jeopardy to resident health or safety; a pattern of widespread actual harm that is not immediate jeopardy; or a widespread potential for more than minimal harm, but less than immediate jeopardy, with no actual harm *(CMS State Operations Manual Provider Certification)*.

substantial compliance a level of compliance with the requirements of participation such that any identified deficiencies pose no greater risk to resident health or safety than the potential for causing minimal harm. Substantial compliance constitutes compliance with participation requirements *(CMS State Operations Manual)*.

REVIEW QUESTIONS

Knowledge-based Questions

1. What two primary agencies regulate long-term care facilities?

2. What are the primary reimbursement categories for care of residents in long-term care facilities?

3. Who determines how long-term care facilities are reimbursed under the Medicaid program?

4. What are the principal uses of the MDS 2.0 in the long-term care industry? (a) By the individual provider? (b) By the state agency? (c) By CMS?

5. What are some of the strategic quality indicators that a long-term care facility should monitor as an ongoing presurvey tool and risk management tool?

6. What is the single most important content characteristic of a care plan in a long-term care facility that is subject to federal regulations?

Application-based Questions

1. How is ICD-9 coding of relevance to the long-term care setting?

2. What would be determining factors in selecting an automated system for the minimum data set?

3. Why is there a greater focus on concurrent documentation monitoring in the long-term care setting as compared to evaluating documentation in the closed medical record?

Web Activity

Go to the CMS MDS 2.0 Manuals and Forms Web site at http://cms.hhs.gov/medicaid/mds20/man-form.asp. Click on the hyperlink for Chapter 1, "Resident Assessment Instrument." Scroll through the chapter until you find the form entitled

MINIMUM DATA SET (MDS)—VERSION 2.0
FOR NURSING HOME RESIDENT ASSESSMENT AND CARE SCREENING
FULL ASSESSMENT FORM

1. According to information printed on the form, the assessment is to reflect the patient's status during a certain number of days before the completion of the form. What time frame does the patient status reflect?

2. What is the alphabetic section that includes diseases and diagnosis codes?

Case Study

You are the consultant for a long-term care facility that has recently undergone a long-term care survey in which the facility received several deficiencies for noncompliance with federal requirements. The most significant deficiency involved a noted pattern (7 of 10 examples reviewed in the surveyor sample) in which comprehensive assessments (MDS) were not completed within the required time frame (within 14 days of admission). In addition, surveyors identified that there was no documentation to support that the triggered resident assessment protocols were being used in the assessment and care-planning process. This resulted in related quality of care deficiencies for failure to adequately assess and manage urinary incontinence and psychosocial needs. In three additional examples, surveyors identified that residents had experienced a significant change in condition without evidence of a new assessment being done. Within the statement of deficiencies, surveyors noted that the director of nursing stated that she was unaware that assessments had not been done. It was also noted that the nursing staff stated they did not understand what the resident assessment protocols were, and they were unaware of the federal criteria for determining when a significant change had occurred. The administrator of this facility has called you to help develop a plan to correct these deficiencies.

1. What would be your recommendations for overall system evaluation and revision?
2. What would be your recommendations for staff education?
3. How could the facility medical records designee be utilized to prevent similar problems from occurring in the future?

References and Suggested Readings

[ALTHA] Acute Long Term Hospital Association. (No date). [Online]. http://www.altha.org [2003, July 5].

[CMS] Centers for Medicare and Medicaid Services. (2002a). Appendix P: Survey protocol for long term care facilities—Part II: Guidance to surveyors—long term care facilities. *State Operations Manual.* [Online]. http://cms.hhs.gov/manuals/pub07pdf/AP-P-PP.pdf [2003, July 3].

[CMS] Centers for Medicare and Medicaid Services. (2002b). Appendix R: Resident assessment instrument for long term care facilities. *State Operations Manual.* [Online]. http://cms.hhs.gov/manuals/pub07pdf/AP-Q-R.pdf [2003, June 30].

[CMS] Centers for Medicare and Medicaid Services. (2002c). Long-term care hospital PPS. [Online]. http://cms.hhs.gov/providers/longterm/background.asp [2000, July 7].

[CMS] Centers for Medicare and Medicaid Services. (2002d). Part 2—The certification process. *State Operations Manual.* [Online]. http://cms.hhs.gov/manuals/pub07pdf/part-02.pdf [2003, July 2].

[CMS] Centers for Medicare and Medicaid Services. (2002e). Part 7—Survey and enforcement process for SNFs and NFs. *State Operations Manual.* [Online]. http://cms.hhs.gov/manuals/pub07pdf/part-07.pdf [2003, June 30].

[CMS] Centers for Medicare and Medicaid Services. (2002f). Prospective payment system for long-term care hospitals: Implementation and FY 2003 rates. *Federal Register, 67* (169), 55954–56090.

[CMS] Centers for Medicare and Medicaid Services. (2002g). RAVEN: CMS's MDS Data Entry Software. [Online]. http://cms.hhs.gov/medicaid/mds20/raven.asp [2002, July 5].

[CMS] Centers for Medicare and Medicaid Services. (2002h). *Revised Long-Term Care Resident Assessment Instrument User's Manual: Version 2.0.* [Online]. http://cms.hhs.gov/medicaid/mds20/man-form.asp [2003, June 30].

[CMS] Centers for Medicare and Medicaid Services. (2003a). Data assessment and verification project. [Online]. http://cms.hhs.gov/providers/psc/DAVE/DEFAULT.ASP [2003, July 5].

[CMS] Centers for Medicare and Medicaid Services. (2003b). Nursing Home Compare. [Online]. http://www.medicare.gov/NHCompare/home.asp [2003, July 5].

[CMS] Centers for Medicare and Medicaid Services. (No date). Consolidated billing for skilled nursing facility (SNF) residents claims billed to Medicare carriers or DMERCS by physicians, non-physician practitioners, and suppliers. *Medicare Learning Network.* [Online]. http://www.cms.hhs.gov/medlearn/snfcode.asp [2003, July 2].

Kongstvedt, P. (1993). *The Managed Health Care Handbook.* Gaithersburg, MD: Aspen.

Liu, K., Baseggio, C., Wissoker, D., Maxwell, S., Haley, J., and Long, S. (2001). Long-term care hospitals under Medicare: Facility-level characteristics. *Health Care Financing Review, 23* (2), 1–18.

National Case-Mix Reimbursement and Quality Conference, San Antonio, Texas, February 2, 1996.

Sullivan, J. G. (1996, March). Long term care on trial. *Contemporary Long Term Care,* p. 46.

Key Resources

Acute Long Term Hospital Association
1055 North Fairfax Street, Suite 201
Alexandria, VA 22314
Phone: 703-299-5571
Fax: 703-299-5574
http://www.altha.org

American Association of Homes and Services for the Aging
2519 Connecticut Ave., NW
Washington, DC 20008
Phone: 202-783-2242
Fax: 202-783-2255
http://www2.aahsa.org

American College of Health Care Administrators
300 N. Lee St., Suite 301
Alexandria, VA 22314
Phone: 703-739-7900 or 888-88-ACHCA
Fax: 703-739-7901
http://www.achca.org

American Health Care Association
1201 L Street, NW
Washington, DC 20005
Phone: 202-842-4444
Fax: 202-842-3860
http://www.ahca.org

Assisted Living Facilities Federation of America
11200 Waples Mill Road, Suite 150
Fairfax, VA 22030
Phone: 703-691-8100
Fax: 703-691-8106
http://www.alfa.org

Joint Commission on Accreditation of Healthcare Organizations
(See Chapter 1 for contact information.)

National Association for Directors of Nursing Administration in Long Term Care
(NADONA/LTC)
10101 Alliance Road, #140
Cincinnati, OH 45242
Phone: 800-222-0539
Fax: 513-791-3699
http://www.nadona.org

National Association of Long Term Hospitals
c/o Behar & Kalman, Attorneys at Law
Six Beacon Street
Boston, MA 02108
Phone: 617-227-7660
Fax: 617-227-4208
Email: info@nalth.org
http://www.nalth.org

Chapter *11*

Rehabilitation

Terry Winkler, MD
Ann H. Peden, MBA, RHIA, CCS

Learning Objectives

Upon successful completion of this chapter, you should be able to:

1. Identify and describe the various levels of rehabilitative care.
2. Describe the major accrediting agencies for rehabilitation.
3. List the members of a multidisciplinary rehabilitation team.
4. Describe key features of the inpatient rehabilitation facility prospective payment system (IRF PPS).
5. Explain classification systems used to grade severity of injury/disability and relate them to outcome measures.
6. Define basic rehabilitation terms and distinguish between the concepts of impairment, disability, and handicap.
7. Review sample forms used to track a person's progress in rehabilitation.
8. Appreciate current trends in rehabilitation.

SETTING	DESCRIPTION	SYNONYMS/EXAMPLES
Acute Care Hospitals	Inpatient facilities that provide acute medical care	Community hospitals Regional or tertiary care centers
Long-Term Rehabilitation Units	Inpatient rehabilitation programs that provide long-term therapies after acute illness/injury issues are resolved	Rehabilitation institutes Supportive living centers Long-term acute care Transitional living centers
Freestanding Rehabilitation Centers	A center for rehabilitation when the facility stands alone and is not physically part of another health care center	Physical therapy clinics Rehabilitation centers
Subacute and Skilled Rehabilitation Programs	Inpatient rehabilitation for patients who are progressing too slowly to meet criteria for standard rehabilitation programs	Nursing home rehabilitation Skilled nursing facilities
Outpatient Rehabilitation	Programs where therapy is provided but patient does not stay overnight	Day treatment centers Work hardening programs Occupational rehabilitation Chronic pain treatment centers Therapy clinics
Home Health Rehabilitation	Rehabilitation services provided to patients in their home by a home health care agency	Area Agency on Aging Various county health department programs Hospital-owned/operated home health National home health agencies

Introduction to Setting

Rehabilitation is the development of a person to the fullest physical, psychological, social, vocational, avocational, and educational potential consistent with his or her physiological or anatomic impairment and environmental limitations. Rehabilitation should begin when the patient enters a hospital with an injury or illness that is going to result in some limitations of the patient's functional status. The end result of comprehensive rehabilitation should be increased independence, increased overall functional status, and improved quality of life.

Types of Rehabilitation Settings

Rehabilitation is a continuum of care that begins with the patient's stay in the acute care hospital setting, continues throughout the postacute hospital phase, and, in many cases, continues through outpatient treatment. The types of rehabilitation facilities have expanded greatly in recent years. From 1985 to 1990, the number of rehabilitation beds increased from 16,498 to 26,640 (DeLisa, 1993). Rehabilitation is now provided in numerous types of settings.

Acute Rehabilitation

Acute rehabilitation units in hospitals are the most common settings and have more than doubled since around 1990. These rehabilitation wards usually have a set number of beds, ranging from 10 to 30, designated in one ward of a hospital, where patients are transferred for their acute care rehabilitation. Length of patient stays can vary from two to four weeks. When a patient is medically stable and has reached his maximum short-term improvement, he is then transferred to a different setting based on his needs at that point.

Long-Term Acute Care (LTAC)

Long-term acute care (LTAC) facilities provide services to the patient who has an acute illness superimposed on chronic disability or for medically complicated patients. These facilities bridge the gap between acute hospitals and rehabilitation programs. (For more information on long-term acute care, see Chapter 10.)

Postacute Rehabilitation

Postacute rehabilitation is provided in long-term rehabilitation units to which patients are transferred after acute rehabilitation to undergo long-term therapies to maximize their functional status. Generally, patients undergoing postacute rehabilitation are those with brain injuries, strokes, or higher-level spinal cord injuries. Length of patient stays can vary from four weeks to six months or more. Patients being transferred to postacute rehabilitation centers have stabilized medically and acute medical issues related to their illnesses or traumas have been resolved. The patient is felt to have reached a point where he or she can benefit from an intensive inpatient rehabilitation program and should be able at that point to participate in at least three hours of therapy per day to be an ideal candidate. In most cases, the patient will be discharged from the postacute facility to home, perhaps with additional outpatient services or home services. An alternative discharge plan would be to a transitional living center. The patient's equipment needs will have been met and all family members and/or caregivers trained to assist the patient to return to the community.

Freestanding Rehabilitation Hospitals

In the 1990s, several national corporations were created to operate rehabilitation hospitals. These facilities are freestanding, but usually in proximity to larger medical centers to guarantee a referral base. **Freestanding rehabilitation hospitals** include both acute rehabilitation centers and postacute rehabilitation centers.

Rehabilitation Provided in Skilled Nursing Settings

Subacute rehabilitation centers are usually located in a wing of a nursing home or a hospital and serve a skilled-level patient. These facilities can accommodate a patient with multiple problems, or older patients who are progressing more slowly than would be acceptable in an acute or postacute rehabilitation setting.

Due to economic factors, patients are being discharged earlier from the hospital, which has resulted in some patients being discharged who are not yet completely recovered and are unable to care for themselves. In many instances, due to age, multiple medical problems, or other factors, the patient may not be considered a good candidate for acute rehabilitation or postacute rehabilitation centers. If it is felt, however, that the patient would still continue to make some progress given proper rehabilitation, then this patient is an ideal candidate for subacute rehabilitation or skilled-level rehabilitation. Subacute rehabilitation centers serve the population of patients who would benefit from inpatient rehabilitation but do not meet the criteria for rehabilitation admissions and acute or postacute centers.

Outpatient Rehabilitation Facilities

Most rehabilitation centers, whether acute, postacute, or subacute, have outpatient components. In addition, some freestanding outpatient rehabilitation facilities are independent and not affiliated with larger hospitals. These facilities provide therapies and rehabilitation strategies to patients who do not require hospitalization or overnight stays. Most commonly, these facilities provide care to workers' compensation or sports injuries and/or services to patients who have progressed through acute and postacute rehabilitation facilities.

Home Health Care Rehabilitation

Home health care agencies provide rehabilitation services to the "homebound" patient who does not require hospitalization and who is unable to obtain transportation to an outpatient rehabilitation facility. The definition of homebound is that it is substantially difficult for the patient to be mobile in the community. This is interpreted differently from agency to agency and in different regions.

Types of Caregivers

A **rehabilitation team** can be organized along a multidisciplinary approach, meaning team members evaluate the patient in their specific discipline, or in an interdisciplinary approach, which means that the team members work together approaching a problem in a synergistic fashion to solve the specific problem for the patient. An interdisciplinary approach, used in goal setting, problem solving, and coordination of treatment, provides a more cost-effective and nonfragmented treatment to the patient and is generally considered to be the best approach. The interdisciplinary approach also improves patient learning because all team members are reinforcing the learned concepts to approach the specific problems of the patient.

Several clinical specialists might be part of a patient's rehabilitation team. These include the physiatrist, occupational therapist, physical therapist, speech pathologist, psychologist, social worker, and rehabilitation nurse as well as vocational rehabilitation counselors, recreational therapists, kinesiotherapists, music therapists, audiologists, and chaplains.

Physiatrist

A **physiatrist**, or physical medicine and rehabilitation physician, is generally the head of the rehabilitation team. A physiatrist is a physician who has completed four years of approved residency training after medical school in physical medicine and rehabilitation. The American Academy of Physical Medicine and Rehabilitation is the specialty board for physiatry and is recognized by the American Board of Medical Specialties. Physiatry is a small specialty, with some states having as few as a half-dozen physiatrists. However, the specialty has been in existence for some time, with the first specialty boards being given in 1947.

Occupational Therapist

An **occupational therapist (OT)** has completed four years of college training in an OT program and is accredited by the American Occupational Therapy Association (AOTA). Occupational therapists address several areas in their rehabilitation of a patient. These include activities of daily living (ADLs), such as dressing, bathing, grooming, toileting, and transfers. OTs also are the members of the team who focus on upper extremity movement and function, including fine motor control and hand-eye coordination. For example, they may fashion various splints for the upper extremity to preserve range of motion and improve function. OTs also address higher cognitive skills and community skills, such as homemaker chores, driving, and money handling.

Occupational therapists assist in evaluating future equipment needs such as wheelchairs, cushions, and bathtub benches, and assist in recommendations for home modifications.

Physical Therapist

The **physical therapist (PT)** is a member of the rehabilitation team who has completed four years of college training and a PT program and is certified by the American Physical Therapy Association (APTA). The physical therapist is the member of the team who is primarily responsible for improving the patient's strength, range of motion, balance, and mobility. The physical therapist specializes in appropriate strength and endurance exercises, assisting in controlling pain, providing skin care treatment, and providing modalities (such as ultrasound, diathermy, hot packs, and whirlpool treatments). When providing rehabilitation to injured workers, the physical therapist will teach proper lifting techniques, offer ergonomic suggestions, and conduct work hardening programs and functional capacity evaluations. Work hardening programs are outpatient treatment programs that assist an injured worker in maximizing his strength, range of motion, and functional status. They improve a worker's chances of returning to the job and avoiding future injuries. These treatment programs try to simulate activities that the worker would have to do in the workplace. A functional capacity evaluation is a formalized series of tests, usually with some parts computerized, that helps the physician determine what is a safe level of lifting, pushing, toting, bending, and climbing to which an injured worker would be able to return.

Speech and Language Pathologist

The **speech and language pathologist** has a bachelor's or master's level of education and is certified by the American Speech, Language, and Hearing Association. The speech pathologist evaluates and treats the patient who has aphasias, apraxias, dysarthrias, dysphasias, communication disorders, and cognitive deficits. A speech pathologist would primarily be concerned with three broad areas: (1) swallowing problems, (2) communication problems, and (3) cognitive deficits.

Psychologist

A **psychologist** has a Ph.D. level of training and should be certified by the American Psychological Association (APA). The primary role of the psychologist is to assist the newly disabled person and his or her family in adjustment to the disability and to develop a relationship of cooperation between the patient and the rehabilitation team. The psychologist has two primary roles in the rehabilitation team: (1) testing to identify problem areas in cognition or behavior on which the rehabilitation team should focus, and (2) counseling for the patient and his or her family members. When the person performing these roles has a master's degree instead of a doctorate, the position is usually termed "counselor," "specialist," or "clinician," rather than "psychologist."

Social Worker

The **rehabilitation social worker** should have specific training and knowledge in the area of social work and can be accredited by the National Association of Social Workers. The social worker assists the rehabilitation team by providing background information about the patient and his or her family situation, and in coordinating funding resources for the patient. The social worker also assures a smooth transition from the rehabilitation program back to the community.

Rehabilitation Nurse

The **rehabilitation nurse** is an RN who has completed a two-year or four-year accredited nursing program, is licensed in the state in which he or she practices, has completed additional training in rehabilitation nursing, and is certified by the Association of Rehabilitation Nurses. The rehabilitation nurse plays a key role in the patient's rehabilitation by teaching the patient information about proper bowel and bladder management programs and skin care. The rehabilitation nurse is also responsible for teaching the patient about medications, their indications, and side effects. This nurse teaches the patient about the most common complications and problems associated with a disability and how to monitor them, such as deep vein thrombus, skin breakdown, or heterotopic ossification.

Kinesiotherapist

The **kinesiotherapist** has received specialized training in the proper techniques to maximize range of motion, strength, balance, and gait, which is similar to the physical therapist's role with the rehabilitation team.

Other Health Care Workers

Numerous other health care professionals can contribute to the rehabilitation team, including vocational rehabilitation counselors, recreational therapists, music therapists, audiologists, and chaplains.

Rehabilitation programs vary in which members of the rehabilitation team are essential, depending on the setting of the rehabilitation, the type of facility, and the types of rehabilitation patients that are accepted. In general, core members of the rehabilitation team for almost any program would include the physiatrist, occupational therapist, physical therapist, and speech pathologist as a minimum. An inpatient program would also require a rehabilitation nurse and a social worker. The ratio of therapists to patients is critically important. The therapist should not be required to have more than approximately four to six hours of hands-on therapy time per day to allow the opportunity for adequate medical record documentation by the therapist and staffing time.

Types of Patients

Numerous diseases and injuries lead to a variety of disabling conditions. These disabilities can be divided into several general categories, including patients who require rehabilitation to treat injuries or disorders that are orthopedic, neurologic, medical, pediatric, or involve the management of acute or chronic pain or sensory impairment. Patients requiring orthopedic rehabilitation have injuries such as fractured hips, total joint replacements, multiple fractures, amputations, or soft tissue injuries. Pain management patients include those with acute pain and chronic pain, such as back pain or cervical pain, cumulative trauma disorders, or reflex sympathetic dystrophy. Patients with neurologic injuries or diseases include those who have conditions such as stroke, traumatic brain injuries, spinal cord injuries, multiple sclerosis, or muscular dystrophy. A sensory-impaired patient has hearing or visual disabilities. Medical disabilities include chronic obstructive pulmonary disease (COPD), myocardial infarction, diabetes mellitus and its complications, and cancer.

Pediatric rehabilitation patients are generally viewed as a separate category because of their special needs. These patients are often considered to be habilation patients rather than rehabilitation patients. Conditions that are commonly treated include cerebral palsy, spina bifida, and various genetic disorders. Similarly, the aged population often has different rehabilitation issues and goals, and tends to be treated in a geriatric rehabilitation setting such as subacute rehabilitation.

Because of the subspecialization required by rehabilitation team members, rehabilitation hospitals or programs tend to evolve around specific types of injuries. For example, there are rehabilitation centers that treat only brain injuries, spinal cord injuries, or burn survivors.

Spinal cord injury treatment centers have evolved to treat the 7,000 to 10,000 new cases of spinal cord injury each year in the United States. There are model system spinal cord injury treatment centers that specialize in treating the spinal cord–injured patient, such as Craig Hospital in Englewood, Colorado, Rehabilitation Institute of Chicago, Texas Institute of Rehabilitation in Houston, and Shepherd Rehabilitation Center in Atlanta. There are 16 regional model system spinal cord injury treatment centers that are funded by grants from the National Institute of Disability Research, a branch of the National Institutes of Health (NIH).

Similarly, there are rehabilitation centers that focus on traumatic brain injury (TBI), such as Timber Ridge Ranch in Bentonville, Arkansas; the Greenery in Dallas, Texas; and Rancho Los Amigos in Downy, California. It is estimated that approximately 50,000 to 75,000 people per year in the United States have severe traumatic brain injury. There are four to five times as many who have mild to moderate TBI.

It has been estimated that approximately 14 percent of Americans have a disability; this is approximately 35 to 43 million people with disabilities. Of these individuals with a disability, as many as one-third have functional limitations that can be classified as severe.

Understanding proper terminology regarding this population is important. The World Health Organization (WHO) developed an international standard of definitions for terms that are used to discuss individuals with functional limitations. **Impairment** is any loss or abnormality of a psychological, physiologic, or anatomic structure or function. **Disability** is any restriction or lack resulting from the impairment of the ability to perform an activity in a manner or within the range considered normal for a human being. **Handicap** is a disadvantage for a given individual resulting from an impairment or a disability that limits or prevents the fulfillment of a role that is normal (depending on age, sex, social, and cultural factors) for that individual. Stated differently, the impairment might be the disease or diagnosis; the disability is how the impairment (i.e., the disease or diagnosis) affects the person. Finally, the handicap is an interaction between the impairment or disability and the person's socioeconomic environment. In other words, how does the problem affect the person's life? What functional limitations or problems are posed by the impairment or the disability? For example, amputation of a distal segment of the index finger and the long finger of a hand would result in an impairment (i.e., partial amputation of digits) and some disability (decreased range of motion, decreased grip strength). In most situations, this injury would not result in a major handicap. Given some rehabilitation and time, the individual would learn how to adapt quite well to a relatively minor impairment. Now suppose that the individual is a concert classical pianist. The handicap is overwhelming in this situation, and the person would be totally disabled at pursuing his or her occupation.

Consider an example of an individual with a spinal cord injury resulting in paraplegia. This person then attends college, medical school, and residency training to become a rehabilitation physician. The impairment is spinal cord injury with paraplegia; the disability is a mobility impairment with an inability to walk. However, in this situation the handicap is mild or moderate because the hospital is an accessible environment and the individual is able to practice rehabilitation medicine in the environment of a hospital. Remember that the handicap is defined by the socioeconomic environment and the interaction of the impairment. The same individual would be severely handicapped if he were a tree surgeon or a mountain climber.

Durable Medical Equipment Commonly Used

Assistive devices fall into many different categories depending on the type of function the device is intended to supplement or augment. They can be divided into several broad categories: orthotics, prosthetics, ambulation aids, wheelchairs, and high-tech assistive devices such as computers. Refer to Table 11-1 for examples of the various types of durable medical equipment used in rehabilitation.

Orthotics

An **orthotic device** is an external appliance or brace that can supplement an extremity's function or improve stability and positioning. Orthotics have been in existence for more than 300 years and come in a variety of shapes, sizes, and styles from leather to metal to polyethylene plastics. The most commonly seen is a spinal brace, either cervical or lumbar. Cervical orthoses are commonly prescribed after trauma to the cervical spine, such as a motor vehicle accident, or after surgery. A variety of devices are available from the Philadelphia collar, which is a soft foamlike collar that provides very little restriction of head movement and serves only as a proprioceptive reminder to the person to limit range of motion, to the halo, which is placed by the surgeon and provides the greatest level of stability for an unstable cervical

Table 11-1   Examples of Durable Medical Equipment Used in Rehabilitation

Device	Definition	Examples
Orthotics	An orthopedic appliance to support, align, prevent, or correct deformity or to improve function	AFO, KAFO, WHO, neck, back or spine braces*
Ambulation aids	A device to provide stability and support for walking	Straight cane, walker, quad cane, crutches
Prosthetics	A device to replace a missing body part	Mechanical arm or leg, artificial eye, dentures, myoelectric arms
Wheelchairs/mobility devices	A wheeled chair to provide mobility when ambulation is difficult or not possible	Standard wheelchair, power wheelchair, power scooter
High-technology assistive devices	Computer to control environments and control wheelchairs	Kurzweil readers, Peachtree control systems

*AFO (ankle-foot orthosis); KAFO (knee-ankle-foot orthosis); WHO (wrist-hand orthosis)

spine. The most commonly seen cervical orthosis is a SOMI-type brace, named for the body part that it contacts (sternal occipital mandibular immobilizer).

Similarly, thoracolumbar orthoses come in a variety of styles and shapes, the most common being the Jewett brace, which provides support in the upper sternal, midthoracic, and lower anterior abdominal area, and a chair-back type brace that resembles a straight-back chair with straps to keep it positioned properly on the back. For scoliosis, the Milwaukee brace is most commonly used to limit the progression of the scoliotic spine. Thoracolumbar orthoses tend to be named for the city in which they were developed.

Several devices exist to stabilize or assist function of an upper extremity that has impairment. These devices can be static or dynamic. A static device assists in positioning; the dynamic orthosis assists in replacing some function. A sling suspension orthosis, or ball-bearing feeder orthosis, assists a quadriplegic who has limited strength in the upper extremities, allowing this person to perform functional activities such as feeding himself. A Cock-up splint, or flexor hinge splint, can be used in the C6 quadriplegic to replace the lost pinch grasp between the forefingers and the thumb.

Extremity orthoses are named for the body part with which they interact. For example, an orthosis that crosses the wrist and hand is a WHO (wrist-hand orthosis). One that goes over the back of the leg and around the bottom of the foot is an AFO (ankle-foot orthosis). If that same brace extends up the leg and just above the knee, it is a KAFO (knee-ankle-foot orthosis).

The most common lower-extremity orthotic is an AFO to replace weakened muscles in the leg and prevent the foot from dropping when ambulating. An additional brace that is commonly seen is the Swedish knee cage, which is used in athletes who have suffered injury to the ligaments in their knee.

Ambulation Aids

Ambulation aids provide additional stability and support for an individual who has trouble walking. These range from a straight cane to a walker. Wheels may be added to the walker to allow the person to move at a faster pace without having to pick the walker up. A variety of canes exist from a straight cane to a quad cane, a device that has four feet to broaden the base of support. Crutches, such as wooden axillary crutches, are commonly used. A Lofstrand (forearm) crutch is commonly used, and sometimes platform crutches are required depending on the person's functional level.

Prosthetic Devices

Prosthetic devices are divided into upper-extremity and lower-extremity devices. A **prosthesis** is a device that is designed to replace a missing extremity or partially missing extremity. Prosthetics are divided into several categories: mechanical prostheses (body-powered prostheses), which are the most common; myoelectric prostheses, which are high-tech and use a series of electric motors to replace the missing action; and cosmetic prostheses, which improve appearance for social reasons and are usually less functional than body-powered or myoelectric prostheses. Lower-extremity amputations are much more common than upper-extremity amputations. Amputations are further defined by the level of amputation. A major body joint is used to make this distinction. For example, if the person is missing a portion of the hand and wrist, the amputation is said to be a BE (below-the-elbow) amputation. If the amputation is above the elbow, it is an AE amputation. In the lower extremity, if it is below the knee, it is a BKA (below-the-knee) amputation. Above the knee is an AKA amputation.

A variety of prosthetic devices are available depending on the functional status and age of the patient. Terminology regarding prosthetics is presented in a standardized form. The prosthetic device is described based on the type of suspension, the type of skeleton, the type of joint, and the type of terminal devices. For example, a below-the-knee prosthesis is a PTB (patellar tendon-bearing) socket endoskeleton. The ankle is specified as a multiaxis or single-axis ankle, and the type of foot is a SACH foot, Flex foot, or Seattle foot. Upper-extremity prosthetics terminology is presented in the same fashion. A description of the socket that fits over the amputated extremity, the type of skeleton support (endoskeleton or exoskeleton), the type of joint, and the type of terminal device is described.

Wheelchairs

Many different types and styles of wheelchairs exist. The choice depends on the patient's age, size, and intended use of the device. There are two general categories for wheelchairs: manual wheelchairs and power wheelchairs.

Manual wheelchairs are divided into lightweight sports-type wheelchairs and standard wheelchairs. A number of companies manufacture both; the most common companies are Quickie, InvaCare, and E&J. The lightweight sports-type chairs are used by those who pursue an active lifestyle, whereas the standard chairs are more commonly seen in hospitals, nursing homes, and are often used by the elderly population.

Power wheelchairs (they should not be referred to as "electric chairs") and mobility devices are available and manufactured by the same companies as manual wheelchairs. A variety of configurations are available depending on the functional status of the person. Chairs are available that bring the person to a standing position or that lay the person down, or tilt him or her in space if these functions are required. Chairs are also available that have ventilator support. Extremely advanced power wheelchair control systems are available now, such as the Peachtree system, which has a sensory array behind the chair user's head and movement of the head controls the chair. Looking to the left will make the chair turn left and looking to the right will make it turn right.

Computer Technology

There has been an explosion of computer technology designed to assist the disabled person. **Environmental control units (ECUs)** are now available that allow a person who has limited mobility to run many functions in the home such as turning on lights, using appliances, and opening and closing doors and windows. Recently there have been many devices on the market that allow the disabled person greater access to the computer. Prior to this time, computer technology was limited to individuals who had hand dexterity and could type on a keyboard. Now computers can be run with a variety of switching systems such as an eye-blink switch, an infrared beam that is able to catch a reflex from the eye, head control systems such as Head Master by Ultraphonics, and voice recognition systems such as Dragon NaturallySpeaking®.

Computer systems are available to assist visually impaired people. These devices are able to scan print and convert it to spoken language, such as a Kurzweil reader. Augmentative communication devices are available to replace speech for individuals who are unable to communicate verbally.

Regulatory Issues

Medical rehabilitation is both medical and rehabilitative in nature. The dual nature of medical rehabilitation has resulted in two independent accreditation options. The Joint Commission on Accreditation of Healthcare Organizations (JCAHO) and the Commission for Accreditation of Rehabilitation Facilities (CARF) are the nationally recognized agencies that review care. The Centers for Medicare and Medicaid Services (CMS) also has regulations affecting rehabilitation services. The *Code of Federal Regulations* contains *Conditions of Participation* for comprehensive outpatient rehabilitation facilities (CORFs) and for clinics and other agencies providing outpatient physical therapy and speech-language pathology services. In addition, because inpatient rehabilitation facilities have their own prospective payment system for Medicare, CMS has outlined criteria that an inpatient facility must meet to be classified as a rehabilitation hospital. State licensure agencies generally use these regulations and criteria as basic components in the process of licensing rehabilitation facilities. Other criteria for state licensure may vary from state to state.

Joint Commission on Accreditation of Healthcare Organizations

The Joint Commission on Accreditation of Healthcare Organizations (JCAHO) has exact standards that are intended to promote quality and improve outcomes in rehabilitation at all levels of medical care. In order to receive Medicare reimbursement, a facility must have a JCAHO accreditation. JCAHO no longer has specific guidelines for rehabilitation facilities or rehabilitation units in an acute care hospital. The standards of JCAHO have become more "rehabilitation-like," though, and focus on outcomes and outcome management, and apply to all settings of the inpatient and outpatient areas of patient care. The identification of duplication of requirements for JCAHO and CARF standards has resulted in the two accrediting bodies surveying facilities simultaneously through a cooperative accreditation initiative. Facilities (currently freestanding only) that have been jointly surveyed by JCAHO and CARF report improved satisfaction with the new process, and the two agencies continue to work toward improving their processes.

Commission for Accreditation of Rehabilitation Facilities

The Commission on Accreditation of Rehabilitation Facilities (CARF) standards and criteria for full accreditation are comprehensive and specific in regard to the rehabilitation care of patients. CARF accreditation is difficult to attain; thus, many rehabilitation centers fail to apply for CARF accreditation. The quality of care in a rehabilitation program, however, is markedly affected by meeting the standards of CARF. In the managed care market, the insurance companies seek out CARF-accredited programs to ensure the best patient care.

The standards (Section 5.A, Standards 9–16) for the rehabilitation program require the medical director to be a physical medicine and rehabilitation physician (physiatrist) or a physician who is qualified by virtue of his or her training and experience in rehabilitation and who is board certified in his or her area of specialty and has the appropriate experience and training necessary to provide rehabilitation physician services through one of the following:

1. Formal residency in physical medicine and rehabilitation
2. A fellowship in rehabilitation for a minimum of one year
3. A minimum of two years of experience in providing rehabilitation services for patients

The rehabilitation physician has the responsibility for the care of the patient who has the potential for continuing, unstable, or complex medical conditions or must make arrangements for the care to be provided through other physicians (consults). There are three categories of complexity of programs described in the CARF standards with the intensity of medical care relative to each level.

Centers for Medicare and Medicaid Services (CMS)

The Centers for Medicare and Medicaid Services (CMS) promulgate regulations affecting several types of rehabilitation providers. There are *Conditions of Participation* for comprehensive outpatient rehabilitation facilities (CORFs), outpatient physical therapy providers, and rehabilitation hospitals and units

One set of CMS regulations provides criteria that determine whether a hospital or unit can be classified as an inpatient rehabilitation facility. A hospital that meets the criteria can receive Medicare reimbursement under the **inpatient rehabilitation facility prospective payment system (IRF PPS)** rather than under the diagnosis related group (DRG) system of reimbursement applied to short stay acute care hospitals. One of the criteria, informally termed the "75 percent rule," defines the types of conditions that should comprise the caseload of a rehabilitation hospital. The 75 percent rule has been in effect since 1983, when it was used to determine whether a hospital or unit was exempt from the DRG-based inpatient prospective payment system. After implementation of the IRF PPS in 2002, CMS suspended enforcement of the 75 percent rule in order to evaluate whether changes were needed in the regulation. The study commissioned by CMS showed that the majority of IRFs did not meet the criteria specified in the 75 percent rule. Rehabilitation providers strongly opposed re-institution of the old rule and urged CMS to repeal or revise the 75 percent rule (AMRPA, 2003). A new rule, published on May 7, 2004, expands the types of conditions that would be considered and also gives facilities until 2007 to achieve the 75 percent caseload. The conditions that count toward the 75 percent are as follows:

(A) Stroke.

(B) Spinal cord injury.

(C) Congenital deformity.

(D) Amputation.

(E) Major multiple trauma.

(F) Fracture of femur (hip fracture).

(G) Brain injury.

(H) Neurologic disorders, including multiple sclerosis, motor neuron diseases, polyneuropathy, muscular dystrophy, and Parkinson's disease.

(I) Burns.

(J) Active, polyarticular rheumatoid arthritis, psoriatic arthritis, and seronegative arthropathies resulting in significant functional impairment of ambulation and other activities of daily living that have not improved after an appropriate, aggressive, and sustained course of outpatient therapy services or services in other less-intensive rehabilitation settings immediately preceding the inpatient rehabilitation admission or that result from a systemic disease activation immediately before admission, but have the potential to improve with more intensive rehabilitation.

(K) Systemic vasculidities with joint inflammation, resulting in significant functional impairment of ambulation and other activities of daily living that have not improved after an appropriate, aggressive, and sustained course of outpatient therapy services or services in other less-intensive rehabilitation settings immediately preceding the inpatient rehabilitation admission or that result from a systemic disease activation immediately before admission, but have the potential to improve with more intensive rehabilitation.

(L) Severe or advanced osteoarthritis (osteoarthrosis or degenerative joint disease) involving two or more major weight-bearing joints (elbow, shoulders, hips, or knees, but not counting a joint with a prosthesis) with joint deformity and substantial loss of range of motion, atrophy of muscles surrounding the joint, significant functional impairment of ambulation and other activities of daily living that have not improved after the patient has participated in an appropriate, aggressive, and sustained course of outpatient therapy services or services in other less-intensive rehabilitation settings immediately preceding the inpatient rehabilitation admission but have the potential to improve with more intensive rehabilitation. (A joint replaced by a prosthesis no longer is considered to have osteoarthritis, or other arthritis, even though this condition was the reason for the joint replacement.)

(M) Knee or hip joint replacement, or both, during an acute hospitalization immediately preceding the inpatient rehabilitation stay and also . . . one or more of the following specific criteria:

  (1) The patient underwent bilateral knee or bilateral hip joint replacement surgery during the acute hospital admission immediately preceding the IRF admission.

  (2) The patient is extremely obese with a Body Mass Index of at least 50 at the time of admission to the IRF.

  (3) The patient is age 85 or older at the time of admission to the IRF (CMS, 2004, pp. 25775–25776).

The health information department has an important role to play in ensuring data quality so that the percentage of patients falling into the various condition categories can be accurately calculated.

CMS also requires that the hospital have a full-time director of rehabilitation who "is a doctor of medicine or osteopathy, is licensed under state law to practice medicine or surgery, and has had, after completing a one-year hospital internship, at least two years of training or experience in the medical management of patients requiring rehabilitation services" (Excluded hospitals: Classification, 2002), or is board certified in physiatry, neurology, neurosurgery, orthopedic surgery, or rheumatology. Other services needed in a rehabilitation hospital are rehabilitation nursing, physical therapy, occupational therapy, speech therapy, social or psychological services, and orthotic and prosthetic services.

CMS requires that the rehabilitation hospital have a preadmission screening procedure to determine whether a prospective patient is likely to benefit from inpatient rehabilitation. Figure 11-1 is an example of part of a patient database form that collects pertinent functional information about the patient to help define areas of functional deficit and thus assist in goal development. Each inpatient selected for admission must have a plan of treatment established with a multidisciplinary team approach. Team conferences during which the plan is reviewed are held at least every two weeks (Excluded hospitals: Classification, 2002).

Medical Directors

Accrediting agencies and third-party payers strongly advocate that the medical director of a rehabilitation facility be a board-eligible or board-certified physiatrist. In cases where a physiatrist is not available, then board-eligible or board-certified neurologists or orthopedists may serve in the interim.

Documentation

As in all health care facilities, there are specific guidelines regarding the documentation that must be completed in a patient's medical records. It is not the purpose of this chapter to cover this topic in its entirety; refer to other chapters in this text for basic medical record documentation guidelines. This chapter focuses on additional or specific documentation requirements in the rehabilitation facility as it applies to specific sections of the records.

The admission history and physical includes a functional history. The functional history should cover the patient's functional status before the onset of the illness or injury. If the person had a preexisting disability and is now returning to rehabilitation because of a change in condition, then a discussion of the patient's functional status before the onset of the new illness or change is required. The functional history addresses activities of daily living, required assisted devices, reliance on other caregivers, and a discussion of community mobility.

The history also includes a discussion of equipment that the person has at home. A full description of braces, orthoses, prosthetics, or durable medical equipment is required. Also included is a description of the type of vehicle the individual has, because this will affect in many ways the type of wheelchair that can be prescribed for the patient.

The social history must include a discussion of available family members or caregivers, a description of the home (i.e., multilevel, single level, number of steps at entrance, is the bathroom accessible, etc.), educational status, employment status, and previous hobbies, in addition to standard social history information, such as alcohol and drug abuse.

COX HEALTH SYSTEMS
Springfield, MO

Bar Code

PATIENT DATA BASE
PHYSICAL REHABILITATION UNIT

Patient Sticker

Rehab Problem/Diagnosis_____   Initial Evaluation Date_____   Expected Admit Date_____
Patient Address (City/State)_____   Date of Onset_____
TO BE COMPLETED AT PREADMIT   INFORMANT: ☐ SELF   ☐ OTHER:_____

I.   Status Prior to Admission:

How were you doing the following activities at home?	Preadmission*	Current* (prescreening)
1. Grooming (care of hair, teeth, nails, face)		
2. Dressing (shirts, underwear, pants, shoes/socks on/off)		
3. Walking (inside/outside/distance/device		
4. Cooking (home/out/microwave/self/others		
5. Bathing (indep/assist, tub/shower, sink/equip)		
6. Toileting (indep/assist, equip)		
7. Housekeeping (indep/services)		
8. Transportation (self/others, where[Dr./store/church/beauty shop])		
9. Animal/pet care (self/others, describe)		
10. Caregiver responsibilities (who/how many/freq./what)		
11. Medication management (equip/self/others)		
12. Business mgmt (POA/family/self/decision maker)		
13. Swallowing		
14. Bowel/Bladder Management		
15. Communication		
16. Memory Problems		
17. Safety		

* **Key for Independence or Assistance scale: I** = 100% independent;   **S** = Supervision (requires no more help than standby cueing or coaxing); **Min** = expends 75% or more of the effort; **Mod** = expends 50-75% of the effort; **Max** = expends 25-50% of the effort; **D** = dependent, expends less than 25% of the effort

II.   Description of Home: ___ house ___ apartment ___ trailer ___ retirement home ___ nursing home

Number of floors	Stairs inside home? ___ Yes ___ No How many? _____	Steps to gain access to home?___ Yes ___ No	Number	Floors carpeted? ___ Yes ___ No	Which rooms?
Are hallways carpeted? ___ Yes ___ No	Type of carpet ___ Low ___ Medium ___ High ___ Shag			Are there throw rugs or area rugs? ___ Yes ___ No	

Comments:_____
_____

_____
recorder signature   date

\forms\ptdbase2.doc

page 1/6

Figure 11-1   An excerpt from a patient database that covers all CARF criteria. This form promotes interdisciplinary assessment of the patient. (Courtesy Cox Health Systems, Springfield, MO.)

<table>
<tr>
<td>Bar Code</td>
<td>COX HEALTH SYSTEMS
Springfield, MO

PATIENT DATA BASE
PHYSICAL REHABILITATION UNIT</td>
<td>Patient Sticker</td>
</tr>
</table>

III. TO BE COMPLETED AT PRESCREENING: INFORMANT: ☐ SELF   ☐ OTHER:_____

1. Do you live alone? ___ Yes ___ No   With whom?:_____

2. Expected assistance and/or limitation from person living with you:_____
_____

3. Expected assistance from persons outside your home:_____
_____

4. Who will perform the following activities?
   a. Meal Preparation_____
   b. Cleaning/Washing dishes_____
   c. Heavy Housework (scrubbing, floors, cleaning bathrooms, washing laundry, ironing, yard work, etc.)
   _____
   d. Light housework (dusting, folding/putting clothes away, etc.)_____
   e. Shopping_____
   f. Child care_____
   g. Driving_____
   h. Other areas of concern: (farming, etc.)_____

5. What was/is your occupation?_____
   a. How long have you been there?_____
   b. What do you do?_____
   c. Is it full or part time?_____
   d. Is it days or nights?_____

6. Referral Source_____ Episode_____ Patient/Family Tour: Date_____
   Referring Physician_____ Other Acute Care Physician(s)_____
   Program: Evaluation   Limited Services   Comprehensive
   Services Requested: PT / OT / SP / PSY / NPSY / REC / RN / NUT / MSW / PM
   ELOS: _____ Patient Goals: _____
   Trauma: Yes   No   Recommendations:_____ Date_____

IV. Did you have any in home or community services assisting you before this hospitalization?
_____
_____

                                             _____
                                              recorder signature   date

Figure 11-1 *(Continued)*

<table>
<tr><td>Bar Code</td><td>COX HEALTH SYSTEMS
Springfield, MO

PATIENT DATA BASE
PHYSICAL REHABILITATION UNIT</td><td>Patient Sticker</td></tr>
</table>

TO BE COMPLETED WITHIN 2 HOURS OF ADMISSION TO REHAB UNIT:

INFORMANT: ☐SELF ☐OTHER:_____

V. Medical Database

Admission Time:_____Informant:_____Relationship (if not patient)_____

Family Physician _____Person to be contacted in case of emergency:_____

Relationship:_____Phone: day(____)_____night:(_____)_____

ADMISSION VITAL SIGNS: T_____ P_____ R_____ BP_____ L R Height_____ Weight_____ kg lb. Type scale _____

Reason for admission: (patient's own words)_____

List and give dates of pertinent surgeries, serious illnesses or injuries, depression / emotional problems:_____

Cardiovascular:_____

Endocrine:_____

Renal:_____

Respiratory:_____

Flu/Pneumonia immunizations up to date? ____Yes ____No

Have you ever had a blood transfusion? ____Yes ____No   Reaction: ____Yes ____No

Describe:_____

Medications brought to hospital
____Yes ____No

Disposition of medications:
____Home ____Pharmacy ____Bedside

ALLERGIES:(meds, foods, skin, resp, etc.):
____ None ___ Allergy band

List Allergy and reaction: __

_____

_____

_____

_____

LATEX ALLERGY SCREEN:
____ History of multiple catheterizations
____ Occupational exposure to latex
____ Allerg to kiwi, avocado, banana, potato

List Medications: Pills, Patches, Inhaler, O2, etc. ( ) NONE ( ) Unavailable	Dose & how taken: P.O., Injected, Inhaled	Time of last dose

VI. Medical History:

a. How has your overall health been in the past year?_____

b. What pharmacy do you use?_____

c. Do you take your medicines as prescribed?_____

d. Do you utilize anything to help organize your medications (pill organizer)?_____

e. Do you have a family doctor that follows your care?_____

f. Do you use alcohol? Yes____ No____   Intake (daily/weekly)_____ Quit_____

g. Do you use tobacco? Yes____ No____ Type_____pks/day_____

    # years_____ Quit? Yes____ No____ When? _____

h. Do you use street drugs? Yes____ No____ Type_____ Amt./Freq._____

i. Do you wear glasses / contacts? Yes____ No____   For Distance_____ For Reading_____

j. Do you have visual problems not treated by glasses?_____

k. Do you have a hearing aid?_____ Do you wear your hearing aid?_____

l. Do you have any cultural or spiritual beliefs that we need to be aware of that would affect your care?_____

_____

\forms\ptdbase2.doc

page 3/6

Figure 11-1   (*Continued*)

COX HEALTH SYSTEMS
Springfield, MO

Bar Code

Patient Sticker

PATIENT DATA BASE
PHYSICAL REHABILITATION UNIT

m. How long has it been since your vision/hearing has been tested?_____
n. Who do you see for your eye exams?_____ hearing_____
o. Do you wear dentures?_____
p. Do you have chewing problems?_____

Communicable Disease Screening: Recent exposure to infectious disease?   ____Yes ____No

  MRSA: (Check those that apply):
  _____Known MRSA positive   _____Has open wound
  _____from nursing home or other hospital   _____IV drug user
  _____hospitalized or on antibiotic therapy for 14 days or more within 30 days
  If "yes" on any of above MRSA questions, please culture according to policy for MRSA screening.
  CULTURE: Date:_____   Time:_____   Site:_____

  TB   (Check those that apply):   **Hepatitis A**   (Check those that apply):
  Family member with TB?   ____Yes   ____No   Family member with Hep A?   ____Yes   ____No
  Exposed to anyone with TB ____Yes   ____No   Exposed to anyone with Hep A? ____Yes   ____No
  Positive skin test: ____Yes   ____No

VII. General Nutrition / Swallowing Screen

a. What type of diet are you on?_____
b. Do you follow your special diet recommendation?_____
c. Prescribed snacks:_____
d. Recent weight change: ____Loss   ____Gain   _____pounds over _____weeks / months
e. Reason for weight change_____
f. Do you take any vitamins or minerals?   Yes____ No____
g. Swallowing Screen: _____Normal _____See "Dysphagia Consult" Protocol, #s 1,2,6,9,12
h. Patient currently on swallowing program? Yes____ No____

VIII. Elimination

IX. Sleep/Rest Patterns: (Ask patient to describe sleeping pattern/problems and check/complete those that apply.)

  No difficulty_____ Hours per night_____ Naps_____ Sleep aids_____
  History of insomnia_____ Normal sleep time frame_____
  History of orthopnea_____ Sleep apnea_____ Number of pillows_____
  Comments:_____
  What time do you go to bed?_____ Time you get up?_____
  Do you get up in the night?_____ Reason?_____
  Do you take a nap during the day?_____ What time?_____

X. Integumentary Status:

Mark drawing with appropriate
  letter at exact location:
  A - Amputation   L - Laceration
  B - Burn   O - ostomy
  BR - Bruise   P - pressure
  D - Dry patches   R - Rash
  DS - Dressing   S - scar
  I - incision   W - wound

Stages of breakdown:
  O - potential
  1 - Reddened
  2 - Disruption / Ulceration
  3 - Complete destruction of skin
      layers (exposed fat, muscle, bone)
  4 - invasion by ulceration of bone
      structure

Front   Back

Other Comments/descriptions:
_____
_____
_____
_____
_____
_____
_____

If stage 1 or greater, pull skin care flow
sheet and take a picture.

Circumference Measurements:
  Thigh (18 cm above patella)
    Left_____ Right_____
  Calf (13 cm below patellar tendon)
    Left_____ Right_____

\forms\ptdbase2.doc   page 4/6

Figure 11-1   (*Continued*)

COX HEALTH SYSTEMS
Springfield, MO

PATIENT DATA BASE
PHYSICAL REHABILITATION UNIT

Bar Code

Patient Sticker

PAIN ASSESSMENT: Document history of pain and associated symptoms. Make current pain assessment on the Patient Care Record.

_____

_____

_____

_____

XI. Health Care Directive:

It is mandated by law that we ask, "Do you have an Advance Directive or Durable Power of Attorney for health care?"
____Yes   ____No

If "yes", we need a copy for the chart. If "no" is checked, information was given regarding Self Determination Act.   ____Yes

RN Signature_____ **Date**_____ **Time**_____

TO BE COMPLETED WITHIN 2 TO 24 HOURS OF ADMISSION TO REHAB UNIT:

INFORMANT: ☐ SELF   ☐ OTHER:_____

XII. Description of Home:

Description of Bedroom:

Is there room for walker to maneuver? ____Yes ____No	Explain:
Is there room for commode seat, dressing chair? ____Yes ____No	Explain:
Description of bed: ___High ___Low ___Single ___Double ___Waterbed	S.O. sleep in same room? ____Yes ____No
Other areas of concern:	

Description of Bathroom

Do you have?: ____Tub ____Walk-in shower(no threshold)	____Shower stall ____Tub/Shower Combo ____Grab bars		
Do you have glass doors or a curtain? ____Glass Doors ____Curtain	Do you prefer to take : ____shower ____bath	Do you have hand-held shower attachment? ____Yes ____No	
Is bathroom on the same floor as bedroom? ____Yes ____No	Is toilet standard height? ____Yes ____No	Comment:	
Is there a supported sink or tub adjacent to toilet? ____Yes ____No	If so, can the supported sink/tub be used for getting on/off the toilet? ____Yes ____No		
Is there room for a walker or wheelchair to maneuver to toilet? ____Yes ____No	Do you have a non-slip surface in the tub/shower? ____Yes ____No	How wide is the bathroom door?_____	
Do you have any other equipment for the bathroom? Explain:	Other areas of concern:		

Where are your phones located?_____

Do you have a portable phone?   ____Yes   ____No

Do you have: ____ Rotary   ____ Touch-tone   ____ Memory redial

Do you have lifeline?   ____Yes   ____No

Describe the chair or couch you usually sit in: ____ Straight chair   ____Recliner   ____ Couch

Occupational Therapist Signature_____ **Date**_____

Figure 11-1   (*Continued*)

	COX HEALTH SYSTEMS	
Bar Code	Springfield, MO	Patient Sticker
	PATIENT DATA BASE	
	PHYSICAL REHABILITATION UNIT	

DISCHARGE PLANNING

XIII.   Emotional/Social:

1. Which family members do you see most frequently?_____
2. How often do you see them?_____
3. What activities do you do with your family?_____
4. Does your spouse / significant other / family work?_____
  a.   What do they do?_____
  b.   Is it full time or part time?_____
  c.   Is it days or nights?_____
5. Have you had recent episodes of depression or anxiety that persist for more than a few days?_____
6. Have you required services of a mental health professional (psychologist/psychiatrist) ?_____
   If so , for what?_____
7. What medications have you taken for emotional or psychiatric problems?_____
   For what purpose?_____   For how long?_____
8. Do you have to have things "just so" or in perfect order?_____
9. Would you describe yourself as easy-going, quick tempered, high strung, or happy-go-lucky?_____
10. Have you had any major stressors in your life in the last year?_____
   _____
11. How do you handle stress?_____
   _____

To be completed within 24 - 72 hours of admission to Rehab Unit:

   INFORMANT: ☐ SELF   ☐ OTHER:_____

XIV.   Financial/Community Resources

a.   Who manages your financial affairs at home?_____
b.   If it is you, is there someone who could assist you if needed?_____
c.   Have you had financial issues in the past in regards to health care?_____
d.   Purchasing medications_____   Purchasing equipment_____
e.   What is your understanding of how Medicare / private insurance pays for your hospital rehab stay?_____
   _____

XV. Social History

1. Education
  a.   What is the highest grade you completed in school?_____
  b.   Did you like school?_____
  c.   How well did you do in school?_____
  d.   Do you have difficulties reading or writing?_____
2. Family
  a.   ____ Married   ____ Single   ____ Widowed   ____ Divorced   ____Previous marriage
  b.   Do you have children? ____ Yes ___ No   Any children living in your home? ____ Yes (How many?____)   ____ No

XVI.   Hobbies / Leisure Activities

a.   What do you do for fun?_____
b.   List your three favorite things to do
   1._____
   2. _____
   3. _____
c.   Who do you spend recreational time with?_____
d.   Do you   ____travel   ____fish   ____garden   ____woodwork
        ____sports   ____eat out   ____other
e.   Do you enjoy?:   ____church activities   ____crafts   list types: _____
        ____television   ____cards/games   other:_____

Social Worker Signature_____   **Date**_____

\forms\ptdbase2.doc   page 6/6

Figure 11-1   *(Continued)*

The physical examination includes a comprehensive neurologic and musculoskeletal exam, adequate documentation of the condition of the skin, and a description of interventional devices such as a catheter, feeding tube, or tracheostomy. The neurologic exam includes cranial nerves, motor strength, reflexes, and sensory nerves. It also includes a mention of the patient's cognitive status, speech, and language capabilities. The examination must clearly describe the functional status of the individual both cognitively and physically. The musculoskeletal exam should document the range of motion of all joints and extremities, note contractures, amputations, or missing body parts, and indicate the presence or absence of complications such as deep vein thrombosis or heterotopic ossification.

The physiatric history and physical diagnosis section includes standard medical diagnoses as well as functional rehabilitation diagnoses. For example, a spinal cord–injured patient's admission diagnoses may be (1) T9 spinal cord injury, (2) decreased strength and endurance, and (3) dependence for ADL activities. Stating the functional limitations or problems in the diagnostic sections helps focus the rehabilitation team on the primary issue of concern that has led to the rehabilitation treatment.

CARF guidelines specify that the history should contain a statement in the patient's own words as to what his or her goals are for the rehabilitation stay. This section includes a specific discussion of goals as they relate to the interdisciplinary team. For example, a physician notes that occupational therapy is to focus on dressing, bathing, grooming, and equipment needs, or that physical therapy is to address decreased strength, transfer skills, balance, and range of motion. The plan section is specific and outlines the goals in quantitative terms for the entire rehabilitation team. The plan is concluded with a statement of the estimated length of stay for the hospitalization.

In summary, the history and physical by the physician should provide identification of presenting problems, goals and expected benefits, initial estimated time frames for accomplishing goals, and services needed. The individual's pathological diagnosis, impairment, and functional limitations must be thoroughly discussed in the physician history and physical.

The physician is required to document team conferences on the patient. Team conferences are conducted on a weekly basis. In this conference, all members of the health care team sit down to discuss the patient's problems and their progress in rehabilitation. In general, the physician documents in each of the areas of concern the comments that the interdisciplinary team makes regarding the patient's progress. In addition, the team conference sets short-term goals to be accomplished by the next team conference.

The discharge summary includes a discussion in quantifiable terms of the patient's functional status at the time of admission and his or her functional status at the time of discharge, and should reflect the patient's progress or lack of progress. Recommendations regarding equipment needs or home support services are specifically addressed in the discharge summary.

The discharge recommendations and a discharge conference should be held with the patient and/or responsible family members. The discharge summary and recommendations should contain specific warnings or limitations for the patient. Safety issues and other concerns should be discussed, such as driving, preparing meals, and the need for attendant care.

The physical therapist and occupational therapist as well as other disciplines are required to document daily notes regarding their treatment, interactions with the patient, and the results. This documentation should be made in functional terms and clearly be related to the specific goals identified for the hospitalization. The number of hours the patient has actually participated in therapy should be clearly indicated in the therapist's documentation. Figure 11-2 provides an example of a form used in documentation by a therapist. This figure illustrates one way of summarizing the occupational therapist's findings and recommendations for discharge. It allows comparison of admission findings with discharge findings and assists in documenting the patient's improvement.

Nursing documentation includes information about the patient's skin status; knowledge of medications, uses, and side effects; information regarding the patient's functional status in terms of self-care and skin care; and documentation of the patient's knowledge regarding common complications given the disability.

CARF-accredited facilities are required to have a set of policies that clearly address how the rehabilitation patient may gain access to his or her own records. In addition, there must be documentation that the patient has been provided with orientation to the rehabilitation facility, which includes a statement of the organization's mission and philosophy, participation in goal setting, and a patient's rights and responsibilities list.

CARF further requires that individual program planning be performed and documented. The plans must be individualized, establish the goals and objectives for the admission, and incorporate the unique strengths, needs, abilities, and preferences of the person served. There must be documentation that the patient understands the goals, and it must reflect the person's informed choice.

Functions of the interdisciplinary team that must be documented in the records include (1) the assessment of the persons served; (2) determination, modification, and implementation of the individual plan and the discharge plan of the person served; (3) provision of direct services consistent with needs; (4) active participation in conferences regarding the person served; (5) promotion of interdisciplinary functions and mutual support among all members of the team; and (6) promotion of the program's evaluation and treatment philosophy. Medical records systems can be established in such a way to meet these requirements and minimize the number and types of forms required. Examples are provided later in the chapter.

The rehabilitation assessment must document (1) identification of strengths, abilities, needs, and preferences (SNAP) of the patient; (2) desired outcomes and expectations of the patient; (3) outcomes anticipated by the interdisciplinary team; (4) the use of assistive technology as needed; and (5) the use of assessment findings to direct the development of the individual's plan.

Reimbursement and Funding

Equitable reimbursement for rehabilitation cannot be made on the basis of diagnosis related groups (DRGs), because many factors other than those considered by the DRG system determine the patient's functional level and thus the recovery of the patient. In other words, two patients with an identical diagnosis can have different functional

‖‖‖‖‖‖‖‖‖‖‖‖‖

OTD

Patient Sticker

COX HEALTH SYSTEMS
Springfield, Mo
OCCUPATIONAL THERAPY
EVALUATION/DISCHARGE SUMMARY

Diagnosis: _____

Medical History: _____

Precautions: _____

Prior Level of Functioning: _____

Communication/Hearing: _____ Hand Dominance: Right_____ Left_____

MUSCULOSKELETAL: RIGHT   LEFT

	PROM		AROM		STRENGTH		PROM		AROM		STRENGTH	
	INITIAL	D/C	INITIAL	D/C	INITIAL	D/C	INITIAL	D/C	INITIAL	D/C	INITIAL	D/C
SHO flex/ext												
ab/add												
hor ab/add												
int/ext rot												
ELBOW												
flex/ext												
WRIST												
flex/ext												

OTHER _____

EDEMA/TONE _____

PAIN No Pain 0 1 2 3 4 5 6 7 8 9 10   Worst Possible Pain

	RIGHT		LEFT		KEY:	+ = WNL
	INITIAL	D/C	INITIAL	D/C		- = IMPAIRED
GRIP	#	#	#	#		U = UNABLE TO ASSESS
3 JAW PINCH	#	#	#	#		S = SAME AS INITIAL
LATERAL PINCH	#	#	#	#		0 = ABSENT
9 HOLE PEG	sec	sec	sec	sec		NA = NOT ASSESSED

= pounds

SHO = Shoulder
HOR = Horizontal

	RIGHT		LEFT	
SENSORY	INITIAL	D/C	INITIAL	D/C
Light Touch				
Stereognosis				
Sharp/Dull				
Proprioception/Kinesthesia				

PERCEPTION/VISION	INITIAL	D/C
Body Scheme		
Neglect		
Tracking		
Spatial Relations		

HOME ACCESSIBILITY: _____

PRIOR EQUIPMENT USE: _____

POTENTIAL EQUIPMENT NEEDS: _____

VOCATIONAL/SOCIAL: _____

WHITE COPY - Patient's Medical Chart   YELLOW - Department Copy   PINK - Leave on chart until original in chart then discard
CPS 430 11/90; Revised 10/96 page 1 of 3

Figure 11-2   An excerpt from an evaluation/discharge summary for occupational therapy. (Courtesy Cox Health Systems, Springfield, MO.)

Occupational Therapy Eval/Discharge Summary   Patient Sticker

SELF CARE SKILLS: KEY: 7. COMPLETE INDEPENDENCE
                                      6. MODIFIED INDEPENDENCE   3. MODERATE ASSIST (Pt Does 50%)
                                      5. SUPERVISION   2. MAXIMAL ASSIST (Pt Does 25%)
                                      4. MINIMAL (Pt Does 75%)   1. TOTAL ASSIST (Pt Does 0%)

BALANCE: Sit/Stand Initial: _____   _____

    Discharge: _____   _____

MOBILITY: Bed/W/C Initial: _____   _____

    Discharge: _____   _____

TRANSFERS: Initial: _____   _____

    Discharge: _____   _____

FEEDING: Initial:_____   _____

    Discharge: _____   _____

GROOMING: Initial: _____   _____

    Discharge: _____   _____

DRESSING: Initial: _____   _____

    Discharge: _____   _____

BATHING: Initial:_____   _____

    Discharge: _____   _____

TOILETING: Initial: _____   _____

    Discharge: _____   _____

PROB SOLVING: Initial: _____   _____

    Discharge: _____   _____

MEMORY: Initial: _____   _____

    Discharge: _____   _____

SAFETY/JUDGEMENT: _____   _____

    Discharge: _____   _____

ASSESSMENT:

    Strengths:_____

    Needs:_____

    Abilities:_____

    Preferences:_____

    Comments:_____

PROBLEM LIST

____ ↓ 'd Functional Transfer Skills	____ Abnormal Tone	____ ↓'d Safety Awareness
____ ↓ 'd Functional Mobility	____ Edema	____ ↓ 'd Functional Positioning
____ ↓ 'd Self-Care Skills	____ ↓ 'd Awareness of Affected UE	____ ↓'d Endurance/Activity Tolerance
____ ↓ 'd ROM/Contractures	____ ↓ 'd Visual Field/Vision	____ ↓ 'd Home/Community Skills
____ ↓ 'd UE Strength	____ ↓ 'd Sensory Awareness	____ ↓ 'd Safe Home Environment
____ ↓ 'd Functional Use of Rt UE/Lt UE	____ ↓ 'd Perceptual Skills	____ Other _____
____ ↓ 'd Fine/Gross Motor Coordination	____ ↓'d Cognitive Skills	

WHITE COPY - Patient's Medical Chart   YELLOW - Department Copy   PINK - Leave on chart until original in chart then discard
CPS 430 11/90; Revised 10/96 page 2 of 3

Figure 11-2   (*Continued*)

Occupational Therapy Eval/Discharge Summary   Patient Sticker

OTD

TREATMENT PLAN

____Functional Transfer Training   ____Normalization of Tone   ____Positioning Training

____Functional Mobility Skills   ____Orthotic/Splinting   ____Energy Conservation/Work Simplification

____Self-care Retraining   ____Edema Control Techniques   ____Household/Community Skills Training

____Therapeutic UE Exercises   ____Sensory Re-education   ____Home Safety Training

____Neuro. Re-education   ____Visual /Perceptual Retraining ____Home Visit

____Functional Activities   ____Cognitive Retraining   ____Other:_____

____Patient/Family Education   ____Community Reintegration   _____

PATIENT/FAMILY GOALS:_____

Patient will be seen BID, 5 days/week and daily on Saturday based on pt needs, for the following plan of care:

INITIAL/SHORT TERM GOALS:

1._____TIME FRAME:_____

2._____TIME FRAME:_____

3._____TIME FRAME:_____

4._____TIME FRAME:_____

5._____TIME FRAME:_____

LONG TERM GOAL(S):

1._____

2._____

POTENTIAL FOR REHAB:_____ ELOS:_____

THERAPIST:_____DATE:_____

FOR DISCHARGE USE ONLY

RECOMMENDATIONS/REFERRALS:_____

_____

PATIENT/FAMILY EDUCATION/HOME PROGRAM/SERVICES PROVIDED:_____

_____

_____

EQUIPMENT/DME ISSUED/RECOMMENDED:_____

_____

THERAPIST:_____DATE:_____

WHITE COPY - Patient's Medical Chart   **YELLOW** - Department Copy   **PINK** - Leave on chart until original in chart then discard
CPS 430 11/90; Revised 10/96 page 3 of 3

Figure 11-2   (*Continued*)

problems and handicaps based on a host of factors. (Recall the previous discussion of the definitions of *impairment, disability,* and *handicap.*) These factors include age, weight, gender, comorbidities, psychological factors, premorbid personality, educational status, and occupation, to name a few. Implemented in January 2002, the Medicare inpatient rehabilitation facility prospective payment system (IRF PPS) does consider more than the patient's diagnoses and procedures, but it does not take into account every factor that affects the patient's recovery.

Under the IRF PPS, a rehabilitation hospital is reimbursed for each patient admission. Patients are placed into one of 100 **case-mix groups (CMGs)**, which determines the payment the facility will receive from Medicare. The factors that influence the assignment of a case into a particular CMG include rehabilitation impairment categories (RICs), functional measurements, age, and comorbidities. ICD-9-CM codes determine the RICs, which group cases that are similar in clinical characteristics and resource use. Functional measures that influence CMG assignment are motor and cognitive scores. Some CMG categories also consider the patient's age. Finally, comorbidities, or secondary diagnoses, affect CMG assignment and are classified into three categories, or tiers, based on whether the costs are considered high, medium, or low (CMS, 2003). Ninety-five of the 100 CMGs will be subject to 4 weights—the 3 that reflect comorbidities and 1 for patients with no comorbidities. The IRF PPS has increased emphasis on ICD-9-CM coding because the CMG payment is influenced by RICs, which correspond to certain categories of ICD-9-CM codes, and also by comorbidities, which are reported directly as ICD-9-CM codes.

In addition, a length of stay is assigned to each CMG under the payment system. Providers know that these lengths of stay are merely averages, and many patients have longer or shorter lengths of stay than the time outlined in the regulations. However, CMGs have required rehabilitation hospitals to give attention to the length of time it takes to treat patients. See Figure 11-3 for an excerpt from the CMG table demonstrating the assignment of relative weights and average lengths of stay for selected CMGs (CMS, 2001).

The CMG assignment is based on information recorded on the patient assessment tool: the **Inpatient Rehabilitation Facility Patient Assessment Instrument (IRF-PAI)**

EXAMPLES OF RELATIVE WEIGHTS FOR CASE-MIX GROUPS (CMGs)

CMG	CMG description (M=motor, C=cognitive, A=age)	Relative weights				Average length of stay			
		Tier 1	Tier 2	Tier 3	None	Tier 1	Tier 2	Tier 3	None
0101	Stroke; M=69–84 and C=23–35	0.4778	0.4279	0.4078	0.3859	10	9	6	8
0102	Stroke; M=59–68 and C=23–35	0.6506	0.5827	0.5553	0.5255	11	12	10	10
0103	Stroke; M=59–84 and C=5–22	0.8296	0.7430	0.7080	0.6700	14	12	12	12
0104	Stroke; M=53–58	0.9007	0.8067	0.7687	0.7275	17	13	12	13
0105	Stroke; M=47–52	1.1339	1.0155	0.9677	0.9158	16	17	15	15

Figure 11-3 Examples of relative weights for case-mix groups (CMGs). (CMS, 2001, August 7, p. 41394.)

(see Figure 11-4). This tool captures all of the information necessary to assign a CMG, including codes for up to 10 comorbidities. The IRF-PAI must be completed upon the patient's admission and again at discharge, with the admission and discharge data transmitted together after the patient has been discharged. The data from the IRF-PAI must be **encoded** (i.e., entered into a specified computer program) before transmission. CMS published an assessment schedule in the IRF PPS rule that specifies dates by which the admission and discharge assessments must be performed, encoded, and transmitted. There is a 25 percent penalty deducted from the IRF PPS payment for data transmitted more than 10 calendar days late (CMS, 2001).

Information Management

Information Flow

The medical record is initiated during admission to the rehabilitation care system and is maintained as an interdisciplinary unit. Each member of the interdisciplinary team records observations on a daily basis. If the treatment areas are in separate parts of the hospital, then the medical record goes with the patient to the treatment areas.

Coding

The system utilized for diagnostic coding is ICD-9-CM. The codes most frequently reported include those that classify neurologic conditions, musculoskeletal disorders, and amputations. Diagnoses encountered frequently in rehabilitation include neurogenic bladder, fibromyalgia, decubitus ulcer (or pressure sore), spasticity, urinary tract infection, cerebral palsy, and below-the-knee amputation.

Physicians use *Current Procedural Terminology (CPT)* for reporting services provided. Rehabilitation physicians generally address a host of issues on a follow-up visit, frequently utilizing time spent in counseling and coordination of care or complexity of medical decision making as major criteria for coding evaluation and management services. Other common rehabilitation services that would be coded are trigger point injections, motor point blocks, final reports and ratings, medical management conferences, and physician review of care plan.

For inpatient rehabilitation facilities, the ICD-9-CM coding rules differ for the IRF-PAI and the facility's billing form, the UB-92. Unlike the UB-92, the IRF-PAI does not capture the principal diagnosis, but reports the etiologic diagnosis instead. For example, consider the case of a patient who had previously suffered an intracerebral hemorrhage treated at an acute care hospital and who was subsequently admitted to the IRF for rehabilitation for the late effects of the hemorrhage. For the UB-92, the IRF would report the principal diagnosis as a "V code" for admission for rehabilitation. However, on the IRF-PAI, the code for intracerebral hemorrhage would be reported as the etiologic diagnosis. No V code would be reported on the IRF-PAI, and intracerebral hemorrhage would not be reported on the UB-92 (Trela, 2002).

INPATIENT REHABILITATION FACILITY - PATIENT ASSESSMENT INSTRUMENT

Identification Information*

1. Facility Information
   A. Facility Name
   _____
   _____
   _____

   B. Facility Medicare
      Provider Number _____

2. Patient Medicare Number _____

3. Patient Medicaid Number _____

4. Patient First Name _____

5A. Patient Last Name _____

5B. Patient Identification Number _____

6. Birth Date _____ / _____ / _____
                MM / DD / YYYY

7. Social Security Number _____

8. Gender (1 - Male; 2 - Female) _____

9. Race/Ethnicity (Check all that apply)
   American Indian or Alaska Native   A. _____
   Asian   B. _____
   Black or African American   C. _____
   Hispanic or Latino   D. _____
   Native Hawaiian or Other Pacific Islander E. _____
   White   F. _____

10. Marital Status _____
    (1 - Never Married; 2 - Married; 3 - Widowed;
     4 - Separated; 5 - Divorced)

11. Zip Code of Patient's Pre-Hospital Residence _____

Admission Information*

12. Admission Date _____ / _____ / _____
                    MM / DD / YYYY

13. Assessment Reference Date _____ / _____ / _____
                               MM / DD / YYYY

14. Admission Class _____
    (1 - Initial Rehab; 2 - Evaluation; 3 - Readmission;
     4 - Unplanned Discharge; 5 - Continuing Rehabilitation)

15. Admit From
    (01 - Home; 02 - Board & Care; 03 - Transitional Living;
     04 - Intermediate Care; 05 - Skilled Nursing Facility;
     06 - Acute Unit of Own Facility; 07 - Acute Unit of Another
     Facility; 08 - Chronic Hospital; 09 - Rehabilitation Facility;
     10 - Other; 12 - Alternate Level of Care Unit; 13 – Subacute
     Setting; 14 - Assisted Living Residence)

16. Pre-Hospital Living Setting _____
    (Use codes from item 15 above)

17. Pre-Hospital Living With _____
    (Code only if item 16 is 01 - Home;
     Code using 1 - Alone; 2 - Family/Relatives;
     3 - Friends; 4 - Attendant; 5 - Other)

18. Pre-Hospital Vocational Category _____
    (1 - Employed; 2 - Sheltered; 3 - Student;
     4 - Homemaker; 5 - Not Working; 6 - Retired for
     Age; 7 - Retired for Disability)

19. Pre-Hospital Vocational Effort _____
    (Code only if item 18 is coded 1 - 4; Code using
     1 - Full-time; 2 - Part-time; 3 - Adjusted Workload)

Payer Information*

20. Payment Source
    A. Primary Source _____

    B. Secondary Source _____

    (01 - Blue Cross; 02 - Medicare non-MCO;
     03 - Medicaid non-MCO; 04 - Commercial Insurance;
     05 - MCO HMO; 06 - Workers' Compensation;
     07 - Crippled Children's Services; 08 – Developmental
     Disabilities Services; 09 - State Vocational Rehabilitation;
     10 - Private Pay; 11 - Employee Courtesy;
     12 - Unreimbursed; 13 - CHAMPUS; 14 - Other;
     15 - None; 16 – No-Fault Auto Insurance;
     51 – Medicare MCO; 52 - Medicaid MCO)

Medical Information*

21. Impairment Group _____   _____
                      Admission Discharge
    Condition requiring admission to rehabilitation; code
    according to Appendix A, attached.

22. Etiologic Diagnosis _____
    (Use an ICD-9-CM code to indicate the etiologic problem
    that led to the condition for which the patient is receiving
    rehabilitation)

23. Date of Onset of Impairment _____ / _____ / _____
                                 MM / DD / YYYY

24. Comorbid Conditions; Use ICD-9-CM codes to enter up to
    ten medical conditions

    A. _____   B. _____

    C. _____   D. _____

    E. _____   F. _____

    G. _____   H. _____

    I. _____   J. _____

Medical Needs

25. Is patient comatose at admission? _____
                                      0 - No, 1 - Yes

26. Is patient delirious at admission? _____
                                       0 - No, 1 - Yes

27. Swallowing Status _____   _____
                      Admission Discharge

    3 - Regular Food: solids and liquids swallowed safely
        without supervision or modified food consistency
    2 - Modified Food Consistency/ Supervision: subject
        requires modified food consistency and/or needs
        supervision for safety
    1 - Tube /Parenteral Feeding: tube / parenteral feeding
        used wholly or partially as a means of sustenance

28. Clinical signs of dehydration _____   _____
                                  Admission Discharge

    (Code 0 – No; 1 – Yes) e.g., evidence of oliguria, dry
    skin, orthostatic hypotension, somnolence, agitation

*The FIM data set, measurement scale and impairment
codes incorporated or referenced herein are the property of
U B Foundation Activities, Inc. © 1993, 2001 U B Foundation
Activities, Inc. The FIM mark is owned by UBFA, Inc.

OMB-0938-0842 (expires: 07-31-2005)

Figure 11-4   Inpatient Rehabilitation Facility Patient Assessment Instrument (IRF-PAI).
(Reprinted with permission of UB Foundation Activities, Inc.)

INPATIENT REHABILITATION FACILITY - PATIENT ASSESSMENT INSTRUMENT
Page 2

Function Modifiers* | **39. FIM™ Instrument***

Complete the following specific functional items prior to scoring the FIM™ Instrument:

	ADMISSION	DISCHARGE
29. Bladder Level of Assistance (Score using FIM Levels 1 - 7)	☐	☐
30. Bladder Frequency of Accidents (Score as below)	☐	☐

7 - No accidents
6 - No accidents; uses device such as a catheter
5 - One accident in the past 7 days
4 - Two accidents in the past 7 days
3 - Three accidents in the past 7 days
2 - Four accidents in the past 7 days
1 - Five or more accidents in the past 7 days

Enter in Item 39G (Bladder) the lower (more dependent) score from Items 29 and 30 above.

	ADMISSION	DISCHARGE
31. Bowel Level of Assistance (Score using FIM Levels 1 - 7)	☐	☐
32. Bowel Frequency of Accidents (Score as below)	☐	☐

7 - No accidents
6 - No accidents; uses device such as an ostomy
5 - One accident in the past 7 days
4 - Two accidents in the past 7 days
3 - Three accidents in the past 7 days
2 - Four accidents in the past 7 days
1 - Five or more accidents in the past 7 days

Enter in Item 39H (Bowel) the lower (more dependent) score of Items 31 and 32 above.

	ADMISSION	DISCHARGE
33. Tub Transfer	☐	☐
34. Shower Transfer	☐	☐

(Score Items 33 and 34 using FIM Levels 1 - 7; use 0 if activity does not occur) See training manual for scoring of Item 39K (Tub/Shower Transfer)

	ADMISSION	DISCHARGE
35. Distance Walked	☐	☐
36. Distance Traveled in Wheelchair	☐	☐

(Code items 35 and 36 using: 3 - 150 feet; 2 - 50 to 149 feet; 1 - Less than 50 feet; 0 – activity does not occur)

	ADMISSION	DISCHARGE
37. Walk	☐	☐
38. Wheelchair	☐	☐

(Score Items 37 and 38 using FIM Levels 1 - 7; 0 if activity does not occur) See training manual for scoring of Item 39L (Walk/Wheelchair)

*The FIM data set, measurement scale and impairment codes incorporated or referenced herein are the property of U B Foundation Activities, Inc. ©1993, 2001 U B Foundation Activities, Inc. The FIM mark is owned by UBFA, Inc.

39. FIM™ Instrument*

	ADMISSION	DISCHARGE	GOAL
SELF-CARE A. Eating	☐	☐	☐
B. Grooming	☐	☐	☐
C. Bathing	☐	☐	☐
D. Dressing - Upper	☐	☐	☐
E. Dressing - Lower	☐	☐	☐
F. Toileting	☐	☐	☐
SPHINCTER CONTROL G. Bladder	☐	☐	☐
H. Bowel	☐	☐	☐
TRANSFERS I. Bed, Chair, Whlchair	☐	☐	☐
J. Toilet	☐	☐	☐
K. Tub, Shower	☐	☐	☐

W - Walk
C - wheelChair
B - Both

	ADMISSION		DISCHARGE		GOAL
LOCOMOTION L. Walk/Wheelchair	☐	☐	☐	☐	☐
M. Stairs	☐		☐		☐

A - Auditory
V - Visual
B - Both

	ADMISSION		DISCHARGE		GOAL
COMMUNICATION N. Comprehension	☐	☐	☐	☐	☐
O. Expression	☐	☐	☐	☐	☐

V - Vocal
N - Nonvocal
B - Both

	ADMISSION	DISCHARGE	GOAL
SOCIAL COGNITION P. Social Interaction	☐	☐	☐
Q. Problem Solving	☐	☐	☐
R. Memory	☐	☐	☐

FIM LEVELS
No Helper
7 Complete Independence (Timely, Safely)

6 Modified Independence (Device)

Helper - Modified Dependence
5 Supervision (Subject = 100%)

4 Minimal Assistance (Subject = 75% or more)

3 Moderate Assistance (Subject = 50% or more)

Helper - Complete Dependence
2 Maximal Assistance (Subject = 25% or more)

1 Total Assistance (Subject less than 25%)

0 Activity does not occur; Use this code only at admission

OMB-0938-0842 (expires: 07-31-2005)

Figure 11-4 (*Continued*)

INPATIENT REHABILITATION FACILITY - PATIENT ASSESSMENT INSTRUMENT
Page 3

Discharge Information*

40. Discharge Date _____/_____/_____
    MM / DD / YYYY

41. Patient discharged against medical advice? _____
    (0 - No, 1 - Yes)

42. Program Interruption(s) _____
    (0 - No; 1 - Yes)

43. Program Interruption Dates
    (Code only if Item 42 is 1 - Yes)

    A. 1st Interruption Date   B. 1st Return Date

    [   ]   [   ]

    MM / DD / YYYY   MM / DD / YYYY

    C. 2nd Interruption Date   D. 2nd Return Date

    [   ]   [   ]

    MM / DD / YYYY   MM / DD / YYYY

    E. 3rd Interruption Date   F. 3rd Return Date

    [   ]   [   ]

    MM / DD / YYYY   MM / DD / YYYY

44A. Discharge to Living Setting _____
    (01 - Home; 02 - Board and Care; 03 - Transitional
    Living; 04 - Intermediate Care; 05 - Skilled Nursing
    Facility; 06 - Acute Unit of Own Facility; 07 - Acute Unit of
    Another Facility; 08 - Chronic Hospital; 09 - Rehabilitation
    Facility; 10 - Other; 11 - Died; 12 - Alternate Level of Care Unit;
    13 - Subacute Setting; 14 - Assisted Living Residence)

44B. Was patient discharged with Home Health Services? _____
    (0 - No; 1 - Yes)
    (Code only if Item 44A is 01 - Home, 02 - Board and Care,
    03 - Transitional Living, or 14 - Assisted Living Residence)

45. Discharge to Living With _____
    (Code only if Item 44A is 01 - Home; Code using 1 - Alone;
    2 - Family / Relatives; 3 - Friends; 4 - Attendant; 5 - Other

46. Diagnosis for Interruption or Death _____
    (Code using ICD-9-CM code)

47. Complications during rehabilitation stay
    (Use ICD-9-CM codes to specify up to six conditions that
    began with this rehabilitation stay)

    A. _____   B. _____

    C. _____   D. _____

    E. _____   F. _____

Quality Indicators

RESPIRATORY STATUS
(Score items 48 to 50 as 0 - No; 1 - Yes)

	Admission	Discharge
48. Shortness of breath with exertion	_____	_____
49. Shortness of breath at rest	_____	_____
50. Weak cough and difficulty clearing airway secretions	_____	_____

* The FIM data set, measurement scale and impairment codes
incorporated or referenced herein are the property of U B
Foundation Activities, Inc. ©1993, 2001 U B Foundation Activities,
Inc. The FIM mark is owned by UBFA, Inc.

Quality Indicators

PAIN
51. Rate the highest level of pain reported by the patient within
    the assessment period:
    Admission: _____ Discharge: _____

    (Score using the scale below; report whole numbers only)

    0   1   2   3   4   5   6   7   8   9   10
    | | |
    No   Moderate   Worst
    Pain   Pain   Possible Pain

Pressure Ulcers

52A. Highest current pressure ulcer stage
    Admission _____ Discharge _____

    (0 - No pressure ulcer; 1 - Any area of persistent skin
    redness (Stage 1); 2 - Partial loss of skin layers (Stage
    2); 3 - Deep craters in the skin (Stage 3); 4 - Breaks in
    skin exposing muscle or bone (Stage 4); 5 - Not
    stageable (necrotic eschar predominant; no prior
    staging available)

52B. Number of current pressure ulcers
    Admission _____ Discharge _____

PUSH Tool v. 3.0 ©

SELECT THE CURRENT LARGEST PRESSURE ULCER TO
CODE THE FOLLOWING. Calculate three components (C
through E) and code total score in F.

52C. Length multiplied by width (open wound surface area)
    Admission _____ Discharge _____

    (Score as   0 - 0 cm²; 1 - < 0.3 cm²; 2 - 0.3 to 0.6 cm²;
    3 - 0.7 to 1.0 cm²; 4 - 1.1 to 2.0 cm²; 5 - 2.1 to 3.0 cm²;
    6 - 3.1 to 4.0 cm²; 7 - 4.1 to 8.0 cm²; 8 - 8.1 to
    12.0 cm²; 9 - 12.1 to 24.0 cm²; 10 - > 24 cm²)

52D. Exudate amount
    Admission _____ Discharge _____
    0 - None; 1 - Light; 2 - Moderate; 3 - Heavy

52E. Tissue type
    Admission _____ Discharge _____
    0 - Closed/resurfaced: The wound is completely
    covered with epithelium (new skin); 1 - Epithelial
    tissue: For superficial ulcers, new pink or shiny tissue
    (skin) that grows in from the edges or as islands on the
    ulcer surface. 2 - Granulation tissue: Pink or beefy
    red tissue with a shiny, moist, granular appearance.
    3- Slough: Yellow or white tissue that adheres to the
    ulcer bed in strings or thick clumps or is mucinous.
    4 - Necrotic tissue (eschar): Black, brown, or tan
    tissue that adheres firmly to the wound bed or ulcer
    edges.

52F. TOTAL PUSH SCORE (Sum of above three items – C,
    D and E)
    Admission _____ Discharge _____

SAFETY   Admission   Discharge

53. Balance problem   _____   _____
    (0 - No; 1 - Yes)
    e.g., dizziness, vertigo, or light-headedness

                                                 Discharge
54. Total number of falls during
    the rehabilitation stay   _____

OMB-0938-0842 (expires: 07-31-2005)

Figure 11-4   (*Continued*)

The World Health Organization (WHO) publishes the *International Classification of Functioning, Disability and Health (ICF).* [An earlier version of this publication was known as the *International Classification of Impairments, Disabilities and Handicaps (ICIDH)*]. The *ICF* classifies disability concepts by body functions and structure, activities and participation, and environmental factors (World Health Organization, 2001).

Computer Systems

Computer systems are used administratively in rehabilitation facilities in much the same manner as in other types of health care facilities. However, inpatient rehabilitation facilities have the unique requirement to submit IRF-PAI data to fiscal intermediaries. CMS provides software called IRVEN (Inpatient Rehabilitation Validation and Entry) free of charge to facilities that wish to use it to submit the IRF-PAI data. Vendors and other organizations also license software for submission of IRF-PAI data and often include other capabilities, such as the ability to transmit ORYX data to JCAHO or the ability to benchmark performance against peer facilities.

National Databases

National databases on spinal cord injury and traumatic brain injury are examples of systems that provide efficient large-scale collections of data that facilitate research in rehabilitation and promote uniform treatment, thereby leading to improved functional outcomes.

The National Spinal Cord Injury Data Base is maintained in Birmingham, Alabama, and collects its data from the Model Spinal Cord Injury System. The model system's uniform database is the largest longitudinal data set on spinal cord injury in the world and has collected data since June 1973. Information is collected on 472 variables in each spinal cord injury case, and the model system's database captures approximately 15 percent of all new spinal cord injury cases in the United States.

A similar national database is maintained on traumatic brain injury. Due to the multiple types of brain injuries, it is much more difficult to compare brain injury data than to compare spinal cord injury data.

Other databases track all admissions to rehabilitation units and therapy clinics. A variety of data is collected related to demographics, diagnosis, and outcomes. Specific information collected and amount varies by providers.

Classification Systems Used in Rehabilitation

Numerous classification schemes have developed for both spinal cord–injured individuals and traumatic brain–injured individuals. It is extremely important that a standardized nomenclature system be utilized to facilitate research in spinal cord injury and brain injury.

American Spinal Injury Association Classification System

The international standards for neurologic and functional classification of spinal cord injury have been developed by the American Spinal Injury Association in cooperation with the International Medical Society of Paraplegia. This system of classification standardizes the neurologic motor and sensory examination. It further requires that the diagnosis be stated, giving both a sensory and motor neurologic level and a qualifying statement regarding the completeness of the spinal cord injury. For definitions utilized in the development of classification systems, see Table 11-2.

Besides the classifications of tetraplegia, paraplegia, tetraparesis, and paraparesis, spinal cord injuries must be further classified as to whether they are complete, meaning there is total absence of sensory and motor below the level of the lesion, or incomplete, meaning there is partial preservation of sensory and/or motor functions below the neurologic level of injury.

Of the incomplete spinal cord injury syndromes, several can and do occur with a high degree of frequency and have been assigned to specific nomenclature. These are

Table 11-2 Standardization Classification System Definitions.

Classification	*Definition*
Tetraplegia (or quadriplegia)	Spinal cord injury of the cervical level that leads to neurologic and functional damage of the upper extremities and the lower extremities
Paraplegia	Impairment or loss of motor and/or sensory function in the thoracic, lumbar, or sacral segments of the spinal cord affecting the lower extremities only
Tetraparesis or paraparesis	A relative weakness of the extremities (tetraparesis) or the lower extremities (paraparesis) but not complete paralysis
Central cord syndrome	A lesion occurring in the central region of the spinal cord at the cervical level that produces greater weakness in the upper extremities than in the lower extremities
Brown-Sequard syndrome	A lesion that produces a greater motor and proprioception loss ipsilateral and a contralateral loss of sensitivity to pinprick and temperature
Anterior cord syndrome	A spinal lesion that is vascular in origin and produces a loss of motor function, a deficit in sensitivity to pinprick and temperature while preserving proprioception
Conus medullaris syndrome	This injury occurs when there is damage to the conus of the spinal cord resulting in an areflexic bladder and bowel and lower extremities
Cauda equina syndrome	Injury to the lumbosacral nerve roots inside the neurocanal before exiting to the peripheral nerves, resulting in an areflexic bladder and lower extremities

defined in Table 11-2. Central cord syndrome is more common in the elderly population. Brown-Sequard syndrome is said to occur when there is a relative hemisection of the spinal cord with the contralateral side of the spinal cord being preserved. Others are anterior cord syndrome, conus medullaris syndrome, and cauda equina syndrome. The American Spinal Injury Association also publishes a handbook of spinal cord injury classification and nomenclature. See the "Key Resources" section of this chapter for information on how to obtain this document.

It is crucial that accurate spinal cord injury classification be performed by physicians who are caring for spinal cord–injured people so that physicians who come in contact with the patient later will be able to accurately determine if there has been a change in the neurologic status of the patient.

Traumatic Brain Injury Classification Systems

Traumatic brain injury classification systems have evolved, and two primary systems are useful in rehabilitation. One is the Glasgow Coma Scale used early after injury in the emergency room (ER) and in the first few days of hospitalization. The other is the Rancho Los Amigos Levels of Cognitive Function Scale, which is useful in communicating the patient's recovery from traumatic brain injury.

The Glasgow Coma Scale measures three areas: eye opening on a scale of 4 to 1, best motor response on a scale of 6 to 1, and verbal response on a scale of 5 to 1. The range for a Glasgow Coma Scale is 3 to 15. The lowest score possible is 3; a person dead on arrival at an ER would score a 3. The Glasgow Coma Scale scores recorded at the arrival to the ER and on the second, third, fourth, and seventh postinjury days are extremely predictive of the patient's outcome. Glasgow Coma Scale scores of 8 or less are associated with poor outcomes (see Figure 11-5).

The Rancho Los Amigos Scale goes from 1 to 8. A level of 1 or 2 is consistent with a coma or a near-coma state. A level 8 is purposeful and appropriate behavior. The Rancho Los Amigos Scale is extremely beneficial in communicating to other members of the rehabilitation team the patient's level of recovery, and thereby infers what level of treatment is appropriate at that point. In general terms, once a patient has reached level 6 or above, he or she is ready for discharge to home. However, the patient may continue to require some outpatient services. A person who has a Rancho Los Amigos Scale of 3 or less is not considered an inpatient rehabilitation candidate and would be better served in a coma stimulation program (see Figure 11-6).

Self-Care Assessment Scales

A number and variety of tools have been developed to assist in assessing the functional status of the patient in areas addressing bathing, grooming, toileting, and so forth. Some common scales include the Katz index, the Barthel index, and functional independent measures. Deciding which functional assessment tool is most useful depends on the individual institution and patient population that is served.

GLASGOW COMA SCALE

Best Eye Response (4)

1. No eye opening
2. Eye opening to pain
3. Eye opening to verbal command
4. Eyes open spontaneously

Best Verbal Response (5)

1. No verbal response
2. Incomprehensible sounds
3. Inappropriate words
4. Confused
5. Orientated

Best Motor Response (6)

1. No motor response
2. Extension to pain
3. Flexion to pain
4. Withdrawal from pain
5. Localizes pain
6. Obeys commands

Figure 11-5 The Glasgow Coma Scale. Reprinted with permission from Elsevier. (*The Lancet*, 1974, Vol. 2, Teasdale and Jennett, p. 81, "Assessment of coma and impaired consciousness.")

    I. No response
   II. Generalized response to stimulation
  III. Localized response to stimuli
   IV. Confused and agitated behavior
    V. Confused with inappropriate behavior (nonagitated)
   VI. Confused but appropriate behavior
  VII. Automatic and appropriate behavior
 VIII. Purposeful and appropriate behavior

Figure 11-6 Rancho Los Amigos Levels of Cognitive Function Scale. (Courtesy Rancho Los Amigos Medical Center, Downey, CA, Adult Brain Injury Service.)

Functional Independence Measure Scores

The functional independence measure (FIM™) instrument evolved from a task force of the American Congress of Rehabilitation Medicine and the American Academy of Physical Medicine and Rehabilitation, and has established itself as an extremely reliable and valid instrument to document the severity of disabilities as well as outcomes in rehabilitation (FIM™ is a trademark of the Uniform Data System for Medical Rehabilitation, a division of UB Foundation Activities, Inc.). FIM is the most commonly used measure of independence, and, due to its reliability and validity, it has been incorporated into the IRF-PAI (see page 2 of the IRF-PAI in Figure 11-4). FIM scores are issued in 13 motor areas and 5 cognitive areas. The motor areas include self-care (e.g., eating, grooming, bathing, dressing, and toileting), sphincter control (e.g., bowel and bladder management), mobility transfers, and locomotion. The cognitive areas include comprehension, expression, social interaction, problem solving, and memory.

Each area receives a score that ranges from 1 to 7. A score of 1 means that the individual requires total assistance, and 7 means that the individual is totally independent. In any given functional category, a score of 1 to 5 means that the patient requires the assistance of another person for that function.

FIM is a highly reproducible and reliable measure of the patient's independence. The FIM scores are repeated on a routine basis to help document the progress or lack of progress of the patient in rehabilitation. If FIM scores do not show an improvement, then the treatment plan must be reevaluated and the patient's plan of treatment modified to meet current needs, or the patient must be placed at maximum medical improvement and discharged from rehabilitation. All members of the rehabilitation team should receive specific training in the proper way to assess the patient and assign FIM scores.

FIM is an excellent technique for almost all rehabilitation problems, including traumatic brain injury, spinal cord injury, stroke, amputations, and medical disability. The reason FIM works well for the various types of disabilities is because it is a measure of the functional status of the patient irrespective of the etiology of the disability.

There are some subsets of patients in which FIM does not work well, including patients who are progressing extremely slowly, or pediatric patients. A separate scale called WEE-FIM® has been developed for pediatric patients.

FIM scores or some other reliable, reproducible measure of functional outcome is required in rehabilitation. It allows the rehabilitation interdisciplinary team to (1) assess functional improvement of the patient and response to the treatment plan; (2) document functional status and thereby needs for discharge planning; (3) establish the beneficial role of the rehabilitation service; (4) justify the treatment and cost incurred; (5) allow rapid communication of a patient's functional status to other interested parties such as third-party payers or other rehabilitation teams that may become involved in the patient's score; and (6) standardize the nomenclature system regarding functional outcome.

Quality Improvement and Program Evaluation Systems

The primary product of rehabilitation is improvement in the patient's functional status. There are three components of quality care: appropriateness of care, technical competence with which the care was given, and patient dignity and involvement. Quality assessment may be done on a multidisciplinary basis by monitoring the different departments and outcomes. For example, an increase in ADL skills can be used to measure quality of services provided by the occupational therapy department; an increase in physical functioning indicates an improved outcome for the physical therapy department; and an increase in cognitive and emotional adaptation by the patient and the family can be used to assess the quality of services by the psychology staff. Quality of outcome is also viewed in terms of the absolute level of independence by the patient, a reduction in the need for caregivers, and the setting to which the patient was discharged.

FIM scores lend themselves readily to quality and outcome measurements. In addition, costs can be analyzed in light of changes in FIM scores. For example, a patient's FIM score could improve from 50 to 75—a gain of 25 points—after several weeks of rehabilitation. If the cost of providing rehabilitation services during that time period was $25,000, then the cost per point-change in FIM score would be $1,000 for that patient.

Program evaluation systems are best organized along diagnostic and functional groups such as general inpatient medical rehabilitation and stroke, spinal cord injury, or traumatic brain injury. Program evaluation and assessments of quality in outcome should continue after discharge. The patient should be seen for a follow-up visit to determine how he is functioning at home, which is the true indicator of the effectiveness of the rehabilitation program.

Risk Management and Legal Issues

The rehabilitation team, its records, and physiatrists are often called on to provide information regarding the disability, functional status, and future needs of an individual with a handicapping condition. This is entirely understandable because the rehabilitation team is the primary caregiver for individuals who have permanent injuries and disabilities. Some of these people have been injured as a result of a motor vehicle accident, work-related injury, or malpractice. The rehabilitation professional is responsible for maximizing the quality of life and functional status, and follows the individual over a lifetime to meet his or her needs related to the injury and the disability. As a result, the physiatrist is frequently called on to render opinions in these areas as an expert witness. The physiatrist is uniquely qualified to provide this service to his or her patient because of the specific training in recovery from injuries, an understanding of the natural history of the disease process, and a working knowledge of the types of equipment and supplies necessary to maximize functional status and preserve health.

The rehabilitation medical records, FIM scores, discharge recommendations, medications, and equipment recommendations are useful to help prepare a **life care plan.**

A life care plan is a "dynamic document based upon published standards of practice, comprehensive assessment, data analysis, and research, which provides an organized concise plan for current and future needs with associated cost, for individuals who have experienced catastrophic injury or have chronic health care needs" (IALCP, No date, p. 1). The life care plan is developed on an individualized basis given that person's unique presentation. It lists the items required over a lifetime for the individual, their cost, and the frequency of replacement. This document serves as a medical legal document that may guide court decisions regarding a settlement. The document could also be used as a guide to provide future medical services for the individual.

Medicare Set-Aside Trust

In 2001, CMS addressed guidelines regarding settlement of claims for individuals with work-related injuries, or injuries covered under other general liability insurance plans. The objective was to ensure that third-party payers do not shift the responsibility for payment of medical services to Medicare (Lump-sum payments, 2002). CMS guidelines require a life care plan be used to assess future medical care in cases where a high level of future care is likely to be required.

Role of the Health Information Manager

The health information professional in a rehabilitation setting may manage traditional types of services related to the creation, development, storage, and retrieval of the patient record and patient information, and as in other settings, has an important part to play in obtaining and maintaining accreditation of the rehabilitation facility. In addition, the health information manager may assist in selecting or developing appropriate forms to track patient outcomes and may work with others to develop and implement quality improvement programs. The health information manager may monitor rates of complications, early discharges, or failures to improve, and present findings that can help target processes for improvement. Some of the trends described in the next section call for the skills of a health information manager. For example, the health information professional may help in the development of **care paths**. A care path is a document outlining the interventions planned and the outcomes expected during each phase of rehabilitation for a particular type of case, and is described in more detail in the section on "Trends" that follows.

Trends

Acute Rehabilitation versus Skilled Nursing

Since 1990, a continuum of nonhospital-based postacute rehabilitation facilities has evolved, which has been driven by economic factors in the American health care delivery system. Earlier discharges from the hospital have resulted in patients being discharged who are unable to care for themselves. Skilled rehabilitation facilities provide a cost-effective, economic system that allows the patient to develop a functional level of independence that would make returning home safe. The level of care offered by rehabilitation units in skilled nursing facilities is generally more cost-effective for older patients who often cannot participate in the intensive rehabilitation programs offered at more acute levels of care. The resulting trend has been toward increasing the number of skilled rehabilitation beds and decreasing the number of acute inpatient rehabilitation beds.

Outpatient Rehabilitation

The same market forces that are driving subacute rehabilitation care are also increasing the demand for outpatient rehabilitation. The cost savings are substantial when rehabilitation services—PT, OT, and speech pathology—can be provided in an outpatient setting. The number of outpatient rehabilitation settings and freestanding rehabilitation clinics has continued to increase in the twenty-first century.

Independent Living

As a result of CMS guidelines regarding reimbursements, individuals who have limiting conditions that reduce their functional status have had little option except discharge to nursing homes. State policy has been influenced by federal policy that provides three-to-one matching funds from the federal government to the state government if the individual resides in a nursing home. A movement has been underway in the disabled community and is gaining momentum and the attention of policy makers in Washington, D.C., to divert some portion of those federal funds to independent living programs. These programs will be specifically designed to provide support services to the individual at the level required to keep the person in his or her home, resulting in decreased morbidity and mortality for the patient and increasing the likelihood that the disabled person will be employable. The independent living movement will continue to progress because of its cost-effectiveness and because health care delivery systems will need to adapt strategies that promote independent living. It will be a challenge for health information management specialists to develop systems of documentation that promote good health care in the independent living situation.

Technology

There is a rapid explosion of technology in rehabilitation. Computer systems are being developed that may some day replace lost vision, and computer-assisted ambulation systems are becoming much more functional and smaller. Robotic devices are now in existence and are able to supplement the missing function of upper extremities. This technology is in its infancy and will continue to grow.

Small pacemaker neurostimulation devices (Neuro-Control) are now commonly implanted in the brachial plexus to replace lost motor function in the upper extremities, and similar devices can be used to cause a neurogenic bladder to function appropriately.

Persons with above-the-knee amputation now have an option of using the C-leg prosthesis, a computerized prosthesis that increases safety while allowing infinite variability in walking cadences.

Care Paths

Care pathways are evolving tools that allow a physician or health care delivery team to provide high-quality, effective care in a systematic fashion. A properly prepared care path will provide overall guidance for the patient's care. Figure 11-7 shows an excerpt from a care path.

Care paths can be beneficial in numerous ways:

1. Standardization of care
2. Efficient resource utilization
3. Enhancement of effectiveness of the interdisciplinary team
4. Decreased length of stay and cost
5. Automation of the medical record

Care paths allow a rehabilitation team to readily recognize if a person is not progressing as expected. When care paths are adequately planned and developed, redundant documentation and redundant forms in a record system are eliminated. The care paths themselves serve as educational tools for the staff members as well as the patient.

Care paths are expensive to develop. They take a tremendous amount of effort on the part of the rehabilitation team; typically from 1.5 to 2.5 years are required due to the complex nature of neurologic injuries and rehabilitation. The individual team members who serve on the care path committee must have a keen insight into the process of rehabilitation and recovery in order to develop an adequate care path. Care paths may stifle or reduce creativity or produce a relative resistance to changes or trends within the field and must be monitored closely and updated frequently in order to be effective. A major drawback is the tendency of individuals to view variances from the care path as a deviance below some standard of care. A **variance** is simply any event that falls outside the expected course of recovery and outcome as outlined in the care path.

Health information managers will be called on to assist rehabilitation programs in developing and updating care paths for specific types of disabilities. These care paths will serve as standard protocol for treatment for the uncomplicated patient. Care paths must be developed specifically for each institution in which they are used and must be approved by the medical staff involved. When the care path mentions a specific protocol such as PT protocol or OT protocol, there is a very specialized protocol that has been developed in these areas that must be readily available to all members of the health care team. Variances are measured in three areas: patient variance, provider variance, and system variance. Care paths are extremely difficult to develop in rehabilitation because of the variety of functional problems associated with a given disability.

An effective care path permits documentation by exception. When the care path adequately describes the patient's rehabilitation course, the team members may use

RNPATH

COX MEDICAL CENTERS
Springfield, MO. 65807
CAREPATH TOTAL KNEE REHAB

Code Status: _____

PATIENT STICKER

	ADMIT ORDERS	EVALUATION PHASE LEVEL I –Date_____		Admit FIM (1st 24 hours)
		INTERVENTIONS	OUTCOMES	
PRECAUTIONS (falls, infections, behavior, cardiac, siezures, anticoag., swallowing, diet, weight-bearing,, Adv. Directive, Diabetes)	Wt.bearing:_____ Anticoagulation:_____ _____ Continue TEDS SCDs if currently in use CPM if currently in use	Anticoagulation precautions Fall precautions	Free of complications that prohibit participation in therapies	
DIAGNOSTICS (special procedures/tests)		Anticoagulation labs	Therapeutic levels maintained	
TREATMENTS	Ice pack prn operative knee Drsg. change PRN	Ice packs prn per patient Gravity stretch with meals Ankle pumps/quad sets b.i.d.	Pt. utilizes ice for control of pain/swelling	
CONSULTS (orthotics / vocational / Dr.)				
NUTRITION	Diet _____	Dietary Screen	Appropriate diet and adequate intake	
DISCHARGE PLANNING	Social Services	Verify patient's discharge needs	Patient and team agree on DC plan and site Proposed DC site_____ Proposed DC Plan_____	
SELF-CARE	OT Eval & Treat May shower; keep wound dry; no tub bath Bowel Protocol	Evaluate toilet transfer: FIM____ Provide appropriate equipment Introduce Adaptive Equipment Bowel Management Protocol	Transfer to BSC/toilet ≥FIM 3 Patient maintains regular bowel habits	1. Eating (OT/RN) _____ 2. Grooming (OT/RN) _____ 3. Bathing (OT/RN) _____ 4. Dressing UE (OT/RN) _____ 5. Dressing LE (OT/RN) _____ 6. Toileting (OT/RN) _____ 7. Bladder mgmt.(RN) _____ 8. Bowel mgmt. (RN) _____
ACTIVITY / MOBILITY	Protocol Total Knee Rehab (PT) Activity: Up as tolerated	Bed / chair transfers FIM ____ Follow Level I PT protocol	Ambulate 40' SBA in P.T. ≥FIM 1 Wheelchair used to therapies, bathroom, etc. ROM:_____	9. Bed/Chair (PT/OT) _____ 10. Toilet (OT/RN) _____ 11. Tub/Shower (OT/RN) _____ 12. Walk/W/C (PT) _____ 13. Stair ↑↓ (PT) _____
COGNITION / COMMUNICATION		Cognitive Screen per OT/RN	Comprehension, expression, problem-solving & memory ≥FIM 5	MOTOR SUBSCORE _____ 14. Comprehension (RN) _____ 15. Expression (RN) _____
PSYCHOSOCIAL ADJUSTMENT		Monitor patient/family adjustment Review patient/family goals for discharge needs	Communicates needs/concerns to staff Social Interaction ≥ FIM 5	16. Social Interaction (MSW) _____ 17. Problem Solving (OT) _____ 18. Memory (OT) _____
EDUCATION		Introduce orientation manual, education manual, patient path	Verbalizes understanding of purpose of rehab program Verbalizes understanding of precautions	TOTAL ADMIT FIM _____

_____   _____
      physician signature   *date*

SIGNATURE LOG: RN_____   OT_____
(Signature indicates completion of   MSW_____   PT_____
level/attendance at staffing)   Prog. Mgr. _____   Other _____
MAY PROGRESS TO NEXT LEVEL, Team Leader_____   Date_____
✧ indicates key criteria to advance to next level
CPS-1142-1/97

Figure 11-7   An excerpt from a care path for total knee rehabilitation. (Courtesy Cox Health Systems, Springfield, MO.)

COX MEDICAL CENTERS
Springfield, MO. 65807
CAREPATH TOTAL KNEE REHAB

Code Status:

	LEVEL II - SKILLS ACQUISITION PHASE Date(s)		PATIENT STICKER
	INTERVENTIONS	**OUTCOMES**	**TEAM CONFERENCE FIM** Date:_____
PRECAUTIONS (falls, infections, behavior, cardiac, siezures, anticoag., swallowing, diet, weight-bearing, Adv. Directive, Diabetes)	Anticoagulation precautions Fall precautions	Free of complications that prohibit participation in therapies	1. Eating _____ 11. Tub/Shower Tsfr. _____ 2. Grooming _____ 12. Walk/W/C Tsfr. _____ 3. Bathing _____ 13. Stair ↑↓ _____
DIAGNOSTICS (special procedures/tests)	Anticoagulation Labs	Therapeutic levels maintained	4. Dressing UE _____ MOTOR SUBSCORE _____
TREATMENTS	Ice packs prn per patient Gravity stretch with meals Ankle pumps/quad sets b.i.d.	Pt. utilizes ice for control of pain/swelling	5. Dressing LE _____ 14. Comprehension _____ 6. Toileting _____ 15. Expression _____
CONSULTS (orthotics/ vocational /Dr.)			7. Bladder Mgmt. _____ 16. Social Interaction _____
NUTRITION	Diet___ _____	Appropriate diet and adequate intake	8. Bowel Mgmt. _____ 17. Problem Solving _____
DISCHARGE PLANNING	Identify potential follow-up needs Determine need for home eval	Patient/family verbalize potential needs for discharge/follow-up	9. Bed/Chair Tsfr. _____ 18. Memory _____ 10. Toilet Tsfr. _____ FIM TOTAL _____

			GOAL FIM	CURRENT FIM
SELF-CARE	OT evaluate dressing and bathing ADL training Issue adaptive equipment for ADL's as appropriate Self-med Level II Monitor bowel status	Toileting Tasks ≥FIM 4 Toilet transfers ≥FIM 4 Completes simple grooming from W/C, FIM 5 Bathes at preferred location ≥FIM 3 Calls for meds at appropriate time	1. Eating (OT/RN) 7 2. Grooming (OT/RN 5 3. Bathing (OT/RN) 3 4. Dressing UE (OT/RN) 5 5. Dressing LE (OT/RN) 3 6. Toileting (OT/RN) 4 7. Bladder mgmt.(RN) 5 8. Bowel mgmt.(RN) 5	1. Eating (OT/RN) _____ 2. Grooming (OT/RN) _____ 3. Bathing (OT/RN) _____ 4. Dressing UE (OT/RN) _____ 5. Dressing LE (OT/RN) _____ 6. Toileting (OT/RN) _____ 7. Bladder mgmt.(RN) _____ 8. Bowel mgmt.(RN) _____
ACTIVITY / MOBILITY	Level II PT Protocol - gait & transfer training Begin curb training TKA exercise group	✧Ambulates to bathroom Ambulates on even surfaces 50+ feet SBA – FIM 2 ✧ All transfers ≥FIM 4 ↑↓ curb with min A ≥FIM 1 ROM:_____	9. Bed/Chair (PT/OT) 4 10. Toilet (OT/RN) 4 11. Tub/Shower (OT/RN) 1 12. Walk/W/C (PT) 2 13. Stair ↑↓ (PT) 1	9. Bed/Chair (PT/OT) _____ 10. Toilet (OT/RN) _____ 11. Tub/Shower (OT/RN) _____ 12. Walk/W/C (PT) _____ 13. Stair ↑↓ (PT) _____
COGNITION / COMMUNICATION			MOTOR SUBSCORE 49 14. Comprehension (RN) 5 15. Expression (RN) 5	MOTOR SUBSCORE _____ 14. Comprehension (RN) _____ 15. Expression (RN) _____
PSYCHOSOCIAL ADJUSTMENT	Monitor pt/family adjustment for concerns -- ongoing Review patient path / DC goals	Pt. compensates for limitations; willing to learn new way of functioning. Patient verbalizes understanding of and is in agreement with program goals	16. Social Interaction (MSW) 5 17. Problem Solving (OT) 5 18. Memory (OT) 5	16. Social Interaction (MSW) _____ 17. Problem Solving (OT) _____ 18. Memory (OT) _____
EDUCATION	Introduce P.T. home exercise program Educate patient on current meds /self med program & pain control Initiate wound care education	Needs assist with home program Verbalizes pain relief methods Verbalizes understanding of normal surgical wound characteristics	TOTAL FIM 74	TOTAL FIM _____

SIGNATURE LOG:
(Signature indicates completion of level/attendance at staffing)

RN_____ OT_____
MSW_____ PT_____
Prog. Mgr._____ Other_____

MAY PROGRESS TO NEXT LEVEL, Team Leader_____ Date_____

✧ indicates key criteria to advance to next level

CPS-1142-1/97 Page 2 of 5

Figure 11-7 *(Continued)*

the care path to indicate the patient's progress by making notations on the care path when each point of the care path is met. Additional documentation is required only when there is a variance or when the patient does not meet the criteria of the care path. In a system where documentation by exception is utilized, noting the variances that occur is extremely important because such documentation:

1. Allows individualization of the care
2. Requires judgment and team planning
3. Legitimizes documentation by exception
4. Facilitates improvement in performance of the rehabilitation team

It is extremely important for the health information management specialist to be involved in the development of care paths because the care path in some situations is the documentation of the care given. In a well-planned care path where documentation by exception has been utilized, there is little or no duplication in the medical record. Staff time spent in documentation can realistically be cut by two-thirds in such a system.

Although documentation by exception is being used successfully, some have expressed concern that there could be a tendency to minimize documentation of variances. Also, weaknesses in the care path could lead to weaknesses in documentation. Therefore, a facility using documentation by exception must emphasize the importance of thoroughly documenting all variances and the development of extensive, detailed care paths. Furthermore, whenever there is any doubt that the care path is adequate to document a given situation, the caregiver should provide documentation in addition to that provided in the care path.

Summary

Rehabilitation is a continuum of care that spans the entire gamut of disabling conditions, involves all age groups, and is provided in numerous types of health care settings. The field is experiencing enormous growth and evolving trends at a rapid rate. It will be challenging for the health care information specialist to assist in developing medical record systems that improve the quality of care and enhance full team interdisciplinary communication. In addition, as the care pathways evolve to a management by exception level, the health care information specialist's role will be crucial to ensure that adequate documentation is present and that the lines of responsibility and chains of command are well maintained.

Key Terms

acute rehabilitation unit   a designated unit in a hospital where patients can be transferred for rehabilitation after treatment for the original acute illness or injury. Length of stay in these units is typically two to four weeks.

ambulation aids   devices that provide additional stability and support for an individual who has trouble walking.

care path a detailed and extensive document outlining the interventions planned and the outcomes expected during each phase of rehabilitation for a particular type of case. In some facilities, the care path is used for documenting certain events and outcomes that occur during rehabilitation.

case-mix group (CMG) any of 100 categories into which an inpatient rehabilitation stay can be classified based on data submitted on the IRF-PAI. The CMG is determined by factors such as rehabilitation impairment category (RIC), functional measurements, age, and comorbidities

disability a restriction or lack resulting from an impairment of the ability to perform an activity in a manner or within the range considered to be normal for a human being.

documentation by exception providing thorough documentation for events that fall outside the normal course of rehabilitation outlined in a care path, while using notations on the care path to document the events that follow the expected course.

encoding with regard to the IRF-PAI, encoding refers to using a specified computer program to enter data that will subsequently be transmitted to the Centers for Medicare and Medicaid Services (CMS).

environmental control units (ECUs) equipment that allows a person who has limited mobility to perform many functions in the home, such as turning on lights, using appliances, and opening and closing doors and windows.

freestanding rehabilitation hospitals inpatient rehabilitation facilities that may operate both acute and postacute rehabilitation units.

handicap a disadvantage for a given individual resulting from an impairment or a disability that prevents or limits fulfillment of a role that is normal for that individual.

impairment a loss or abnormality of a psychological, physiologic, or anatomic structure or function.

Inpatient Rehabilitation Facility-Patient Assessment Instrument (IRF-PAI) an instrument used to gather data regarding each patient stay that will be used to determine the payment for that stay under the Medicare inpatient rehabilitation facility prospective payment system.

inpatient rehabilitation facility prospective payment system (IRF PPS) the prospective payment system by which inpatient rehabilitation facilities are paid for services provided to Medicare beneficiaries. Each patient stay is categorized into a case-mix group (CMG) that determines the payment that will be received by the facility from Medicare.

Inpatient Rehabilitation Validation and Entry (IRVEN) software provided by CMS for entry of IRF-PAI data.

kinesiotherapist a person with specialized training in the proper techniques to maximize range of motion, strength, balance, and gait.

life care plan a dynamic document that details current and future health care needs based on published standards of practice.

occupational therapist (OT) a therapist who has completed an educational program accredited by the American Occupational Therapy Association at the bachelor's level or higher. OTs address activities of daily living, upper extremity movement, higher cognitive, and community skills, among other areas of rehabilitation.

orthotic device   an external appliance or brace that can supplement an extremity's function or improve stability and positioning.

physiatrist   a physical medicine and rehabilitation physician.

physical therapist (PT)   a therapist who has completed an educational program accredited by the American Physical Therapy Association at the bachelor's level or higher. PTs help patients improve their strength, range of motion, balance, and mobility, among other things.

postacute rehabilitation   rehabilitation involving long-term therapies to maximize functional status. Lengths of patient stay in postacute rehabilitation can vary from four weeks to six months or more.

prosthesis   a device designed to replace a missing extremity or partially missing extremity.

psychologist   a person trained in psychology at the doctoral level who is certified by the American Psychological Association. In rehabilitation, a psychologist tests patients to identify problems in cognition or behavior and counsels the patient and family. A master's-level counselor may also perform some of these duties.

rehabilitation nurse   a registered nurse who has received training and credentialing as a rehabilitation nurse.

rehabilitation social worker   a member of the rehabilitation team who has specific training and knowledge in the area of social work and who may be certified by the National Association of Social Workers. The social worker provides background information on the patient and family, coordinates funding resources, and helps the patient with the transition back to the community.

rehabilitation team   an interdisciplinary team made up of numerous allied health professions.

speech and language pathologist   a rehabilitation team member with a bachelor's or master's level of education who is certified by the American Speech, Language, and Hearing Association. The speech pathologist evaluates and treats patients with swallowing problems, communication problems, and cognitive deficits.

variance   an event or condition that does not follow the expected course of recovery or the expected outcome as outlined in the care path.

REVIEW QUESTIONS

Knowledge-based Questions

1. Define the term rehabilitation.

2. List and describe three various levels of rehabilitative care.

3. List and describe the two ways of organizing rehabilitation teams.

4. Which method of organization for rehabilitation teams is generally considered best and why?

5. List the various medical and other specialists that might be part of a rehabilitation team.

6. List the major categories of disabling conditions.

7. List and give the World Health Organization's definitions of three major terms used to discuss individuals with functional limitations.

8. List, define, and give examples of the five main classes of durable medical equipment used in rehabilitation.

9. List two voluntary accrediting agencies for rehabilitation facilities.

10. What are some of the CMS criteria for inpatient rehabilitation facilities?

11. List the functions of the interdisciplinary team that must be documented in a patient's medical records under CARF guidelines.

12. List the five items the rehabilitation assessment must document under CARF guidelines.

13. Briefly describe the inpatient rehabilitation prospective payment system (IRF PPS).

14. What are FIM scores and how are they used?

15. List six advantages rehabilitation teams reap from using FIM scores.

16. Discuss recent changes in the delivery system of rehabilitative care.

17. What are some of the advantages and disadvantages of using care paths?

18. What roles will the health information manager play in rehabilitation facilities in the future?

Application-based Questions

1. Why is accreditation by CARF important to rehabilitative facilities and their patients? What role will the health information manager play in the CARF accreditation process for his or her rehabilitative facility?

2. What challenges might the health information manager face when implementing care pathways into the rehabilitative care delivery system at his or her facility?

Web Activity

Visit the AHIMA Web site at http://www.ahima.org. If you are a member of AHIMA, log on to the Communities of Practice (CoPs) and visit one of the communities related to rehabilitation, such as the "Rehabilitation Facilities/Units" community or the "Coding (SCC): Physical Medicine and Rehabilitation" community. Within the community you selected, click on some of the links, resources, or discussion threads. Write a brief description of what you learned in this community.

If you are not a member of AHIMA, type the term "rehabilitation" into the "Site Search" blank and look at one or more of the documents returned in response to your query. Write a brief description of what you learned from the documents you reviewed.

Case Study

In monitoring for various complications at XYZ Rehabilitation Hospital, Mary Moore discovers that in many instances patients with deep vein thrombosis or pressure sores are being admitted to the hospital with those conditions. Because rehabilitation cannot proceed until these medical conditions are resolved, these patients may be discharged from rehabilitation to another type of care after a short stay and later readmitted to rehabilitation. Or these conditions may prolong the patient's length of stay in the rehabilitation facility. Mary plans to report these findings to the quality improvement committee.

What recommendations might the committee make regarding these findings? What role can Mary play in improving this situation?

References and Suggested Readings

[AMRPA] American Medical Rehabilitation Providers Association. (2003, May 27). Action Alert. [Online]. http://www.amrpa.org/PDF_Files/052703_Action%20Alert_LoBiondo_75%25_Rule%20_Bill.pdf [2003, July 15].

American Spinal Cord Injury Association. (1990). *Standards for Neurological Classification of Spinal Cord Injured Patients.* Atlanta: American Spinal Cord Injury Association.

American Spinal Cord Injury Association. (1996). *International Standards for Neurological and Functional Classification of SCI.* Chicago, IL: American Spinal Cord Injury Association.

Braddom, R. (Ed.). (2001). *Physical Medicine and Rehabilitation* (2nd ed.). Philadelphia: W. B. Saunders.

[CMS] Centers for Medicare and Medicaid Services. (2001, August 7). Prospective payment system for inpatient rehabilitation facilities; final rule. *Federal Register, 66* (152), 41315–41430.

[CMS] Centers for Medicare and Medicaid Services. (2002). *IRF-PAI Training Manual.* [Online]. http://cms.hhs.gov/providers/irfpps/irfpai-manualint.pdf [2003, July 14].

[CMS] Centers for Medicare and Medicaid Services. (2003). *Medicare Inpatient Rehabilitation Facility Prospective Payment System Training Manual.* [Online]. http://cms.hhs.gov/medlearn/inpatref.asp [2003, July 12].

[CMS] Centers for Medicare and Medicaid Services. (2003, May 16). Inpatient rehabilitation facility prospective payment system for FY 2004; proposed rule. *Federal Register, 68* (95), 26785–26837.

[CMS] Centers for Medicare and Medicaid Services. (2004, May 7). Medicare program; changes to the criteria for being classified as an inpatient rehabilitation facility; final rule. *Federal Register, 69* (89), 25752–25776.

[CMS] Centers for Medicare and Medicaid Services. (No date). Chapter 28: Prospective payments. *Provider Reimbursement Manual: Part I.* [Online]. http://cms.hhs.gov/manuals/pub151/PUB_15_1.asp [2003, July 2].

Conditions of Participation: Comprehensive Outpatient Rehabilitation Facilities, *Code of Federal Regulations*, Title 42, Pt. 485, Subpart B, 1996 ed.

Conditions of Participation for Clinics, Rehabilitation Agencies, and Public Health Agencies as Providers of Outpatient Physical Therapy and Speech-Language Pathology Services, *Code of Federal Regulations*, Title 42, Pt. 485, Subpart H, 1996 ed.

DeLisa, J. A., and Gans, B. M. (1993). *Rehabilitation Medicine: Principles and Practice* (2nd ed.). Philadelphia: J. B. Lippincott.

Excluded hospitals: Classifications, *Code of Federal Regulations*, Title 42, §412.23, 2002 ed.

Granger, C.V., Hamilton, B.B., and Sherwin, F.S. (1986). *Guide for Use of the Uniform Data Set for Medical Rehabilitation*. Buffalo, NY: Uniform Data Systems for Medical Rehabilitation.

Hagen, C., Melkmus, D., and Durham, P. (1979). *Levels of Cognitive Function: Rehabilitation of the Head Injured Adult: Comprehensive Physical Management*. Downey, CA: Professional Staff Association, Rancho Los Amogos Hospital.

Hospital Services Subject to and Excluded from the Prospective Payment System, *Code of Federal Regulations*, Title 42, Pt. 412, Subpart B, 1996 ed.

[IALCP] International Academy of Life Care Planners (No date). [Online]. Introduction. *Standards of Practice*. http://www.internationalacademyoflifecareplanners.com/life_care_planning_guidelines.html#intro [2003, July 15].

Lump-sum payments, *Code of Federal Regulations*, Title 42, §411.46, 2002 ed.

Manley, B. (2003). Workers compensation settlements with Medicare set-aside arrangements: Problem solving the issues. *Journal of Life Care Planning, 2* (1), 25–31.

Stover, S., DeLisa, L., and Whiteneck, G., (1995). *Spinal Cord Injury: Clinical Outcomes from the Model Systems*. Gaithersburg, MD: Aspen Publishers, Inc.

Trela, P. (2002). Inpatient rehabilitation PPS presents new challenges, opportunities. *Journal of the American Hospital Information Management Association, 73* (1), 48A–48D.

World Health Organization. (2001). *International Classification of Functioning, Disability and Health (ICF)*. Geneva, Switzerland: World Health Organization

Key Resources

American Academy of Physical Medicine and Rehabilitation
One IBM Plaza, Suite 2500
Chicago, IL 60611-3604
Phone: 312-464-9700
Fax: 312-464-0227
http://www.aapmr.org

American Medical Rehabilitation Providers Association
1710 N Street, NW
Washington, DC 20036
Toll-Free: 888-346-4624
Phone: 202-223-1920
Fax: 202-223-1925
http://www.amrpa.org

American Spinal Injury Association (ASIA)
345 East Superior St., Room 1436
Chicago, IL 60611
Phone: 312-238-6207
Fax: 312-238-0869
or
2020 Peachtree Road, Northwest
Atlanta, GA 30309
Phone: 404-355-9772
Fax: 404-355-1826
http://www.asia-spinalinjury.org

Commission on Accreditation of Rehabilitation Facilities (CARF)
(See Chapter 1 for contact information.)

International Academy of Life Care Planners
114 NW Fifth Street
Ankeny, IA 50021
Phone: 800-531-5146
Fax: 515-965-1286
http://www.internationalacademyoflifecareplanners.com

Joint Commission on Accreditation of Healthcare Organizations
(See Chapter 1 for contact information.)

National Institute on Disability Research and Rehabilitation (NIDRR)
U.S. Department of Education
400 Maryland Ave. SW
Washington, DC 20202
Phone: 202-205-8134
http://www.ed.gov/offices/OSERS/NIDRR

National Institute of Neurological Disorders and Stroke
Office of Scientific and Health Reports
P.O. Box 5801
Bethesda, MD 20824
Phone: 301-496-5751
Phone: 1-800-352-9424
http://www.ninds.nih.gov

Chapter 12

Home Health Care

Kim A. Boyles, MS, RHIA
Gwen D. Smith, RHIA

Learning Objectives

Upon successful completion of this chapter, you should be able to:

1. Explain the basic operations of a home health care company and identify potential future trends of the industry.
2. Discuss the importance of data collection, analysis, and reporting to be competitive in the current managed care environment.
3. Identify the types and services of home health care agencies.
4. List the advantages of home health care.
5. Explain the growth of home health care.
6. List the agencies or organizations that develop standards for home health care.
7. Explain the purpose of the Outcome and Assessment Information Set (OASIS).
8. Discuss the importance of outcome-based quality improvement (OBQI) and outcome-based quality management (OBQM) in the home care setting.

SETTING	DESCRIPTION	SYNONYMS/EXAMPLES
Home Health Care	A service to the recovering, disabled, or chronically ill person, providing for treatment and/or effective functioning in the home environment (NAHC, 1992)	Home care, visiting nurses, visiting staff

Introduction to Setting

Home health care by definition is a service to the recovering, disabled, or chronically ill person, providing for treatment and/or effective functioning in the home environment (NAHC, 1992). Services provided to patients and their families may be either medical or nonmedical.

Throughout this chapter and in the real world, the term **home health care** is synonymous with home care, visiting nurses, and visiting staff. Home care is an alternative to some procedures and treatments of the traditional hospital or clinic setting. Although it may seem to be a new means of delivering care to patients, it has been around for years. The concept of caring for a very ill patient at home was common in earlier days but was not considered an industry.

Since then, there has been rapid growth in the home care market. The probable reasons for this growth are cost savings, technology, and advances in patients' right to choose. With the implementation of the inpatient prospective payment system, government regulations have forced hospitals to contain their costs, compelling them to utilize other methods to deliver care to their patients. Developing and utilizing home care are solutions to minimizing hospital expenses while maintaining continuity of care.

Advances in medical equipment allow patients to receive treatment in the home versus a visit to the hospital or a stay within a long-term care facility. For example, intravenous (IV) drip bags are now portable and can be used to administer IV treatments, such as pain medication and antibiotics, within a patient's home.

Many patients choose to receive their treatments at home because it gives them a greater sense of independence and comfort, which are vital aspects in healing many disease processes. If the patient's condition warrants home care, it is important for the patient, the hospital, and the home care provider to realize that the selection of the agency is the patient's choice.

Types of Patients

Home visitation services are provided to those individuals identified by a physician as having a medical necessity for skilled services. Some payer sources, such as Medicare and many private insurance companies, require the patient be **homebound** (i.e., confined to the home except for infrequent or relatively short absences) to receive home health services; however, not all payers have this requirement. Patient referrals can be received from a variety of services, such as hospital discharge planners, patients, patients' physicians, insurance companies through their case management programs, preferred provider organizations (PPOs), and health maintenance organizations (HMOs).

Usually a staff person from the home care agency works with the patient's physician to begin the patient's action plan for **home care visits**. The preliminary work includes identifying the types of services that should be provided to the patient, how often, and special orders, to ensure continuity of care for the patient.

Types of Caregivers

Many services can be offered to homebound patients. A facility can be selective in what it offers to its patients; however, an agency has a competitive advantage in the home care market if it offers a variety of services. The following discussion explains some of the available home health care options. Most options are paid by Medicare and third-party payers, with a few exceptions.

Skilled Nursing Services

Skilled nursing services employ health care personnel with a variety of skill levels. Individuals employed by these services may include nurses trained in medical-surgical nursing, intravenous therapy, enterostomal therapy, psychiatric or mental health, maternity, or restorative nursing. The level of nursing care used depends on individual patient need.

Home health aides are also employed by skilled nursing services. A home health aide is a certified staff person who is able to enhance patient care by assisting with activities of daily living, such as checking vital signs, bathing, grooming, preparing meals, and shopping.

Specialty Services

Home health care also encompasses a range of specialty services, again depending on the level of care required by the patient. These services may include the following **disciplines**: physical therapy, occupational therapy, speech-language pathology, medical social services, nutrition services, respiratory therapy, patient transportation, respite care, homemaking services, medical equipment, and Meals on Wheels.

Physical therapists establish a home maintenance program for the patient, assisting with exercise routines and ambulating devices. Occupational therapists assist the patient to become independent with personal care duties, such as dressing, bathing, and other normal activities of daily living. Speech-language pathologists assist patients who suffer from a stroke or adverse effects of feeding tubes or endotracheal tubes. Speech-language pathologists teach proper swallowing techniques, word formation, and word enunciation.

Medical social services help patients and family members cope with a patient's disease process through placement and involvement with community services. They also help find appropriate resources and make suggestions for long-range planning.

Nutrition services are not typically covered by Medicare, but patients always have the option to privately pay for special assistance with dietary needs. However, Medicare does pay for skilled nurses who monitor the patient's diet during a home care treatment period, and it also pays for teaching those who need help with special feeding equipment.

For special respiratory conditions, respiratory therapists teach techniques to increase efficiency in the lungs, such as pursed-lip breathing, and safety precautions when using oxygen equipment in the home.

Patient transportation services will pick up patients and transport them to their desired destination, such as the physician's office. This service is available for those who are willing to pay the fee.

Respite care is a fee-for-service not paid by Medicare. Those delivering respite care relieve the primary caregiver of his or her duties for an extended time. During this time, the respite caregiver monitors the patient as the caregiver would. Respite care simply allows the primary caregiver to have some free time.

Durable medical equipment, such as a wheelchair or hospital bed, is leased or purchased to aid in the healing of the patient within the home setting. The use of durable medical equipment in the home is covered under Medicare Part B. If co-insurance is used, the patient pays a deductible and 20 percent of the bill.

Meals on Wheels is a charitable organization that provides food services for those unable to leave the home.

Regulatory Issues

Home care institutions may be not-for-profit or they may be proprietarily owned. They can operate as stand-alone companies, often referred to as freestanding. They can also participate in a partnership or operate as an **affiliate** to another institution, often a hospital. In the latter case, the home care headquarters can be physically separate from its affiliate or they can be affiliate based.

There are only a few accrediting and certifying agencies that home care organizations need to consider:

- **Joint Commission on Accreditation of Healthcare Organizations (JCAHO)**
- National League for Nursing's **Community Health Accreditation Program (CHAP)**
- Medicare/Medicaid—the latter is sometimes referred to as medical assistance
- Individual state licensing requirements

In 1997, the Centers for Medicare and Medicaid Services (CMS, formerly known as the Healthcare Financing Administration, or HCFA), offered **"deemed status"** to home health agencies that had been accredited by JCAHO or CHAP. "Deemed status" means that the voluntary accrediting agency's standards (e.g., JCAHO's or CHAP's standards) are deemed to be equivalent to the standards found in the Medicare and Medicaid Programs' *Conditions of Participation* **(MCOP)**. Deemed status exempts the accredited home health agency from routine surveys under the MCOP.

Joint Commission on Accreditation of Healthcare Organizations

JCAHO has been in existence since 1951 and is currently the largest accrediting body in the health care industry. It established its Home Care Accreditation Program in 1988. The scope of accreditation for home care encompasses many types of organizations, such as Medicare-certified home health agencies, hospices, private duty, durable medical equipment companies, and infusion therapy companies.

JCAHO is a well-known accrediting body for those in the home care industry. To receive the JCAHO seal of approval, an agency must apply for a survey and prepare to be evaluated on performance, functions, and processes aimed at improving patient **outcomes**, or end results. An evaluation is done by JCAHO with qualitative and quantitative **standards** or rules. JCAHO publishes its home care standards in the *Comprehensive Accreditation Manual for Home Care*, which is updated yearly.

Community Health Accreditation Program

The Community Health Accreditation Program (CHAP) was founded in 1965 and is the only accrediting body dedicated exclusively to quality home, community, and public health care. It is a subsidiary of the National League for Nursing and focuses on improving community-based health care through voluntary programs.

JCAHO and CHAP have collaborated in an effort to decrease overlaps within their business operations. JCAHO now recognizes and accepts the accreditation process, findings, and decisions of CHAP for home care institutions.

Four key principles for all CHAP standards are as follows:

1. The organization's structure and function consistently support its consumer-oriented philosophy and purpose.
2. The organization consistently provides high-quality services and products.
3. The organization has adequate human, financial, and physical resources effectively organized to accomplish its stated purpose.
4. The organization is positioned for long-term viability.

The following CHAP manuals are available to aid an institution in receiving the CHAP seal of approval:

- *Core Standards*
- *Service-Specific Standards*

- *Self-Study*
- *CHAP Standards Packages*
- *Benchmarks for Excellence in Home Care*

Medicare/Medicaid

The **Centers for Medicare and Medicaid Services (CMS)** is a federal agency within the Department of Health and Human Services. It was created in 1977 to administer the Medicare and Medicaid programs. CMS maintains its headquarters in Baltimore, Maryland, and has 10 regional offices nationwide. The headquarters administers the national direction of the Medicare and Medicaid programs while the regional offices provide CMS with the local presence necessary for quality customer service and oversight.

CMS mainly acts as a purchaser of health care services for the Medicare and Medicaid beneficiaries. Four key principles for Medicare/Medicaid standards are:

1. Assuring that Medicare and Medicaid are properly administered by their contractors and state agencies
2. Establishing policies for the reimbursement of health care providers
3. Conducting research on the effectiveness of various methods of health care management, treatment, and financing
4. Assessing the quality of health care facilities and services

Medicare/Medicaid manuals, interim manual instructions, and Medicare transmittals are distributed to intermediaries, carriers, CMS regional offices, federal agencies, state agencies, and congressional offices. Medicare providers may contact their carrier and/or intermediary to obtain copies of Medicare/Medicaid manuals and transmittals or obtain them from the CMS Web site.

The **National Association for Home Care (NAHC)** also offers supplemental information for Medicare-certified home care providers.

- *A Provider's Guide to the Medicare Home Health Survey and Certification Process*
- **HIM-11** *Coverage Guide for Field Staff*

Documentation

The primary reasons for documentation, whether electronic or hard copy, are to maintain an accurate record on all care and services provided to the patient and to meet all regulatory requirements in order to obtain reimbursement.

For Medicare-certified agencies, the Medicare *Conditions of Participation* (MCOP or COP) for Home Health Agencies specify certain documentation requirements. If an agency is interested in becoming JCAHO accredited, JCAHO has its own list of documentation requirements. As mentioned before, both organizations produce manuals that follow specific standards of content, time frames, and authorized staff. Additionally, the American Health Information Management Association (AHIMA) has published an excellent reference book, *Documentation and Reimbursement for Home Care and Hospice Programs*, containing documentation strategies and examples of the necessary forms (Abraham, 2001).

There are three forms developed by CMS that are very important in home care. These are the CMS 485, CMS 486, and CMS 487 forms. The *Home Health Certification and Plan of Care*, also known as the **485**, certifies the patient's need for home health services (see Figure 12-1). The 485 also outlines the patient's plan of care, which must be established by his or her attending physician. This document includes pertinent diagnoses, types of services, frequency and duration of visits, medication and treatments, safety measures, durable medical equipment (DME), nutritional requirements, functional limitations, allergies, mental status, prognosis, activities of daily living, goals, rehabilitation potential, and discharge plans.

The patient's physician must review, update, and recertify (if necessary) the plan of care at least every 60 days. This time frame is often referred to as the patient's **certification period**. **Recertification** can continue every 60 days until the patient is discharged from services.

An addendum or a **487** is completed when the information does not fit on the 485. A **486** is a medical update of the patient information.

Another important document for home care is the **initial baseline assessment**, which is completed on the first visit. The document should include the patient's present illness, significant past history, review of all systems/physical assessment, medications, psychological, social, and economic factors, emergency plans, and skilled nursing performed that day.

Based on the initial assessment and the patient's needs, the skilled nurse develops a **care plan** that includes goals, objectives, and those responsible for completing this plan.

An authorized staff person, determined by state law, takes verbal orders from the patient's physician. He or she must document, date, and sign the order. The order must also be signed by the physician and returned to the home care agency within a certain time frame, determined by state law. This includes the patient's discharge summary.

Skilled nursing services must be supervised by a registered nurse and documented at appropriate intervals, determined by state law. Home health aide services require supervisory visits by the registered nurse and documentation at appropriate intervals, determined by state law.

Additional documents include the patient database, hospital discharge information, patient bill of rights, advance directives, DNR (do not resuscitate) orders, medication and treatment sheet, all initial baseline assessments and progress notes, problem list, critical paths, teaching guides, and discharge summary.

A **source-oriented record** is the traditional way a record is organized in sections according to patient care departments and/or disciplines. Within each section, the

Department of Health and Human Services Centers for Medicare & Medicaid Services				Form Approved OMB No. 0938-0357

HOME HEALTH CERTIFICATION AND PLAN OF CARE

1. Patient's HI Claim No.	2. Start Of Care Date	3. Certification Period	4. Medical Record No.	5. Provider No.
		From: To:		

6. Patient's Name and Address

7. Provider's Name, Address and Telephone Number

8. Date of Birth	9. Sex ☐M ☐F	10. Medications: Dose/Frequency/Route (N)ew (C)hanged

11. ICD-9-CM	Principal Diagnosis	Date
12. ICD-9-CM	Surgical Procedure	Date
13. ICD-9-CM	Other Pertinent Diagnoses	Date

14. DME and Supplies	15. Safety Measures:
16. Nutritional Req.	17. Allergies:

18.A. Functional Limitations

1 ☐ Amputation	5 ☐ Paralysis	9 ☐ Legally Blind
2 ☐ Bowel/Bladder (Incontinence)	6 ☐ Endurance	A ☐ Dyspnea With Minimal Exertion
3 ☐ Contracture	7 ☐ Ambulation	B ☐ Other (Specify)
4 ☐ Hearing	8 ☐ Speech	

18.B. Activities Permitted

1 ☐ Complete Bedrest	6 ☐ Partial Weight Bearing	A ☐ Wheelchair
2 ☐ Bedrest BRP	7 ☐ Independent At Home	B ☐ Walker
3 ☐ Up As Tolerated	8 ☐ Crutches	C ☐ No Restrictions
4 ☐ Transfer Bed/Chair	9 ☐ Cane	D ☐ Other (Specify)
5 ☐ Exercises Prescribed		

19. Mental Status:

| 1 ☐ Oriented | 3 ☐ Forgetful | 5 ☐ Disoriented | 7 ☐ Agitated |
| 2 ☐ Comatose | 4 ☐ Depressed | 6 ☐ Lethargic | 8 ☐ Other |

20. Prognosis: 1 ☐ Poor   2 ☐ Guarded   3 ☐ Fair   4 ☐ Good   5 ☐ Excellent

21. Orders for Discipline and Treatments (Specify Amount/Frequency/Duration)

22. Goals/Rehabilitation Potential/Discharge Plans

23. Nurse's Signature and Date of Verbal SOC Where Applicable:	25. Date HHA Received Signed POT

24. Physician's Name and Address	26. I certify/recertify that this patient is confined to his/her home and needs intermittent skilled nursing care, physical therapy and/or speech therapy or continues to need occupational therapy. The patient is under my care, and I have authorized the services on this plan of care and will periodically review the plan.
27. Attending Physician's Signature and Date Signed	28. Anyone who misrepresents, falsifies, or conceals essential information required for payment of Federal funds may be subject to fine, imprisonment, or civil penalty under applicable Federal laws.

Form CMS-485 (C-3) (02-94) (Formerly HCFA-485) (Print Aligned)

Figure 12-1   CMS-485, Home Health Certification and Plan of Care.

forms are arranged according to date. The major advantage to the source-oriented format is that it organizes reports from each source together, thus making it easy to determine the assessment, treatments, and observations a particular discipline has provided. One disadvantage of the source-oriented format is that it is not possible to quickly determine all of the patient's problems. It is also difficult to determine all of the treatments being provided for the patient at a given time.

The **problem-oriented record** provides a systematic method of documentation to reflect logical thinking on the part of the person directing the care of the patient. The individual directing the care of the patient defines and follows each clinical problem individually and organizes the problems for solution. The record must contain four basic components: database, complete problem list, initial plans, and progress notes.

Advantages to this format are that the individual directing the patient care is required to consider all the patient's problems in total context. The record clearly indicates the goals and methods in treating the patient. Medical education is facilitated by the documentation of logical thought processes.

A disadvantage of the problem-oriented record is that the format usually requires training of the professional staff. Also, for this chart format to be effective, the professional staff must be convinced of the system's worth.

In an **integrated** format, the information is organized in strict chronological order. The forms from the various sources are intermingled. An advantage to this format is that the information included reads like a book, providing a clear picture of the patient's illness and response to treatment. However, it is difficult to compare similar information (e.g., fasting blood sugar levels) over a period of time. It also proves difficult for each discipline to quickly determine its treatment regimen and patient outcome.

Outcome and Assessment Information Set (OASIS)

The **Outcome and Assessment Information Set (OASIS)** is a group of data items designed to establish a means of systematic measurement of patient home health care outcomes. Outcomes, for the purpose of OASIS, measure changes in a patient's health status between two or more time points.

OASIS data items address sociodemographic, environmental, support systems, health status, functional status, and health service utilization characteristics of the patient. The data is collected at the start of care, every 60 days on a follow-up OASIS, and at discharge. It is important to note that the OASIS data elements alone are not a complete and comprehensive assessment tool and must be incorporated into a comprehensive patient assessment. For example, the OASIS data elements do not include such things as vital signs, home safety issues, wound measurements, and so on.

Regulatory Overview

Only home health agencies that participate in the Medicare program are required to follow the OASIS regulations, as stated in the Medicare *Conditions of Participation*. An

OASIS assessment should be performed on all patients who are adult (over age 18), nonmaternity, and receiving skilled care. The JCAHO also has requirements and standards that address improving organization performance, which can be met by using OASIS processes. In addition, state and Medicare surveyors have access to OASIS-generated quality reports, which they may review before an agency's survey. Some reports may be used in the survey process, and surveyors will expect agencies to show how they use OASIS data reports for quality monitoring. These quality improvement and quality management uses of OASIS are described later.

Reporting of OASIS Information

There are several methods for gathering and reporting the OASIS information. Some home health agencies may be fully computerized and gather all of their information electronically in the field and then transmit the data. Others may gather the information on paper and manually enter the data into a computer file, which is called encoding. Others may gather the data on paper and scan the information into a computer.

Data is also submitted in a variety of ways. Some agencies have purchased software specifically for the OASIS data and its transmission; others have elected to use software available at no charge from CMS. The software available from CMS is called Home Assessment Validation and Entry (HAVEN) and was developed to provide home health agencies with software for data entry, editing, and validation of OASIS data.

The Medicare *Conditions of Participation* detail the time frames for completion and transmission of the OASIS data. Generally, the data must be encoded and "locked" within seven days of the assessment. During this seven-day time frame, the data must be analyzed for accuracy and edited, if needed. Once the data elements have been locked, which prevents subsequent editing and ensures stability of the data, it can be batched in a submission file and transmitted to the state agency.

CMS requires that the data be electronically transmitted at least monthly. Transmissions may occur more frequently at the discretion of the home health agency. Data must be transmitted by the end of the month following the date of collection. For example, an assessment completed in February would have to be transmitted by the end of March. There is no specific date on which the agency must transmit the data, which allows agencies to develop schedules that best meet their needs.

Once the data has been transmitted to the state agency, the home health agency must monitor the state reports for initial and final validation of the submission. If any errors or exceptions occur, the home health agency will receive a message in the final validation report, and errors must be corrected and resubmitted.

Reimbursement and Funding

When a home care agency receives a request to service a patient, it accepts the responsibility to determine the patient's financial eligibility. A patient may be insured by

Medicare, Medicaid, private/third-party payer, or willing to issue payment personally. Some institutions may also have a fund established for those uninsured and unable to submit payments.

Upon completion of services and documentation, a bill is submitted and payment to the home care institution is based on the following:

- Medicare—a home care agency is paid a specific dollar amount for a 60-day period based on the patient's Home Health Resource Group (HHRG), as described in the following section on the Prospective Payment System (PPS).

- Medicaid—a home care agency is paid based on a rate determined by the state legislature. This rate varies with each state.

- Private insurance—a home care agency is paid based on a percentage of charges.

Medicare Prospective Payment System

On October 1, 2000, the Home Health Prospective Payment System (HHPPS) became effective and changed the way home care agencies were reimbursed for Medicare patients. This system was implemented to promote the same efficiencies and cost savings experienced when Medicare payments to hospitals were converted to a prospective payment system.

Under the new payment system, home care agencies are paid a predetermined amount of money that may vary for each 60-day episode of care, depending on the severity of the patient's illness and the services required. Once the assessment of the patient has been performed and the OASIS completed, the Home Health Resource Group (HHRG), which is based on the answers to 21 of the OASIS questions, can be determined. The HHRG is represented by an alphanumeric code indicating severity.

Patients are assessed in three areas to determine the HHRG: clinical (C), functional (F), and service utilization (S):

- *Clinical dimension*: Evaluates the patient's medical status by assessing primary diagnosis, vision, level of pain, presence of ulcers or wounds, dyspnea, urinary and bowel status, need for infusion, and behavior.

- *Functional dimension*: Assesses the patient's ability to perform activities of daily living (ADLs), such as dressing, bathing, toileting, transferring, and ambulation.

- *Service utilization*: Determines what level of service the patient is likely to need based on location at the time of the home care referral (e.g., home, hospital, rehabilitation or skilled nursing facility), and whether there will be a need for 10 or more therapy visits in the next 60 days.

There are 80 HHRGs, which range from C0F0S0 on the low end to C3F4S3 on the high end, with payment amounts ranging from approximately $1,000 to $5,900. Payments are adjusted to accommodate area wage differences.

Before submitting the claims to Medicare, the HHRG must be converted to a Health Insurance Prospective Payment System code (HIPPS). HIPPS codes are also alphanumeric, but unlike the HHRG are made up of five alpha characters and one numeric position.

Payments for the 60-day episodes are made in two installments, the first when a Request for Anticipated Payment (RAP)* is submitted to Medicare, and the second when the final claim is filed. Patients are covered for an unlimited number of episodes as long as they continue to meet the Medicare criteria for skilled care.

There are some exceptions to the 60-day episode payment as follows:

- *Low Utilization Payment Adjustment (LUPA)*—If a patient receives 4 or fewer visits in a 60-day episode, payment will be made by the visit.
- *Significant Change in Condition (SCIC,* pronounced "sic")—Patients who have a significant and unexpected change in their condition during the 60-day episode will have an adjustment in their payment rate.
- *Partial Episode Payment (PEP)*—Occasionally a patient may transfer to another agency for care, in which case the first agency would only receive payment for the part of the episode it actually provided care to the patient. When the patient starts receiving care from the new agency, they begin a new episode.
- *Outliers*—Occur when the provision of care to a patient results in unusually high costs to the home care agency. Payment adjustments are made for a portion of the costs above the set threshold.

With the implementation of the prospective payment system, home care agencies have had to evaluate how they provide care to their patients and balance quality care with the efficiency and cost-saving measures the new payment method requires.

Payer Mix

An agency may have 70 percent of its patients insured by Medicare, 20 percent by Medicaid, and 10 percent by other third-party payers. This ratio is considered the agency's **payer mix**.

This ratio is very important for the financial security of the company. Government programs, such as Medicare and Medicaid, focus on paying for care on the basis of agency or industry costs. Other third-party payers generally pay on the basis of charges, which can be higher than costs and are set by the agency.

Financial Stability

Within the federal government, CMS and the Department of Health and Human Services administer the Medicare program. They manage the program through

---

*Note that the same acronym, RAP, carries two different meanings in long-term care and in home health care. (See Chapter 10.)

rules and regulations described within the Medicare *Conditions of Participation*. At the state level, the fiscal intermediary, such as Blue Cross, carries out these rules and regulations.

Each agency must submit a yearly cost report to its fiscal intermediary for review. This report includes such things as operating costs, number of visits, and payer mix. Upon review of this report, a rate is determined for cost reimbursement adjustment.

A good business practice is to keep **fixed costs** as low as possible. Fixed costs do not change when the volume of services changes. In a service industry such as home health, rent and utilities are examples of fixed costs. **Variable costs** vary in proportion to the services provided. For example, when visits increase in number, the costs associated with visits, such as labor costs and transportation costs, also increase.

Medicare coverage issues also affect the financial stability of the agency. With regard to Medicare, both Part A and Part B apply. The home health care agency is reimbursed for nursing and other patient care through Part A. However, durable medical equipment is covered under Part B. What is not covered by Medicare?

- Twenty-four-hour care at home (unless it is only necessary for one day)
- Prescription drugs (exceptions may apply to drugs administered by a pump)
- Meals delivered to the home
- Homemaker services such as shopping, cleaning, and laundry, except that home health aides may do a small amount of these chores at the time they are providing covered services
- Personal care provided by home health aides, such as bathing, toileting, or providing help in getting dressed, *if* this is the only care needed. Medicare classifies this personal care as "custodial" because it could be provided safely and reasonably by people without professional skills and training. However, when skilled services are needed, personal care is covered.

There is a potential for the financial side of an agency to be **audited**. The possible reasons are a cost report that needs further investigation, a high volume of services, or a history of a high denial rate. However, *if* claims are submitted properly, as stated in guidelines, and documentation exists to support the reimbursement, such as the physician review of the plan of care every 60 days, an audit is not a serious risk to the agency.

A **denial** occurs when a bill amount to Medicare is no longer considered a receivable to an agency. The process begins with Medicare noticing an area in the delivery of care that does not follow guidelines, such as excessive utilization of a particular service. Medicare then requests documentation. If documentation does not support the utilization, a denial is issued. An agency may appeal by sending further documentation as well as written justification. Medicare ultimately submits or denies payment. Most agencies have a low denial rate.

Information Management

Coding and Classification

Coding classification includes diagnosis, procedural, and physician procedural office codes. Diagnosis and procedural codes are classified within ICD-9-CM and physician procedural office codes are classified within CPT.

ICD-9-CM

International Classification of Diseases, 9th Revision, Clinical Modification (ICD-9-CM) coding is required for home care agencies to receive payment. Codes are usually assigned upon completion of the initial assessment and may be updated with each certification period.

Home care coding generally follows the traditional ICD-9-CM coding conventions. Just as the diagnoses and procedures coded for the hospital must be relevant to the hospital care provided, diagnoses and procedures coded for home care should be relevant to the care provided within the home.

The home care principal diagnosis is the diagnosis most related to the plan of care and is recorded on the 485. If the principal diagnosis has changed by the time of the next recertification (60 days later), the code for the new principal diagnosis is recorded on the 485. Other diagnoses that affect home care are also coded since several codes may be required to indicate the seriousness of the patient's condition and to explain the care provided in the home (Miller, 1996).

ICD-9-CM procedure codes are also recorded on the 485. Medicare requires that ICD-9-CM procedure codes be recorded for hospital procedures that have a bearing on the home care provided (Miller, 1996). For example, a patient who has undergone a laparotomy in the hospital may have a postoperative wound that needs dressing changes. The hospital laparotomy is therefore relevant to the home care plan and should be coded.

Before the fall of 2003, V and E codes were not accepted on the OASIS forms. However, with the implementation of the transactions and code sets standards of HIPAA, OASIS forms are now required to accept V and E codes. When the OASIS reports a V code as the primary diagnosis, a non-V code that can be used to determine the applicable HHRG must be submitted as a payment diagnosis.

With the implementation of the PPS in home health, accurate coding has become more important because of the impact of coding on reimbursement and the resulting increased potential for fraud and abuse.

Durable medical equipment (DME) companies are also required to use ICD-9-CM codes for proper payment. The codes must correspond to the type of equipment being billed for per patient. For example, a fractured hip would support the use of ambulating devices, and a respiratory condition would support the use of oxygen equipment.

CPT

The physicians who do care planning can use Current Procedural Terminology (CPT) codes. These are available for the physician to use to bill for care plan oversight. These codes were implemented in 1995 to allow physicians to bill for time spent discussing a patient's care with home health personnel and in the development of a care plan. Physicians must keep their own records documenting the time spent per patient on care plan oversight because time spent provides the basis for payment.

Data and Information Flow

Data collection generally begins upon the referral of the patient to home care. During the initial and subsequent home visits, home care staff members collect data using paper-based systems or computer-based systems that utilize laptop or handheld computers. Data is transmitted to the home care agency's office by manual or electronic means. When the patient is discharged from home care, the complete record is maintained in a central location, in either paper or electronic format.

Computer Systems

Most home care agencies manage data through some type of database management system. Some agencies use their own homegrown systems and others use systems available from various health care information systems vendors. Information system vendors specializing in home care systems generally offer the ability to manage information concerning referral, census, OASIS reporting, medication profiles, orders, scheduling, Medicare certification and recertification, progress and visit notes, and other data and documentation (Anderson, 1999).

Data Sets

Previous discussion of the OASIS data set has described its documentation and reimbursement features. The OASIS data elements were developed, tested, and refined over a 10-year period through an extensive research and demonstration program funded by CMS. The Center for Health Services Research in Denver, Colorado, developed the OASIS and maintains its copyright. However, the Center permits the free use of OASIS by home care providers and related organizations. This extensive data set is approximately 17 pages when printed. See Figure 12-2 for an excerpt from the OASIS in its paper format (Centers for Medicare and Medicaid Services, Online).

Quality Improvement and Utilization Management

Quality Improvement

Outcome measures are the heart of outcome-based quality improvement (OBQI) and outcome-based quality management (OBQM), which are systematic approaches

Outcome and Assessment Information Set (OASIS-B1)

Items to be Used at Specific Time Points

Start of Care --- Home Health Patient Tracking Sheet, M0080-M0825

    Start of care—further visits planned

Resumption of Care -- M0080-M0825

    Resumption of care (after inpatient stay)

Follow-Up -- M0080-M0100, M0175, M0230-M0250, M0390, M0420,
                                                 M0440, M0450, M0460, M0476, M0488, M0490, M0530-
    Recertification (follow-up) assessment   M0550, M0610, M0650-M0700, M0825
    Other follow-up assessment

Transfer to an Inpatient Facility------------------------------- M0080-M0100, M0830-M0855, M0890-M0906

    Transferred to an inpatient facility—patient not discharged from an agency
    Transferred to an inpatient facility—patient discharged from agency

Discharge from Agency — Not to an Inpatient Facility

    Death at home-- M0080-M0100, M0906
    Discharge from agency--- M0080-M0100, M0200-M0220, M0250, M0280-M0380,
                                                 M0410-M0820, M0830-M0880, M0903-M0906

Note: For items M0640-M0800, please note special instructions at the beginning of the section.

CLINICAL RECORD ITEMS

(M0080) Discipline of Person Completing Assessment:

      ☐ 1-RN   ☐ 2-PT   ☐ 3-SLP/ST   ☐ 4-OT

(M0090) Date Assessment Completed: __ __ /__ __ /__ __ __ __
                                            month day   year

(M0100) This Assessment is Currently Being Completed for the Following Reason:

    Start/Resumption of Care
    ☐ 1 – Start of care—further visits planned
    ☐ 3 – Resumption of care (after inpatient stay)
    Follow-Up
    ☐ 4 – Recertification (follow-up) reassessment **[Go to *M0175*]**
    ☐ 5 – Other follow-up **[Go to *M0175*]**
    Transfer to an Inpatient Facility
    ☐ 6 – Transferred to an inpatient facility—patient not discharged from agency **[Go to *M0830*]**
    ☐ 7 – Transferred to an inpatient facility—patient discharged from agency **[Go to *M0830*]**
    Discharge from Agency — Not to an Inpatient Facility
    ☐ 8 – Death at home **[Go to *M0906*]**
    ☐ 9 – Discharge from agency **[Go to *M0200*]**

© 2002, Center for Health Services Research, UCHSC, Denver, CO
OASIS-B1 (12/2002)
1

Figure 12-2 Excerpt from Outcome and Assessment Information Set. (OASIS is the intellectual property of the Center for Health Services Research, Denver, Colorado. It is used with permission.)

DEMOGRAPHICS AND PATIENT HISTORY

(M0175) From which of the following **Inpatient Facilities** was the patient discharged <u>during the past 14 days</u>? **(Mark all that apply.)**

☐ 1 - Hospital
☐ 2 - Rehabilitation facility
☐ 3 - Skilled nursing facility
☐ 4 - Other nursing home
☐ 5 - Other (specify) _____
☐ NA - Patient was not discharged from an inpatient facility **[If NA at SOC/ROC, go to *M0200;* If NA at Follow-Up, go to *M0230*]**

(M0180) Inpatient Discharge Date (most recent):

__ __ / __ __ / __ __ __ __
month day   year

☐ UK - Unknown

(M0190) Inpatient Diagnoses and ICD-9-CM code categories (three digits required; five digits optional) <u>for only those conditions treated during an inpatient facility stay within the last 14 days</u> (no surgical or V-codes):

Inpatient Facility Diagnosis	ICD-9-CM
a. _____	(__ __ __ . __ __)
b. _____	(__ __ __ . __ __)

> **Effective 10/1/2003**
>
> List each Inpatient Diagnosis and ICD-9-CM code at the level of highest specificity for only those conditions treated during an inpatient stay within the last 14 days (no surgical, E-codes, or V-codes):
>
> | Inpatient Facility Diagnosis | ICD-9-CM |
> |---|---|
> | a. _____ | (__ __ __ . __ __) |
> | b. _____ | (__ __ __ . __ __) |

(M0200) Medical or Treatment Regimen Change Within Past 14 Days: Has this patient experienced a change in medical or treatment regimen (e.g., medication, treatment, or service change due to new or additional diagnosis, etc.) within the last 14 days?

☐ 0 - No **[If No, go to *M0220*]**
☐ 1 - Yes

(M0210) List the patient's **Medical Diagnoses** and ICD-9-CM code categories (three digits required; five digits optional) <u>for those conditions requiring changed medical or treatment regimen</u> (no surgical or V-codes):

Changed Medical Regimen Diagnosis	ICD-9-CM
a. _____	(__ __ __ . __ __)
b. _____	(__ __ __ . __ __)
c. _____	(__ __ __ . __ __)
d. _____	(__ __ __ . __ __)

> **Effective 10/1/2003**
>
> List the patient's Medical Diagnoses and ICD-9-CM codes at the level of highest specificity for those conditions requiring changed medical or treatment regimen (no surgical, E-codes, or V-codes):
>
> | Changed Medical Regimen Diagnosis | ICD-9-CM |
> |---|---|
> | a. _____ | (__ __ __ . __ __) |
> | b. _____ | (__ __ __ . __ __) |
> | c. _____ | (__ __ __ . __ __) |
> | d. _____ | (__ __ __ . __ __) |

Figure 12-2   *(Continued)*

home health agencies use to continuously manage and improve the quality of care they provide. Home health agencies are able to access reports on outcomes for their patients through their state agency, and thus compare their results to the national reference, enabling them to identify areas of strengths and weaknesses in their patient outcomes. OBQI/OBQM requires precise, uniform measures, which can only be obtained from standardized data items. The OASIS was designed to provide the necessary standardized data elements to measure outcomes.

In all health care areas, including home health, outcomes are of interest and importance to many parties. Payers want to know how the patients they insure are benefiting from the dollars they spend on care. On the federal level, outcomes have been stressed in changes to regulations. And, as previously mentioned, accrediting and licensing programs are focusing on outcomes. Consumers and their representatives are requiring outcome information from care providers. And last, but not least, home health agencies have always been concerned with measuring their performance relative to other providers.

While gathering, encoding, and submitting the OASIS data may seem to be an end in itself, it is merely the means to achieve outcome measurement and only the beginning of the process. OBQI/OBQM is fundamentally a two-stage process. First, the data must be gathered in a uniform manner (OASIS). This results in a report showing the agency's performance in terms of outcomes relative to the national sample. During this first step, risk adjustment occurs through grouping or statistical methods to compensate for the potential influence of case mix variables that can affect outcomes. Risk adjustment is done by the state agency for some data elements. Reports may be printed with and/or without the risk adjustment. In the second step, the agency would select target outcomes for enhancement, evaluate care for the target outcome, develop a plan of action to change the care, and finally monitor the outcome to see if the desired gains had been accomplished (see Figure 12-3). CMS has established a Quality Improvement Organization (QIO) for each state. These organizations are available to assist agencies with understanding the OBQI/OBQM process, selecting a target outcome, and developing action plans.

One added advantage of a fully developed OBQI/OBQM program is that agencies are able to move into the domain of managing resources for the explicit purpose of gaining the best outcome. Agencies can improve outcomes in areas of inadequate performance, reinforce outcomes in areas in which they do well, and maintain outcomes in areas where performance is acceptable. By managing outcomes in this way, resources are naturally affected. Staffing patterns as well as frequency of services can be altered with a clear bottom-line assessment of the impact that such alterations have on patients. In the long run, this allows agencies to enhance their quality of care, yet manage their resources to become more cost effective, an important goal under the new prospective payment system.

Utilization Management

Utilization management focuses on monitoring the increase and decrease in utilization of services provided to patients. For example, a patient may be receiving skilled nursing services for a terminal disease. Offering social and mental health services to such a patient is typical for proper utilization.

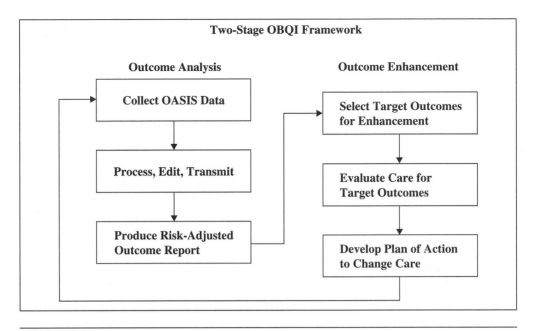

Figure 12-3   Two-Stage OBQI Framework. (From the Centers for Medicare and Medicaid Services' *Outcome-Based Quality Improvement (OBQI) Implementation Manual*, p. 2.4.)

A home care agency may have separate written plans for quality improvement and utilization management. It seems the plans that produce the best results combine the efforts of all information-based areas: quality improvement, utilization management, risk management, information management/systems, and finance. These areas have a common interest: to improve processes that have an impact on the agency's internal and external customer base and to be competitive in price and quality of service within the market of home care.

HIM professionals are increasingly and successfully taking on quality improvement and utilization management duties/roles considering their clinical knowledge and ability to develop tools and reports from the large repositories of clinical data.

Risk Management and Legal Issues

Risk Management

Risk management, in general terms, is a program that monitors the liability and accountability of home care services delivered to its customers. The areas at risk are measured through clinical analysis by way of incident reporting and financial analysis through the agency's insurance policy. Typically the health information manager will manage the incident reporting to minimize the risk of injury to patients, visitors, and employees and to delineate procedures for reporting and follow-up of incidents. Health information managers are rarely involved with the financial analysis and insurance policies.

An **incident** or **unusual occurrence** is defined as any happening that is not consistent with the routine operations of the agency or routine care of a particular patient. Key elements of the procedure for reporting incidents include the following:

- Establish time frames for reporting and evaluation of the occurrences.
- Establish reporting of occurrences as a positive means of improving the delivery of quality care as opposed to a punitive performance evaluation.
- Record only the facts.
- Narrative description should be written in the first person and recorded by the employee who witnessed or experienced the occurrence.
- Incident reports should not be maintained with the medical record; however, the chart should be documented regarding the occurrence, reflecting the continuation of the treatment provided to the patient.
- Categorize occurrences and utilize reports to identify trends and patterns.
- Share the reports with the appropriate committees, such as the quality improvement committee, to improve processes that are risks and potential risks to the company.

Satisfaction Committee

Another form of proactive risk management is to utilize a satisfaction committee to monitor customer satisfaction issues. During the initial visit all patients/caregivers should be informed and presented with the patient bill of rights, which includes the toll-free state department of health hotline number and the agency's contact number if there is a problem. This allows patients/caregivers to express concerns and grievances regarding patient care.

Customers include patients and their primary caregivers, physicians, and insurance companies. The committee should monitor issues for all customers and try to resolve them in a timely manner while maintaining continuity of care for patients.

Legal Issues

Legal issues are important for all departments of home care and are handled best if done proactively. The human resource department is legally required to have certain information on file for new employees. Following is a general list of items to complete when bringing on new employees:

- Past employment—dates, employer, salary, and work performance
- Education—license in particular profession
- Criminal background
- State driver's license
- Credit check for finance employees

The most common requirements for licensed professionals (check with your particular state requirements) are as follows:

- Cardiopulmonary resuscitation (CPR)—each staff person should be certified when hired and is typically recertified once every two years.
- **Occupational Safety and Health Administration (OSHA)**—in-services are implemented to provide a safe work environment for employees. Safety topics include ergonomics, first aid, and bloodborne pathogens. OSHA in-services are typically done annually.
- Universal precautions should be practiced at all times.
- Safety in the community should be practiced at all times.
- JCAHO requires the original license of all professional staff to be a part of their personnel file.

Other common in-services required by all home care employees are the following:

- Body mechanics is required and usually completed annually.
- Confidentiality in-services are required at the time of hire and recommended to be done annually.

Policies and Procedures

The health information manager ordinarily develops, or at least updates, particular policies related to medical record procedures. Following is a recommended list of certain policies for review and approval by the agency's legal council:

Advance Directives
Release of Medical Information
   General Treatment
   Alcohol and Drug Treatment
   HIV/AIDS Treatment
   Mental Health Information
Procedure for Responding to Subpoena and Court Orders
Procedure for Do Not Resuscitate Orders

Role of the Health Information Management Professional

HIM positions within home care are still considered nontraditional; however, this career path is becoming more common for recent graduates. The role can be very rewarding considering it usually extends beyond medical records. HIM home care positions require knowledge of finance, quality improvement, utilization review, and information systems.

Now more than ever, agencies must make good use of the information available to them to survive and thrive in the data-driven world of home care. Health information managers can play a key role in developing, implementing, and maintaining effective information systems for home care. Becoming familiar with the home care market and how to be competitive within that market provides HIM professionals with another arena in which to demonstrate their skills in managing information and making that information useful.

Trends

Several new types of programs for the delivery of health care in the home have developed in recent years. Among these innovations are home-based primary care and disease management programs (Turk, Parmley, Ames, and Schumacher, 2000). Physicians have also shown increased interest in house-call training, education, and practice. In the realm of technology, telemedicine programs for the home will likely expand because of the potential benefits these provide to both patients and providers (Leff and Burton, 2001). Home care providers should strive to make effective use of technology without losing the personal touch that homebound patients require. Certainly, the 21st century holds both promises and challenges for the home care industry.

Summary

The health care industry continues to evolve to offer quality care at a reasonable level of operating cost. Also, rules and regulations placed on hospitals have provided and will continue to provide opportunities for the home care industry to grow.

This rapid growth has forced home care providers to be creative in their business planning to make their agency stand out among the rest. HIM professionals can contribute greatly to the future business planning of home care, considering their training and ability to couple the clinical side with the technical side of management of information.

Key Terms

485   a document facilitating a patient's orders for home care on CMS form number 485 entitled Home Health Certification and Plan of Care. This plan of care must be established and reviewed, at least once every 60 days by the patient's attending physician.

486   updates to the 485 are placed on this particular CMS document.

487   a supplemental form that holds any additional information that does not fit on the 485.

affiliate   an associate or member of a particular business.

audit   a formal way of checking financial and other records.

care plan   an outline for patient care based on an initial assessment and the patient's specific needs that includes goals, objectives, and those responsible for completing the plan.

Centers for Medicare and Medicaid Services (CMS)   a federal agency within the Department of Health and Human Services. Its main focus is to administer the Medicare and Medicaid Programs. Formerly known as the Health Care Financing Administration (HCFA).

certification period   the billing period for which a physician's home care order is valid for patient treatment; 60 days; a time frame in which a patient's physician must review, update, and recertify (if necessary) a patient's plan of care.

Community Health Accreditation Program (CHAP)   an accrediting subsidiary of the National League for Nursing focusing on improving the quality of community-based health care through voluntary programs, including an accreditation program. Meeting CHAP standards provides an home health agency with deemed status with regard to the Medicare *Conditions of Participation*.

deemed status   a status conferred by the Centers for Medicare and Medicaid Services (CMS) to health care providers who meet the voluntary standards of an accrediting organization whose standards have been determined by CMS to be the equivalent to the Medicare *Conditions of Participation* in that particular category. An organization with deemed status is no longer subject to routine surveys under the Medicare *Conditions of Participation*.

denials   lack of payment for home visits/treatments due to noncompliance with governing rules and regulations.

disciplines   specialty services offering a variety treatments for patients; physical therapy, maternity services, and medical social services.

durable medical equipment (DME)   medical equipment provided to the patient within the home environment.

fixed costs   costs that do not change in proportion to changes in volume of services. Office rent and utilities are examples of fixed costs in home health.

HIM-11   a reference to CMS's Publication 11, the *Home Health Agency Manual*, which includes information about coverage of home health services under Medicare, along with other policies and procedures.

homebound   when an individual is physically or mentally limited with regard to the number of absences from his/her home per calendar month.

home care visit   medical and nonmedical treatments provided to patients within the privacy and comforts of their own homes.

home health aide   a certified staff person who is able to enhance the patients care by assisting with the patients activities of daily living, such as checking vital signs, bathing, grooming, meal preparation, and shopping.

home health care   service and treatment provided in the home environment to a recovering, disabled or chronically ill person to improve health or effective functioning.

incident/unusual occurrence   any happening that is not consistent with the routine operations of the agency or routine care of a particular patient.

initial baseline assessment   a document that is completed on the first visit to the patient's home. The document should include the patient's present illness, significant past history, review of all systems/physical assessment, medications, psychological, social, and economic factors, emergency plans, and skilled nursing performed that day, and incorporate the required OASIS data elements.

integrated record   a record in which the information is organized in a strict chronological order.

Joint Commission on Accreditation of Healthcare Organizations, Home Care Accreditation Program (JCAHO)   promotes quality in home care by accrediting a variety of organizations that provide home care services. Meeting JCAHO standards provides a home health agency with deemed status with regard to the Medicare *Conditions of Participation*.

Medicare *Conditions of Participation* (MCOP)   federal regulations with which home health agencies must comply in order to participate in the Medicare program. In addition to other regulations, the MCOP outline documentation requirements for Medicare-certified home health agencies.

National Association for Home Care (NAHC)   an association for organizations and individuals who provide health care and supportive services on an outreach basis to patients in their homes.

Outcomes and Assessment Information Set (OASIS)   a data set requirement under Medicare's *Conditions of Participation*. Medicare-certified home health agencies collect and use OASIS data when evaluating adult, nonmaternity patients. The intent of OASIS is to make the *Conditions of Participation* more patient-centered and outcome-oriented while providing home care agencies with more flexibility to operate their programs. It also measures treatment outcomes and provides individual agencies with the ability to compare themselves to the national data set.

Occupational Safety and Health Administration (OSHA)   an organization that develops criteria meant to provide a safe work environment for all employees.

outcome   end result or consequence; the patient's health and functional status after a period of treatment.

payer mix   a ratio of an agency's various patient insurers and third-party payers.

per visit basis   a unit of measure in home health care for evaluating costs, scheduling, and productivity; often the unit of payment for services.

problem-oriented record   a record organized by the patient's problems; the problem-oriented record follows each clinical problem individually and provides a systematic method of documentation to reflect logical thinking on the part of the one directing the care of the patient.

recertification   additional physician orders after the 60-day certification period.

skilled nursing services   nursing services offered to patients based on their individual needs, such as trained medical-surgical nursing, intravenous therapy, enterostomal therapy, psychiatric or mental health, maternity, or restorative nursing.

source-oriented record   a record organized in sections according to patient care departments and/or disciplines.

standards   rule used as a basis of comparison for measuring quantitative or qualitative value.

variable costs   costs that vary in proportion to the volume of service provided.

REVIEW QUESTIONS

Knowledge-based Questions

1. Identify a few services that home care agencies deliver.

2. Who are the accrediting bodies that develop the standards for home care?

3. Define a certification period.

4. Explain the importance of documentation and coding for proper reimbursement.

5. What is the OASIS and what is its purpose?

6. Explain how Medicare reimburses home care agencies for the provision of care to patients.

Application-based Questions

1. Compare and contrast home care coding with hospital inpatient coding.

2. As home care agencies implement efficiencies to increase their potential profitability under the Medicare PPS, what are some of the issues and concerns they face?

Web Activity

Visit the "Home Health Information Resource for Medicare" Web site at http://www.cms.hhs.gov/providers/hha/. Select a link to one of the many topics available on this page. Which link did you select? Describe information about home health care that was available through the link you selected.

Case Study

Mary Jones is the Health Information Supervisor at Somewhere Home Care, which is Medicare certified. As required by Medicare, her agency has been completing and submitting OASIS data to their state. They have been accessing their patient data through their OASIS reports available from the state, as well as monitoring and documenting visit patterns/frequency by the clinicians in the agency. In addition, they have been monitoring the cost of supplies utilized per patient.

In reviewing their financial data, Mary's director has indicated the agency has performed marginally under the Medicare Prospective Payment System. They would like to improve their financial performance and have met with the leadership team of the agency to discuss a possible plan of action. In the meeting with their leadership team, one item discussed at length was the change the Medicare PPS has had on their reimbursement. Instead of being paid by the visit, they are now paid a set amount of money for the provision of care over a 60-day period. Currently the agency has not implemented the usage of any Clinical Pathways.

Mary has some statistics available to her to assist the director with formulating a plan. These include:

- The number of patients the agency has had in each HHRG classification since the implementation of Medicare PPS on 10/01/00
- The number of visits (by clinician type; i.e., RN, LPN, HHA, PT, OT, SLP) made to each patient for each 60-day episode of care
- The average number of visits made to patients in each HHRG classification
- Financial data, including reimbursement amounts for each HHRG and the agency specific costs per each visit type
- Primary diagnosis for each patient
- OASIS outcome reports printed for OBQI/OBQM showing how the agency has performed in outcomes as compared to other agencies in the country
- Payer mix report, which shows the percentage of patients the agency has in each payer source (i.e., Medicare, Medicaid, Commercial Insurance, Private Pay, etc.). At Somewhere Home Care, 65 percent of their patients are covered by Medicare.

Investigation into care plans and visit patterns indicate there is wide fluctuation in visit patterns between clinicians. Patients who fall into the same HHRG category, who should basically be very similar, have widely varying visit ranges.

Based on the above information and scenario, answer the following questions:

1. What are some significant factors Mary and her director should consider about their payment sources as they evaluate their financial performance?
2. What statistical data available to Mary would be most helpful in developing an action plan?
3. Where should Mary focus her clinical and medical record expertise?

References and Suggested Readings

Abraham, P. R. (2001). *Documentation and Reimbursement for Home Care and Hospice Programs.* Chicago, IL: American Health Information Management Association.

Anderson, E. (1999). Case study: Viewing the EHR in health services organizations. In G. F. Murphy, M. A. Hanken, and K. A. Waters (Eds.). *Electronic Health Records: Changing the Vision* (pp. 42–52). Philadelphia, PA: W. B. Saunders Company.

Campbell, M. (September 1995). Homeward bound: Growth in home care industry opens door for HIM professionals. *Journal of the American Health Information Management Association, 66,* 54–58.

Centers for Medicare and Medicaid Services (2002). *Outcome-Based Quality Improvement (OBQI) Implementation Manual* [Online]. http://www.cms.hhs.gov/oasis/obqi.asp [2003, June 16].

Centers for Medicare and Medicaid Services. (No date). *OASIS Data Sets* [Online]. http://www.cms.hhs.gov/oasis/oasisdat.asp [2003, June 14].

Community Health Accreditation Program. (1993). *Standards of Excellence for Home Health Organizations.* New York: Community Health Accreditation Program.

Frawley, K. A., and Asmonga, D. (March 1995). Medicare coverage of home health services. *Journal of the American Health Information Management Association, 66,* 10.

Home Care Report. (March–April 1997). Volume 6, issues 3 and 4. Totowa, NJ: W. D. Cabin & Associates.

Joint Commission on Accreditation of Healthcare Organizations. (1997). *Comprehensive Accreditation Manual for Home Care.* Oakbrook Terrace, Illinois: Joint Commission on Accreditation of Healthcare Organizations.

Leff, B., and Burton, J. R. (2001). The future history of home care and physician house calls in the United States. *Journals of Gerontology Series A—Biological Sciences & Medical Sciences, 56* (10), M603–M608.

Miller, S. (1996). *Documentation and Information Management in Home Care and Hospice Programs.* Chicago, IL: American Health Information Management Association.

National Association for Home Care. (1992). *How to Choose a Home Care Agency.* Washington, DC: National Association for Home Care.

National Association for Home Care. (1995). *Uniform Data Set for Home Care and Hospice.*

Turk, L., Parmley, J., Ames, A., and Schumacher, K. L. (2000). A new era in home care. *Seminars for Nurse Managers, 8* (3), 143–150.

Key Resources

Community Health Accreditation Program, Inc.
39 Broadway, Suite 710
New York, NY 10006
Phone: 800-656-9656 or 212-480-8828
Fax: 212-480-8832
http://www.chapinc. org

Joint Commission on Accreditation of Healthcare Organizations
(See Chapter 1 for contact information)

National Association for Home Care
228 Seventh Street, SE
Washington, DC 20003
Phone: 202-547-7424
Fax: 202-547-3540
http://www.nahc.org

Chapter 13

Hospice

Karen M. Staszel, RHIA
Teresa Sherfy, RHIT

Learning Objectives

Upon successful completion of this chapter, you should be able to:

1. Describe the hospice patient.

2. Define the term hospice and describe the difference between hospice care and traditional acute care.

3. Describe the composition and role of the interdisciplinary team in providing hospice care to patients, families, and significant others.

4. Define the four reimbursement levels of hospice care—routine home care, respite care, pain and symptom management, and continuous care—and discuss components of appropriate documentation of these levels of care.

5. Describe the use of hospice benefit periods, reimbursement caps, and per diem versus per service payments.

6. Describe the roles played by volunteers in hospice care and issues relating to the volunteer documentation in the medical record.

7. Discuss the capture of clinical visit information to track the cost of hospice care.

8. Discuss the Medicare *Conditions of Participation* relating to hospice care.

9. Describe a utilization review plan in the hospice setting.

10. Discuss bereavement care and documentation following the death of the hospice patient.

SETTING	DESCRIPTION	SYNONYMS/EXAMPLES
Patient's Residence	The majority of hospice programs provide patient care in the patient's place of residence, which may include the patient's home, a relative's or friend's home, a nursing home, or a senior citizen complex.	
Nursing Home or Hospital	Some hospices contract with major hospital complexes and/or nursing homes to establish hospice units or wings. The hospice wing then becomes the patient's place of residence. These units are used primarily when patients have nobody in their place of residence who can help care for them, or if they are too sick to leave the existing facility and can just be transferred to another wing, or for respite care.	Hospice inpatient unit, ICU (inpatient care unit), care center, hospice wing.
Stand-alone Hospice	Some hospice programs build their own facilities. These facilities are not associated with an existing hospital or nursing home. Similar to nursing home and/or hospital beds, the bed in the stand-alone hospice becomes patients' place of residence. Again, these facilities are used primarily when there is nobody at home to help care for the patient, or for respite care.	Freestanding hospice, hospice inpatient unit, hospice care center, ICU (inpatient care unit). Depending on the state requirements, hospices may license these facilities as nursing homes, adult foster care homes, or freestanding hospice units (if the state has a category for them).

Introduction to Setting

The history of **hospice** can trace its roots along the same timeline as the history and development of the hospital. Charitable, religious organizations and individuals were caring for not only the sick and diseased throughout history, but also the dying and those grieving for them. *Hospice* is a French word derived from the Latin *hospitium*, which was a place in which a guest was received. This is very similar to the Latin *hospitalis*, meaning "of a guest," and *hospes*, meaning "a guest," from which hospital is derived. It was not until 1967, however, when Dame Cicely Saunders opened St. Christopher's Hospice in London, that caring for the dying patient was recognized and developed as a philosophy and practice. The time period it appears was especially ripe for the emergence of the hospice discipline:

> A hundred years ago, doctors cured only a few patients because they lacked the powerful medical tools that exist today. With the advent of safer surgery and the enormous advances in therapeutics, doctors have apparently developed the power to remove problems and effect cures. The relentless pursuit of cures for more and more diseases can lead the blinkered into believing that care of those who are incurable is less important. (Corr and Corr, 1983)

Most hospice programs provide patient care in the patient's **place of residence**, which could be the patient's home, a relative's or friend's home, a nursing home, or a senior citizen complex. In addition to providing care in the patient's place of residence, some hospice programs have built their own facilities and/or contracted with major hospital complexes and/or nursing homes, to establish hospice units or wings. The hospice facility or the hospice wing then becomes the patient's place of residence.

Types of Patients

The Terminally Ill

Hospices provide **palliative care** or symptom management rather than **curative therapy** to patients considered **terminally ill**, with a life expectancy of less than six months. Terminal diseases range from congenital disorders of children to multiple sclerosis, end-stage renal, respiratory, and cardiac diseases, AIDS (Acquired Immune Deficiency Syndrome), cancer, and a host of other illnesses. Symptom management includes not only methods to relieve chronic pain and other physical results of the disease process, but it also helps relieve the emotional and mental stress of the dying process. Hospices use nonnarcotic analgesics, narcotic analgesics (titrated to manage pain, not cause mental confusion), frequent changes of position, back rubs, massage, oxygen, tranquilizers, antidepressants, music, conversation, and companionship to relieve terminal symptoms. Hospices do not routinely use X-rays, transfusions, chemotherapy, radiation therapy, intubations, cardopulmonary resuscitation (CPR), or any other therapy that would be considered curative. In general, a hospice allows patients to live as symptom-free as possible, and enables them to lead as meaningful a life as they wish for the remainder of their illness.

Significant Others

In the acute care setting, the focus of care is on treating the patient. Hospice philosophy, on the other hand, recognizes that the dying process is difficult not only for the patient, but also for the patient's family and significant others. Thus hospice care focuses not just on the needs of the patient, but also on the physical, emotional, and mental states of those around the patient. This is such an important part of a hospice treatment plan that the National Hospice and Palliative Case Organization (NHPCO) states, "The unit of care in hospice is the patient/family." Treatment plans and options are discussed with the patient and with family members; goals are written for the patient and family members.

Types of Caregivers

The Interdisciplinary Team

The hospice is similar to other patient care settings in managing the treatment plan using an **interdisciplinary team**. The difference, however, is in the composition of the hospice interdisciplinary team. The team is led by a physician, either a hospice-employed physician or the patient's attending physician, who can elect to continue following the patient. The remaining members include, but are not limited to, a nurse, social worker, pastoral or other counselor, and a bereavement coordinator. Some hospices may also include a volunteer or the volunteer coordinator, a pharmacist, or a home health aide as part of the interdisciplinary team.

The nurse acts as the case manager and coordinates changes to the care plan with other members of the team. The social worker provides psychosocial evaluation and social resources that can be utilized by the patient and family. The pastoral or other counselor offers spiritual support and comfort. The bereavement coordinator prepares the patient and family for the impending death and provides grief support to the family after the patient's death. **Volunteers** who receive special hospice training offer companionship, comfort, transportation, light housekeeping, and even direct patient care (depending on their professional qualifications). The pharmacist works with the nurse and attending physician to provide adequate symptom relief. The home health aide is assigned by the nurse and the attending physician to provide bathing, shampooing, other personal care, light housekeeping, and other nonskilled treatments such as dressing changes.

Primary Caregivers

The fact that most hospice care is provided in the patient's home requires that a member of the patient's immediate family and/or friends act as a **primary caregiver**. Members of the patient's interdisciplinary team visit the patient a few times per week, possibly more often depending on the patient's condition. The team, however, is not with the patient 24 hours per day, so the team members must teach the primary caregiver to give treatments, medications, and baths, and to watch for changes in the patient's condition, when hospice personnel are not present.

If the patient can no longer live alone and does not have anyone who can act as the primary caregiver, the hospice has two options. If the hospice has its own facility, or contracts with a nursing home or hospital for a hospice unit, the patient could be placed in a bed there. The staff on these units act as primary caregivers under the direction of the staff and treatment plan of the hospice. The hospice can also arrange to have volunteers and/or home health aides provide additional hours of care in the patient's home if necessary.

Regulatory Issues

Licensure and Accreditation

A hospice program is licensed by the state in which it is located. In many states, licensure regulations closely follow the Medicare *Conditions of Participation*.

A licensure issue that has recently been in the forefront for many hospices in the United States is regulation of stand-alone facilities, or hospice facilities that are not directly affiliated with a larger hospital system. These stand-alone facilities have inpatient beds that can be used by hospice patients for management of acute symptoms and/or as a residence if there is not someone in their home to help care for them. In many states, these facilities would need to be licensed and regulated as nursing homes, because there is no other licensure category available. Many hospices feel that the nursing home standards are not applicable to hospice care and do not recognize the significant differences in hospice treatment protocols. One example is the requirement in nursing homes to monitor the amount of food eaten by a patient. In hospice, the terminal patient usually does not eat within the final stage (**active phase of dying**) before death. There is very little necessity to monitor food intake.

The National Hospice and Palliative Care Organization (NHPCO) publishes a book of standards that can be utilized by hospices to validate the quality of care provided. The NHPCO, however, does not require hospices to be certified or accredited under these standards to date and has no survey process similar to other regulating and accrediting organizations. Staff at the NHPCO are available for questions or concerns regarding interpretation of NHPCO standards and the *Conditions of Participation*.

The Joint Commission on Accreditation of Health Care Organizations (JCAHO) publishes hospice standards as part of its home care standards. The publication is entitled *The Comprehensive Accreditation Manual for Home Care*. The number of hospices seeking accreditation from JCAHO increases every year; however, many hospices are still not accredited because of the high cost of the survey application and preparation process. For this reason, this chapter specifically addresses the *Conditions of Participation* that all hospices (usually regardless of size) need to meet in order to receive reimbursement under the Medicare program (and any other third-party reimbursement subsequently).

The *Conditions of Participation* standards describe regulations pertaining specifically to Medicare patients; however, most third-party payers refer back to the *Conditions of Participation* when evaluating acceptability of hospice election for their clients. In addition, the *Conditions of Participation* are utilized by state regulators to assess hospice programs for licensure, making the *Conditions of Participation* the main standards that hospices follow.

Hospice Medicare Benefit

Throughout the Medicare *Conditions of Participation*, using hospice coverage is referred to as "electing the hospice benefit." Hospice is reimbursed under Part A for Medicare patients. Upon election of the Hospice Medicare Benefit, Medicare will pay for no other Part A services that are related to the patient's hospice (terminal) diagnosis. The hospice benefit literally is a benefit for patients, because hospice coverage includes all services: clinical staff, medications, durable medical equipment, oxygen, supplies, lab work, and therapy. If a patient decides to **revoke** hospice coverage, because he or she would like to return to aggressive treatment rather than palliative treatment, the patient returns to regular Medicare coverage.

Certification

To be eligible to elect hospice coverage under Medicare, the patient must be entitled to Medicare Part A and be certified as terminally ill. An individual is considered to be terminally ill if he or she has a medical prognosis of six months or less if the illness runs its normal course. The Benefits Improvement Protection Act of 2000 clarified that this certification "shall be based on the physician's and medical director's clinical judgement regarding the normal course of the individual's illness" (P. L. 106-554, 2000, p. 501).

Health information management (HIM) department staff members are not usually responsible for obtaining the oral certifications, as these must be obtained from a clinical staff member (usually a registered nurse), but they may have significant involvement in obtaining the written certification statements. Many outside physicians (not employed by the hospice) choose to follow their own patients within the hospice program. Either way, the certification must be signed by both the certifying physician and the hospice medical director. Before the Balanced Budget Act of 1997 (P. L. 105-33), hospices were required to have these certifications signed no later than eight calendar days after election. This eight-day requirement was lifted in 1997, and hospices are now required to have written certification before submission of a claim to Medicare. Hospices focus significantly on this process of obtaining the certification statements in order not to affect reimbursement, which based on the regulations cannot be paid without both signatures, within the required time frame. Fiscal intermediaries for Medicare reimbursement have begun more actively requesting copies of hospice patient medical records, and have requested the return of payment when the above signatures were not in place.

The Hospice Medicare Benefit is structured into benefit periods, the first of which begins on the date of election. The Balanced Budget Act of 1997 also revised regulations relating to these benefit periods. Patients now have three benefit periods: an initial 90-day period, a subsequent 90-day period, followed by an unlimited number of 60-day periods. Before 1997, patients leaving hospice care in their final period had exhausted their benefit and could not receive hospice care under Medicare again. Patients can now revoke or leave hospice care and return at a later time with no risk to their Medicare coverage. Patients must continue to be eligible for hospice care at the beginning of each new period. This process is described later in this chapter.

Election of Hospice Care

Medicare regulations require that the patient or his or her legal representative sign an election statement at the time of admission to hospice care. The election statement must include specific requirements described in the Medicare *Conditions of Participation*. The statement must identify the hospice. It must contain a statement that acknowledges that the patient understands the palliative nature of hospice care and that standard coverage for Medicare services related to the patient's terminal diagnosis is waived. The statement must have an effective date and be signed by the patient or legal representative.

The HIM department must ensure that if the election statement is signed by the patient's legal representative, there is documentation (power of attorney, legal guardian, patient advocate) in the medical record reflecting that this person is indeed the legal representative. Many hospice programs in the past have assumed that if the person signing is the patient's primary caregiver, then no other proof is necessary. As an authorization for release of medical information is evaluated for validity, so should the signature on the election form. The HIM department must provide significant clinical education in this area.

Revocation

A patient may revoke the election of hospice care at any time. There must be a revocation form signed by the patient and filed with the hospice stating that the patient loses the remaining days in the current benefit period and the effective date of the revocation. The effective date may not be earlier than the date on which the form is signed by the patient.

The HIM department needs to ensure that the statement is received and filed in the medical record. Upon revocation of Medicare hospice coverage, the patient resumes regular Medicare coverage and loses all remaining days within the election period. To elect hospice care again, the patient would be admitted in the subsequent election period. Monitoring the election periods to ensure correct billing practices may be the responsibility of the HIM department or the billing department staff. Verification of the validity of the signature on this form is also appropriate.

Change of Designated Hospice

The patient may change (transfer) hospices once during each benefit period without needing to revoke. A statement must be filed with the hospice from which care has been received and with the new hospice. The statement must indicate the date the change is effective and must be signed by the patient.

The statement must be filed in the patient's medical record. Verification of the signature is again appropriate. It is important to establish the actual date of change and coordinate it with the other hospice.

Contracting with Other Facilities

When care is provided to hospice patients in contracted hospitals or nursing homes, the hospice must maintain professional management of the patient's plan of care.

The HIM department is responsible for obtaining documentation from these facilities. It is important to coordinate with clinical staff the signing of a patient authorization to obtain this information from the treating facility. Most hospitals and/or nursing homes will not provide copies of this information without an authorization even if the hospice program still considers these patients as active hospice patients. It is important that the HIM director is involved in the establishment of any contract with a hospital and/or nursing home that will provide acute treatment to hospice patients, so that the issue of obtaining copies of medical records on hospice patients can be addressed.

Plan of Care

A plan of care must be established for all hospice patients. The plan of care must include the following components per Medicare *Conditions of Participation*:

1. Assessment of patient needs
2. Identification of services to be provided
3. The scope and frequency of services required to meet the needs of the patient and families
4. Schedule for regular reviews and updates by the interdisciplinary team

Many hospice programs design a form specifically for an interdisciplinary team meeting and retain this form in the medical record. If the patient's attending physician is not a hospice employee, it will be necessary to document the physician's participation in development and maintenance of the interdisciplinary plan of care. This can be done through documentation of physician orders, clinical staff documenting conferences with the patient's attending physician, and/or communicating with the attending physician regarding the patient's status and the updates made to the plan of care. It is also important that the plan specify the interval until the next review. This information can also be added to the written plan of care kept in the medical record.

Informed Consent

Hospice is required to obtain an informed consent that specifies the type of care and services that may be provided. The HIM department must ensure that the signature on the informed consent is valid and any associated documentation of personal representative status is included in the medical record.

Quality Assurance

Hospices must have a quality assurance program that monitors and reviews the quality of care provided, including inpatient services. Information documented in the medical record and/or collected by HIM department staff can be the primary source of quality review activities. HIM department staff should work closely with clinical staff to provide ongoing documentation, to review feedback, and to identify cases to be evaluated.

Volunteers

A unique regulation in the Medicare *Conditions of Participation* is the requirement for volunteers. Hospices must document volunteer hours in both administrative and patient care activities in an amount that equals 5 percent of the total patient care hours of all paid and contract staff.

To substantiate that volunteers provide direct patient care, HIM department staff should participate in volunteer orientation programs to provide basic documentation guidelines. Volunteer staff may or may not be clinically oriented. They may never have documented in a patient's medical record, so basic education on the do's and don'ts of documentation is very important. The capture of volunteer hours may or may not be an HIM department function. The capture of volunteer hours is made easier with the use of volunteer logs, completed by all volunteers regardless of the functions being performed. The log documents the name of the volunteer, the patient seen or activity performed, the number of hours and minutes, and any miles driven if applicable. The data can then be captured in a spreadsheet program or hospice software program. The number of hours of volunteer time is then compared to overall paid staff time in direct patient care to determine if the 5 percent criterion has been met.

Patient Records

Hospices must establish and maintain a medical record for every patient receiving hospice care. Services provided by all disciplines should be documented and included in the patient record. Signatures and dates are required for all entries. The record should include a minimum of the following:

1. Initial and subsequent assessments
2. Plan of care including interdisciplinary team updates
3. Identification data
4. Consents
5. Authorizations
6. Election forms
7. Pertinent medical history
8. Complete documentation of all services

Records must be evaluated to determine if all progress notes have been signed appropriately. In addition, records should be easily accessible. They could be filed numerically or alphabetically depending on patient volume.

Documentation

As stated previously, most hospice care is provided in the patient's place of residence. Clinical staff members (nurses, social workers, home health aides) visit the patient's home at least once every two weeks, probably even more depending on the condition of the patient. Their visit length varies depending on the condition of the patient and the needs of the family. The patient may or may not be seen by a physician during the entire hospice stay. If the patient has an attending physician outside the hospice, the patient may go to the physician's office if well enough. The hospice physician may only visit in an emergency situation or if the patient does not have an attending physician. The nurse acts as the case manager, coordinating care from all disciplines and communicating changes in the patient's condition with the physician.

Overall, the hospice medical record contains significant *nonphysician* documentation and is *nonintegrated*; all disciplines document separately on their own progress notes, primarily because all disciplines do not visit the patient at the same time and integrated notes would be difficult to manage. The hospice should establish a standard time frame in which the clinical staff must have each visit documented. Many hospices require clinical staff to document their visits within 24 hours of the actual visits; others hospices may provide longer time frames. Regardless of the standard, it is critical that it be routinely enforced to ensure that the medical record of each patient is current. This is extremely important when the primary nurse (or other primary team member) is not available (such as on a weekend or during vacations). If necessary documentation (or physician orders) is missing, then quality patient care is lacking. The HIM department should take an active role in this process by routinely evaluating current charts for documentation.

Historically, many hospice programs left ongoing clinical notes in the patient's home. Periodically, or upon the death of the patient, progress notes were sent to the HIM department for filing. Over time, many hospices have eliminated this practice due to confidentiality and continuity of care. The open medical record at the hospice is only as current as the most recent note documented and subsequently filed.

This practice can create several problems for HIM department staff. The first is timeliness of visit documentation. If not monitored, some clinical staff members may not keep current in documentation practices. In order to facilitate documentation, progress notes should be created as check-off forms. As much as possible, the clinician should be allowed to check a box for an appropriate assessment, rather than writing a sentence (see Figure 13-1).

Later, the clinician can add progress notes using the check-off assessment as a guide. Offering the ability for clinical staff to dictate progress notes can also reduce time spent in documentation. Some hospices are also providing clinical staff with laptop or palmtop computers with specific software to utilize for progress note documentation. This may or may not save time in progress note documentation depending on the computer skills of the user, but may, by linking the information in the laptop

---

HOSPICE OF SOUTHERN ILLINOIS, INC.

PATIENT NAME _____   PATIENT NUMBER_____   DATE _____
                                                         am   am
DIAGNOSIS_____   TIME IN____ pm TIME OUT____ pm

VITAL SIGNS
B/P_____Pulse_____
Resp_____Other _____

ACTIVITY
☐ Up Ad Lib
☐ Needs Assist
☐ Total Care
☐ W/C ☐ Geri Chair
☐ Bedfast

MENTAL STATUS
☐ Alert
☐ Oriented
☐ Disoriented
☐ Confused
☐ Drowsy
☐ Lethargic
☐ Withdrawn
☐ Agitated/Anxious
☐ Unresponsive

NUTRITION
☐ Solid foods
☐ Soft foods
☐ Liquids
☐ Other _____
☐ Dysphagia
Appetite
☐ Good ☐ Fair ☐ Poor

ORAL CAVITY
☐ Pink ☐ Thrush
☐ Dry
☐ Other_____

SKIN
☐ No Difficulty
☐ Rough, Dry/Scaly
☐ Skin Tears
    Location_____
☐ Rash/Itching
    Location_____
☐ Bruising Site

☐ Active Decubitus
    Size_____
    Location_____
☐ Edema
    Location_____
    Pitting (Circle)
    0 +1 +2 +3 +4
TURGOR
☐ Good ☐ Fair ☐ Poor
COLOR
☐ WNL   ☐ Pallid
☐ Cyanotic ☐ Ashen
☐ Jaundice ☐ Flushed
☐ Mottled

RESPIRATORY
☐ No Problem Assessed
Description_____
Apnea_____/Sec
☐ Dyspnea
    ☐ At Rest
    ☐ With Exertion
O₂ @_____L
☐ N/C
☐ Mask
☐ Continuous
☐ PRN

COUGH
☐ Seldom
☐ Frequent
☐ Intermittent
☐ Dry
☐ Productive
☐ Sputum
    Color_____

URINARY
☐ WNL
☐ Incontinent
☐ Catheter
    Size_____
Output_____
Color_____

BOWELS
☐ Regular
☐ Incontinent
☐ Diarrhea
☐ Constipation
☐ Elimination Aids

☐ Colostomy
LBM _____
Bowel Sounds
☐ Absent ☐ Present

GASTROINTESTINAL
☐ No Problem
    Assessed
☐ Abdominal pain
☐ Distention
☐ Ascites
☐ Nausea
☐ Vomiting

MEDICATION SCHEDULE REVIEWED
☐ Yes ☐ No

CAREPLAN CHANGES NECESSARY
☐ Yes ☐ No

VISIT ☐ On-call Visit
           ☐ Routine Nursing Visit

CURRENT PAIN RATING
☐ Pt report   ☐ C/G report
☐ Nurse Assmt
    circle one
0 1 2 3 4 5 6 7 8 9 10

Number of B/T in 24 hours _____

☐ Declined Medication Change

Meds re-orders/New Orders
_____
_____
_____
_____
_____
_____

Problems
_____
_____
_____
_____

Interventions
_____

Freq Changes (discuss with CSM)
☐ Nsg   ☐ HHA

PATIENT/CAREGIVER COMMENTS _____

PROGRESS NOTES_____
_____
_____
_____
_____
_____
_____
_____
_____
_____
_____

TEACHING/EDUCATION Instructions given to ☐ Patient ☐ Caregiver ☐ NH Staff ☐ Other
Subjects:_____
_____

HHA SUPERVISORY VISIT   ☐ Direct   ☐ Indirect
☐ Following POC   ☐ Following Assignment Sheet   ☐ Courteous/Cooperative   ☐ Quality of Care   ☐ Documentation
Patient/Caregiver Response _____

Overall HHA Evaluation   ☐ Satisfactory   ☐ Unsatisfactory

Staff Signature_____   Visit Verification Signature_____
8/25/99 Rev 8/2003
N:\HSI Forms\Pagemaker\nsg note340.1.p65\tms

Nursing Visit Note

Form # NSG 340.1
2 Part

Figure 13-1   Nursing Visit Note. (Courtesy of Hospice of Southern Illinois, Inc., Belleville, Il.)

computer with a larger network, provide more continuity of patient care. The benefits of laptop computers would need to be extensively researched by the organization. Ultimately, regardless of the system used, HIM department staff should periodically monitor open charts to verify timeliness of documentation.

A **hospice inpatient unit** can take two forms. The hospice can contract with a nursing home or a hospital to utilize designated beds or a wing of the facility for hospice patients. The patients are often already in the facility and are identified by the staff as hospice appropriate. The nursing home or hospital staff contacts the hospice to admit the patient. In this method, the facility where the patient is staying continues to maintain a medical record. The hospice creates and maintains a separate medical record. There will be overlap. Physician orders and interdisciplinary care plans will come from the hospice. The hospice nurses will continue to visit the patient on a regular basis, as in the patient's home. Once the patient dies or is discharged, the hospice will supplement the patient's record by taking copies of portions of the facility's medical record (just the portion during the time the patient was in hospice). Critical to this program is the negotiation of the contract. Administrators as well as staff must know all aspects of the contract relating to caring for the patient. HIM personnel should ensure that they are involved in this process in order to obtain portions of the medical record after the patient's death and to understand the flow of the documentation.

The second way in which a hospice can be considered an inpatient unit is if it has its own inpatient facility. Patients are admitted directly to the facility, although they may have been referred from a hospital or nursing home. In this facility, all care is given around the clock by hospice employees. The medical record created here is similar to a hospital or nursing home record with periodic assessment of the patient's condition. Unlike home care documentation, inpatient documentation can use integrated progress notes. All disciplines document on the same set of progress notes.

Regardless of the setting, a physician must certify that the patient is terminally ill, with a life expectancy of six months or less, if the disease follows its normal course. This physician can be the patient's attending physician or the hospice physician. The certification statement can be incorporated onto a review of the patient's previous history obtained by the nurse upon initial physical assessment. In this way, the certifying physician can verify history given by the patient about the illness. The statement could also be incorporated onto the initial orders for treatment to reduce the amount of paperwork needing the signature of an outside physician. In either case, the hospice medical director (or a designee) must also sign the same statement. It is important that the HIM staff determine the most effective method to obtain the statement promptly and reduce time spent by the medical staff to sign paperwork.

At the time of admission to the hospice program, a nurse visits the patient in the place of residence to perform an initial assessment. At this time, the nurse completes a history of the patient's illness, performs a physical examination, and evaluates the appropriateness of the patient for hospice care. If the nurse assesses that the patient is hospice appropriate, the interdisciplinary care plan will be started. Initially, this will be nursing care plans, and if necessary, volunteer and home health aide care plans.

The nurse will then notify the additional members of the team (social work, therapy, chaplaincy, bereavement), who will initiate their care plans. The interdisciplinary care plan is developed from a compilation of the individual care plans initiated by each discipline. The nurse (or case manager) is responsible for coordinating the compilation of the care plans and communicating them to the attending physician. The interdisciplinary team usually meets every two weeks, or more or less, often depending on the hospice. During the meeting, each active patient is discussed, care plans are reviewed, the hospice physician may recommend new orders, and specific problems may be addressed. These reviews are documented for each individual patient on a specific interdisciplinary team conference form (which includes the compilation of care plans to form the interdisciplinary care plan) filed in the patient's medical record. The interdisciplinary care plan may or may not change depending on the condition of the patient.

It is necessary to indicate which team members are present at each meeting. All team members can sign in for each meeting, and this sign-in sheet can be retained for future review, or each team member can sign the individual team conference forms for each active patient. Depending on the number of active patients, the second method may be too time-consuming for the team members. It is important that the interdisciplinary care plan be filed in the patient's medical record, even if the patient dies before an actual team meeting. This care plan will be a focus area for most inspectors, who will clearly evaluate the presence of interdisciplinary communication.

The home health aide provides basic, nonskilled care for patients, and may or may not be required in every case. It is the nurse's responsibility to determine the need for a home health aide, including frequency and scope of the visit (what is to be performed). What is to be performed may depend on the skills of the aide. Many states have initiated testing for home health aides. The aide must demonstrate certain skills to become certified. Hospices hiring certified home health aides can at least be assured of a minimum skill level. Once the case manager has determined that an aide is required, a home health aide care plan is initiated. It is important that a *written* home health aide care plan is filed in the medical record. On the care plan, the case manager provides specific instructions for tasks to be performed, the frequency of the tasks, as well as any potential complications (or signs and symptoms) of which the aide should be aware. The home health aide must then document completion of the individual tasks according to the specified frequency as documented by the case manager.

It is the responsibility of the case manager to supervise the services provided by the home health aide. This supervision must be documented in the medical record. The case manager must assess the skills of home health aides by watching them provide services to the patient and/or family, as well as evaluating the patient/family's assessment of the home health aide's services. The case manager can usually document this supervision within routine progress notes or on a separate supervisory visit note. The case manager can rotate the assessments to include one visit with the home health aide to assess his or her skills with the next visit without the home health aide to discuss the aide's skills with the patient and family. In addition, the nurse should be ensuring that the home health aide care plan is being carried out as specified for each visit, which can be accomplished by requiring the case manager to cosign visit records completed by the home health aide. This procedure will also help further document supervision of the home health aide.

The nurse may also identify additional services needed by the patient and family that cannot be adequately covered or provided by paid hospice staff, including companionship, shopping, transportation to the doctor, or respite for family members. The case manager may initiate a request for volunteer services and begin the written volunteer care plan (again including scope and frequency of the services required). The hospice volunteer coordinator is then responsible for locating active volunteers who are willing to provide the requested services. Though the regulations do not require a specific documentation of supervision of volunteer services, the case manager should ensure that the volunteer care plan is being carried out effectively.

Volunteers are required to document all contact with hospice patients, including telephone calls. To help volunteer staff complete documentation in a timely manner, most hospices have volunteer offices and/or space available for volunteers to come in and document, or allow the volunteer to document at home, but provide self-addressed envelopes for the volunteer to mail in progress notes. The volunteer coordinator should take an active role to ensure that all visits made are documented by volunteer staff. The HIM department can also help in this process by open and closed chart review.

Upon the death of the hospice patient, all active care plans as well as the interdisciplinary care plan are closed. If the death is in the patient's home, a registered nurse makes a death visit. A death in an institutional setting such as a nursing home or hospital may not require the services of a hospice nurse. Depending on the state, and individual cities and counties, a home death may require opening a medical examiner's case file. In addition, state laws may specify who can legally pronounce a patient dead. The hospice usually notifies local police departments or the coroner's office that there is a hospice patient residing in their district, so that upon the patient's death ambulances and police cars do not come with sirens blaring. This is important for the well-being of the family. Regardless of the specific legal requirements, the nurse must document all steps clearly in the medical record, including (but not limited to) notification of the medical examiner (if applicable) with the corresponding case number, notification of local police, the time the patient was pronounced dead (which may be different from the time of the patient's actual death), contact with a funeral home to pick up the patient's body, as well as the condition of the family and significant others present. A death visit may be from two to four hours depending on the condition and request of the family. In addition to documentation of the death visit, the nurse should also complete a discharge summary documenting all care plans opened and their method of resolution. Resolution may be death of the patient or specific problems that were addressed previously.

After the death of the patient, bereavement services are available to the patient's family and any significant friends for up to one year following the death. The bereavement coordinator may have been working with the family before the patient's death to initiate potential care plans. The bereavement staff then tailors a bereavement program according to the needs and wants of family and friends. This may run from the initial bereavement assessment visit only, in which the family and/or friends want no additional contact from the hospice, to families and friends who require regular visits. The medical record is not considered complete without bereavement assessment and bereavement notes. Because of the lengthiness of the bereavement period, the record is usually analyzed, coded, and filed in a permanent location without complete bereavement documentation. As bereavement notes are written, they are added to the record in the permanent file throughout the one-year bereavement period. It is important that HIM department staff continuously monitor the status of bereavement activities to ensure that all bereavement documentation is contained in the patient's medical record.

Reimbursement and Funding

The Medicare *Conditions of Participation* provide four levels of hospice care (Figure 13-2). All levels of hospice care must be directed by the interdisciplinary team, and the medical record must document the need for each required level of care. The most common is *routine home care*. Routine home care occurs when a patient is receiving routine (or nonproblematic) care in the place of residence.

MEDICARE CONDITIONS OF PARTICIPATION - LEVELS OF HOSPICE CARE

- **ROUTINE HOME CARE**

  — A patient is at "home" and is not receiving continuous care.

- **GENERAL INPATIENT CARE**

  — A patient receives general inpatient care in an inpatient facility for pain control or acute or chronic symptom management that cannot be managed in other settings.

- **CONTINUOUS CARE**

  — A patient receives hospice care consisting predominantly of nursing care on a continuous basis at "home." Must be at least eight hours to be reimbursed at the continuous care rate.

- **INPATIENT RESPITE**

  — A patient receives care in an approved facility on a short-term basis.

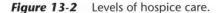

Figure 13-2   Levels of hospice care.

Respite care provides an interval of rest for the primary caregiver and is provided to hospice patients in an approved (or contracted) facility (e.g., a nursing home, hospital, or hospice inpatient unit). Respite is provided on an occasional basis, for not more than five days at a time. The regulations are not specific on the definition of "occasional," but they do require hospices to evaluate families who require frequent respite periods to determine if the patient more appropriately belongs in a nursing home or inpatient hospice. When respite services are not provided by the hospice, but in a contracted facility, the hospice maintains a separate medical record from the facility providing the services. The nurse, social worker, home health aide, and hospice physician continue to visit the patient and provide services as if the patient were still at home. The contracted facility staff members act as the primary caregivers when hospice staff members are not there. The medical record must clearly indicate the need for respite services and also when and where the services are being provided. The hospice must obtain copies of the corresponding medical record from the facility providing respite care (if not the hospice itself) and incorporate these medical records in the current hospice medical record.

General inpatient care occurs when a patient receives care in an inpatient facility (a hospice inpatient unit or a facility contracted by the hospice) for pain control or acute or chronic symptom management that cannot be managed in the patient's place of residence. Situations include pain that could not be controlled in the home with titrated doses of medication and requiring IV or nerve block therapy, or hemorrhaging from a tumor site. Again, the hospice interdisciplinary team is in charge of the plan of care, even if the services are provided by a nursing home or inpatient hospital. In addition, the *Conditions of Participation* require a hospice nurse to visit a patient daily when the patient is receiving general inpatient care. The medical record must clearly indicate this information. Medicare limits the number of inpatient days (including general inpatient and respite) to 20 percent of the total patient care days. As with respite care, the hospice maintains its own medical record, and the medical record from the facility providing general inpatient care must be obtained and incorporated into the hospice medical record.

Continuous care occurs in the patient's place of residence when a patient requires continuous care for a minimum of 8 hours in a 24-hour period. Continuous care must be predominantly nursing care, although home health aides may also participate. An example of the need for continuous care includes the hours before the patient's actual death (the active phase) in which the family is not able to handle the emotional stress of waiting alone or is not able to handle the patient's physical symptoms. The medical record must document at least hourly progress notes confirming the presence of continuous care.

The levels of hospice care are directly related to the way hospices receive reimbursement. Medicare (Part A), Medicaid, and most commercial insurance companies reimburse hospice care on a *per diem* basis or each day the patient is enrolled in a hospice program. This is in contrast to a *service-based* reimbursement (utilized for some non-hospice home care) in which an agency receives payment based on services provided by clinical staff. Per diem payments are paid regardless of whether any services (visits by clinical staff) are actually given each day. Each level of hospice care is reimbursed at a different per diem rate. Once again, the Balanced Budget Act of 1997 changed the way all levels of care are reimbursed by Medicare. Hospices must now submit claims indicating the Metropolitan Statistical Area (MSA) code based on the geographic location of the patient. Claims are paid based on the physical geographic location of the patient. These rates are published annually by the Centers for Medicare and Medicaid Services (CMS).

Medicare rates are fixed by CMS. Medicaid rates are controlled by the individual state; and other commercial insurers, such as Blue Cross, may have their own hospice per diem rates. The hospice per diem includes not only visits by hospice clinical staff (nurses, social workers, home health aides, and chaplains; only the hospice physician can bill separately from the per diem) but also medications (relating to the hospice diagnosis, e.g., pain medication for bone cancer, but not necessarily insulin for long-term diabetes), durable medical equipment, laboratory work, oxygen, supplies, and bereavement services. When the patient expires, reimbursement stops, even though the family and friends may be receiving bereavement services for up to one year. The insurers state that the per diem rate has been calculated to include bereavement support. If the patient is seen by the attending physician during the hospice admission, the physician can continue to bill under Medicare Part B (and separately for other insurers as well).

Upon admission to a hospice program, the *patient* signs an "election of the hospice benefit" statement. This statement not only indicates that the patient is invoking the hospice benefit (through Medicare Part A, Medicaid, and most other commercial insurers), but also states that all other services related to the patient's hospice diagnosis, such as skilled home care, inpatient hospitalization, and nursing home care, are not to be paid by the insurer to any other agency. This is an important aspect of hospice reimbursement, especially when a hospice patient receives respite care or general inpatient care in a nursing home or inpatient hospital setting. If a hospice does not have its own inpatient facility, it must *contract* with an approved (at least meeting the *Conditions of Participation*, licensed) nursing home and/or inpatient hospital to provide respite and pain and symptom management. The contract stipulates that only the hospice can bill Medicare (and other insurers) for hospice care. The hospital or nursing home can charge the patient (or an insurance company or even the hospice) for room and board only, but cannot bill for the hospice services (even if services are provided by its staff) according to the election statement. As described previously, the hospice patient is still managed by the hospice interdisciplinary team regardless of the setting for care. The incentive for a nursing home or inpatient hospital to sign such a contract with a hospice would be to fill beds that might otherwise be vacant to receive room and board payments.

In addition to the levels of hospice care, the *Conditions of Participation* also describe three benefit periods.

As described previously, the benefit periods are currently one 90-day period, a second 90-day period, and an unlimited number of 60-day periods. The hospice must evaluate the patient at the end of each benefit period to determine if the patient is still considered hospice appropriate or continues to have a limited life expectancy. The premise for hospice care is that the patient has a life expectancy of six months or less, so it should be unnecessary for most hospice patients to stay beyond the second benefit period. At the end of each benefit period, if the patient is still considered hospice appropriate, the hospice medical director (or physician designee) must recertify the patient as requiring hospice care. Evaluating that the patient still has a limited life expectancy can be difficult in some diagnoses (congestive heart failure, chronic obstructive pulmonary disease, Alzheimer's disease) because not every diagnosis follows a usual path. To assist hospices in determining life expectancy, the National Hospice and Palliative Care Organization has released a series of papers developed by various clinicians outlining signs, symptoms, laboratory testing, and examination results that may indicate limited life expectancy for various diagnosis groups (renal, cardiac, respiratory, mental). These can be used to develop a specific worksheet for the different diagnosis groups, which can be used by the nurse in consultation with the patient's attending physician (or the hospice physician) to determine if a patient should be recertified for hospice care. The recertification statement signed by the hospice physician could be added to the worksheet, which should be filed in the medical record. The medical record will then clearly indicate the process that was used to determine that the patient is still considered hospice appropriate.

If the hospice finds, according to available criteria and analysis, that the patient no longer has a limited life expectancy, it is the hospice's responsibility to discharge the patient from the hospice benefit. It is important that the hospice determines as soon as possible in the first benefit period that the patient may not be hospice appropriate for further benefit periods, because once a patient is discharged within a benefit period, he or she loses all subsequent days not used within that benefit period. Some insurance companies may have reimbursement caps and/or day caps for hospice care. The insurance company may only pay up to 180 days for hospice coverage, eliminating the unlimited benefit periods for hospice coverage, or it may only pay a designated dollar amount as a lifetime maximum for hospice services. It is important for hospice insurance verification staff when negotiating with commercial insurers to determine if any of these caps are in place.

The hospice patient can also choose not to continue with hospice services. The patient's terminal condition may improve slightly and/or the patient and family may choose to seek more aggressive treatment (such as chemotherapy). If the patient chooses to stop receiving hospice services, the patient may revoke the hospice benefit. Discharge (other than death) is initiated by the hospice; revocation is initiated by the patient. In both circumstances, the patient loses the remainder of days within the current benefit period. If the patient chooses to be readmitted to a hospice, he or she will be readmitted in the next consecutive benefit period. It is critical for HIM departments to monitor the level of care and benefit period status of all admitted patients on a daily basis to ensure that billing is correct. This process can be accomplished through completion of the daily census and cooperative communication with clinical staff.

Information Management

Information management in hospice has much in common with all other health care settings. There is a master patient index, diagnosis index, and physician index. Data contained in medical records is abstracted and utilized for quality improvement, reimbursement, and statistics. This section describes some of the differences in information management that make hospice unique.

Data and Information Flow

The start of any database in hospice begins with the first contact a patient or potential patient has with the hospice, either from the patient or family, a physician, a hospital, or a nursing home. The hospice admissions area can capture the name of the patient, demographic information, diagnosis, referring physician, and all other elements of a standard minimum data set on a paper referral form or in a computerized information system. Many patients and families are not ready for hospice initially, so every contact may not always result in an admission, but many return after time to the hospice for admission, so it is important to retain information from these initial contacts to make any subsequent contact easier.

Once the hospice determines that a patient is to be admitted, a nurse is assigned to the case. The nurse visits the patient at home and performs a history and physical assessment, which further verifies the appropriateness of the patient for hospice. At this visit, the nurse also obtains patient/legal representative signatures on the election of hospice, medical and financial consents, and any other appropriate paperwork. Simultaneously, or just before this visit, the hospice obtains verbal certification from the patient's attending physician verifying that the patient has a limited life expectancy, obtains information about the patient's primary diagnosis and related diagnoses, determines if the patient's attending physician wants to continue "following" the patient (or would prefer the hospice physician to act as the attending), and obtains any initial physician orders for medication. The medical record begins with a paper referral form or face sheet, the history and physical, consents, and initial physician's orders. The HIM department can begin a computerized database with information abstracted from this initial documentation, including the date of admission, benefit period, and level of care, which can be tracked for a daily census and reimbursement.

The nurse coordinates the assignment of additional hospice personnel, social workers, home health aides, the hospice physician, and volunteers, and begins the interdisciplinary care plan. The medical record, now housed at the hospice, will be expanded to include the hospice physician's assessment, social work assessment, home health aide assignment of duties, additional physician orders, and an attending physician/hospice medical director signed certification of terminal illness. As various clinical staff members make assigned visits to the patient, and physician orders change, they will be added to the medical record at the hospice. At least every two weeks, the interdisciplinary team will meet as a group to discuss the care of the patient; the record will document these meetings as appropriate.

The HIM staff may review the record concurrently for signatures, but will need to concentrate more on ensuring that all visits made by clinical staff members are documented and filed in the medical record. Many hospices and home care agencies require their clinical staff to complete a daily log, documenting which patients have been visited, the length of the visit, and associated mileage, which is usually reimbursable to the employee (see Figure 13-3).

Clinical staff could attach all progress notes to their corresponding logs, which could be turned into HIM on a daily basis. HIM department staff can then verify that a progress note exists for each patient visit made; those visits missing progress notes could be addressed with the specific staff member immediately. In addition, data from the mileage logs, including name of clinical staff member, name of patient(s) visited, date of visit, length of visit, associated mileage, and type of visit made (assessment visit versus routine visit), could be abstracted into an information system. This will begin a resource utilization tracking database. If supplies are dispensed during a patient visit, documentation on a requisition form or on the progress note could also be abstracted, if included with the progress note and activity log.

Upon the death (or discharge) of the patient, all open interdisciplinary care plans are closed, the nurse documents a discharge summary (summarizing all care plans initiated, actions taken, and results), and the bereavement assessment is documented. The HIM department at this point should complete a qualitative analysis of the medical record and abstract additional pertinent information (such as ICD-9-CM codes for symptoms and complications addressed in care plans), date of death (or discharge), and location of death (or reason why the patient was discharged, e.g., revocation, hospice discharge, or transfer to another program). Depending on the state and city of death, the HIM department may also be responsible for initiating the death certificate or providing information to a funeral home to complete the death certificate. This is especially true if a hospice-employed physician has been acting as the patient's attending physician. The death certificate may require the signature of the hospice physician. Upon final analysis by the HIM department, the medical record can be filed in an appropriate permanent location waiting for the bereavement progress notes.

Coding and Classification

The primary requirement for hospice admission is the certification of the patient's attending physician that the patient has a limited life expectancy (six months or less). The per diem reimbursement (unlike the prospective payment system used in acute care hospitals) is based solely on the care level and the benefit periods, not on the patient's diagnosis. This reimbursement perspective makes hospice diagnosis coding different from other settings. The hospice medical record does not include significant

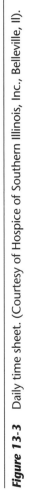

Figure 13-3 Daily time sheet. (Courtesy of Hospice of Southern Illinois, Inc., Belleville, Il).

FINANCIAL CLASS CODES

M   Medicare
W   Medicaid
V   Per Visit
P   Per Diem
R   Non-Reimbursable
C   Champus
B   Black Lung
O   Other

SERVICE CODE

1   RN (Registered Nurse)
2   LPN (Licensed Practical Nurse)
3   HHA (Home Health Aide)
4   SS (Social Services)
5   CNSL (Counseling Services)
6   SUPP (Supportive Services)
7   VL (Volunteer Services)
8   VLP (Volunteer Professional

VISIT/NONVISIT CODE

11   Client Contact, Assessment
12   Client Contact, Visit
13   Client Contact, Preadmission
16   Client Contact, Continuous Home Care
17   ClientContact, Phone Call
18   Bereavement
19   Client Contact, Documentation
21   Meetings, Team meetings
22   Community Education

Administrative

23   Administrative/Office Time
24   Meetings, Inservices and Supervision
25   Orientation and Education
26   Marketing/Fundraising

Team meetings include Interdisciplinary Team meetings, morning report and all other patient care meetings.

Community Education includes time spent by HSI staff doing education to the community, contracted facilities or other healthcare providers.

Meetings and Inservices includes staff meetings and inservices provided in house by PIT or other outside presenters and supervisory visits.

Orientation and Education includes new employee orientation and educational conferences and workshops attended outside of the HSI offices.

Visit time is defined as the time actually spent with the patient or caregiver.

S=start
F=finish

PAY CODES

R   Regular Time
V   Vacation
S   Sick
P   Personal
H   Holiday
B   Bereavement
J   Jury duty
C   Pager Time

Time Increments (Time spent)

.25 =	8 to 22 minutes
.50	23 to 37 minutes
.75	38 to 52 minutes
1.00	53 to 67 minutes

10/2002 Revised 3/2003
N:\daily time sheets\daily activity log legend revision.doc\tms

Figure 13-3   (*Continued*)

laboratory findings, radiological reporting, or any other ancillary services that could be used to "diagnose" the patient. The hospice medical record may include copies of medical records from a hospital if the patient is a direct transfer, or if the patient may not have been to a hospital recently, with the only information about the patient's diagnosis coming from the physician's office medical records. It is important that the hospice attempt to obtain copies of as many recent medical records as available on the patient to aid in the coding of the principal diagnosis, but in the end, the assignment must be the reason the patient has a limited life expectancy.

ICD-9-CM

International Classification of Disease, 9th Revision, Clinical Modification (ICD-9-CM) coding principles should be followed in the assignment of diagnosis codes; however, the specificity of coding may be limited depending on what information is available. To hospice clinical staff, it does not matter if the patient has lung cancer of the lower lobe, lung cancer of the upper lobe, lung cancer of the bronchus, and so forth. It only matters that the patient has terminal lung cancer and is treated accordingly. It is not necessary in hospice to obtain or document the specificity required in ICD-9, or for the diagnosis related group (DRG) system. This is not to imply that HIM coders should not try to be as specific as possible in the coding assignment; it merely indicates that there is not an incentive for the information to be available. It is important that HIM professionals attempt to alter this perception, because a database is being created by insurance carriers and Medicare with these limited diagnosis codes, and eventually the database may be used to create a prospective payment system for hospice.

The hospice medical record is significantly nursing documentation. Hospice coding staff should evaluate nursing documentation to look for complications or symptoms that the nurse is trying to manage. Symptoms such as pain (of any body location), constipation (which is a direct result of pain medication such as morphine), respiratory distress, and fatigue are all acceptable to code in hospice. In addition, complications such as urinary tract infections, decubitus ulcers, open wounds or hemorrhage of tumor sites, and thrush are all coded. The coding of these additional signs and symptoms helps build a diagnosis database that can be used to evaluate not only the quality of care given (how many catheter patients develop urinary tract infections) but also the components to the care of various diagnosis groups (such as end-stage respiratory diseases).

CPT

Physicians who are *employed* by the hospice can also bill for their services. Depending on the location of the patient, either in the home or in an inpatient facility, the current procedure terminology (CPT) evaluation and management codes can be used to bill for hospice physician services. Hospice coders should discuss the CPT evaluation and management codes with hospice physicians to educate them on their correct use.

If a hospice physician performs a procedure, such as a paracentesis (which is common in patients who have abdominal cancers), ICD-9-CM and CPT can be utilized to assign procedure codes. HIM department staff should coordinate the assignment of procedure codes with hospice billing staff to ensure that physician services are appropriately reimbursed.

Computer Systems

The decision to computerize any database, whether in a hospital or a hospice, is very important and requires careful analysis and thought before purchase. In hospice, benefits of a computerized database or clinical information software include online registration of all patients, electronic billing, resource utilization, donation tracking (hospices receive many monetary and other donations that should be tracked), minimum patient data set, order entry tracking, and online documentation of progress notes. The number of applications is only limited by the imagination and expertise of the users.

Currently there are two main hardware options for computer implementation. The first is the use of a mainframe or central computer. There are hospice clinical information systems that use a mainframe architecture. Several issues must be addressed before the purchase of a mainframe system. Mainframe systems are usually more costly than local-area network systems or personal computer–based systems. Mainframe systems usually require the expertise of a programmer to retrieve nonstandard reports and information. Mainframe systems may not allow immediate access to data; they may need to be "downed" at certain times to update the database with newly entered information. Mainframe systems have more power to capture and store large volumes of information than a local-area network. They may be more effective at integrating financial and clinical information in one database. All of these elements should be evaluated by the hospice.

The second and more popular option is to utilize a local-area network. A local-area network is less expensive and can be expanded from a one-user system to a multiuser system over time. A local-area network does not usually require the expertise of a programmer, depending on the software. There are currently many hospice software vendors that use local-area networks. Software on a local-area network is usually Windows compatible, which opens up a wide range of possibilities for integrating with financial software, billing software, and spreadsheet and word-processing software. Once the choice of hardware is made, then searching for a vendor for hospice clinical information software is the next step. There are not as many hospice software vendors as are available for hospitals. Many hospice software vendors combine a hospice component with a skilled home care system, or offer hospice software with a skilled home care component, because many hospices are dually certified to provide both types of care. As the hospice market expands, more vendors will become available.

The newest trend in computer hardware and software for hospice and skilled home care is the use of the laptop or palmtop computer, which can be used to record progress notes at the patient's bedside. Bedside terminals have been widely used in acute care settings, and the use of laptops or palmtops in home care is increasing every year. One problem that clinical staff has most often is getting progress notes documented. The use of the laptop with progress note capability is an effort to reduce documentation time. In addition, the laptop, if linked to a network, could obtain daily schedules of all visits to be made and could be utilized to capture date, length of visit, patient visited, and mileage, virtually eliminating the need for a daily activity log.

There have been mixed reviews in the hospice industry about the use of the laptop. Clinicians who are computer literate and comfortable with a keyboard or even a pen-based system have no problem. However, clinicians who are not computer literate have a great deal more trouble adapting to this system. For these staff members, hand documenting progress notes is probably faster. Some hospices have reported that laptop computers do not save time but do provide more continuity of care and improve documentation. The hospice organization must decide what is best for its needs. In another effort to help clinicians provide more timely documentation, some hospices allow staff to dictate progress notes on handheld recorders or on more expensive dictating systems. These notes are then transcribed on a word-processing program, printed, signed by the dictator, and filed in the medical record. As with the laptop computers, some clinicians are comfortable dictating, but others cannot organize their thoughts well enough. Providing staff with a standard outline of a progress note on a business card will aid them in organizing their notes.

Data Sets

Several data sets should be captured and maintained within the hospice. These include patient data, resource data, and census data.

Patient Data

Patient information should include as a minimum those data elements in a standard minimum data set. In addition, the hospice will also want to capture the name of the primary caregiver and any other significant family members (for bereavement tracking), the referral source (this is useful to aid marketing staff), where the patient is or was employed, religion, directions to the home, funeral home, language spoken, location of death, and reason for discharge. The National Hospice and Palliative Care Organization requests significant statistical information about the patient population from each hospice on a yearly basis. In addition, many hospices are involved with grant writing to obtain additional funding for programs, also requiring significant descriptions of the patient population to be served.

Resource Data

Resources are all those clinical staff members and vendors who provide services to a patient. Because hospice is reimbursed on a per diem basis, it is critical that the hospice monitor its actual cost per patient versus reimbursement per patient. A resource database can help provide this information. Resource data and resource utilization should capture the name and specialty (registered nurse, social worker, etc.) of all clinical staff members; the names of all vendors, such as durable medical equipment, pharmacy, and supplies; all durable medical equipment dispensed to the patient and associated costs to the hospice; all supplies dispensed to the patient and associated costs to the hospice; the date, clinician, mileage, type of visit, and length of visit on every patient; other clinician time associated with the patient including telephone calls, interdisciplinary team conferences, and staff conferences; the cost of clinician time using salary plus benefits to obtain a cost per hour; cost of mileage reimbursement; and all medications and associated costs dispensed to the patient. The contents of the resource data set can be utilized in combination with the patient data set to provide total costs per patient, total costs by diagnosis, and total costs by resource. In addition to costs, staff hours by patient, staff hours by diagnosis, and staff hours by resource are examples of other reports that can be created to monitor resource utilization.

Census Data

Census data include the number of admissions, discharges, transfers, and the number of patients under the care of the hospice on a given day. Other statistics that should be captured include patient days, average length of stay, and average daily census not only for the patients but also by insurance, by age group, and by location (nursing home, inpatient hospital, home care). Many agencies request census information on a yearly basis from each hospice, and the hospice itself monitors census status.

Hospices may also want to create databases or ensure that hospice software contains data elements for the following:

- *Donations*, including type and amount of all monetary and nonmonetary donations, donors, and relationship to any previous patients. (This is useful for fundraising efforts.)
- *Bereavement*, including names and current addresses of bereaved family members, associated patient and date of patient's death, and status of bereavement efforts (active or inactive).
- *Volunteers*, including names and addresses, training dates, evaluation dates, cost savings attributable to volunteers, special skills (e.g., barber or nurse), availability (days, evenings, weekends), and status (active or inactive).

Ultimately, it is better to collect too much information at least initially than to not collect enough. Once the data entry document is filed, it is very time-consuming to retrieve it and go back later to capture the information.

Quality Improvement and Utilization Management

Quality Improvement

In general, hospices evaluate quality of care similarly to other health care settings. Patient, family, and physician satisfaction surveys are a key method of evaluating quality of care provided by hospice staff. The satisfaction surveys are geared toward evaluating responses to the specific services offered to patients/families/physicians by the hospice (Did you find volunteers helpful?) as well as regulatory requirements (Did you receive a copy of the patient's rights?). It is important that hospices attempt to obtain satisfaction surveys from living patients. It is not enough to send a patient satisfaction survey to the family after the patient's death. A patient satisfaction survey should allow the patient to respond. Hospices also have formal quality improvement committees with a documented quality improvement plan. Similar to a hospital, the quality improvement committee requires quality improvement programs within each hospice division or department. Certain departments may report the results of their quality improvement efforts on a quarterly or yearly basis, whereas other departments (e.g., nursing) may report quality improvement results more often.

Quality improvement in the hospice medical record department takes the form of two distinct operations. One is monitoring the contents of the medical record to ensure compliance with federal, state, and local accrediting agencies (and JCAHO); the second is ensuring the integrity of all data abstracted and captured on computer.

The medical record department evaluates the contents of each medical record, ensuring compliance with all appropriate regulations. In addition, the review should also monitor compliance to the contents of care plans. If the home health aide's care plan says that the patient should be shampooed at each visit, the record should document that this activity was performed. If the nurse's care plan states that the patient is to be educated on the cleaning of a wound, the medical record should document that this education was performed. There is debate at most agencies about whether care plan compliance review is a medical record department function or a nursing peer review function. Nursing peer review tends to justify decisions and documentation because the reviewing nurse too closely identifies with the practicing nurse. Medical record review by trained health information professionals looks at the documentation much more objectively. This perspective may need to be emphasized within the organization.

As mentioned previously, medical record departments also have the responsibility of ensuring that all visits made by clinical staff have also been documented. This can be done concurrently utilizing clinical staff daily activity logs to verify the presence of documentation associated with a visit, or this process can be done upon death (or discharge) of the patient by pulling the daily activity logs at the back end. It is recommended, from a quality perspective, that clinical staff turn in activity logs with associated progress notes on a daily basis, which will ensure that the medical record is accurate and current at all times. The longer the interval for the documentation of progress notes, the less likely the clinician will document an accurate or complete note.

Medical record departments should continuously monitor all clinicians to determine who is in compliance and who is not. Hospice and home care tend to be high-pressure, high-burnout working environments for clinical staff, with staff turnover high in some areas. Closely monitoring staff compliance to documentation ensures that medical records are not left incomplete as a result of staff resignation.

Because of the number of outside physicians who continue to follow patients through the hospice, medical record documentation review also encounters many occasions when it is necessary to obtain progress notes and/or signatures from outside physicians, for example, on physician telephone orders (which will be the majority of orders in the medical record unless given by a hospice-employed physician), physician certification of terminal illness, and any related physician office documentation to supplement the hospice medical record. The Medicare *Conditions of Participation* require the original signature (as opposed to a faxed signature or stamp signature) on all documentation, so it is necessary to make a copy of the document and send the original document to the physician for an original signature. The medical record department should create a "tickler" file or log indicating which originals have been sent out and then carefully monitor the log to ensure the originals are returned in a reasonable amount of time (7 to 10 days). The physician's office should be contacted or visited (marketing personnel or volunteers are options) to determine the status of any originals not returned. The original medical record should not be filed as complete without these documents.

The second quality improvement operation, computerized data integrity, may be considered secondary to medical record compliance review in some agencies; however, with the growing statistical requirements from all types of agencies (Medicare, JCAHO, Medicaid, National Hospice and Palliative Care Organization, local state hospice organization, insurance companies, managed care agencies), this operation is just as critical. Data entry operations should be continuously monitored for accuracy. Data should be evaluated not only for accuracy but also validity.

Utilization Management

Hospice utilization management evaluates three areas: appropriateness of admission (Is the patient terminally ill?); continued stay review at the second and subsequent benefit periods; and appropriateness of level of service (routine home care versus general inpatient care). A utilization management committee is appropriate to monitor trends and statistics regarding review functions. The National Hospice and Palliative Care Organization's publications describing factors that *may* indicate limited life expectancy by diagnosis group can help identify appropriateness of admission and aid in the recertification of continued stay. However, these guidelines need clinical interpretation and should be used in conjunction with a physical examination and evaluation of the patient and family situation to fully determine appropriateness. It is because of this difficulty in predicting terminal illness that it is recommended that admission review and continued stay review be performed by a nurse. The medical record staff can aid in tracking the results and/or initiating a worksheet, but with limited criteria (unlike more specific acute care criteria) for determining appropriateness, it would be difficult for nonclinical staff to predict the status of the terminal illness.

Evaluating appropriate level of care can be performed concurrently before initiating a level of care transfer, or retrospectively by reviewing the closed medical record. Because respite and continuous care tend to be requested by the family rather than initiated by the clinical staff, it may be helpful to evaluate these cases retrospectively to determine if any other course of action could have been taken to alleviate patient and/or family stress (such as the placement of additional volunteers or home health aides in the home more frequently). General inpatient care should have clear criteria for use and should be reviewed concurrently. However, many times it is difficult to determine if a symptom is related to the terminal illness, for example, the patient who falls at home and breaks a hip. The patient's principal diagnosis is lung cancer. On initial review, the broken hip is probably not related to the terminal illness, but upon admission to the hospital, bone metastases in the hip are found that contributed to the break.

Hospices can also benefit from the use of a severity system. The Karnofsky scale is a good example, rating level of functioning on a scale of 100 to 0, with 100 meaning no evidence of disease and 0 meaning death. A sample of the Karnofsky Scale is shown in Figure 13-4. It is expected that all hospice patients will continue to decline and eventually die, but evaluating the severity of their illness on admission would provide valuable statistics related to resource utilization, so that one nurse would not always be assigned the most severely ill patients. The most severely ill patients die sooner, affecting overall length of stay. Statistical monitoring and trending of severity could help plan an effective diagnosis case mix.

Risk Management and Legal Issues

The fact that most hospice care is provided in the patient's home could increase the risk of possible lawsuits significantly, not only from the possibility of the clinical staff being injured at the patient's home, but also because clinical staff must function virtually independently. Nobody other than the patient and/or family is with the clinician during an examination, which can culminate in a "we" versus "they" scenario—"but the nurse said"; "but the family said." At this time, hospice has remained relatively lawsuit-free, although the potential exists. Many families and friends are so thankful that hospice was there to help them that thoughts of lawsuits are not in their mind. However other families argue over the concept of hospice—"you're letting our mom die"—so the hospice ends up in the middle. Other families argue over an estate, and in their grief, may also place hospice in the middle.

It is with this risk that clinical staff need to be educated on the importance of obtaining proper consent for admission and procedures. Many hospice patients are unable to consent for themselves and have appointed personal representatives.

Karnofsky Performance Status Scale		
Definitions	*Rating (%)*	*Criteria*
Able to carry on normal activity and to work; no special care needed.	100	Normal no complaints; no evidence of disease.
	90	Able to carry on normal activity; minor signs or symptoms of disease.
	80	Normal activity with effort; some signs or symptoms of disease.
Unable to work; able to live at home and care for most personal needs; varying amount of assistance needed.	70	Cares for self; unable to carry on normal activity or do active work.
	60	Requires occasional assistance, but is able to care for most of his or her personal needs.
	50	Requires considerable assistance and frequent medical care.
Unable to care for self; requires equivalent of institutional or hospital care; disease may be progressing rapidly.	40	Disabled; requires special care and assistance.
	30	Severly disabled; hospital admission is indicated although death not imminent.
	20	Very sick; hospital admission necessary; active supportive treatment necessary.
	10	Moribund; fatal processes progressing rapidly.
	0	Dead

Figure 13-4 "Karnofsky Performance Status Scale" (p. 109) from *Oxford Textbook of Palliative Medicine* (1993) edited by Doyle, D. et al. (By permission of Oxford University Press.)

Clinical staff should verify that someone is actually a personal representative by reviewing proper legal documents. A progress note can document that these papers were seen, or a copy of the documents can be filed in the medical record. If no representative has been assigned, clinical staff should be educated to help the family obtain personal representative status. The patient should, however, be the first to sign consents; an "X" is appropriate if witnessed. If the patient is unable to sign, the medical record should document why the patient was unable to sign (patient in a coma, patient has Alzheimer's disease). Clinical staff truly want to help patients/ families, and in doing this, they tend to overlook that the patient is a widower with four sons. All they want to do is get help for the patient, but they must be educated to verify which of the four sons is appropriate to consent for their father.

Upon the death of the patient, the medical record department may get requests from insurance companies or attorneys to settle a claim or probate the patient's estate. No copies of the medical record should be released without proper authorization from the assigned representative of the estate. Documentation verifying representative status should be requested and kept in the medical record. Requests for copies of medical records may also come from family members, usually in dispute of a will or insurance claim. It is important that medical record department staff speak with the family about their request. Because of the nature of hospice care, many family members are angry, hurt, and upset by the death of their family member and are trying to seek some closure. Many of them feel that a copy of the medical record may help them do this, to understand why their family member died. Sometimes, just by talking with family members, medical record staff can gently discuss with them the difficulty in obtaining a medical record (authorization by representative of the estate, etc.). If the family is still adamant, it is important that the medical record be reviewed to ensure that no negligence or complaint was voiced by the patient or family. Remembering that the care plans are the standard of care, all care plan documentation should be reviewed to verify proper completion and proper compliance by the patient.

Another area requiring continued education is the documentation of telephone calls and interdisciplinary communication. All Medicare and JCAHO surveyors expect to see interdisciplinary communication documented in the medical record, but even more important are the legal ramifications of not documenting telephone calls and interdisciplinary communication. As an example, if a hospice does not have its own pharmacy, it is necessary to order medications from an outside pharmacy. The nurse may place the order by telephone; if the telephone call is not documented, and it is the weekend and the primary nurse is not available, another nurse might order the medications again. Another example may be that a home health aide visits the patient for a daily bath and the patient complains of severe pain. The aide documents on her progress note that the patient complained of pain, but does not communicate this with the nurse. The patient suffers, until finally the primary caregiver calls the nurse later that evening wondering when pain relief is coming. Both are examples of the importance of telephone calls and interdisciplinary communication. Provide all clinicians with adequate supplies of blank progress notes.

Role of the Health Information Management Professional

The HIM professional in hospice must be the documentation expert on all documentation standards from all accrediting and licensing agencies. This responsibility may be difficult because hospice is traditionally dominated by nursing staff, who also feel that they are the documentation experts. The HIM professional needs to continually offer workshops to clinical staff in basic documentation techniques (including how to correct an error, telephone call documentation, legal viewpoint on documentation,

documentation requirements of accrediting and licensing agencies). Gradually, nursing and other clinical staff will gain respect for the HIM professional. In addition to documentation expert, the HIM professional should also volunteer to create and revise medical record forms; a good working knowledge of word-processing or spreadsheet software will make this job easy. A forms committee can coordinate form usage and revision. If the HIM professional starts the committee, it is likely that he or she might be the chairperson.

Another role for the HIM professional is that of data manager. Assertiveness in offering to retrieve information at meetings and team conferences is a way to build a reputation as a data manager. The HIM professional can offer to complete statistical reports requested by agencies and compile and distribute a daily census. The admissions or discharges or patient days for a period of time can be graphed. The HIM professional can look at trends and describe them to others. Again, it is important to be assertive in telling people what an HIM professional is able to do. Many hospices are not yet as sophisticated as hospitals in their interpretation and evaluation of data and need an expert who can educate them.

Other areas in which the HIM professional should be involved are as a member or chairperson of a utilization review committee or a quality improvement committee, as an advisory board member for the hospice, or as a coalition organizer of other hospice HIM staff in the area or across the state.

Trends

In the future, hospice will be challenged by issues related to:

- Decreasing length of stay
- OIG scrutiny of hospice care provided to nursing home residents
- HIPAA privacy
- Expansion of the palliative care specialty
- Increased computerization

In the past several years, hospices across the nation have experienced a sharp decline in the average length of stay for hospice patients to the point that one- and two-day lengths of stay are becoming commonplace. Because of the per diem reimbursement provided by Medicare, finding ways to increase average length of stay is a constant challenge facing hospices. Education of both the health care community and the lay community on the benefits of involving hospice sooner will be the key to changing this trend.

The Office of the Inspector General (OIG), which is the arm of the Department of Health and Human Services charged with investigating and monitoring the Medicare and Medicaid programs, has been scrutinizing hospice care provided to nursing home residents for several years. The OIG has questioned whether hospice services provided to nursing home patients are equivalent to services provided to home patients and whether the services qualify for equal reimbursement. Hospices across the nation along with the NHPCO are working to maintain the reimbursement and eligibility for hospice care for nursing home residents.

The Health Insurance Portability and Accountability Act (HIPAA) of 1996 has changed the face of health information privacy across the health care continuum. As mentioned earlier in this chapter, hospice treats the patient and family as one unit of care. Hospices are now challenged with changing their internal policies and procedures to tighten this unit and ensure that HIPAA privacy standards are met.

Many hospices have expanded their scope of practice to include palliative care services that can be provided to patients who are not eligible for hospice benefits. Members of the hospice team work together to provide comfort care through the control of pain and symptoms for patients who are chronically ill or have chronic pain and symptom issues. Certifications are now available for both physicians and nurses in the specialty of hospice and palliative care.

An expanded need for data management and information management personnel will occur. The use of computerized patient records, laptops and/or palmtops, telemedicine, and the Internet requires expertise that many health care professionals do not have. HIM professionals will continue to be in high demand, with their skills in document management, computerization, privacy, and statistical management.

Summary

Hospice care for terminally ill patients is significantly different from the care provided in other health care settings. It is the only health care setting in which the focus of care is not on curing the patient. It is with this philosophy in mind that the HIM professional must also realize that his or her role will be unique. What is significant about coding in hospitals, outpatient facilities, skilled home care, and other facilities relying on a prospective payment system for reimbursement will not apply in hospice. The high volume of requests from insurance companies, attorneys, and patients requesting medical records to the degree that a correspondence service is needed to help process the requests will not be significant in hospice. Finally, we spend a multitude of time learning and trying to understand the medical staff, their committees, their governance, their handwriting, their signatures, and even their dictation, which we can unlearn in hospice. Thus, as hospice forges a new role in the provision of health care, the HIM professional must also forge a new role in hospice.

Key Terms

active phase of dying   hospice staff refer to the patient as being "active." This is usually the last 24 to 48 hours before the patient's death, but can begin up to two weeks before the patient's death. This period is marked by shutting down of the body functions (low or no urinary output, more secretions, possible significant respiratory congestion, the "death rattle," mottling or blotching of the skin of the extremities). The patient stops eating, may stop drinking, may not be able to swallow or have difficulty swallowing, may become restless and confused, and may be unresponsive. Some patients may have all of these symptoms, others just some, but for the most part the death of the patient can be anticipated.

bereavement (bereaved, bereave)   suffering the death of a loved one. Refers to the time immediately following the death of the patient. In hospice, clinical staff help family and significant others through this period for up to one year, and longer if requested by the patient's family and friends.

curative therapy   any medical therapy given for the purpose of curing disease.

hospice   a facility or a program designed to provide a caring environment to meet the physical and emotional needs of terminally ill patients and their families and significant others.

hospice inpatient unit   a hospice with a specific set of beds either in its own building or as a wing of a hospital or nursing home, providing round-the-clock clinical staff to care for terminally ill patients. These units provide respite care, pain and symptom management, and/or routine home care for patients who have nobody in their home to help care for them.

interdisciplinary team   a patient care team made up of two or more clinical disciplines—usually a nurse, social worker, home health aide, physician, pastoral or other counselor, volunteer, therapist, and dietitian—who plan for the care of the terminally ill patient.

palliative care   the opposite of curative therapy. Clinical measures are taken to reduce the intensity of disease symptoms, rather than providing a cure for the disease. Hospice tries to reduce the intensity of such symptoms as pain, nausea, and anxiety with a variety of pharmacological and nonpharmacological methods.

place of residence   wherever the patient is currently living—his or her own home, a relative's home, a senior citizen's complex, a nursing home, assisted living, etc.

primary caregiver   the person designated to provide care for the patient when hospice staff is not available. This can be any relative, a spouse, a friend, a significant other, a paid caregiver, an adult child, or any other person. The primary caregiver provides a range of care depending on his or her comfort level, from giving medications to changing dressings to emptying catheter bags.

revoke (revocation)   performed by a hospice patient (or family or legal guardian) to give back or annul his or her hospice benefit. Once a patient has revoked the hospice benefit, the patient returns to routine Medicare or other commercial insurance benefits and loses all remaining days in the current benefit period.

terminally ill   a limited life expectancy, usually less than six months.

volunteer   a person who provides a service (clerical, clinical, companionship, etc.) without any monetary or other reimbursement.

REVIEW QUESTIONS

Knowledge-based Questions

1. True or false: Hospice takes care of only cancer patients.

2. Provide examples of how hospice tries to relieve terminal symptoms for patients.

3. List the members of an interdisiplinary team in hospice.

4. What is the role of the primary caregiver?

5. Describe how a Medicare patient elects to receive hospice care.

6. Describe the role that volunteers play in hospice care.

7. Discuss bereavement services provided by hospice.

8. Describe the four levels of hospice care described in the Medicare *Conditions of Participation*.

Application-based Questions

1. Provide examples of some of the data that can be collected by hospices.

2. Describe components of a hospice utilization review program.

Web Activity

Visit the National Archives and Records Administration (NARA) Public and Private Laws database at the following URL: http://www.gpoaccess.gov/plaws/index.html
    Click "browse" under "previous Congresses" then select the *105th Congress*. Scroll down or search for Public Law 105-33 (Balanced Budget Act of 1997). Click on either the text or PDF link to this law. Find the section of the law that deals with hospice care benefits periods. What is this section number?
    As a follow-up to the preceding activity, review federal regulations in the *Code of Federal Regulations* by visiting http://www.gpoaccess.gov/cfr/index.html
    Follow these steps to find the appropriate section of the regulations:

- Click the link to the "Browse" feature.
- Scroll down and check the most recent revision of Title 42, "Public Health."
- Scroll down and click the "Continue" button.
- Hospice regulations are found in Part 418 of Title 42, so click on the range of "Parts" that includes 418.
- When this range of "Parts" appears, click on the specific link to Part 418, "Hospice Care."

- Click on either the text or PDF link to the section that corresponds to "Condition of Participation—Central Clinical Records" (Section 418.74).

How might you use each of these documents as a hospice health information manager?

Case Study

A 66-year-old woman and her two daughters present themselves at the hospice. The woman's attending physician suggests that she investigate hospice as a health care alternative. The woman has breast cancer with bilateral mastectomies and has recently been found to have metastases to the liver. Her physician has stated that she could have additional chemotherapy, but that her liver cancer may not respond. At this point, other than mild pain, she is able to get around relatively well. She is not sure she wants to have additional chemotherapy; it made her terribly ill the first time. Her daughters and their families (both have two children; all are under the age of 10) are her only close relatives. She has been divorced since her first mastectomy. One daughter lives 5 minutes away; the other daughter lives 40 minutes away. Upon further discussion with the daughters, the first daughter wants only what her mother wants, and will support whatever decision she chooses; the second daughter wants her mother to have the additional chemotherapy no matter what and cannot understand why anyone would "just give up." You are the admission representative:

1. What would you tell this woman and her daughters about hospice?
2. What problems do you anticipate this family having?
3. How would you respond to the second daughter's comment that hospice is "just giving up"?
4. Is this patient appropriate for hospice?

References and Suggested Readings

Abraham, P. R. (2001). *Documentation and Reimbursement for Home Care and Hospice Programs.* Chicago, IL: American Health Information Management Association.

Corr, C., and Corr, D. (1983). *Hospice Care Principles and Practice.* New York: Springer Publishing Company.

Home Health and Hospice Standards. (1995). Chicago, IL: Joint Commission on the Accreditation of Healthcare Organizations.

Hospice care, *Conditions of Participation, Code of Federal Regulations*, Title 42, Pt. 418, 2003 ed.

Miller, S. C. (1996). *Documentation and Information Management in Home Care and Hospice Programs.* Chicago, IL: American Health Information Management Association.

P. L. 105-33. (1997). Balanced Budget Act of 1997.

P. L. 106-554. (2000). Appendix F. Medicare, Medicaid, and SCHIP Benefits Improvement and Protection Act of 2000.

Standards of a Hospice Program of Care. (1993). Arlington, VA: National Hospice and Palliative Care Organization.

Key Resources

Hospice Association of America
228 Seventh Street, SE
Washington, DC 20003
Phone: 202-546-4759
http://www.hospice-america.org

Joint Commission on Accreditation of Healthcare Organizations
(See Chapter 1 for contact information.)

National Hospice and Palliative Care Organization
1700 Diagonal Road
Suite 625
Alexandria, VA 22314
Phone: 703-837-1500
Fax: 703-837-1233
http://www.nhpco.org

Chapter 14

Dental Care Settings

Cheryl L. Berthelsen, PhD, RHIA
Denise D. Krause, MA, MS
Francis G. Serio, DMD, MS

Learning Objectives

Upon successful completion of this chapter, you should be able to:

1. Identify the different practitioners associated with dental care and describe their roles.
2. Describe documentation requirements specific to the practice of dentistry.
3. Explain the importance of the medical history in dentistry.
4. Discuss the potential impact of managed care on dental practices.
5. Describe utilization management strategies used in dentistry.
6. Identify specific risks associated with dentistry and strategies to manage the risks.
7. List the information needs of the dental office.
8. Identify the important components of a dental computer system.
9. Describe potential career opportunities for HIM practitioners.

SETTING	DESCRIPTION	SYNONYMS/EXAMPLES
Dental Office	A private practice facility where patients receive dental care	
Dental Clinic	A department within a larger health organization where patients receive dental care	Within a community health center Within a dental school Within a VA medical center Within a prison Within a local government health department
Dental School	A school within a university where dentists and dental hygienists are educated and trained.	

Introduction to Setting

Dental practitioners may treat patients in a variety of settings. Whenever a patient receives a dental examination or treatment, a dental record is created. Each setting poses unique problems and challenges in the provision of dental care for patients, the type of documentation generated, and the management of dental records.

Care Settings

Solo Dental Practice

A **solo dental practice** is owned and operated by one dentist. The dentist owns or leases the office building or suite and all the necessary equipment and furniture to run the business. The solo-practice dentist usually employs at least a receptionist and a dental assistant, and may also hire an office manager to oversee the day-to-day business operations of the practice. Dentists may employ a full-time dental hygienist or contract with a hygienist to come to the office one or two days per week to provide either routine preventive care or definitive periodontal treatment. Some dentists elect to perform routine cleanings themselves.

Although the solo-practice dentist is responsible for his or her patients 24 hours a day, in reality the dentist is not often called when the practice is closed. Occasionally, a patient may need a prescription for an antibiotic or pain medication, but the instances in which a dentist has to meet a patient at the office during off-hours are rare.

The solo-practice setting has been remarkably stable over the years despite increasing competition. Figure 14-1 contains information about the practice setting of dentists in the United States in 1994 (Lazar, 1997). These percentages have changed little over the past 10 years. Solo-practice dentists sometimes rent space in their offices to another practicing dentist to supplement office income or hire a newly licensed dentist to work

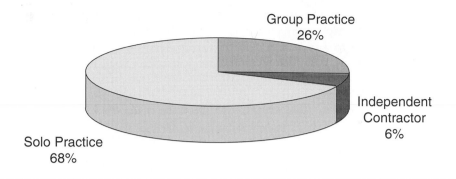

Group Practice
26%

Independent
Contractor
6%

Solo Practice
68%

Figure 14-1 Practice setting of dentists in 1994. (Graphic created by C. Berthelsen, based on data from Lazar, 1997.)

as an associate. The associate receives only a portion of the fees collected for work performed, and the remainder of the fee reimburses the practice for use of office and equipment. The solo-practice dentist is responsible for maintaining dental records of all patients treated. Dental records for patients of tenant dentists who rent space on evenings and weekends are the responsibility of the tenant, not the dentist–owner of the practice. When the solo practitioner retires, he or she must store and maintain the dental records of patients as long as state statute dictates. If a dentist sells the practice, the dental records usually transfer to the dentist buying the practice, as these patient records constitute the majority of the value of the practice.

Group Dental Practice

A **group dental practice** is composed of two or more dentists practicing together. The group of dentists is usually incorporated as a legal entity, and the corporation owns and operates the business rather than the individual dentists. Ownership of the corporation may be shared equally among the owner–dentists, or there may be one or two major owners with the remaining dentists as minor owners. The amount of money each dentist earns from the business is based on how well the business did as a whole and the percentage of ownership in the corporation instead of individual productivity. There may be bonuses based on individual productivity. A group practice may also be composed of two or more dentists who share office expenses and equipment but are not incorporated. They practice as a group to benefit from sharing the expenses of running the business, but income belongs to the dentist who treated the patient and generated the fees.

Group dental practices may be composed of dentists practicing in the same specialty (orthodontists) or different specialties (general dentists plus an endodontist, periodontist, and prosthodontist). Multiple specialties allow the dentists to refer patients needing specialty care to a dentist within the group rather than to an outside practice. Single specialty groups use the same type of equipment and instruments and can share them. Multispecialty groups need a wide variety of instruments specific to the specialties involved. Dentists within the group practice usually share on-call service for each other to deal with patient emergencies. Dental records of patients of group practices are usually filed and maintained together. The records are available to any dentist in the group seeing a patient during an emergency appointment. It is the corporation's responsibility to store and maintain the dental records.

Clinics in Academic Institutions

All universities that have a school of dentistry to educate and train dentists have clinics for patients to receive dental treatment. Dental care is provided by dental students under close supervision of faculty who are licensed dentists. Patients are charged significantly reduced fees for dental care, but the treatment may take many more visits to complete than in a private dental office. Schools that educate and train dental hygienists may be associated with a dental school or may be independent and have their own training clinics. The care provided to patients at a dental hygiene clinic is limited to procedures that a dental hygienist is allowed to perform by state licensure rules.

The dental records generated in academic settings serve purposes beyond the documentation of care provided. They are important evidence of the student's progress toward and preparation for graduation and licensure. Most states require dental students and dental hygiene students to complete a certain number of specific dental treatments and procedures before they are eligible to take state board licensing examinations. Dental records of patients who these students treated are material to proving their eligibility for licensure. Dental records in academic settings are also important to research. Faculty is involved in the discovery of treatment modalities, diagnostic tests, restorative materials, prostheses and anesthetics, as well as the invention of new devices, instruments, and equipment. New methods of preventing dental decay and periodontal (gum) disease are being studied and proven at major dental schools throughout the world. Dental records within these institutions are important to that progress.

Third-Party Organizations

Dentists and patients may participate in a variety of third-party organizations to assist in the payment for dental services. For more detail on these organizations, see the "Reimbursement" section of this chapter. In most instances of third-party payment, the care is provided in the dentist's private office, although there are separate dental clinics for some health plans in certain parts of the country.

Acute Care Hospital

Large academic medical centers and acute care hospitals may have an associated dental clinic or dental emergency room. Patients served in this setting may be victims of trauma who have sustained an injury to face or teeth (alone or in addition to other types of injuries), or patients requiring general anesthesia for dental treatment. Dental treatment may be provided in the emergency room, as an inpatient, or as outpatient surgery. Dental records of these treatments may be filed with hospital records for an inpatient or maintained separately for emergency room or outpatients. Storage and maintenance of these dental records are the responsibility of the associated institution.

Many of these hospitals also provide outpatient dental care through a general dental residency program. Care is provided by graduate dentists who are receiving advanced training in general dentistry from a group of attending dentists. These dental records are maintained by the dental clinic or may be part of the hospital's general medical record.

Other Settings

There are many other settings where dental treatment may be provided and dental records created and maintained. Prisons usually have dental clinics to care for inmates. Veterans Affairs (VA) hospitals also have dental clinics to serve the dental needs of veterans. Active military bases usually have dental clinics associated with the base hospital or medical clinic. Some colleges and universities have dental clinics to care for dental needs of students. Community health centers may also provide both routine and emergency dental care for its patients. The storage and maintenance of dental records are the responsibility of the entity operating the clinic, not the dentists providing the care.

Types of Patients

Children and Adolescents

Dentistry has changed for children in the twenty-first century. The use of fluoride has made a tremendous impact in the prevention of dental **caries** in children. The National Institute of Dental Research estimates that 60 percent of children aged 2 to 9 are caries-free in their primary dentition and 55 percent of children aged 5 to 17 are caries-free in their permanent dentition (Kaste et al., 1996).

Early childhood caries, also known as nursing caries or baby bottle tooth decay (BBTD), is a problem for infants and toddlers. Children who are allowed to go to bed at night with a bottle filled with liquid other than water develop caries in their **primary teeth**. A study of Head Start children across 5 southwestern states found that 24 percent of all children had BBTD (Barnes et al., 1992). Unfortunately, the public has not been well educated about this problem. A study of midwestern college students found that only 39 percent of respondents had heard of BBTD and 32 percent of those thought it was a fictional health problem (Logan et al., 1996). A 1991 study on inappropriate infant bottle feeding for Healthy People 2000 found that 95 percent of children 6 months to 5 years old had used a bottle and 20 percent of them were put to bed with a bottle with contents other than water (Kaste and Gift, 1995). More than 8 percent of children 2 to 5 years old still used a bottle, thus highlighting the need for widespread education on the risks of bottle feeding.

Chipping, fracturing, and loss of primary and permanent teeth caused by falls and accidents are common. A child typically begins to lose primary teeth at ages 5 to 7. When development is delayed, dental intervention may be needed to ensure the eruption of healthy permanent teeth. The dentist may need to pull stubborn primary teeth that fail to come out on their own. Many American children and adolescents receive orthodontic treatment (braces to straighten teeth). Orthodontic and palatal deformities caused by thumb-sucking or persistent use of pacifiers is also a problem requiring corrective orthodontia and sometimes surgery.

Adults

Adults generally have more dental disease than children and require costly restorations. Many children from 1950 to 1970 had teeth filled with a variety of materials to treat dental caries. As adults, these restorations gradually fail, requiring replacement by larger and larger fillings and eventually **root canal therapy (RCT)** and prosthetic **crowns**. The National Institute of Dental Research estimates that 57 percent of the elderly and 21 percent of the 18-to-64 age population have root caries. Adults also develop gingivitis and periodontal disease. If untreated, teeth loosen and eventually fall out. A missing tooth, from trauma or decay, can cause problems. The empty space in the adult's mouth allows teeth to shift, changing the way the person bites and chews. Bony tissue in the mandible and maxilla can erode, making prosthetic restoration difficult. Adults also suffer chips, fractures, and loss of teeth from falls, accidents, and assaults. Some adults seek dental treatment for solely cosmetic reasons. Cosmetic dentistry includes dental implants for missing teeth, orthodontia to straighten teeth, and inlays to cover badly stained teeth.

Pregnant Females

The dentist needs to be very careful about inadvertently exposing the developing fetus to radiation from **radiographs** (X-ray films). Female patients of child-bearing age are routinely questioned about the possibility of being pregnant before radiological exams are performed. Routine dental cleaning and checkups are very important for pregnant women. The stress and nutritional demands on their bodies increase the incidence of dental caries. Although dental treatment can be safely performed on pregnant women, in the second trimester, some choose to wait until after delivery to have teeth repaired.

The Elderly

As more individuals live longer lives, they are more likely to keep most, if not all, of their teeth. This retention of teeth has changed the approach to treatment for the elderly, with an emphasis on prevention and maintenance of the natural dentition. While at one time the loss of teeth meant having to use complete removable dentures that were often unstable, significant progress in the use of dental implants has allowed people to have a stable dentition, either of crowns and bridges or of implant stabilized and retained dentures.

The living situations of the elderly can have a great effect on oral health and disease. Those who live independently are generally in good physical health and also enjoy good oral health. Those with chronic illnesses or those in dependent living situations may have many oral health problems. One study of VA patients found only 6 percent of healthy, independent-living patients were edentulous, and those who had teeth were missing an average of 4.5 teeth. But 49 percent of the patients living in the VA nursing home or those hospitalized for illness were edentulous, and those who had teeth were missing an average of 12 teeth with 5 decayed teeth (Loesche et al., 1995).

The problem of lack of proper dental care and oral hygiene for nursing home residents is well documented. Figure 14-2 demonstrates the prevalence of dental health problems among nursing home residents in the state of Washington (Kiyak et al., 1993).

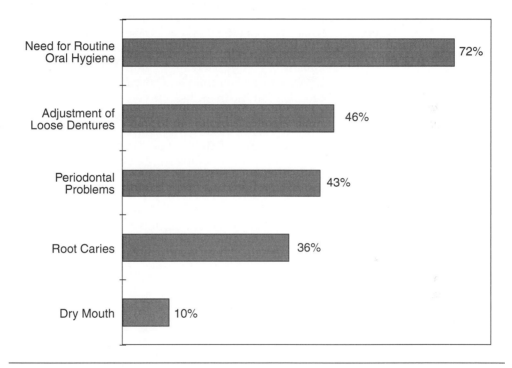

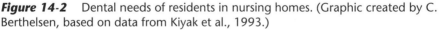

Figure 14-2 Dental needs of residents in nursing homes. (Graphic created by C. Berthelsen, based on data from Kiyak et al., 1993.)

Patients with Special Problems

Patients who are developmentally challenged pose special problems when they need dental care. These patients may not cooperate with the dentist and may be unable to understand simple commands such as "open your mouth." More functional individuals may be able to cooperate for a short time, but may be unable to sit still long enough for the needed treatment. Nevertheless, they still need preventive and restorative dentistry to maintain optimum health. Major restorative treatment for these patients is generally carried out under deep sedation or general anesthesia, which may preclude treatment at a typical dental office and require admission to an outpatient surgery facility.

Individuals with mental illness can be difficult for the dentist to treat. Patients suffering hallucinations and uncontrolled psychosis may be unable to cooperate with the dentist. They may be treated normally if well controlled on proper psychotropic medications. However, the dentist must be aware of what medications the patient takes to avoid interaction with anesthetic drugs used in dentistry. Psychotropic medications can cause drowsiness, drooling, extremely dry mouth, excessive salivation, nervousness, uncontrolled movements of the tongue, muscle rigidity, and nasal congestion requiring mouth breathing. These side effects may cause discomfort to the patient undergoing dental treatment and difficulties for the dentist.

Patients who are physically challenged may not be easy to treat. Deformities may make sitting in the dental chair very uncomfortable. Paralysis may impair the patient's ability to sit or balance in a normal dentist chair. A hearing-impaired patient may not be able to hear the dentist's commands. These patients should be treated in a setting that can adapt to their handicap or disability.

Patients with serious medical illnesses may also pose special problems to the dentist. A patient with severe heart disease may suffer angina or elevated blood pressure while at the dentist's office. Patients may be on portable oxygen tanks, feeding tubes, or a central line for intravenous fluids. Neurologic disease (Parkinsonism) may cause uncontrollable head shaking and tongue movements. Stroke survivors may be less able to control swallowing or have minimal gag reflex. Care must be taken when treating these patients. A thorough understanding of the patient's medical problems and associated symptoms is important. The patient's medical and dental history should always be available for the dentist to review when treating the patient.

Types of Providers

General Dentists

A **dentist** usually completes four years of college and four years of dental education before becoming licensed to practice. A dentist earns either a DDS or DMD degree. A general dentistry practice focuses on a wide range of dental treatments and procedures and can treat young and old patients. The general dentist is much like a family practice physician, taking care of the dental health of all members of the family, providing periodic checkups and cleanings, and monitoring the condition of teeth and gums. The general dentist is allowed to perform almost all dental procedures appropriately trained to perform according to state license but many choose to refer patients to specialty dentists for the more complex care.

Dental Specialties

There are nine dental specialties recognized by the American Dental Association. They are dental public health, endodontics, oral and maxillofacial radiology, oral and maxillofacial surgery, oral pathology, orthodontics, pediatric dentistry, periodontics, and prosthodontics. While several of these specialties are recognizable to most people, public health dentists, oral pathologists, and oral and maxillofacial radiologists usually practice in institutional settings.

An **orthodontist** is a dentist who specializes in straightening teeth. Many orthodontists complete two years of specialty education following the four years of dental school to prepare for their specialty. Orthodontic treatment may be medically necessary or cosmetic. Patients are usually referred to an orthodontist by a general dentist for a consultation, and treatment begins when appropriate. Orthodontists use radiographs, impressions of the patient's teeth and bite, and a variety of orthodontic appliances (braces, retainers, bands and brackets bonded to teeth, headgear) to accomplish the goal of straightening teeth. Patients undergoing treatment see their orthodontist regularly over a period of several years. The dental record is important to the orthodontist to monitor the progress of treatment and must be available for reference every time the patient is seen.

A **periodontist** is a dentist who specializes in treating the tissues surrounding and supporting the teeth. Periodontists study three years beyond regular dental school to prepare for practice in their specialty. Periodontal disease begins as an inflammation of the **gingiva** and can progress to abscesses around the teeth and infection of the jawbones. As the disease progresses, the victim develops **loss of attachment (LA)** of teeth. The teeth become loose and are eventually lost. Although periodontal disease is preventable, it is still quite prevalent among Americans. Studies during 1988–1991 indicate that more than 90 percent of Americans over 12 years of age had experienced some clinical LA. The LA increases with age, with 15 percent of Americans showing moderate or severe LA. Periodontal disease is treated by removing the bacterial plaque (the causative agent of the disease) and the calcified calculus deposits on the teeth. Depending on the severity of the disease, surgery or the use of antibiotics may be necessary. The key is to prevent the buildup of plaque and the initiation of disease in the first place. Patients are usually referred to the periodontist by a general dentist.

An **endodontist** is a dentist who specializes in treating the inside of the tooth, the nerve and pulp. An endodontist performs root canal therapy to remove the dying or dead tissue from the root canal system found within the tooth. The patient may complain of severe toothache or a tooth that is very sensitive to anything hot or cold—foods, liquids, or breathing cold air. The patient then goes back to the referring dentist or a prosthodontist for restoration of the tooth with a crown. An endodontist may never see the patient again or may treat the patient for problems with a different tooth in the future.

A prosthodontist is a dentist who specializes in replacing missing teeth with a prosthetic device. Full-mouth dentures are required for an edentulous person. Other **prostheses** include partial denture, **bridge** with **pontic**, and dental **implant**.

An oral and maxillofacial surgeon is a dentist who specializes in surgery to the mouth and facial bones. A patient may be referred for oral surgery by a general dentist for removal of a mucocele or a cancerous growth of the mouth or tongue. A patient with **impacted** wisdom teeth (wisdom teeth that will not erupt through the gum) is referred for surgical removal. It is not uncommon for an orthodontist to refer a patient for extraction of teeth before applying braces.

Dental Hygienists

A dental hygienist usually completes two years of special training at a college or university before becoming eligible to take state board examinations for licensure. (The student may earn an A.S. or B.S. degree depending on the length of the education program.) Dental hygienists are licensed to perform some of the same procedures that dentists perform. However, most states do not allow the dental hygienist to establish an independent practice. The hygienist must be under the supervision of a licensed dentist when performing treatments. The hygienist typically performs oral and dental exams, cleans teeth by removing **plaque** and scraping off hardened **calculus**, polishes teeth, and applies fluoride and **sealants** to teeth. Depending on the state, the hygienist may inject anesthetic agents and make and interpret radiographs. The hygienist plays an important role in the prevention of dental disease and is usually responsible for educating the dental patient about good hygiene and dietary habits that promote good oral health. Instructions provided to the dental patient include proper brushing and flossing techniques and recommendations for diet and lifestyle changes. In many dental practices, the hygienist is the professional who collects the patient's medical and dental history, records initial vital signs, and documents important examination findings in the dental chart.

Dental Assistants

A dental assistant may receive formal training at a technical college or may be personally trained by a dentist. Many states do not license dental assistants. The dental assistant's primary role is to assist the dentist in the treatment of patients. The assistant anticipates what instruments will be needed, hands the instruments to the dentist, holds instruments in position in the patient's mouth, and prepares dental materials. The hands of the dental assistant act as the dentist's second pair of hands. The dental assistant may also help the dentist in charting dental exam findings and writing treatment notes. Most dental assistants have limited education and training. Most state laws limit a dental assistant to an assistive role rather than a treating role.

Regulatory Issues

Professionals providing dental care in the United States are regulated by the individual states. Each state is responsible for licensing dentists and dental hygienists who will practice in their state. Although there is no national licensure or credentialing for dental care providers, many states will recognize the license of a dentist from another state through credentialing or reciprocity procedures.

State Licensure

Most states have a board of dentistry that issues licenses to practice. The applicant must provide evidence of adequate training and demonstrate treatment skills through state board examinations. The applicant's personal integrity, mental health, and moral behavior are all evaluated to determine whether the person can safely practice in the state. Licensure is the primary means of protecting the public from incompetent dental practitioners. Dentists may have their licenses suspended or revoked for gross negligence, behavior that endangers a patient, sexual abuse of a patient, dispensing narcotics inappropriately, abusing drugs or alcohol themselves, or mental unfitness. Dentists may also be required to carry adequate malpractice insurance to be licensed to practice.

Drug Enforcement Agency Regulations

Dentists prescribe a variety of medications during treatment of patients. They must adhere to federal and state regulations whenever a controlled substance is involved. A dentist may prescribe narcotic pain relievers, and they are regulated by the same laws that physicians must follow. A dentist must have a valid Drug Enforcement Agency (DEA) number for patients to fill prescriptions for narcotics and other controlled substances at a pharmacy. The DEA number may be revoked if a dentist violates DEA regulations in prescribing narcotics.

Reporting of Adverse Effects of Medications and Dental Materials

Dentists use a variety of substances and materials in their treatment of patients and must report adverse or untoward effects of medications to the manufacturer, just as physicians and hospitals do. They are also supposed to report adverse reactions that patients have to dental materials used in restorations, including allergic reactions to metals and composite resin materials.

Reporting of Physical Abuse

Many spousal batteries occur with blows to the victim's face and teeth. Loosened, broken teeth and facial fractures are often diagnosed and treated by dentists. The dentist is legally obligated to report suspected cases of abuse to law enforcement authorities just as physicians and other health care providers are. Dental records may be used as evidence of repeated trauma indicative of battery or abuse.

Documentation

The typical dental record of a patient visiting a general dentist consists of patient information, the medical and dental history, dental examination and charting, periodontal exam, dental radiographs, and treatment notes. Specialists have additional information appropriate to the kinds of care provided.

Patient Information

The first time a person visits a dental practice, certain identifying information is routinely collected, including name, gender, date of birth, age, marital status, address, home and work phone numbers, and Social Security number. The patient is usually given a form to complete to provide this information. The patient is also asked to provide the name and phone number of his or her personal physician. It may be necessary for the dentist to contact the patient's physician regarding proposed treatment, medication allergies, or medical conditions that affect the patient's dental care. The patient information form typically includes a statement that the patient or parent is asked to sign authorizing and consenting to the dental exam and treatment. Additional information such as employer, insurance carrier, spouse's name, address, phone, and Social Security number is usually obtained to assist the dentist in collecting fees and insurance benefits to pay for care provided. The form may also include an assignment of benefits that allows the dentist to bill the insurance carrier and authorizes the carrier to send payment to the dentist.

Medical and Dental History

A medical history questionnaire is usually given to the patient to complete at the first visit along with the personal information form. The questions are usually answered with "yes" or "no" and cover a wide range of medical symptoms and diseases. Many medical conditions are important in dental disease and treatment, and it is crucial that the dentist be provided with complete and accurate information before caring for a patient. Patients are asked to identify prescription medications they take regularly and the date of their last visit to a physician. The form also asks the patient about the use of recreational drugs, HIV (human immunodeficiency virus) status, and history of hepatitis. Allergies to drugs and substances must be identified. Increasing numbers of health care workers have developed a sensitivity to latex, the material used to manufacture disposable gloves. It is estimated that 12 percent of dental and health care workers are hypersensitive to latex (Safadi et al., 1996). Dental professionals need to identify patients who are hypersensitive to latex so latex gloves are not worn while treating these patients.

A dental history, which is usually part of the medical history form, is also completed by the patient. The patient is asked about dental symptoms, previous dental treatments, and what prompted the visit to the dentist. The form may also contain questions about patients' dental routines at home, whether they are satisfied with the cosmetic look of their smile, and whether they are nervous or anxious about seeing the dentist.

The patient's medical and dental histories are reviewed by the dentist or dental hygienist with the patient. The professional asks further questions about items to which the patient answered "yes" to get a complete picture or clarification. Notes are made on the history form or elsewhere to document additional information provided in the interview.

Head, Neck, and Intraoral Examination

This first part of a routine dental exam evaluates the patient's general health. The dental care professional may take and chart an adult's blood pressure and other vital signs and make a note of the patient's general appearance. Next, the head and neck are examined for any abnormal findings such as enlarged lymph nodes, bruises or cuts on the face, or abnormal-looking growths. Positive findings are noted in the chart. The intraoral exam evaluates the appearance of the patient's mouth, lips, tongue, mucosa inside the cheek, tonsils, palate, and gums. Any abnormal or positive findings are documented in the chart. Growths that appear suspicious may prompt a referral to an oral surgeon. Patients with active cold sores and fever blisters (herpes simplex) should not receive anesthetic injections until the sores are healed to avoid the risk of spreading the herpes infection to facial nerves.

Dental Examination & Charting

The examination next focuses on the patient's teeth. The dentist documents information about each tooth in the patient's chart. This is commonly done using a graphic chart as in Figure 14-3. Every missing tooth and all existing restorations are charted. The chart indicates the surfaces involved, the size, and the material of each filling. Each tooth is visually examined and probed to ascertain whether decay is present or a restoration is cracked or failing. The dental charts of children note which permanent teeth have erupted, which primary teeth are still present, and the condition of the teeth.

Periodontal Examination

The health of the gingiva and supporting tissue of the patient's teeth is evaluated during the periodontal exam. The dentist or hygienist gently inserts a probe between the base of the tooth and the gingiva to measure the depth of pockets around the tooth. Periodontal disease is manifested by deepening pockets around the tooth, receding of the gingiva, and loss of attachment of the tooth. Each tooth is probed at six locations, three on the front surface and three on the tongue surface. Adults typically have a depth of 2–3 millimeters, which is considered normal. If the gums bleed when probed, it may be a sign of early gingivitis. A depth of 4–6 millimeters is worrisome, and a depth of 9 millimeters means the tooth has very little attachment left and will likely be quite loose. Each probe measurement is recorded on a dental chart (Figure 14-4). The probing results are discussed with the patient, and the dental caregiver points out specific teeth that should be flossed and brushed

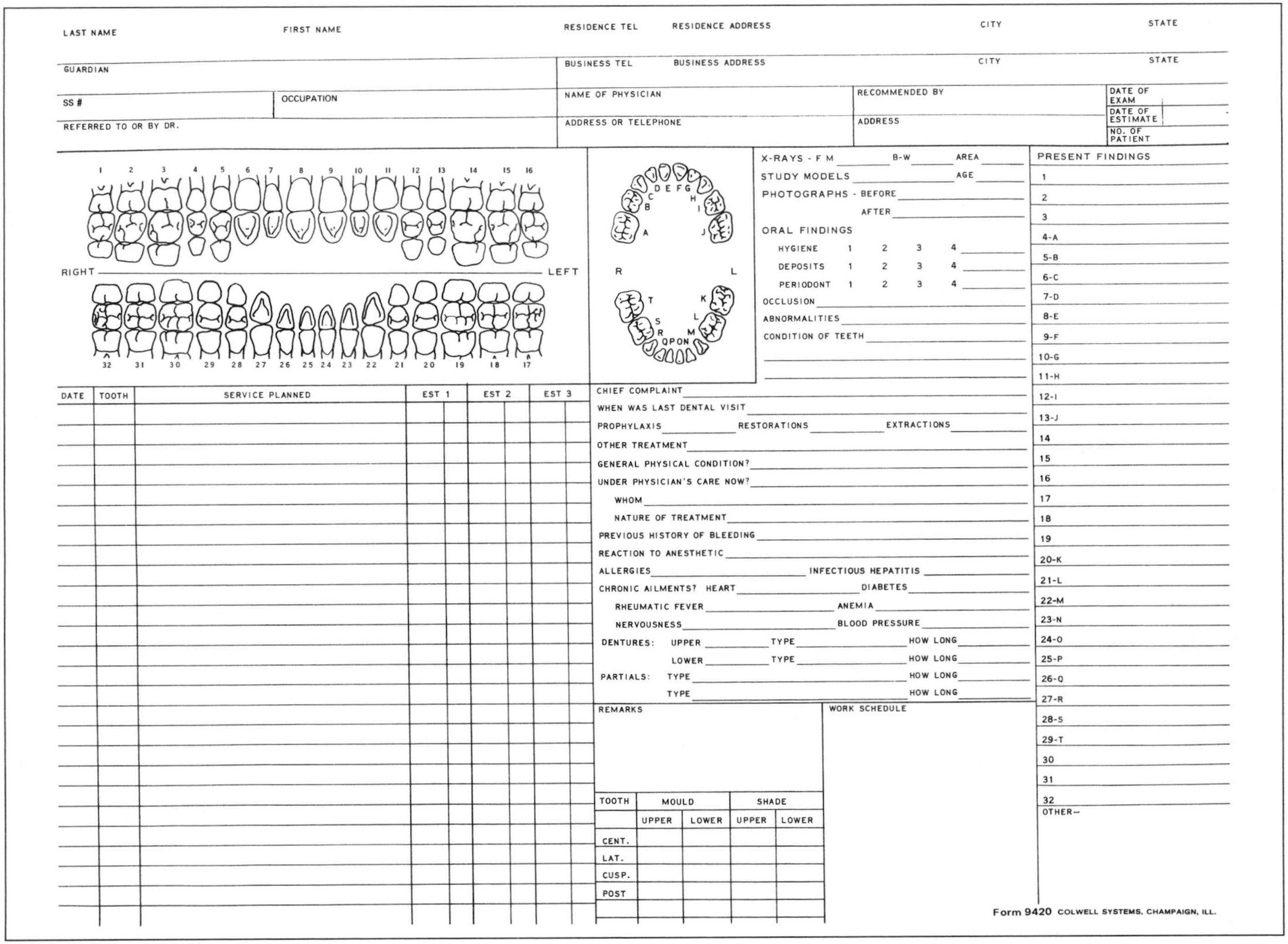

Figure 14-3 Sample dental restoration chart. (Courtesy Colwell Systems, Inc., Champaign, IL.)

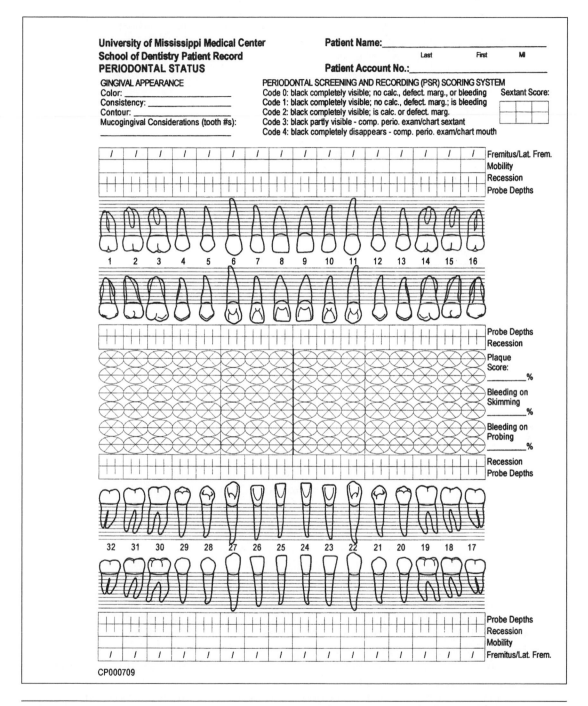

Figure 14-4 Sample periodontal status chart. (Courtesy University of Mississippi Medical Center, Jackson, MS.)

more carefully. A general description of the amount of calculus (hardened plaque) present is noted in the chart. Patients who have regular cleanings and checkups at recommended six-month intervals have a lot less calculus to be scraped off than patients who have not seen a dentist in years.

Dental Radiography and Intraoral Photography

The dentist usually orders dental radiographs during the patient's first visit. They may be full-mouth radiographs (multiple radiographs), a **panoramic radiograph** (all teeth shown on one film), or just bite-wing radiographs of the molars. The radiographs become part of the patient's chart and are usually stored with the chart. Subsequent radiographs can be compared with previous radiographs to monitor progress of decay or identify when a defect first appeared. Radiographs help the dentist confirm or discover the presence of dental disease. Insurance companies may ask the dentist to submit radiographs to verify the necessity of dental treatment. Abnormal lesions on the tongue or mucosa may be photographed using an intraoral camera. New computer imaging technologies now allow dentists to digitize the image of teeth and gums with a tiny video camera on a dental instrument inside the patient's mouth and display the image on a computer screen for the patient to see. The patient can be shown the problem the dentist sees and may be more willing to have the problem fixed.

Treatment Plan

After the dental exam, periodontal exam, and radiographic exam, the dentist outlines a treatment plan for the patient. The patient may just need **prophylaxis** (cleaning of teeth) and application of fluoride to prevent decay. Any decay or pathology found should be treated as soon as possible to minimize damage to the tooth. The dentist tells the patient what needs to be done, and the patient is encouraged to make a return appointment to get the work done. Unfortunately, not all patients are willing to have the work done, and some never return to receive the recommended treatment. Others may get minor restorations but refuse to have an expensive root canal or crown until an unbearable toothache develops.

Treatment Notes

All dental treatment is documented in the patient's dental chart. The dentist notes the type of anesthetic agent used, the type of nerve block and injection approach, the location of decay on the tooth, and the type of material used to restore the tooth after drilling away the decay. This information is important for future dental care. The dentist may find that certain anesthetic agents do not numb the patient's tooth fast enough, long enough, or sufficiently. The dentist makes a note to choose a different agent for this patient the next time.

Legally, it is imperative that the dentist keeps complete treatment notes. If the dentist is called into any legal proceedings, the information in the chart may be critical for the dentist's defense. In a legal context, if something is not written down, it is assumed not to have happened. The surreptitious alteration of documents after the fact is illegal and casts aspersions on the dentist.

Patient Education

Dentistry has made great strides in the prevention of dental caries. This has been accomplished through education, the use of fluoride, changes in diet, and an improvement in personal oral hygiene. Most people now know that they need to brush and floss their teeth daily, cut down on consumption of sugary sweets, and use toothpaste and drinking water that has fluoride to maintain healthy teeth. Another aspect of patient education emphasizes the importance of periodic dental checkups and prophylaxis. Most dentists send patients a postcard reminding them that it is time to come in for a checkup. These notices are important to the patient and to the financial viability of the dental practice.

The current generation of children has a lower prevalence of tooth decay and a higher probability of keeping their teeth for life. As Americans become more health conscious and take better care of their teeth, dentures and false teeth may be a thing of the past.

Diet Evaluation

Some dental practices may perform an evaluation of the patient's dietary habits. Poor nutrition can contribute to dental disease. It is particularly important that adequate calcium is provided in the diet for the calcification of tooth enamel. Children, teenagers, and pregnant and menopausal women are most at risk for softening of the enamel and tooth decay caused by calcium deficiency. If a dietary evaluation is done, it is documented in the patient's chart along with recommendations provided to the patient.

Reimbursement

Dental patients often pay for their own dental care, but many have dental benefits through a third-party plan. The most common form of third-party plan is traditional dental insurance. Under this form of reimbursement, the patient is covered for a percentage of the fee based on the agreement negotiated between the employer and the third-party insurance carrier. The patient is responsible for any deductible and that part of the dentist's fee not covered by the insurance plan. Employers, patients, and dentists may also participate in managed care plans, capitation plans, preferred provider organizations (PPOs), and health maintenance organizations (HMOs). Under these arrangements, the dentist agrees to provide certain services for a set rate of reimbursement from the plan. A patient is responsible for the full fee for any necessary or elective services that are not specifically covered by the plan.

Dental Insurance

American employers have become more conscious of the dental needs of their employees, and many now offer dental insurance in their benefit packages. About 48 percent of the U.S. population has private dental insurance coverage (California Dental Association, 2000). Sometimes dental insurance is optional, and the employee must pay a small premium for coverage. Sometimes it is totally free for the employee with a small premium for the employee's spouse and family. Most dental insurance policies cover checkups and preventive dentistry at 100 percent; filling-type restorations and extractions at 80 percent; and crowns, bridges, and other prosthetics at 50 percent. Orthodontic treatment may be covered at 50 percent to a lifetime maximum of $1,000. Some policies may require the patient to pay a deductible on nonpreventive treatment each year before any treatment is covered, and most have a $1,000 to $2,000 limit of benefits per year.

Dentists generally appreciate treating patients with dental insurance. Collection of fees is simpler and easier for the patient, and many times the dentist can confirm insurance coverage and get the treatment plan approved before beginning it. Dental insurance policies pay the percentages listed based on usual and customary fees. Occasionally the amount the insurance company says it will pay for a certain treatment is lower than what the dentist charges. The patient must pay the difference or the dentist forgives it. Dental insurance payments are processed promptly if submitted correctly.

Dentists participating in a PPO agree to charge the patient only the amount allowed by the insurance company. Dentists agree to the reduced reimbursement because the plan also provides benefits for the dental practice. For example, there may be an increase in the number of patients because insured patients have incentives to receive care from a participating dentist. There may be discounts on the cost of making crowns, bridges, and dentures from a central dental lab for PPO members.

Self-Pay Patients

Most patients must still pay cash directly for their dental checkups and treatments. Dental insurance is rarely available to retired people, and Medicare does not cover dental care for the elderly. The working poor, unemployed, disabled, and elderly have a difficult time paying for dental care. Most self-pay dental patients are those who recognize the importance of good dental health and can afford it or are willing to sacrifice to receive it.

HMO Plans

Many HMOs now include dental care in their plans. The plans vary in what is covered, amount of patient copayment, and availability. It is not uncommon for HMO plans to require patients to schedule routine checkups up to six months in advance to receive care and to provide limited availability for dental emergencies. This is part of the strategy for holding down costs.

Medicare and Medicaid

Medicare does not include any benefits for dental care for the elderly. This segment of the population, with years of wear on their teeth or with no teeth left, is in great need of dental care to improve quality of life. The cost to taxpayers of adding dental coverage for the elderly would likely be prohibitive.

Medicaid offers some dental benefits for children. Preventive checkups and necessary restorations are covered by Medicaid, but the number of dentists accepting Medicaid patients is quite limited. Medicaid coverage for adult recipients is optional by federal regulations, so many state Medicaid programs do not provide coverage for adult dental care.

TRICARE Dental Program

The TRICARE Dental Program (TDP) provides dental benefits for families of active-duty military personnel (Department of Defense, 2003). TDP coverage is generally good and is as acceptable to dentists as dental insurance. (TRICARE replaced the Civilian Health and Medical Program of the Uniformed Services [CHAMPUS], which used to be the source of dental coverage for families of military personnel.)

Veterans Affairs

Dental care is available to veterans at VA medical centers. The patients pay little or no fees for treatment if obtained at the VA facility. There is no billing involved, but the facility must keep track of utilization to adequately staff and budget for the VA dental clinic. Veterans with private dental insurance policies generally obtain dental care through private dental practices rather than at a VA dental clinic.

Information Management

Information is crucial to the practice of dentistry, including information about individual patients, dental equipment and supplies, vendors, dental coverages of each insurance company, new medications and anesthetic agents, new treatment modalities, the epidemiology of dental disease, financial information about the practice, withholding and employment taxes, and more.

Coding and Classification

There are three main coding systems used in dentistry. The American Dental Association (ADA) has a coding system for diagnoses and procedures, the *Current Dental Terminology*, or *CDT-4*. This system is typically used to file dental insurance claims for patients. This coding system is also used by dental schools and dental hygiene training clinics to collect statistical information. Table 14-1 is a list of common ADA codes.

Table 14-1   Common ADA Codes

Code	Description
0140	Limited oral evaluation
0150	Comprehensive oral evaluation
0210	Intraoral—complete series
1110	Prophylaxis—adult
1203	Topical fluoride—child

The *International Classification of Diseases, 9th Revision, Clinical Modification* (ICD-9-CM) diagnosis codes are used by hospitals and medical centers for dental patients treated as inpatients, outpatients, or emergency room patients. ICD-9-CM dental procedure codes are used for inpatients only. HCPCS codes are used to code dental procedures for hospital outpatients and emergency room patients.

Computers in Dentistry

Computers have been used in dentistry primarily for practice management applications, which typically include accounting, patient billing, insurance claim tracking, appointment scheduling, payroll, and patient recall notices. In recent years, computers have been used increasingly for clinical applications as well. As systems and applications for dentistry continue to improve, the use of computers in the dental practice has steadily increased. To illustrate, in 1976, only 1 percent of dentists used computers in their practices and less than 25 percent used commercial computing services. (Arthur Young and Company, 2002). By 2000, 85.1 percent of dentists in the United States used a computer in the dental office, and 48.3 percent of these computers had Internet access (American Dental Association, 2001). Figure 14-5 illustrates the trends of computer usage in the dental practice from 1984 to 2000 (Schleyer et al., 2003).

Practice Management Software

A computer software package to manage a dental practice may include the following modules.

Patient Registration

One of the primary functions of the software is the collection of patients' demographic information, including address, contact numbers, e-mail address, date of birth, insurance information, and possibly a digital photograph for the dental record.

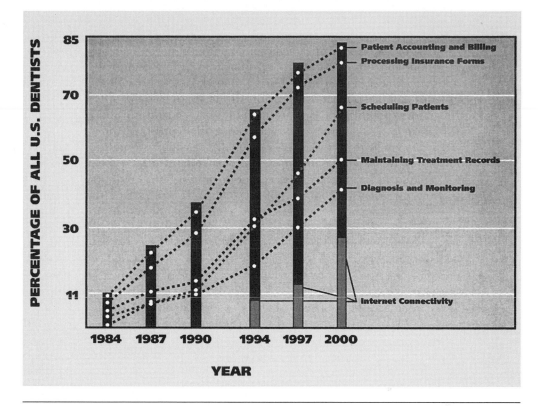

Figure 14-5 Computer ownership, Internet connectivity, and selected computer uses in dental practice in the United States (1984–2000). Data collected from the American Dental Association Survey Center. (Schleyer, T.K.L., Spallek, H., Bartling, W.C., and Corby, P.C. (2003). The technologically well-equipped dental office. *Journal of the American Dental Association, 134,* 30–41. Copyright © 2003 American Dental Association. All rights reserved. Reprinted by permission.)

Appointment Scheduling

The scheduling software should be flexible and fit the way the dental practice operates. It should provide for multiple dentists, multiple chairs, and double booking of patients if implemented in a group practice. The time slots must be variable according to individual practice patterns. One dentist may want to routinely allow an hour for a crown preparation and another may want an hour and a half. Despite the routine time allowed for a procedure, there may be special patients or more complicated procedures that require more than the normal amount of time. The software must allow a standard allotment of time or a custom allotment of time to schedule appointments.

The software must provide easy and flexible query capabilities. The reception-ist may need to answer questions such as: What day is Jane Doe scheduled to come in? What is the next available one-hour slot for Dr. Brown? Which patient can be called to reschedule a later appointment so another patient with an emergency can be seen?

Insurance Billing and Claims Tracking

Insurance patients can compose a large portion of a dentist's practice. The cash flow of the practice will suffer severely if the process of billing and tracking claims is inef-ficient. The insurance claims module should be integrated with the patient accounts module and may be set up for electronic claims submission to third-party payers, thereby reducing paperwork and providing for greater accuracy. The software should be able to identify patients who have received treatment but for whom claims have not yet been submitted, patients who have preauthorization for treatment, claims that have not been paid 30 days after submission, and accounts that have received only a partial payment from the insurance company.

Another important function for dental practices serving large numbers of insur-ance patients is the ability to confirm benefit amounts and patient copayment amounts or deductibles. Dentists prefer to collect copayment and deductible amounts at the time of service rather than to bill the patient after receiving partial payment from the insurance company. If the software identifies this amount at the time of checkout, the patient can be asked to pay the amount at that time.

Patient Accounting Information

Although dentists would like to have all patients pay when treatment is rendered, it is not realistic to believe this will always happen. Patient accounts software should keep track of total charges for the day, total charges for the family, amount paid and when, remaining balance, and age of balance. It should be able to print regular monthly billing statements for accounts with outstanding balances as well as an individual statement on demand and allow insertion of a special message to some or all recipients.

Software should follow accepted accounting principles and provide for closing the month, quarter, and fiscal year. Many dentists contract with an accountant to prepare tax returns and provide financial statements for the business. Accounting software must provide acceptable output and verification of financial matters for the dentist's accountant. Some dentists charge interest on outstanding balances but may request that a special account be exempt from interest charges. The software should be able to charge a specified interest rate on some accounts and none on others.

It is preferred to have patient accounts integrated with scheduling and patient recall. The system can then alert the receptionist when an appointment is being sched-uled for a patient who has an unpaid balance from a previous visit. The system can also send a recall notice to a patient with an outstanding balance with a message that the account needs to be brought up to date before scheduling another appointment.

Patient Recall Reminders

Periodic checkups and teeth cleanings are important for dental heath. Dentists recognize that it is their professional responsibility to encourage patients to have this routine care and send reminders when it is time to be seen again. It is also important to the financial viability of the dental practice to see patients regularly. Practice management software should be able to identify patients who should receive a recall notice and patients who failed to respond to a previous recall notice. The software should be able to print envelopes and perform a mail merge to personalize the recall notices the patients receive. A database should keep track of when patient recalls are due and when they are sent.

Patient Referral

Dentists, particularly specialists, like to know who is referring patients to their practice for care. Software should keep track of who referred each patient, prepare statistical reports based on the referring source and payment source, or compile a list of all patients referred by a specific dentist. The dentist may foster a social relationship with professionals who frequently refer patients.

Practice Reporting

Reporting is an important function of practice management software for monitoring and effectively managing the business. Administrative and clinical reports, providing data about patient account status, provider productivity, appointment utilization, and treatment plan procedures completed or in progress, can be invaluable tools for running a successful dental practice.

Inventory Management

Some software includes the functionality to monitor inventory items, including supplies and equipment. This can make reordering more timely and efficient. The software application may even provide an interface for online ordering.

Electronic Dental Record

The electronic dental record is being more commonly used in dental practices, especially among younger dentists or those establishing new practices. Some software packages for the dental practice store the complete dental record, including digital radiographs, while others are more limited in functionality. The comprehensive electronic dental record stores medical and dental histories and results of dental and periodontal examinations; provides alerts about medical conditions and allergies and the need for antibiotic premedication; and facilitates comparison between previous exams and current exams to aid in monitoring progression of disease. The electronic record should interface seamlessly with digital radiography and imaging software, which provides compact and safe storage of dental radiographs and allows the dentist to share radiographs with a specialist or an insurance company via the Internet.

Computers in dental practice can be enhanced through the use of alternate methods of input such as voice recognition, touch-screen, and pen-based computing. These features may facilitate ease of use by the dentist, hygienist, or dental assistant. Voice recognition may be a particularly promising feature because it allows hands-free data entry. This type of input could also be useful in controlling the spread of infection in the dental office by removing the pen and paper, display, or keyboard as potential vectors for bacteria and viruses.

Computer Hardware and Networking

One computer at the front desk used to be sufficient for the dental practice, but many dental offices now have multiple computers. There may be a computer at each patient chair and in private offices. Determining the layout and specifications of computers depends heavily on the practice management software being used and its specific requirements. Networking the computers allows the computers to communicate with one another, to share practice management and clinical software, to store and back up data in a single central location, and to share hardware resources such as printers, intraoral cameras, or high-speed modems providing Internet access.

Other Technological Devices

Digital cameras are becoming increasingly popular in the dental practice to take photographs for the dental record to help identify the patient or to show before and after treatment photos. *Intraoral cameras* capture images that can be helpful to educate the patient about treatment needs or to show progression of ongoing treatment. *Digital imaging devices* provide an alternative to traditional film X-rays. Digital radiographs can be integrated directly into the patient record and are supposed to decrease exposure to radiation. *Personal digital assistants (PDAs)* are handheld computers that can be used to download appointments or other information from the practice management software or as a reference to drug information.

Application Service Providers

For dental professionals who do not wish to maintain an office network, handle hardware and software upgrades, or be responsible for daily backups of data, an alternative may be to enlist the services of an application service provider (ASP). The dentist would contract with an ASP who, through an Internet connection, would provide the practice management software. The ASP would store the data for the practice, maintain network server equipment, upgrade software applications, and perform daily data backups. An unreliable or slow Internet connection, however, could be extremely detrimental to the well-being of the dental practice.

Quality Improvement and Utilization Management

In small dental practices, a formal quality improvement program or plan is not the focus. However, a wise dentist will continuously try to improve the quality of the service provided. The Dental Society of the State of New York has developed a unique peer review program for quality assurance that stands as a model for other dental societies across the country (Benton and Shub, 1995).

Clinical dental practice guidelines are well developed. A model clinical guideline for general dentists for managing patients with adult periodontitis provides recommendations on the content of the medical, dental, social and habit history; exam, diagnosis, and treatment documentation; and treatment guidelines (Workshop, 1994). Results of a survey in 1995 revealed that, "Seven of the ten primary professional dental organizations have or soon should have some form of practice guidelines" (Shugars and Bader, 1995). Organizations that have published practice guidelines for dentistry are as follows:

- American Academy of Pediatric Dentistry
- American Academy of Periodontology
- American Association of Endodontists
- American Association of Oral and Maxillofacial Surgeons
- American Association of Orthodontists
- American College of Prosthodontists
- American Dental Association

Large dental practices, particularly those associated with managed dental care and HMOs, are more interested in formally measuring quality and using quality indicators. Some suggested quality indicators for managed dental care are as follows.

- How long does it take to get an appointment for a routine checkup and cleaning?
- How long does it take to get an appointment for a new dental symptom?
- How many child and adolescent patients have sealants applied?
- How many third molar extractions are performed?
- How many enrollees received prophylaxis and checkups during the year?
- How many referrals were made to dental specialists?

Utilization of dental services is generally managed by dental insurance plans and HMOs providing dental benefits. The approaches to limiting expenses include the exclusion of benefits for preexisting dental conditions, requiring pretreatment authorization, and actively evaluating the necessity of treatment. Dentists may be required to submit copies of dental records and radiographs to justify the need for treatment. Patients self-manage utilization if large copayments and deductibles are instituted. Most dental plans, however, recognize the importance of preventive care in controlling costs, so they cover semiannual checkups and cleanings. Some plans impose an annual limit to benefits, exclude coverage for cosmetic dental procedures, and require the dentist to use the least expensive restorative method, for example, limiting the use of expensive gold crowns to molars only. Most dental plans do not cover treatment for temporomandibular joint (TMJ) syndrome, cosmetic orthodontia, and experimental dentistry (dental implants).

Overutilization of dental services is rarely a problem with self-pay patients. Excess visits to the dentist do not seem to be common. Some analogies such as "like pulling teeth" and "I'd rather have a root canal" reflect the attitude many people have about a visit to the dentist. However, two areas of potential overutilization have been identified. Many teens and young adults may be having their **wisdom teeth** extracted unnecessarily. The routine use of dental sealants on primary teeth of children is also questionable.

Risk Management and Legal Issues

Injuries to Caregivers and Patients

An important area of risk management is injury to patients and practitioners. Potential for injury includes instrument traumas from needles, drills, and probes. Proper use of a "rubber dam," which isolates the operative field to the tooth undergoing treatment, can help prevent injury to the mouth and tongue. Burns from sterilization equipment and skin injuries from grinders are another area of risk. Proper training of personnel and consistent use of safety measures are important to prevent injuries. There is the potential for the patient or practitioner to suffer foreign body or debris in the eye, which can be prevented if both the patient and dental practitioner wear safety goggles during dental treatment. Another potential risk is for the dental patient to accidentally swallow a foreign body during treating. The natural gag reflex makes it easy for a patient to swallow a cotton roll, bite block, or small object accidentally dropped by the dentist. The rubber dam can be helpful in preventing this problem.

Musculoskeletal injuries to the neck and back from long hours of leaning over dental chairs are occupational hazards in dentistry. Repetitive motion injuries such as carpal tunnel syndrome and ulnar nerve compression are also common. To control risk, education of personnel on these issues is vital. All dental personnel should also protect themselves from contaminants by using standard barrier precautions. These precautions include safety glasses, a mask, disposable gloves, and possibly a full-length gown.

Malpractice and Negligence

It is standard practice for practitioners to routinely use latex gloves and face masks while treating all patients, not just "risky" patients. Practitioners should be very careful when they have open lesions on fingers and hands. Cuts and abrasions can be a source of bacteria to transfer to dental patients. Patients are at low risk of acquiring hepatitis, HIV, and other infections at the dental office. Infections acquired through dental treatment can be the result of negligent and improper procedures in the office.

Patients who have rheumatic heart disease, heart valve problems, or prosthetic joints should be premedicated with antibiotics before undergoing dental treatment to prevent bacterial endocarditis. A dentist who fails to recognize the need for premedication is negligent in treating these patients.

Another area of potential lawsuits is inappropriate or inadequate treatment of a patient's problem. Failure to treat early pulpitis can progress to dental abscess. A patient can suffer the loss of a permanent tooth because the dentist failed to diagnose or adequately treat a tooth early enough to save the tooth.

As in the medical field, adequate documentation is the best defense against malpractice and negligence suits. Dentists should document posttreatment instructions provided to patients, procedures performed, reactions to medications, and complaints of tooth pain and sensitivity. Dentists also need to know the limits of their expertise. Failure to refer a patient to a specialist for complicated conditions can result in malpractice.

Adverse Reactions to Medications and Dental Materials

Dentists should report dangerous and unusual medication reactions to the pharmaceutical company just as physicians do. It is particularly important to document the reaction in the patient's dental record to avoid using the same agent again in the future with that patient. A variety of materials are used in dentistry and become a permanent part of a person's mouth. Adverse reactions to metal and other substances should be carefully evaluated and reported.

In the late 1980s and early 1990s, the subject of mercury poisoning from **amalgam** fillings drew much discussion and consumer concern. Although it has been proven scientifically that amalgam fillings expose the patient to small amounts of mercury over the life of the filling, there is no documented evidence that amalgam fillings cause systemic disease. There are numerous anecdotal reports of neurologic, neuropsychiatric, and allergic disease associated with the presence of dental amalgam, which disappeared when the amalgam was removed. A National Institutes of Health conference in 1991 determined that there was insufficient evidence to consider amalgam fillings a health risk.

Dental Records for Identification of Individuals

Dental records are very useful in the identification of an individual, either dead or alive. Dental records are typically used by the coroner or medical examiner to identify a decedent. In mass disasters, such as airplane crashes and the bombing of the federal building in Oklahoma, dental records may be the only way to confirm the identity of a body. Occasionally, they can be useful in discovering the identity of a patient suffering amnesia.

Role of the Health Information Management Professional

Health information management (HIM) professionals have a unique set of skills that could greatly benefit dental practitioners. Principles of filing and numbering systems, documentation, confidentiality, and good management are all relevant to the practice of dentistry. The growth of managed care and capitation requires education and planning for the financial survival of dental practitioners. There are many opportunities for the HIM professional to share skills with the dental profession.

With the advancement of technology, many dental practices are assessing their needs as they relate to information technology (IT) and their IT infrastructures. What dental software package is the most appropriate for the practice? What other applications might be useful? How do the systems integrate for best business practices? What are the hardware requirements? Is a computer network necessary? If so, how should it be set up? How is electronic insurance filing done? How secure is the data? Many other questions may arise as technology is integrated into the dental practice. The HIM professional could be an invaluable consultant in these areas.

As more Americans receive dental care through managed care plans and insurance, there is a need for individuals with expertise in electronic billing and utilization review. Expertise in quality improvement may be valuable for the compilation of quality indicators and evaluation of patient satisfaction of managed dental care plans. The HIM professional who can manipulate and analyze data using a computer may be invaluable in helping dental practices estimate a capitation amount for a managed care plan.

There are opportunities for HIM careers at dental clinics associated with academic institutions. The information management tasks are very much like those of a large ambulatory care clinic. The management of checking charts in and out, getting paperwork completed, and releasing copies of charts and radiographs are the primary functions. There are also statistics that must be collected and reported on patients seen in the clinic and what procedures each dental student has performed.

HIM professionals can also be involved in the design and selection of dental information systems, particularly as health care becomes more integrated. The goal of a computer-based patient record with a comprehensive, lifetime history of each patient is a relatively new idea for dentistry. The dental profession may need help in understanding the technologies and approaches to integrating data. As dental records and systems become integrated with existing medical records and systems, the development of data dictionaries and combined master patient indexes will become issues.

Trends

Dental Services

The face of dentistry is changing in the twenty-first century. The dentist-to-population ratio is declining after having peaked in 1998. As there are fewer dentists with an increasing general population, and as older individuals continue to keep their natural teeth, the demand for dental services should remain strong for the foreseeable future.

Many of these services will be elective in nature as more people ask for aesthetic dental procedures to improve their appearance. The demand for implant dentistry will also continue to increase as people demand stability for their prostheses and are in a position to afford this type of care.

Many health plans offer dental benefits as an enticement to subscribers. However, the capitation formulas used are sometimes inadequate. If all subscribers used the dental benefits offered, the plan would not be able to cover the costs of the care. To prevent financial disaster, some plans make it difficult for patients to get an appointment for checkups by scheduling them up to six months in advance. Some limit the days and times that first-time patients can be seen and make it inconvenient for the patient to receive the benefits offered. Another method of saving money is not to recommend restorations unless absolutely necessary, thus postponing the care, perhaps until the patient discontinues coverage or transfers to a different plan. None of these methods is in the best interests of the patient. Plans should be carefully scrutinized on the financial viability of the dental benefits offered before dental practitioners join.

Unfortunately, many dentists do not realize the impact of managed care in dentistry and have little comprehension of the information requirements to prepare capitation contracts. A study of attitudes of dentists toward emerging competencies in dental practice found that less than half of the dentists felt that competency in managing information or working in managed care settings was very important (Shugars et al., 1992). Perhaps one reason for this attitude is the general opinion that managed dental care "is certain to grow and become an important part of the dental delivery and financing systems but is unlikely to achieve the dominance that it has in medicine" (Nasser, 1996).

Dental Treatment

Dentistry is one of the few health professions that has successfully discovered how to prevent disease and decrease its financial impact on society. The public has been well educated on the value of fluoridated water and toothpaste, the need to brush and floss regularly, and the value of frequent teeth cleaning and removal of calculus. The number of children and teens with dental caries has greatly decreased, and the number of elderly who still have their own teeth is increasing. The need for dentures is on the decline. New restorative materials, medications, and treatment procedures are being used. New methods of treating periodontal disease, the major cause of tooth loss, are being discovered.

As the American lifestyle becomes more active, there is an increase in dental injuries. A study of emergency room visits to an urban children's hospital found the number of dental emergencies in 1991 was 2.1 times the number in 1982. Almost two-thirds (60 percent) of the dental emergencies were the result of trauma, and 70 percent of those involved trauma to the maxillary anterior teeth (Zeng et al., 1994). Sports dentistry is emerging as a new practice specialty (Padilla and Balikov, 1993). There continues to be great progress in the treatment of dental traumas. Teeth that have been knocked out can be reimplanted. Fractured teeth can be splinted and restored rather than extracted.

Dental implants are still considered experimental. Progress in this area will soon benefit many people who have lost a tooth. Cosmetic dentistry is on the rise. Methods of treating discolored teeth from smoking and coffee are popular. The number of adults undergoing orthodontic treatment has increased.

Another area of progress is dental anesthesia. Some patients can comfortably undergo dental treatment without the use of anesthetic agents through the use of biofeedback, hypnosis, and other techniques. Painless dentistry enhances the acceptability of going to the dentist and thus increases the dental health of Americans.

Another new development in the practice of dentistry is the sale of oral devices. An antisnore device can be obtained from a dentist. It may be the solution to sleepless nights because of a loud, snoring partner. A soft splint called a nightguard, worn in the mouth at night to prevent bruxing or grinding of teeth, offers relief to many sufferers of TMJ syndrome. Dentists have even become involved in making mouth guards for sports. Although outside the realm of traditional dentistry, devices for the mouth available through dentists can improve the quality of life.

Technology in Dentistry

The next important trend is the increase in computerization of dental practices. Electronic billing and benefit confirmation can be important for healthy cash flow. Efficient and convenient handling of appointment scheduling and recall notices provides great financial benefits. The automation of dental practice management is inevitable. Technologies such as digital radiography, intraoral imaging, computer modeling of prostheses, and after-treatment appearances stimulate the interest in computer-based dental records.

Dental Informatics

The new field of dental informatics is mushrooming as dentists are beginning to realize the value of expert systems, automated clinical alerts and warnings, and digital information for clinical practice. Systems have been developed for digital imaging, digital radiology, digital charting, computer-assisted design and manufacture of dental restorations, and diagnostic aids.

Summary

Although not a traditional setting of practice for health information management, opportunities currently exist and future careers are possible in the area of dental care. The knowledge and skills of a health information manager can be applied to the management of dental records. The future electronic health record will be comprehensive and will include dental records. HIM professionals have the knowledge and skills needed to help dentists make the transition from paper to computer records. As progress is made, information managers will need to understand both medical and dental records to manage integrated health information systems. Growth in managed dental care plans will demand better information systems for dentists to manage their dental practices, thus providing opportunities for consulting and careers in managing dental information. This alternate health care setting has great career potential.

Key Terms

amalgam   a silver-colored filling composed of several metals. Amalgams are usually placed on the back teeth (posterior teeth).

bite wing   a radiograph that shows the upper and lower teeth's biting surfaces on the same film. This radiograph shows the portion of the teeth above the gum line.

bridge   a fixed appliance (prosthesis) that replaces missing teeth. A bridge is a series of crowns (abutments and pontics).

calculus   plaque that has hardened. Also known as tartar.

caries   correct technical term for tooth decay.

composite filling   a tooth-colored filling.

crown   full coverage of a tooth when it cannot be restored by a filling.

dentist   a licensed health care professional specializing in the prevention and treatment of disorders of the oral cavity and associated body structures. A dentist possesses either a DDS or DMD degree.

denture   a removable prosthesis (false teeth) that replaces all of the teeth in either the upper or lower jaw.

endodontist   a dentist who specializes in treating diseases or injuries that affect the root tip or nerve of the tooth. The most common procedure is a root canal.

gingiva   the gums.

group dental practice   two or more dentists practicing together.

impaction   an unerupted or partially erupted tooth that will not fully erupt because it is obstructed by another tooth, bone, or soft tissue.

implant   a post that is implanted in the bone. A crown, bridge, or denture is then attached to the implant.

loss of attachment (LA)   the loss of the supporting structure of the teeth that causes the tooth to become loose and that may result in loss of the tooth.

orthodontist   a dentist who specializes in straightening teeth.

panoramic radiograph   a radiograph taken outside of the mouth that shows all the teeth on one film.

periodontist   a dentist who specializes in the treatment of diseases of the gum or bone (supporting structure).

plaque   the sticky film on teeth made up predominantly of bacteria.

pontic   the part of a bridge that replaces the missing tooth.

primary teeth   the baby teeth. Also known as the primary dentition. The baby teeth are replaced by adult teeth (permanent teeth).

prophylaxis   the scaling, cleaning, and removal of calculus.

prosthesis   a fixed or removable appliance to replace missing teeth. Examples are bridges, dentures, and partials. Sometimes single crowns are considered prosthetics.

radiograph   a graphic image produced by the use of radiation.

root canal therapy (RCT)   the nerve of the tooth is removed from the canal inside the root and replaced with a filling material.

sealant   clear application of acrylic placed over the biting surface of the tooth to prevent decay.

solo dental practice   a dental practice owned and operated by one dentist.

wisdom tooth   the third molar; this is the eighth tooth from the center of the mouth to the back of the mouth. Wisdom teeth are often impacted (obstructed from erupting) and have to be extracted.

REVIEW QUESTIONS

Knowledge-based Questions

1. Describe the roles of the dentist, the dental hygienist, and the dental assistant.

2. Why does the dentist need to have a complete and accurate medical history for a patient?

3. What are the typical percentages covered by dental insurance for various types of services?

4. What are the potential risks of injury to dentists or their employees?

5. List several important functional components of a dental practice management system?

6. Why are computer information systems important for managed dental care?

Application-based Questions

1. Compare the frequency and purpose of patient visits to an orthodontist with those to an endodontist. What effect do these differences have on the management and content of dental records?

2. How will the longitudinal, multidisciplinary electronic patient record affect the quality of dental care?

3. Computerization of which functions of a dental practice will have the most impact on the dentist's finances?

4. How could a dentist evaluate the quality of care provided and compare it with other dentists?

5. How is the utilization of dental services different from the utilization of medical services and how do these differences affect utilization management?

6. In general, how can the use of computers in dentistry improve the quality of dental care?

7. What effect will the trend in oral health problems have on the type and number of dental specialists needed in the future?

Web Activity

Visit the American Dental Association's (ADA) Web site at http://www.ada.org . The ADA has several publicly accessible hyperlinks, ranging from professional publications to games and animations for children. Select one or more of these links. Describe how the link you selected can help the public or promote an understanding of the profession of dentistry.

Case Study

Valley Dental Group is composed of three general-practice dentists in the suburb of a large city. The group has a receptionist and an office manager. Most of the group's patients are from families with dental insurance. The benefits and coverages of the insurance policies are different. Some require preauthorization of all restorations whereas others require only preauthorization for crowns, bridges, and dentures. Some policies have a family deductible for all dental care, whereas others have individual deductibles for nonpreventive care only. The usual and customary price that the insurance companies allow for procedures are different so the amount the patient must pay depends on the insurance policy.

The practice needs to organize the way the office handles the information flow to process insurance billing and track payments. Some of the tasks that need to be performed are:

- Verify the patient's insurance company and policy number.

- Keep track of deductible paid so far for family and/or family members.

- Submit insurance claim for services rendered.

- Determine the amount the patient's insurance policy will pay for the procedure.

- Collect the patient's copayment and deductible before the patient leaves the office.

- Follow up on insurance claims submitted that have not been paid.

- Handle claim rejections and bill patient for amount not covered.

- Collect statistics on the number of procedures done, the number of self-payments and insurance payments, the amount paid by insurance, and the number of claims rejected.

- Collect statistics that measure the productivity of each dentist in the group.

Design a system (computer or manual) to accomplish these tasks. (Each student can be assigned a function to design a solution as a class project or students can be assigned one or more parts to do individually.) Avoid duplication of effort and the storing of redundant data in your design. The write-up of the design should include:

1. What information must be collected?

2. How and when will it be collected?

3. How will it be stored and accessed?

4. Describe the procedures to be used to accomplish tasks.

References and Suggested Readings

Barnes, G. P., Parker, W. A., Lyon, T. C., Jr., Drum, M. A., and Coleman, G. C. (1992). Ethnicity, location, age, and fluoridation factors in baby bottle tooth decay and caries prevalence of Head Start children [CD-ROM]. *Public Health Reports, 107* (2), 167–173. Abstract from SilverPlatter File: MedLine Item 92220922.

Benton, R. M., and Shub, J. L. (1995). Peer review. It's good for dentists and patients [CD-ROM]. *New York State Dental Journal, 61* (6), 28–29. Abstract from SilverPlatter File: MedLine Item 95349891.

Brown, L. J., Brunelle, J. A., and Kingman, A. (1996). Periodontal status in the United States, 1988–1991: Prevalence, extent, and demographic variation [CD-ROM]. *Journal of Dental Research, 75* (Spec. No.), 672–683. Abstract from SilverPlatter File: MedLine Item 96176356.

California Dental Association. (2000). Selecting and using dental benefits: A consumer's guide to dental insurance [Online]. http://www.cda.org/public/dentalcare/consumer.htm [2004, January 10].

Department of Defense. (2003, June 16). *TRICARE Handbook.* [Online]. http://www.tricare.osd.mil/TricareHandbook/default.cfm [2003, July 25].

Kaste, L. M., and Gift, H. C. (1995). Inappropriate infant bottle feeding. Status of the Healthy People 2000 objective [CD-ROM]. *Archives of Pediatric and Adolescent Medicine, 149* (7), 786–791. Abstract from SilverPlatter File: MedLine Item 95316126.

Kaste, L. M., Selwitz, R. H., Oldakowski, R. J., Brunelle, J. A., Winn, D. M., and Brown, L. J. (1996). Coronal caries in the primary and permanent dentition of children and adolescents 1–17 years of age: United States, 1988–1991 [CD-ROM]. *Journal of Dental Research, 75* (Spec. No.), 631–641. Abstract from SilverPlatter File: MedLine Item 96176352.

Kehoe, B. (1994, July/August). Special Report: How dentists use their computers. *Dental Practice and Finance*, 58–61.

Kiyak, H. A., Grayston, M. N., and Crinean, C. L. (1993). Oral health problems and needs of nursing home residents [CD-ROM]. *Community Dentistry and Oral Epidemiology, 21* (1), 49–52. Abstract from SilverPlatter File: MedLine Item 93161712.

Lazar, V. (1997). To solo or not to solo. *Journal of American Dental Association, 128* (2), 233–235.

Loesche, W. J., Abrams, J., Terpenning, M. S., and Bretz, W. A. (1995). Dental findings of geriatric populations with diverse medical backgrounds [CD-ROM]. *Oral Surgery, Oral Medicine, Oral Pathology, Oral Radiology, and Endodontics, 80* (1), 43–54. Abstract from SilverPlatter File: MedLine Item 96012668.

Logan, H. L., Baron, R. S., Kanellis, M., Brennan, M., and Brunsman, B. A. (1996). Knowledge of male and female midwestern college students about baby bottle tooth decay [CD-ROM]. *Pediatric Dentistry, 18* (3), 219–223. Abstract from SilverPlatter File: MedLine Item 96379379.

Nasser, F. E., Jr. (1996). Managed care seizes the attention of dentistry [CD-ROM]. *General Dentistry, 44* (2), 154–158. Abstract from SilverPlatter File: MedLine Item 96335743.

Padilla, R., and Balikov, S. (1993). Sports dentistry: Coming of age in the '90s [CD-ROM]. *Journal of the California Dental Association, 21* (4), 27–34. Abstract from SilverPlatter File: MedLine Item 93316138.

Peterson, L. C., Cobb, D. S., and Reynolds, D. C. (1995). ICOHR: Intelligent computer based oral health record [CD-ROM]. *MEDINFO, 8* (Pt. 2), 1709. Abstract from SilverPlatter File: MedLine Item 96174052.

Quattlebaum, Bryan (1995). *Managed Care in Dentistry.* Tulsa, OK: Pen Well Books. An excellent primer on dental managed care.

Safadi, G. S., Safadi, T. J., Terezhalmy, G. T., and Taylor, J. S. (1996). Latex hypersensitivity: Its prevalence among dental professionals [CD-ROM]. *Journal of the American Dental Association, 127* (1), 83–88. Abstract from SilverPlatter File: MedLine Item 96166172.

Schleyer, T.K.L., Spallek, H., Bartling, W.C., and Corby, P.C. (2003). The technologically well-equipped dental office. *Journal of the American Dental Association, 134,* 30–41.

Schoen, M. H. (1992). Dentistry and national health insurance [CD-ROM]. *Current Opinion in Dentistry, 2,* 1–5. Abstract from SilverPlatter File: MedLine Item: 93004823.

Shugars, D. A., and Bader, J. D. (1995). Practice parameters in dentistry: Where do we stand? *Journal of American Dental Association, 126* (8), 1134–1143.

Shugars, D. A., Bader, J. D., and O'Neil, E. H. (1992). Attitudes of dentists toward emerging competencies for health care practitioners [CD-ROM]. *Journal of Dental Education, 56* (9), 640–645. Abstract from SilverPlatter File: MedLine Item 93017358.

Workshop on Quality Assurance in Dentistry (1994). Model clinical guidelines for primary dental health care providers for managing patients with adult periodontitis. *Journal of Dental Education, 58* (8), 659–662.

Zeng, Y., Sheller, B., and Milgrom, P. (1994). Epidemiology of dental emergency visits to an urban children's hospital [CD-ROM]. *Pediatric Dentistry, 16* (6), 419–423. Abstract from SilverPlatter File: MedLine Item 95158186.

Key Resources

American Dental Association
211 E. Chicago Avenue
Chicago, IL 60611
Phone: 312-440-2500
http://www.ada.org/
Professional association for licensed dentists and accreditation body for dental education programs.

American Dental Hygienists Association
444 N. Michigan Avenue
Suite 3400
Chicago, IL 60611
Phone: 312-440-8900
http://www.adha.org
Professional association for licensed dental hygienists and accreditation body for dental hygiene education programs.

Association of Managed Care Dentists
1223 Wilshire Boulevard #483
Santa Monica, CA 90403
Phone: 310-453-3439
http://www.amcd.org
A nonprofit organization whose goal is to provide education, representation, and a forum for communication among dentists.

Chapter *15*

Veterinary Settings

Margaret L. Neterer, MM, RHIA

Learning Objectives

Upon successful completion of this chapter, you should be able to:

1. List at least five similarities between veterinary and human health records.
2. Explain why SNOMED-CT is preferred over SNVDO as a veterinary nomenclature and describe its importance to human and animal welfare in the twenty-first century.
3. Explain the necessity of maintaining records for groups of animals rather than individual animals in particular veterinary care settings.
4. Illustrate the interaction between veterinary and human medicine professionals.
5. Describe the client's rights in information ownership and be able to identify the client in a given situation.
6. Identify key organizations that provide the most current information relating to the practice of veterinary health information management.

SETTING	DESCRIPTION
Veterinary or Animal Medical Center	A facility in which consultative, clinical, and hospital services are rendered and in which a large staff of basic and applied veterinary scientists perform significant research and conduct advanced professional educational programs.
Veterinary or Animal Hospital	A facility in which the practice conducted includes the confinement as well as the treatment of patients.
Clinic	A facility in which the practice conducted is essentially an outpatient type of practice.
Office	A facility where a limited or consultative practice is conducted and that provides no facilities for the housing of patients.
Mobile Facility	A practice conducted from a vehicle with special medical or surgical facilities or from a vehicle suitable only for making house or farm calls. Regardless of mode of transportation, such practice shall have a permanent base of operations with a published address and telephone facilities for making appointments or responding to emergency situations.
Emergency Facility	A veterinary medical service whose primary function is the receiving, treatment, and monitoring of emergency patients during its specified hours of operation. A doctor is in attendance at all hours of operation and sufficient staff is always available to provide timely and appropriate care. Doctors, support staff, instrumentation, medications, and supplies must be sufficient to provide an appropriate level of emergency care. This service may be an independent, after-hours service; an independent 24-hour service; or part of a full-service hospital or large teaching institution.
On-call Emergency Service	A veterinary medical service whose doctors and staff are not on premises during all hours of operation or whose doctors leave after a patient is treated.

Introduction to Setting

The **veterinary** profession is practiced in a variety of care settings. The information presented for the learner in this chapter centers on the veterinary *teaching* hospital, the most probable employment setting.

Types of Patients

The term *patient* in this chapter refers to an **animal**. The animal's owner is the hospital's client.

According to James F. Wilson, DVM, JD, "Animals are usually classified according to species and distinguished as either domestic or wild. Problems occur with simple classifications like this, because certain species or individual animals do not fall neatly into either category. Others fit into both categories based on their use" (Wilson et al., 1988). For our purposes, this discussion distinguishes between domestic animals, including pets, and wild animals.

The domestic animals most commonly treated in veterinary teaching hospitals include small animals such as **canine** (dog), **feline** (cat), and other small animals (birds, parrots, snakes, lizards, hamsters, ferrets, etc.); food animals such as **bovine** (cow), **ovine** (sheep), **porcine** (swine), **caprine** (goat), llamas, and sometimes ratites (ostriches, emus, and rheas); and **equine** (horse).

Wild animals sometimes cared for in the veterinary teaching hospital setting include owls, eagles, hawks, songbirds such as sparrows and cardinals, deer, moose, and bears. These animals are usually cared for under the direction of the staff zoological veterinarian. Wolves or wolf-hybrid dogs are generally not treated in the veterinary teaching hospital because they are unpredictable and could seriously injure a health care provider, the client, or other patients in the health care facility.

Types of Caregivers

The veterinary health care provider diagnoses, treats, corrects, changes, relieves, or prevents animal disease, deformity, defect, injury, or other physical or mental conditions. This includes the prescription or administration of any drug, medicine, biologic, apparatus, application, anesthetic, or other therapeutic or diagnostic substance or technique, and the use of any manual or mechanical procedure for artificial insemination, for testing for pregnancy, or for correcting sterility or infertility or to render advice or recommendation with regard to any of the above (LaFrana, 1995).

The **veterinarian** has received a professional degree from a college of veterinary medicine. Women now comprise 70 to 80 percent of veterinary medicine enrollment. As of October 31, 2002, 43 percent of the American Veterinary Medical Association (AVMA) membership is women (Fagan). There are 32 veterinary schools in the United States and Canada, and 5 foreign schools are also approved by the AVMA. A list of the schools along with each school's address, phone number, accreditation status, a brief history of the program, and names and phone numbers of various administrative individuals are in the *AVMA Directory*.

Similar to medical doctors (MDs) and doctors of osteopathic medicine (DOs), doctors of veterinary medicine (DVMs) or veterinary medical doctors (VMDs) may choose to pursue advanced training and write examinations in specialty boards. These include toxicology, laboratory animal medicine, poultry, **theriogenology** (animal reproduction), anesthesiology, behavior, clinical pharmacology, dermatology, emergency and critical care, microbiology, nutrition, ophthalmology, pathology, preventive medicine, radiology, surgery, zoological medicine, dentistry, and internal medicine with subspecialties in cardiology, neurology, and oncology.

The **veterinary technician** is a graduate of a two- or three-year AVMA-accredited program in veterinary technology or a person so recognized by the board in rules and regulations promulgated to regulate veterinary technicians

(LaFrana, 1995). Information about individual programs is also available in the *AVMA Directory*.

The **veterinary technologist** is a graduate of a four-year AVMA-accredited program in veterinary technology or a person so recognized by the board in rules and regulations promulgated to regulate veterinary technologists (LaFrana, 1995).

The veterinary practice manager is responsible for the veterinary facility's business management including human resource management, financial management, organizational structuring, marketing, and the areas of law, insurance, and ethics. A formal education in areas such as psychology, accounting, marketing, and business management is recommended. The practice manager is eligible for certification as a **certified veterinary practice manager (CVPM)** through the **Veterinary Hospital Managers Association (VHMA)**.

Regulatory Issues

In many ways, the practice of health information management in the veterinary setting is less stressful than in human medicine settings that have multiple layers of government and third-party regulations to address. The obvious lack of detailed regulations often makes it easier to practice health information management because the health information management (HIM) professional is more free to creatively apply trends in human medicine that will work best for health care delivery for patients and procedures in the practice. At times, however, more strict rules force a caregiver to conform and practice good veterinary medicine when various members of the practice are reluctant to relearn procedures or expend money to make necessary advancements.

The actual practice of veterinary medicine is governed by individual state veterinary practice acts. The AVMA has established a model veterinary practice act, which is found in the *AVMA Directory*. This model act provides definitions related to the practice of veterinary medicine (i.e., "Animal," "Licensed Veterinarian," etc.). It also outlines licensing requirements and exceptions, establishes state boards of veterinary medicine, and outlines the processes of license application to practice veterinary medicine, license renewal, discipline of licensees, and the appeals process.

The veterinary practice act may fall under one of a variety of state codes (examples: Public Health Code [Michigan], Business and Professions Code [California], and Education Laws [New York]). A digest of each state's practice act is available in the *AVMA Directory*, along with the name, address, and phone number of the state's board of veterinary medicine or executive officer of the board.

The AVMA establishes guidelines and policy statements for the practice of veterinary medicine through its executive board or House of Delegates. These guidelines are printed annually in the *AVMA Membership Directory and Resource Manual*.

The AVMA's Council on Education is the accrediting body for programs of study in veterinary medicine. Reference to the importance of medical record keeping is found in Standard 4, Clinical Resources: "Medical records must be comprehensive and maintained in an effective retrieval system to efficiently support the teaching, research and service programs of the college" (AVMA, 2003, p. 16). The HIM service may provide the statistics necessary to document the number of patients available to the students in a typical year, to show that there are enough patients to provide quality clinical instruction. The survey forms (Tables 15-1 and 15-2) request data on the **number of accessions**, which include statistics on patient visits, hospitalizations, and field services.

Table 15-1 AVMA Council on Accreditation, Clinical Resources of the Teaching Hospital (Courtesy of AVMA. Used with permission.)

Animal Species	*Number of Patient Visits*	*Number Hospitalized*	*Number of Hospital Days*
Bovine			
Canine			
Caprine			
Equine			
Feline			
Ovine			
Porcine			
Caged Pet Birds			
Caged Pet Mammals			
Avian Wildlife			
Other			

Number of Patient Visits—total number of times the patient visits the hospital (if Buffy visits the hospital 3 times this year, this would count as 3 visits).

Number Hospitalized—number of patients that were hospitalized.

Number of Hospital Days—cumulative days that the total number of patients were hospitalized.

Table 15-2 AVMA Council on Accreditation, Clinical Resources of the Ambulatory/Field Service Program (Courtesy of AVMA. Used with permission.)

Animal Species	*Number of Farm (site) Calls*	*Number of Animals Examined/Treated*
Bovine		
Caprine		
Equine		
Ovine		
Porcine		
Other		

Number of Farm (site) Calls—total number of calls/visits made to farm/operations.

Number of Animals Examined/Treated—number of individual animals examined/treated.

The data collected in these surveys corresponds with data collected by the Association of American Veterinary Medical Colleges (AAVMC) that is used, along with other statistical data, in describing all aspects of academic veterinary medicine. The AAVMC also manages the Veterinary Medical College Application Service (VMCAS), which collects, processes, and distributes applications for admission to veterinary medical colleges.

The **American Animal Hospital Association (AAHA)**, established in 1933, develops and circulates standards for companion animal hospitals. The 2003 standards focus on the facility's patient-centered practice and assist the practice in setting future goals. The final accreditation decision is made at the time of the accreditation visit. The facility either meets the majority of the accreditation points or it does not.

The medical record standards address many areas common to the human health care setting, such as the following:

- Legibility
- Use of standard abbreviations
- Authentication of entries
- Documentation of communications between the health care providers and the client
- Security and confidentiality of electronic records
- Use of a standard nomenclature for recording diagnoses
- Necessity of using medical messaging standards such as Health Level 7 (HL-7) when transmitting electronic medical information

Documentation

Current documentation elements will seem very familiar to the traditional HIM professional. They include the following:

1. Owner (client) identification: name, address, telephone numbers for home and office are minimal; additional information may include names, addresses, and telephone numbers for alternate or co-owners of the animal.
2. Animal (patient) identification: name, identification number if applicable (i.e., tatoo or identification chip), species, breed, date of birth, sex, color, and/or markings
3. Vaccination history of the patient
4. Chief complaint: observations reported by the client
5. Medical history
6. Physical examination, including the current weight of the animal
7. Problem list
8. Diagnostic reports (e.g., laboratory, diagnostic imaging, etc.)

9. Patient-identifiable source data, including photographs, video recordings, audio recordings, diagnostic films, and electrocardiogram tracings

10. Consultation reports, including telephone consultations

11. Prognosis

12. Progress notes recording medical and surgical events should be made in chronological order; communications with the client should be documented, including waiver or deferral of recommended care.

13. Surgical and dental records, including the consent form signed by the client

14. Written discharge summary and instructions

15. Necropsy reports, when applicable. (A **necropsy** is a postmortem examination to determine the cause of death or the character and extent of changes produced by the disease.)

16. Financial records

Standards

The AVMA has produced several policy statements and guidelines that support the maintenance of veterinary health records. The policy statements and guidelines referenced below can be found in the current issue of the *AVMA Directory*.

In April 2001, the AVMA Executive Board approved "Guidelines for Veterinary Practice Facilities," listing 15 general principles of good practice encompassing all aspects of veterinary medicine that should be considered in the development and operation of any practice. Principle 10 reads "Adequate patient and financial records." Unfortunately, "adequate" is not further defined.

The 1998 AVMA Executive Board approved "Guidelines for Veterinary Prescription Drugs," which was amended by the Executive Board in April 1999. This guideline also addresses record keeping:

> Adequate treatment records should be maintained by the veterinarian for at least two years (or as otherwise mandated by law), for all animals treated, to show that the drugs were supplied to the clients with whom a valid VCPR [veterinarian/client/patient relationship] had existed.

This guideline goes on to say that,

> Such records should include the information set forth under *Basic Information for Records (R), Prescriptions (P), and Labels (L)*. This information includes:
>
> a. Name, address, and telephone number of veterinarians (RPL)
> b. Name (L), address, and telephone number of clients (RP)
> c. Identification of animal(s) treated, species, and numbers of animals treated where possible (RPL)

> **d.** Date of treatment, prescribing, or dispensing of drug (RPL)
>
> **e.** Name and quantity of the drug (or drug preparation) to be prescribed or dispensed (RPL)
>
> **f.** Dosage and duration directions for use (RPL)
>
> **g.** Number of refills authorized (RP)
>
> **h.** Cautionary statements, as needed (RPL)
>
> **i.** Expiration date (L)
>
> **j.** Slaughter withdrawal and/or milk withholding times, if applicable (RPL)
>
> **k.** Signature or equivalent (P)

In 1998, the AVMA Executive Board approved the "Position on Pre-signed Certificates of Veterinary Inspection," which states:

> Any veterinarian found guilty of pre-signing or otherwise misusing intra- or inter-state or export certificates of veterinary inspection should have his or her accreditation immediately removed, and all pertinent information should be transmitted to the state board of veterinary medical examiners for a proper hearing. The AVMA believes that the chief animal health official of each state should exercise strict control over the issuing and control of all health certificates of veterinary inspection.

The AAHA has created standards for medical record services that will look and feel more familiar to the student of health information technology or health information management. Records management is also addressed in other AAHA standards, such as those for emergency hospitals. As part of the on-site accreditation process, the health information management professional is asked to pull a record at random with a particular diagnosis or procedure. The record is then reviewed against the standards.

Format

The **problem-oriented medical record (POMR)** format or a combination POMR–source-oriented format is most commonly used in the veterinary teaching hospital. The source-oriented health record is more common in nonteaching hospitals.

A variation of the family-oriented format is also quite common for **herd health** (sometimes referred to as **production medicine** or ambulatory care services) programs in teaching and nonteaching facilities. For instance, rather than generate a separate record on each of the 100 cows examined or treated at Mr. MacDonald's farm on a particular day, the "MacDonald Farm" record would be maintained through the use of specialized forms or electronic formats that enable the health care provider to document treatments on a large number of animals at one time. Figure 15-1 displays a sample format for this "family" record for production medicine (PM) and equine (EQ) patients.

MICHIGAN STATE
UNIVERSITY

MSU Veterinary Teaching Hospital
Production Medicine
East Lansing, Michigan 48824-1314
Appointments: (517) 355-3500   Billing: (517) 353-4957

Nº 05287

WHITE-CLIENT
YELLOW-MED. REC.
PINK-BUS. OFF.

CLIENT _____

CLINICIAN _____
DATE _____
REGFERRING _____
VETERINARIAN _____

TRIP FEE
___ 32011 CHUTE FEE   ___
___ 32110 REFERRAL   ___
___ 32109 REGULAR   ___

EMERGENCY FEE
___ 32211 6 A.M.-8P.M.   ___
___ 32212 8P.M.-6 A.M.   ___

EXAMINATION
___ 35219 A   ___
___ 35220 B   ___
___ 32020 PROF. SERV.   ___
___ _____ ___
___ _____ ___
___ _____ ___

TECHNIQUES

___ 32002 EPIDURAL   ___

___ 32107 TREATMENT   ___
___ _____ ___
___ _____ ___
___ _____ ___

REGULATORY
___ 32317 ANAPLASMOSIS   ___
___ 32319 BOVINE BTV   ___
___ 32321 BRUC. TEST-BOV   ___
___ 32044 CALFHOOD VAC   ___
___ 32047 HEALTH PAPERS   ___
___ 35065 PRV   ___
___ 35064 PRV + BRUC.   ___
___ 32048 SEROLOGY FORMS ___
___ 32049 TB INJ.   ___
___ 32050 TB READ   ___
___ _____ ___
___ _____ ___

SURGERY
___ 32058 CASLICKS
___ 32331 CASTRATE BOV (A)
___ 32332 CASTRATE BOV (B)
___ 32064 CASTRATE PROCINE
___ 32329 DEHORN BOVINE A
___ 32330 DEHORN BOVINE B
___ 35501 DEHORN ELEC C
___ 32031 LAMENESS-BOV. FOOT
___ 32035 LAME-WOOD BLOCK
___ 32075 LDA ROLL
___ 32074 LDA SURGERY
___ 32076 LDA TOGGLE
___ 32082 PROCINE HERNIA
___ 32307 TEAT
___ _____
___ _____
___ _____
___ _____
___ _____

REPRODUCTION/OBSTETRICS
___ 32087 BSE-BULL
___ 35252 BSE-BULL PROGRAM
___ 32302 OB 15 MIN.
___ 32303 OB 30 MIN.
___ 32304 OB 45 MIN.
___ 32305 OB 60 MIN.
___ 35502 PELVIC MEASURE
___ 35214 RP
___ 32097 RECTALS-BOVINE
___ 32101 ULTRASOUND-BOV.
___ 32300 UTERINE INF.
___ 32105 VAGINAL EXAM-FA
___ _____
___ _____

CONSULTATION
___ 32310   0.5 HRS
___ 32311   1.0 HRS
___ 32311   1.5 HRS
___ 32318 FIELD INVESTIGATION
___ 32320 EQUIPMENT
___ _____

PHARMACY/SUPPLIES
___ ___ 24083 BANAMINE/ML   ___
___ ___ 24063 ASPIRIN 240GM   ___
___ ___ 25303 BROWN GAUZE   ___
___ ___ 24149 CAL GLUCONATE   ___
___ ___ 24145 CAL MPK   ___
___ ___ 25001 CATTLEMASTER-4-L5(5)   ___
___ ___ 24220 CYSTORELIN   ___
___ ___ 24262 DEXYTROSE 50%   ___
___ ___ 24469 LA-200 ML   ___
___ ___ 24518 LUTALYSE 10ML/ML   ___
___ ___ 24519 LUTALYSE 30ML/ML   ___
___ ___ 24571 NAXCEL 1GM   ___
___ ___ 24572 NAXCEL 4GM   ___
___ ___ 24509 OTC 100MG/ML/ML   ___
___ ___ 24620 OXYTOCIN 20U/ML/ML   ___
___ ___ 24629 PANMYCIN BOLUS/E   ___
___ ___ 24638 PEN G 100ML/ML   ___
___ ___ 25047 SOMUBAC 10 DS/VL   ___
___ ___ 26666 TRIANGLE 9   ___
___ 35070 SIMPLEX   ___
___ 35221 MAGNET   ___
___ 24943 VENOSET IV SET   ___
___ ___ 25163 VETRAP ROLL   ___
___ ___ 35300 MISC. SUPPLIES   ___
___ ___ _____   ___
___ ___ _____   ___
___ ___ _____   ___

OTHER SERVICES
___ ___ 32010 BANDAGING   ___
___ ___ 32030 LABS.-NON. CLINIC   ___
___ ___ 32051 SAMPLES HANDLING   ___
___ ___ 32052 SAMPLES SHIPPING   ___
___ ___ _____   ___

SUBTOTAL   ___
TEACHING DISCOUNT   ___

TOTAL   ___
NUMBER OF STUDENTS   ___
SPECIES___ NO___ TREATED
___ CONSULTED

COMMENTS _____
_____
_____
_____
_____

O-21781

Figure 15-1 Equine and production medicine records. (Courtesy Michigan State University, Veterinary Teaching Hospital.)

EQ 05080

MSU Veterinary Teaching Hospital
Equine Field Service
East Lansing, Michigan 48824-1314
Appointments: (517) 355-3500   Billing: (517) 353-4957

WHITE-CLIENT
YELLOW-MED. REC.
PINK-BUS. OFF.

CLIENT _____
CLINICIAN _____
DATE _____

TRIP FEE
__ 32208 EMERG. FEE 8AM-5PM   ____
__ 32210 EMERG. FEE 5PM-8AM   ____
__ 32109 REGULAR   ____
__ 32111 STABLE   ____

ANESTHESIA
__ 24004 ACEPROMZINE ML   ____
__ 32006 ADMIN. LOCAL   ____
__ 32007 ADMIN. NERVE BLOCK   ____
__ 34160 CARBOCAINE HCL/ML   ____
__ 25571 DORMOSEDAN ML   ____
__ 24735 ROMPUN 100MG/ML   ____
__ 24814 STADOL 2MG/ML   ____
__ 24913 TORBUGESIC ML   ____
__ 24944 VETALAR ML   ____
__ _____   ____

PHARMACY/SUPPLIES
__ 25305 ADAPTIC DRESSING   ____
__ 25441 AKTROL OPTH.   ____
__ 24048 ANTHELCIDE   ____
__ 24071 ATROPINE OINT   ____
__ 24074 AZIUM ML   ____
__ 24081 BANAMINE PASTE   ____
__ 24080 BANAMINE PK.   ____
__ 24083 BANAMINE INJ./ML   ____
__ 24094 BENZA-PEN INJ./ML   ____
__ 24097 BET. SCRUB OZ   ____
__ 25303 BROWN GAUZE   ____
__ 24141 BUTE 1GM. TAB   ____
__ 24138 BUTE INJ ML   ____
__ 25476 BUTE 4GM PASTE   ____
__ 24184 CHLORO OPTH   ____
__ 25174 COTTON SHEET   ____
__ 25667 DMSO SWEAT   ____
__ 24312 ELASTIKON 3″ ROLL   ____
__ 24326 EQVALAN   ____
__ 24322 EQUIMATE VL   ____
__ 24383 GENT 100MG/ML   ____
__ 24379 GENT. OPTH.   ____

SURGERY
__ 32014 DENT. FLOAT   ____
__ 32016 DENT. WOLF TOOTH   ____
__ 32059 CASLICKS   ____
__ 32342 CASTRATION (B)   ____
__ 32077 LACERATION (A)   ____
__ 32202 LACERATION (B)   ____
__ 32203 LACERATION (C)   ____
__ 32204 LACERATION (D)   ____
__ _____   ____
__ _____   ____

REPRODUCTION
__ 32086 AI-EQUINE   ____
__ 32024 DIAG. UTER. CULTURE   ____
__ 32098 RECTALS   ____
__ 32100 ULTRASOUND   ____
__ 32091 UTERINE BIOPSY   ____
__ 32337 UTERINE INF W/O MED   ____
__ _____   ____

PHARMACY/SUPPLIES
__ 24190 HCG VIAL   ____
__ 24519 LUTALYSE ML   ____
__ 24530 MAXITROL OPTH.   ____
__ 24549 MINERAL OIL OZ.   ____
__ 24591 NOL. OINT OZ.   ____
__ 24608 OPTHOCORT TUBE   ____
__ 24626 PANACUR PASTE   ____
__ 24638 PENICILLIN G ML   ____
__ 25216 PRD FLESH OINT OZ   ____
__ 25379 SMZ 480/TAB   ____
__ 25380 SMZ 960/TAB   ____
__ 24816 STATROL OPTH   ____
__ 24826 STRONGID PASTE   ____
__ 25163 VETRAP ROLL   ____
__ 24950 VETROPOLYCIN   ____
__ 25434 VETROPOLYCIN/HC   ____
__ 35300 MISC. SUPPLIES   ____
__ _____   ____
__ _____   ____
__ _____   ____

EXAMINATIONS
__ 32314 EXAM-/RECHECK   ____
__ 32315 EXAMINATION B   ____
__ 32316 EXAMINATION C   ____
__ 35210 EXAM-INSURANCE   ____
__ 32033 LAMENESS(UNITS)   ____
__ 32339 PREPURCHASE (B)   ____
__ 32045 REG.-HEALTH EXAM   ____
__ 32047 REG.-HEALTH PAPER   ____
__ _____   ____

VACCINATIONS
__ 32344 EQUINE FIVE WAY   ____
__ 32346 PNEUMABORT K   ____
__ 32347 POT. HORSE FEVER   ____
__ 32349 RHINOMUNE   ____
__ 32350 STRANGLES   ____
__ 32352 TETANUS TOXOID   ____
__ _____   ____
__ _____   ____

LAB
__ 32020 DIAG.-FOAL CITE TEST   ____
__ 32030 NON CLINIC LAB   ____
__ 32354 REG. COGGINS   ____
__ _____   ____

PROFESSIONAL
__ 32004 ADMINISTRATION   ____
__ 32010 BANDAGING   ____
__ 32040 PROFESSIONAL SVC.   ____
__ 32066 RADIOGRAPHS BASIC   ____
__ 32205 RADIOGRAPHS ADD.   ____
__ 32053 STOMACH TUBE   ____
__ _____   ____
__ _____   ____

SUBTOTAL _____
CASH DISCOUNT _____
_____
TOTAL _____

NUMBER OF STUDENTS _____
SPECIES ____ NO __ TREATED
_____ (GROUP)

COMMENTS _____
_____
_____
_____

O-20181

Figure 15-1   (*Continued*)

Forms of Documentation

The sophistication of record-keeping formats varies from totally paperless to hand-written 5-by-7-inch cards.

Reimbursement

Out-of-Pocket

Few owners have health insurance for their animals and often make treatment decisions based on how much they can afford to pay out-of-pocket for the animal's care. For this reason, detailed and accurate written cost estimates, together with a signed informed consent, are essential elements in establishing the contractual relationship between the owner and the veterinarian, and become an important part of the veterinary health record. When generated through an electronic record-keeping system, the account can be flagged when the cost of care is reaching the estimated total agreed to by the owner. At that time, the health care provider attempts to reach the owner for authorization to continue beyond the original estimate. If the owner cannot be reached, the health care provider must make the decision of whether to continue testing and/or treating, and must document that decision in the health record.

Veterinary teaching hospital health records generally include the patient's final bill from each episode of care. As mentioned earlier, continuance of treatment sometimes takes into consideration how much the owner can afford to pay out-of-pocket. Along with an understanding of the patient's current medical condition, a review of expenditures made to date will help the owners make the correct decision for themselves and the animal.

Mortality Insurance

The economic value of some horses requires that the owner, or owners, secure mortality insurance on the animal. The insurance company's authorization to euthanize the animal may be more critical than the owner's when the insured animal is ill or injured and euthanasia is a strong option (Wilson et al., 1988). Euthanasia without the insurance company's authorization may lead to the company's refusal to pay the death benefit. Therefore, documentation of the name of the person(s) authorizing the euthanasia, along with their telephone number, the date, and time of verbal authorization(s) in the health record, becomes vital for payment of the death benefit (Wilson et al., 1988).

Pet Health Insurance

As the availability of pet health insurance and veterinary medical and surgical insurance increases, so does the importance of complete, accurate veterinary health records. In the event that the insurance company finds the health record inadequate to justify the claim and refuses to pay for services rendered, the client may choose to take legal action against the veterinarian for the amount of the claim, or seek the assistance of the state's insurance commissioner in resolving the issue (Wilson et al., 1988).

Information Management

Coding and Classification

The ability to easily retrieve information based on diagnoses or procedures is important in veterinary research. There are several systems used for this purpose in the veterinary setting. Coding and classification systems can meet this need as can other methods, such as the use of a controlled vocabulary, which is also described in this section.

SNVDO

The ***Standard Nomenclature of Veterinary Diseases and Operations (SNVDO)*** is based on the *Standard Nomenclature of Diseases and Operations*. The second abridged edition of SNVDO was published in 1976 by the Public Health Service. The nomenclature has been only intermittently maintained over the past 20 years and is still being used in most North American veterinary teaching hospitals.

The diagnosis code in SNVDO consists of three parts: topography (four characters), etiology (four characters), and the structural or function code (one character).

Unlike human medicine coding procedures, there is no emphasis placed on differentiation between principal and secondary diagnoses. The procedure code in SNVDO consists of two parts: The first three characters are an abbreviated topography code and the last two characters depict the procedure performed in that topography.

Through the efforts of several members of the AVMA Committee on Standard Nomenclature and Coding, who were also board members of the **Veterinary Medical Data Base (VMDB)**, it was decided in the early 1980s that the *Systematized Nomenclature of Medicine (SNOMED)* would, with the addition of unique veterinary terms, best meet the veterinary profession's information needs.

SNOMED-CT

The *Systematized Nomenclature of Medicine, Clinical Terms (SNOMED-CT)* was released in 2002 as the latest version of a detailed reference terminology published by SNOMED International, a division of the College of American Pathologists (CAP).

Beginning in 2004, access to the core content of *SNOMED-CT* became available through the National Library of Medicine's (NLM) Unified Medical Language System (UMLS). This open access enabled various interested parties (e.g., vendors, informatics professionals, and health care professionals) to exchange information for improving patient care, creating databases studying public health threats, and conducting research. This permitted the entire health care community to realize the importance of this dynamic nomenclature containing more than 344,000 concepts, 913,000 descriptions or synonyms, and 1.3 million semantic relationships.

Figure 15-2 illustrates *SNOMED-CT*'s CLUE browser interface, which was developed by David Markwell of the United Kingdom and is available from the Clinical Information Consultancy. The excerpt of information shown in Figure 15-2 displays the hierarchical nature of SNOMED-CT, which makes this system extremely powerful, rich, and intricate. It allows the user to enter and/or retrieve data as broadly or with as much granularity as necessary.

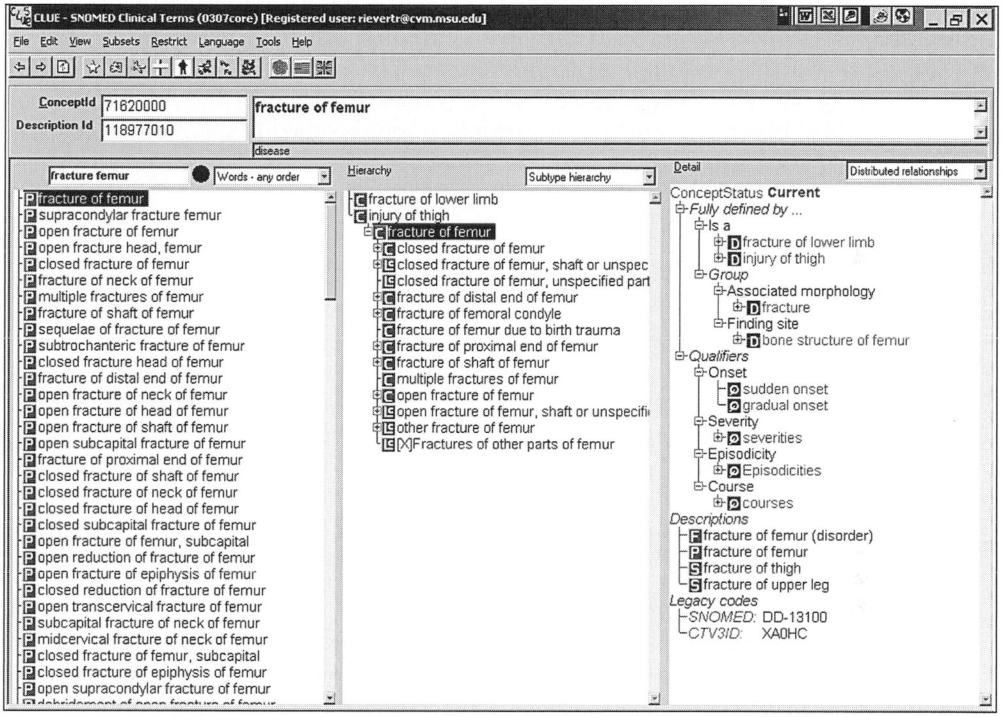

Figure 15-2 The rich detail of SNOMED CT as viewed through the CLUE browser. [This material includes SNOMED Clinical Terms ® (SNOMED CT ®), which is used by permission of the College of American Pathologists. © 2002, 2003 College of American Pathologists. All rights reserved. SNOMED CT has been created by combining SNOMED RT ® and a computer based nomenclature and classification known as Clinical Terms Version 3, formerly known as the Read Codes Version 3, Copyright. SNOMED and SNOMED CT are registered trademarks of the College of American Pathologists. For more information on the CLUE browser, which is available from the Clinical Information Consultancy (CIC), visit the Web site http://www.clininfo.co.uk/clue5].

SNOMED-CT was developed by merging *SNOMED RT* (Reference Terminology) with the United Kingdom's National Health Service (NHS) Clinical Terms Version 3. Before *SNOMED RT*, the *Systematized Nomenclature of Human and Veterinary Medicine (SNOMED International)* or *SNOMED III* had been published in 1993 by the College of American Pathologists. One of the editors, Roger A. Cote, MED, described it as the only multiaxial nomenclature designed and created for indexing, storing, and retrieving information from the computer-based medical record (Cote, 1995).

Kathleen Ellis, RHIT, RN, BS, and Roberta Schmidt, RHIA, health information management professionals for the colleges of veterinary medicine at the University of Illinois and Ohio State University, respectively, along with Jeff R. Wilcke, DVM, MS, DACVCP, the AVMA Secretariat at the Virginia-Maryland Regional College of Veterinary Medicine, have been the leaders in adapting *SNOMED-CT* for use in the veterinary profession. The Secretariat and his staff have created a Web site (http://snomed.vetmed.vt.edu) offering user discussion forums for the purpose of developing standardized usage of the nomenclature in daily practice in the veterinary setting.

(For the most current information on *SNOMED-CT*, refer to Internet link http://www.snomed.org.)

ISIS

The **International Species Information System (ISIS)** is a computer-based, global zoo animal information system that began in 1973 and now has at least 586 member institutions in 72 countries on 6 continents. ISIS collects the age, sex, parentage, place of birth, and circumstance of death on the specimen. It now has data on more than 1.65 million specimens in total. The ISIS organization created the MedARKS (Medical Animal Records Keeping System) software package for each facility to assemble and report its own data. MedARKS includes clinical notes, clinical pathology, anesthesia, an integrated specimen medical history report, along with inventory reports and an interface to the fourth version of ARKS (Animal Records Keeping System).

Free Text

The Veterinary Medical Teaching Hospital of the University of California at Davis has developed its own in-house system whereby there is no coding of diagnoses or procedures. Health care providers enter their findings and recommendations into the information system in English and are then able to retrieve records the same way. A controlled vocabulary has evolved that standardizes the entries, but authors are able to bypass this vocabulary and enter their unique concept in their preferred terminology.

Data Sets

Data Flow

One hundred sixteen data elements are abstracted from the patient's health record by the veterinary HIM professional. The abstract is then submitted electronically to the Veterinary Medical Databases (VMDB), where it is stored for future retrieval by university faculty or administration, representatives of drug companies, breed clubs, pet food producers, and so on. The data may be useful in the process of making an application for a grant proposal, decision making about services to be offered by the health care facility, or marketing of a new product.

VMDB

The VMDB began in 1963 when a group of scientists from the National Cancer Institute (NCI) recognized a common interest in the prevalence of various forms of cancer in animals and met at Michigan State University in East Lansing to discuss how to best collect the data for study. They hypothesized that if data were collected on animal cancer, the study of that data would reveal information that is relevant to the study of cancer in humans. They recognized the necessity of abstracting data from the medical records of veterinary teaching hospitals and decided to modify the *Standard Nomenclature of Diseases and Operations (SNDO)* used for coding human medical records at that time. The resultant nomenclature, SNVDO, has been described previously. This data was gathered into a database at Michigan State University, supported by NCI until 1975, when the principal scientists were planning to retire. NCI representatives wanted to continue to purchase the data, and the participating veterinary schools wished to continue to participate because of the increased interest by faculty to also use the data in teaching and research. Therefore, the American Association of Veterinary Medical Data Program Participants, Inc. (AAVMDPP) was created.

At that time the database was referred to as *VMDP*, the *Veterinary Medical Data Program*. The database was moved to Cornell University in 1975 because of the university's advances in computing capabilities. It remained at Cornell until 1987, when it was relocated to Purdue University and its name was officially changed to *Veterinary Medical Database (VMDB)*, and became an umbrella organization to manage other veterinary databases such as the *Canine Eye Registry Foundation (CERF)*, the *Equine Eye Registration Foundation (EERF)*, a copper toxicosis registry for Bedlington terriers, and a DNA registry for progressive retinal atrophy (PRA). A constitution revision in July 2002 updated the name to reflect these multiple databases: Veterinary Medical Databases (VMDB).

The VMDB is still used heavily by clinicians in veterinary teaching hospitals as a starting point for retrospective studies, teaching, and in scholarly publications. The database does not accommodate herd health or production medicine settings. Clinicians from participating university hospitals may search through their individual school's data, or perform a nationwide or regional search for cases relevant to their topic, at no cost to the user. Outside agencies such as drug companies, pet food producers, and nonparticipating universities are charged for the searches they order.

Maintenance of the Database

Once the patient health record has been completed by the clinician, the diagnoses and procedures are coded by an HIM professional or, in some facilities, by the clinician. The data displayed in Figure 15-3 is abstracted from the patient's record and submitted to the VMDB either electronically or through the traditional mail system.

The VMDB database administrator then runs the data through two edit programs. The *preedit* checks the internal consistency of the current abstract. Examples: Are the species and breed codes consistent? If the animal was spayed, does the abstract record the sex as *female-spay*? If the abstract fails the preedit checks, it is rejected and returned to the submitting institution for error correction and resubmission.

VETERINARY MEDICAL CASE ABSTRACT

Batch _____ Page _____

Patient Number _____   Discharge Date _____   Owners Name _____

Batch _____ Page _____

Institution	Patient Number	Continuation Code	Date of Discharge			Length of Stay (Days)	Attending Clinician	Sex	Species
			Mo.	Day	Year			0 – Litter	0 – Bovine
0 1		0 1						1 – F	1 – Equine
1 2	3 4 5 6 7 8	9 10	11 12	13 14	15 16	17 18	19 20	2 – FS 3 – FU 4 – M 5 – MC 6 – Other/unk.	2 – Porcine 3 – Ovine 4 – Caprine 7 – Feline 5 – Other LA 8 – Avian 6 – Canine 9 – Other SA

21   22

Breed Code   23 24 25

DISCHARGE STATUS
0 – Alive
1 – Died – Necropsy
2 – Died – No Necropsy   26
3 – Euthanasia – Necropsy
4 – Euthanasia – No Necropsy

AGE
0 – 0 to 2 wks.   5 – 2 to 4 yrs.
1 – 2 wks. to 2 mos.   6 – 4 to 7 yrs.
2 – 2 to 6 mos.   7 – 7 to 10 yrs.
3 – 6 to 12 mos.   8 – 10 to 15 yrs.   27
4 – 1 to 2 yrs.   9 – 15 yrs. and older

WEIGHT (POUNDS)

Large Animal
0 – 0 to 3   5 – 300 to 600
1 – 3 to 15   6 – 600 to 1000
2 – 15 to 50   7 – 1000 to 1300
3 – 50 to 150   8 – 1300 and over
4 – 150 to 300

28

Small Animal
0 – 0 to 1   4 – 30 to 50
1 – 1 to 5   5 – 50 to 75
2 – 5 to 15   6 – 75 to 100
3 – 15 to 30   7 – 100 and over

FIRST DIAGNOSIS   29   Initial   Recheck (<)   30 31 32 33 34 35 36 37 38

FIRST OPERATION   79 80 81 82 83

SECOND DIAGNOSIS   39   Initial   Recheck (<)   40 41 42 43 44 45 46 47 48

SECOND OPERATION   84 85 86 87 88

THIRD DIAGNOSIS   49   Initial   Recheck (<)   50 51 52 53 54 55 56 57 58

THIRD OPERATION   89 90 91 92 93

FOURTH DIAGNOSIS   59   Initial   Recheck (<)   60 61 62 63 64 65 66 67 68

FIFTH DIAGNOSIS   69   Initial   Recheck (<)   70 71 72 73 74 75 76 77 78

NON-DIAGNOSTIC   94

0 – Not applicable
1 – Total exam – normal
2 – Bone & joint exam – normal
3 – Sensory organs exam – normal
4 – Reproductive exam – normal
5 – Cardio-vascular exam – normal
6 – Integumentary exam – normal
7 – Other exam – normal
8 – Biologic donor
9 – Other (boarder, etc.)

DIAGNOSTIC PROCEDURES ("X" Appropriate Boxes)

95	Clinical Diagnosis **ONLY**	101	Electrophysiology
96	Gross Pathology	102	Hematology
97	Histopathology	103	Urinalysis
98	Serology	104	Chemistry
99	Microbiology	105	Parasitology
100	Radiology	106	Other not specified

ZIP CODE   107 108 109 110 111 112 113 114 115

DELETION CODE   116

NOTES:

O-14864

VETERINARY MEDICAL CASE ABSTRACT

Figure 15-3   Veterinary medical case abstract. (Courtesy Michigan State University, Veterinary Teaching Hospital.)

When an abstract passes the preedit, it moves into the next editing stage, the *edit-update*, which now compares this current abstract with the existing database, looking for a match in patient identification numbers for that institution. If there is a match with the identification number, several data elements are checked for consistency. For example, are the species, breed, and sex codes consistent with past submissions? If not, the record is rejected. Is the discharge status logical? If the identification number was abstracted as dead or euthanized in the past, but is alive now with a subsequent discharge date, the record is rejected.

Rejected abstracts are reported to the participating institution for correction and resubmission. Once accepted by the VMDB for inclusion in the database, the record is available for reference by users.

NOAH

The AVMA provides the online, interactive **Network of Animal Health (NOAH)** for association members. There are multiple forums as well as a resource center where members can consult with specialists, network with other members, study current legal issues and zoonosis updates, and retrieve Material Safety Data Sheets (MSDS) for their practice.

OFA

The **Orthopedic Foundation for Animals (OFA)** (http://www.offa.org) was established in 1966 to provide registries for standardized evaluation for canine hip and elbow dysplasia. Currently, elbow and patella deformities, craniomandibular osteopathy, autoimmune thyroiditis, congenital heart disease, copper toxicosis in Bedlington Terriers, and various DNA databases are also maintained.

Computer Systems

The listing of vendors of veterinary hospital information systems changes frequently. Refer to Figure 15-4 for a listing of some current vendors of veterinary hospital information systems. Work continues under the auspices of the AVMA's Committee on Veterinary Medical Informatics, through the Standards Subcommittee, to standardize data collection, storage, maintenance, and transmission standards not only within the veterinary profession but to also be able to seamlessly share data with human medicine. AVMA members represent these interests and concerns on behalf of the profession to organizations such as **Health Level 7 (HL7)** and **Logical Observations, Identifiers, Names, and Codes (LOINC)**.

Quality Improvement and Utilization Management

There are no formal requirements for quality assurance or utilization management processes. Informally, however, quality of care is studied each time a veterinary teaching hospital health care provider uses health records for retrospective study in

Company Name	Location	Product Name
Advanced Technology Corp.	Ramsey, New Jersey	VetStar
AltaPoint	Midvale, Utah	
Animal Intelligence Software, Inc.	Silverdale, Washington	
DVMax	New York, New York	
e-Friends for DVMs	Lomita, California	
Elinc Veterinary Practice Management Systems	Plano, Texas	Veterinary Information Assistant (VIA)
Idexx Informatics	Eau Claire, Wisconsin	
ImproMed, Inc.	Oshkosh, Wisconsin	
IntraVet	Dublin, Ohio	
McAllister Software Systems	Piedmont, Missouri	
NuSoft Technologies	Lynden, Washington	
Ross Group	Douglasville, Georgia	Universal Veterinary Information System (UVIS)
University of California School of Veterinary Medicine	Davis, California	
Vetech	Walnut Creek, California	Vetech Advantage

Note: This list may not be complete and is not meant to be an endorsement by the author.

Figure 15-4   Veterinary hospital management information systems.

preparing for a lecture, writing a research grant proposal, or writing an article for a scholarly publication. The outcome of such a review is often discussed during faculty conferences, meetings, or through publication.

Risk Management and Legal Issues

Risk Management

With increasing public awareness of the value of animals in people's lives, litigation, attorney awareness of veterinarians, rising expectations of animal owners, and increasing economic value of some animals, risk management is becoming more important in veterinary health care settings.

Michigan State University has developed an incident report form specifically for use in the veterinary teaching hospital. It is displayed in Figure 15-5. Once completed, it is forwarded to hospital administration and then to the university's risk management office. It is not kept in the patient's health record.

One area of tremendous risk in the veterinary health care setting is patient restraint. The AVMA's Professional Liability Insurance Trust quarterly report, *Professional*

MICHIGAN STATE UNIVERSITY
COLLEGE OF VETERINARY MEDICINE - REPORT OF INCIDENT
(DO NOT FILE WITH MEDICAL RECORD)

PATIENT ID

INSTRUCTIONS:
1. Circle appropriate answers. Write legibly.
2. ALWAYS COMPLETE SECTION I & THE REVERSE SIDE.

SECTION I

INCIDENT DATE: _____
Month-Day-Year

TIME OF INCIDENT: _____
am__ pm__

INCIDENT DAY
01 Monday
02 Tuesday   05 Friday
03 Wednesday   06 Saturday
04 Thursday   07 Sunday

MSU PERSONNEL INVOLVED
01 Anesthesia Technician   06 Veterinarian
02 Anesthesiologist   07 Other _____
03 Animal Technician Student   Department _____
04 Medical Records Staff
05 Veterinary Student   Name/Phone _____

SECTION II - PATIENT DESCRIPTION

SPECIES:
01 Avian   08 Porcine
02 Bovine   09 Other SA
03 Canine   10 Other LA
05 Equine
06 Feline
07 Ovine

GENDER:
01 Female
02 Female-Spayed
03 Litter
04 Male
05 Male-Neutered
06 Other/Unknown _____

DATE OF BIRTH: _____
Month - Day - Year

PATIENT CATEGORY:
01 Inpatient
02 Outpatient
03 Discharged
04 Ambulatory Service
05 Other _____

CONDITION PRIOR TO INCIDENT:
01 Agitated
02 Comatose
03 Depressed
04 Sedated
05 Well
06 Other/Unknown _____

SECTION III- NON-INJURY INCIDENT

FINANCIAL:
01 Billing Problem
02 Disputed fee
SERVICE:
03 Long wait
04 Client property lost/stolen
05 Client complained about staff
CARE:
06 Client challenged dx
07 Client rejected tx
08 Client complained about care
09 Client left AMA
OTHER:
10 Hostile/abusive client
11 Left without being seen
12 Remarks by client
13 Unusual request for medical records
14 Other _____

SECTION IV - COMPLETE FOR INJURY OR POTENTIAL INJURY

EXAMINED AT TIME OF INCIDENT:
Person's Name: _____
01 Veterinarian _____
02 Technician _____
03 Student _____
04 Other _____

AREA INCIDENT OCCURRED:
Bldg: _____
Room #: _____
01 Ambulatory
02 ICU
03 Inside VTH
04 Medical Records Office
05 Outside VTH
06 Parking lot
07 Prep room
08 Radiology
05 Recovery
06 Stairway
07 Stall/cage
08 Stocks
09 Surgery
10 Waiting Room
11 Ward
12 Other _____

OWNER NOTIFIED:

Date: _____

Time: _____

By whom: _____
Not notified____

BODY PART INVOLVED:
01 Abdomen
02 Chest
03 Eye
04 Fore foot
05 Fore leg
06 Head
07 Hind foot
08 Hind leg
09 Neck
10 Tail
11 Not applicable
12 Other _____

SEVERITY OF INJURY:
01 Death
02 Minor
03 Moderate
04 No apparent injury
05 Severe

TYPE OF INJURY:
01 Abrasion
02 Allergic reaction
03 Burn/erythema
04 Concussion
05 Contusion
06 Cut/laceration
07 Edema
08 Fracture/dislocation
09 Hematoma
10 Inhalation, asphyxia, strangulation
11 Puncture
12 Strain/sprain
13 Viscera injury
14 Other _____

TYPE OF INCIDENT:
FALLS:
01 Different level/stairs
02 Found lying on floor
03 From cage/equipment
04 Walking - same level
05 Other _____
MEDICATION:
06 Dosage-wrong amount set up
07 Dosage-wrong amount given
08 Duplication
09 Labeling error
10 Omission
11 Patient ID error
12 Time given error
13 Transcription
14 Transfusion
15 Unordered
16 Unpredicted response
18 Wrong medication
10 Other _____
OTHER CAUSES:
11 Arrhythmia
12 Catheterization
13 Delivery/postpartum
14 Diagnostic error
15 Disappeared/stolen
16 Drawing blood
17 Equipment related
18 Erroneous test report
19 Infection
20 IV or injection
21 Patient ID error
22 Self-caused injury
23 Struck by object
24 Surgery
25 Treatment
26 X-ray
27 Other _____

Figure 15-5 Incident report. (Courtesy Michigan State University, Veterinary Teaching Hospital.)

(ALWAYS COMPLETE THIS SIDE)

Narrative statement of person preparing report. State name(s) and position(s) of person(s) involved, times, immediate action taken and other relevant information. Be brief, but explicit. (Use extra sheet if necessary.)

Attending Veterinarian notified at_____ By_____

Name/Dept./Phone Number of person discovering incident_____ Position_____

Witnesses (include addresses and telephone numbers):

_____

_____

_____

_____

Signature/Phone Number/Department of person completing this report
_____

Veterinarian's findings:

_____

Veterinarian's Signature
_____

Reviewed by and distributed to:

1.   Immediate Supervisor_____Date_____

2.   Chief of Staff_____Date_____

3.   Department Chairperson_____Date_____

4.   Risk Management & Insurance_____Date_____
      372 Administration Bldg.

VET-INC
RM 3/93

Figure 15-5   *(Continued)*

Liability, routinely provides synopses of claims received in the Trust office. The reports of human or patient injury sustained when owners attempt to restrain their ill or injured pets are numerous. When injured while attempting to restrain his or her own animal, the owner's insurance company often sues the veterinarian for recovery of medical costs associated with the incident.

Legal Issues

Determining Who the Client Is

This matter can sometimes be difficult. The legal system generally considers an animal to be a form of personal property. When someone calls to arrange an appointment for an animal or simply presents an animal for examination or treatment, ownership is implied, unless information to the contrary is given. In the large animal setting, the person who actually presents the animal for examination or treatment may be the owner, an agent for the owner, or simply a transporter. The owner(s) may not live in the same state where the animal resides or where the animal is being presented for examination or care. It is important, then, to carefully question the person who presents the animal to accurately document the owner or owners' name(s), address, and phone number on the health record. If the presenter claims to be the agent, does this person have authorization from the owner to seek medical care for the patient and sign consents for treatment?

The above reference to "owners" is another complicated issue. Some animals are owned by multiple people who are classified as co-owners. Some animals, especially horses, may be owned by a syndicate, which is an official association of persons. In these situations, it is wise to have one person identified as spokesperson for the group of owners who is then contacted for consent to treatment. The information system must be able to document these various parties and their relationship to the patient.

Another confusing situation is the relationship between the breeder of the animal and the person who now has possession of the animal. The person with possession may be the "adopted" owner or simply a trainer. Again, careful questioning will produce more accurate records.

Dogs used in the police canine units can also be registered incorrectly if the receptionist is not careful. The animal may actually live with its handler but is the property of the police department. The police department must be named as owner of the animal, with the officer listed as an alternate owner.

Litigation

Debt collection accounts for almost all of the litigation encountered in the veterinary teaching hospital setting today. As discussed earlier, a signed estimate of charges, along with a signed informed consent, are instrumental in collection of practice debts.

Another issue that accounts for some of the work involved in preparing records for court is litigation in *stray voltage* cases. These cases are mainly brought by dairy farmers who contend that the power lines on or near their property affect the milk production in their herd. The veterinary teaching hospital may have provided veterinary services for members of this herd through its production medicine or herd health service and is then asked to produce such records in court.

Prepurchase Examinations

These exams are a particularly interesting part of the daily management of health information in the large animal veterinary teaching hospital. They are common in equine medicine, but are also occasionally still referred to as breeding soundness examinations of cattle, swine, horses, and dogs. The relationship between the examiner, the buyer, the seller, and agents for either the buyer or seller is very complicated. State veterinary boards may address this issue in their regulations. This topic is thoroughly addressed in *Law and Ethics of the Veterinary Profession* (Wilson et al., 1988). In the best interests of the animal, the owner maintains control of the record until the sale is final.

Wildlife Management

This venture is a cooperative one between the federal government and individual states. This is a very broad topic ranging from international law and international agreements to the issuance of permits for importation, exportation, transportation, inspection, and the use of animals in scientific research. Federal regulations also address wildlife rehabilitation facilities, pet stores, and wildlife auctions. For more information in a particular state, contact the Department of Fish and Game or the Department of Natural Resources.

Animal Cruelty

"Studies have shown a correlation between the incidence of animal abuse on the one hand, and child abuse, spousal abuse or mass murder on the other. . . . Animal abusers have a greater propensity of committing acts of violence against humans than those with no history of animal cruelty" (Lacroix, 1998).

With these startling facts in mind, veterinarians and animal health records are becoming vital resources in identifying, documenting, and reporting suspected abuse in order to prevent further injury to the animal, other animals, and humans.

Animal Welfare Advocates

These advocates impress on the veterinary health professional the importance of complete, accurate documentation of the course of the patient's illness and treatment during hospitalization or during its confinement in a research facility. Two types of patient records that the veterinary HIM professional pays particular attention to are the stray animal and the euthanized animal.

Stray Animals

These animals may be presented for treatment before being sent to the local humane society or animal control facility. It is very important to accurately document the date and time of arrival and departure or euthanasia of these animals, in addition to the treatment rendered while hospitalized, so that there is no question or doubt about what transpired during the animal's stay.

Euthanasia

This option is for the owner to consider when the quality of the animal's life is determined to be minimal and/or when the financial obligation outweighs the potential outcome of continued care. Documentation of the consent for euthanasia is best made in writing to verify the relationship of the signer to the animal. It is also important at the time of consent for euthanasia to determine whether the animal has bitten another animal or a human being, because of the potential for rabies exposure. During the discussion between the veterinary health care provider and owner and subsequent signing of the consent for euthanasia, arrangements can be made for payment of the final bill. The actual procedure of euthanasia should then be documented with the time, date, product used, and signature of the veterinary health care provider performing the procedure. This documentation fully verifies that the owner's wishes were carried out and that the animal was not transferred to a new owner or research project.

Change of Ownership

This situation occurs frequently in the veterinary field. It is important to document the change in the animal's health record by having the original owner sign a form verifying no further responsibility for the patient, the transfer of ownership to a new party, and identification on the form of the new owner. The new owner then has access to past health records of the patient for continued care.

Blood Donors

These animals are available to give blood for a transfusion to a patient. They often reside at the hospital to be available on short notice and are often long-term residents whose health records become quite bulky. Detailed blood donation records are maintained as well as health and vaccination updates.

Donations

Donations of animals are sometimes requested by owners who have an animal with a unique condition that, in their opinion, is not worth the financial commitment to treat. The owner may prefer to donate the animal as a teaching model rather than simply euthanizing it. The client is asked to sign a form transferring ownership of the animal to a specific researcher and include the dollar amount value of the animal. This donation can often be used as a tax deduction.

Role of the Health Information Management Professional

The veterinary HIM professional is responsible for establishing and maintaining information collection and retention systems that ensure accurate, complete, timely, and confidential health information for use in continued patient care, legal defense, education, and management decision making. Such records must also support the final bill.

Statistics are compiled and maintained for use by veterinary and human medicine professionals. For instance, each year the veterinary school is asked to submit statistics to the *American Association of Veterinary Medical Colleges*, which then develops a comparative data summary. Data elements collected include number of clients, number of patients, number of accessions, number hospitalized, and number of hospital days. Ambulatory care statistics are also collected on herd health or production medicine services. These statistics include number of farm calls made, number of animals involved, number of animals treated, and number of animals at risk.

Active participation in the **American Veterinary Health Information Management Association (AVHIMA)** helps the HIM professional develop a network for seeking new ideas and support. Unlike the human health care delivery setting where there may be another professional practicing just down the road, the AVHIMA membership is spread across the United States and Canada, usually with only one member in a given state. The use of a listserv keeps members connected and helps them to work through issues on a timely basis. It is very difficult to maintain continuity and momentum within AVHIMA with such distances between members. Active membership in the component state association of the *American Health Information Management Association (AHIMA)* may seem difficult because the patients are very different, but the use of technology and basic roles and functions are not changed, and it is important to maintain those liaisons for professional support and continuing education.

Trends

The electronic health record (EHR) is the major focus in many veterinary teaching hospital settings today. As mentioned earlier in this chapter, the Subcommittee on Standards of AVMA's Informatics Committee was established in March 1995 for the purpose of creating and publishing standards for electronic data collection, maintenance, transmission, and dissemination, a function necessary for the evolution of the EHR.

The integration of SNOMED-CT into the veterinary teaching hospital setting, as well as private practices, runs parallel with the development of the EHR. The increased use of *telemedicine* impacts the veterinary field and the EHR.

Lawsuits are increasing as the public and attorney awareness of the practice and expectation of practice of veterinary medicine increase. Demands are placed on the veterinary profession to answer to animal welfare advocates who wish to ensure the safety and wellness of all animals.

The increasing interest and expanding use of animal health statistics as sentinels in human health necessitates that common data elements can be easily matched between the two professions. Fewer family farms and more *agribusiness* ventures have necessitated more involved record keeping to meet state and federal government regulations.

Veterinary record systems are also used in the detection, tracking, and control of potential bioterrorism agents, many of which have been identified as zoonotic agents. Diseases that threaten human welfare and/or the safety of our food supply, such as the bovine spongiform encephalopathy (BSE) or "mad cow disease," anthrax, the West Nile Virus, and bovine tuberculosis, are also under the purview of the veterinary HIM system.

Animals (canine, equine, marine mammals, etc.) are used by the Department of Defense and by local public safety departments in various capacities. They are trained at great expense in search and rescue or drug or explosives detection, for instance, to serve and safeguard the public, which makes efficient, accurate documentation of their health maintenance as important as the health record maintenance of their handlers.

Summary

Many of the current roles and functions defined for the HIM professional in the traditional human health care delivery setting can be directly applied to the veterinary hospital. If the learners happen to also love animals, whether domestic or wild, they now have the additional basic tools to present themselves to a veterinary teaching hospital, local veterinary hospital, nearby zoo, veterinary hospital information management software vendor, or research facility with an offer of expertise in establishing or maintaining an information system that will also protect the legal and financial interests of the veterinary professionals and the client.

There are at least three benefits the learner can obtain by moving into this setting. Fewer government regulations related to maintenance of health records can be attractive. There is an opportunity to contribute to the field of veterinary science. The last, more subtle benefit is contact with animals, which is often a stress reliever.

Key Terms

American Animal Hospital Association (AAHA)   promulgates standards for companion animal hospitals.

American Veterinary Health Information Management Association (AVHIMA) promotes quality patient care through the management of health information; is the nation's authoritative body on the management of veterinary health information; advances the competency of those working with veterinary health information; advocates for the profession on governmental, education, social, and business issues that affect the management of veterinary health information.

American Veterinary Medical Association (AVMA) the objective of the Association is to advance the science and art of veterinary medicine, including its relationship to public health, biological science, and agriculture. The association provides a forum for the discussion of issues of importance to the veterinary profession and for the development of official positions. The association is the authorized voice for the profession in presenting its views to government, academia, agriculture, pet owners, the media, and other concerned publics (AVMA Constitution, Article II).

animal any animal other than man, including fowl, birds, fish, and reptiles, wild or domestic, living or dead.

animal health technician *see* **veterinary technician**.

bovine cow or ox.

canine dog.

caprine goat.

certified veterinary practice manager (CVPM) with experience, and at least 18 acceptable college or university credit hours pertinent to business management, evidence of 48 hours of continuing education specifically devoted to management, and appropriate references, a veterinary practice manager may apply to the Veterinary Hospital Manager's Association (VHMA) to take the written and oral examinations which, if successfully passed, certifies the individual as a certified veterinary practice manager.

equine horse.

feline cat.

Health Level 7 (HL7) this is the application level, which is the highest level, of the International Standards Organization's (ISO) communications model for Open Systems Interconnection (OSI). HL7 is a standard for data exchange in health care.

herd health veterinary care provided to a group of animals at their residence rather than being transported to the hospital setting.

International Species Information System (ISIS) a computer-based information system for wild animal species in captivity.

Logical Observations, Identifiers, Names and Codes (LOINC) facilitates the exchange and pooling of results or vital signs for clinical care, outcomes management, and research.

necropsy a postmortem examination for determining the cause of death or the character and extent of changes produced by disease.

Network of Animal Health (NOAH) provided by the AVMA to connect AVMA members and professional resources.

number of accessions the total number of times all patients were treated by the facility in a given time period. One patient may have multiple accessions.

Orthopedic Foundation for Animals (OFA) a collection of voluntary orthopedic and genetic diseases databases of animals.

ovine sheep.

porcine swine.

problem-oriented medical record (POMR) a structured approach to patient care developed by Dr. Lawrence Weed in the late 1950s that has four major parts: database, problem list, initial plan, and progress notes/discharge summary.

production medicine the study and care of food animals that produce milk, meat, eggs, etc.

Standard Nomenclature of Veterinary Diseases and Operations (SNVDO) created in 1963 to standardize the collection of veterinary data in a national database.

Systematized Nomenclature of Medicine-Clinical Terms (SNOMED-CT) a multilingual health care clinical reference terminology providing a uniform nomenclature facilitating international sharing and analysis of both human and veterinary health data.

theriogenology the study of animal reproduction.

veterinarian one qualified and authorized to treat disease and injuries of animals.

veterinary of, relating to, or being the science and art of prevention, cure, or alleviation of disease and injury in animals, especially domestic animals.

Veterinary Hospital Managers Association (VHMA) provides individuals who are actively involved in veterinary practice management with a means of effective communication and interaction. Membership is comprised of veterinarians, hospital administrators, practice managers, office managers, and consultants.

Veterinary Medical Databases (VMDB) a national collection system for data from veterinary teaching hospital patient records from the United States and Canada.

veterinary technician knowledgeable in the care and handling of animals, in the basic principles of normal and abnormal life processes, and in routine laboratory and clinical procedures. The technician is primarily an assistant to veterinarians, biological research workers, and other scientists.

veterinary technologist a graduate of a four-year AVMA-accredited program in veterinary technology or a person so recognized by the board in rules and regulations promulgated to regulate veterinary technologists.

REVIEW QUESTIONS

Knowledge-based Questions

1. Which organization provides minimum standards for maintenance of veterinary health records?

2. Why is a written cost estimate so important in veterinary practice?

3. Where would you find the most current advice on how to properly use SNOMED-CT in a veterinary setting?

4. Who authorizes release of information in a prepurchase situation?

5. Briefly explain the operation and uses of the VMDB

Application-based Questions

1. Describe a circumstance when a record would be maintained for a group of animals rather than an individual patient.

2. In the absence of a specific law or state regulation, what source should be consulted for advice in an uncomfortable legal situation if you are employed in a veterinary teaching hospital?

3. Networking and continuing education activities are an important part of keeping up-to-date in a profession. However, the component state associations of the American Health Information Management Association do not offer programs specific to veterinary medicine. How would one keep current in veterinary health information management and still be able to maintain the credential as an accredited record technician or registered record administrator?

Web Activity

Visit the VMDB Web site at http://www.vmdb.org and click on the hyperlink for Health Information Managers. Select one of the topics or articles available for HIM professionals at this site and write a brief summary.

Case Study

Dr. Sands is a veterinary epidemiologist. She wants to compare statistics from a veterinary hospital from the past five years with statistics from the three human medicine hospitals within a 20-mile radius for patients with confirmed diagnoses of any type of lung tumor. The objective is to show that the diagnosis is made in the animal population at the same rate as in the human population in the area and that it is made 6 to 12 months earlier in the animal population. She needs information from the HIM professional on how to retrieve the statistics from the human hospitals.

1. Which species of animal(s) would the HIM professional recommend as giving the best comparison, and why?

2. Besides diagnosis and species, what other data set(s) would be most useful to narrow down the conclusion?

3. How should the HIM professional retrieve the statistics from the local human hospitals?

References and Suggested Readings

American Animal Hospital Association 2003 Standards and Accreditation Manual. (2003). Denver, CO: American Animal Hospital Association.

American Veterinary Medical Association. (2002). *AVMA Membership Directory and Resource Manual* (139th ed.). Schaumburg, IL: AVMA.

American Veterinary Medical Association. (2003). *Accreditation Policies and Procedures of Council on Education: July 2003 Revised.* Schaumburg, IL: AMVA. [Online]. http://www.avma.org/education/coe_policies2k.pdf [2004, January 10].

College of American Pathologists and American Veterinary Medical Association. (1993). *The Systematized Nomenclature of Human and Veterinary Medicine (Introduction).* Northfield, IL: College of American Pathologists.

Cote, R. (1995). *Snomed International: The Structure, Intrinsic Hierarchies and Implicit Logic.* Handout received at the 1995 annual meeting of the American Veterinary Health Information Management Association, Pittsburgh, PA.

Fagan, D. (2002). *RE: AVMA Directory.* Message to: <neterer@cvm.msu.edu>. 8 January 2003; 12:29 EST. Message-ID: (3E1C6005.67E : 5 : 42622). Personal Communication.

Hannah, H. W. (1991). Legal brief: Veterinary medical records—some legal considerations. *Journal of the American Veterinary Medical Association, 198* (1), 67–69.

Harris, P. A. (1991). Insights and updates on veterinary medical recordkeeping practice. *Journal of AMRA, 62*, 32–35.

Lacroix, C.A. *Animal Cruelty and the Role of Veterinarians.* AVMLA Newsletter, American Veterinary Medical Law Association publication IV (1), December 1998.

Wilson, J. F., Garbe, J. L., and Rollin, B. E. (1988). *Law and Ethics of the Veterinary Profession.* Yardley, PA: Yardley Press, Ltd.

Key Resources

American Animal Hospital Association (AAHA)
P.O. Box 150899
Denver, CO 80215-0899
Phone: 303-986-2800
Fax: 303-986-1700
http://www.aahanet.org

American Veterinary Health Information Management
Association (AVHIMA)
Flo Nelson, President of AVHIMA
University of Missouri
Veterinary Medical Teaching Hospital
379 E. Campus Drive
Columbia, MO 65211
Phone: 573-882-0742

Fax: 573-884-7563
E-mail: nelsonfl@missouri.edu

American Veterinary Medical Association (AVMA)
1931 N. Meacham Road, Suite 100
Schaumburg, IL 60173-4360
Phone: 800-248-2862
Fax: 847-925-1329
http://www.avma.org

American Veterinary Medical Association
Professional Liability Insurance Trust
P.O. Box 1629
Chicago, IL 60690-1629
Phone: 800-228-7548
http://www.avmaplit.com

Animal Law & History Web Center
Michigan State University—DCL College of Law
Shaw Lane
East Lansing, MI 48824-1300
Phone: 517-432-6800
http://www.animallaw.info/index.htm

International Species Information System
12101 Johnny Cake Ridge Road
Building A, Room 6
Apple Valley, MN 55124-8151
Phone: 952-997-9500
Fax: 952-432-2757
http://www.isis.org

Internet Resources on Veterinary Epidemiology:
E-mail discussion group: epivet-l@upei.ca
http://epiweb.massey.ac.nz

Netvet
http://netvet.wustl.edu

Network of Animal Health (NOAH)
AVMA
1931 N. Meacham Road, Suite 100
Schaumburg, IL 60173-4360
Phone: 800-248-2862, ext. 696
http://www.avma.org/network.html

Orthopedic Foundation for Animals
2300 Nifong Boulevard
Columbia, MO 65201-3856
Phone: 573-442-0418
Fax: 573-875-5073
http://www.offa.org

Purdue University
Veterinary Medical Databases
VMDB/Lynn Hall
625 Harrison Street
West Lafayette, IN 47907-2026
Phone: 765-494-9548
Fax: 765-494-9981
http://www.vmdb.org

Veterinary Hospital Managers Association, Inc. (VHMA)
48 Howard St.
Albany, NY 12207
Phone: 518-433-8911
Fax: 518-463-8656
http://www.vhma.org

Veterinary Pet Insurance
DVM Insurance Agency
P.O. Box 2344
Brea, CA 92822-2344
Phone: 800-872-7387
http://www.pet-insurance.com

Veterinary Practice Acts
(*Note:* Refer to the most current issue of the *AVMA Directory* for a digest of each state's
veterinary practice act and current contact information.)

Chapter 16

Consulting

Karen Wright, MHA, RHIA, RHIT
Scott Wright, MBA

Learning Objectives

Upon successful completion of this chapter, you should be able to:

1. Identify the advantages and disadvantages of consulting.
2. Assess personal strengths and weaknesses.
3. Recognize the importance of establishing a productive working relationship with the administrative staff of a health care facility.
4. Develop a business plan.
5. Develop action plans.

SETTING	DESCRIPTION	SYNONYMS/EXAMPLES
Acute Care Hospital	Facility that treats patients with acute conditions or the chronically ill who have an acute crisis and require stabilization	Acute care Day surgery center Emergency center Consults 40 hours per week providing coding support, reviewing accounts receivable not billed, and provides education to administrators and medical staff
Veterinary Teaching Hospital	Facility that treats animals with acute conditions or chronically ill animals that have an acute crisis and require stabilization	Vet hospital Animal hospital Consults 20 hours per month providing expertise regarding data collection for research purposes; storage and retrieval of records; and computerized systems utilized to collect health information of animals
Nursing Facility Assisted Living	Facility that provides 24-hour nursing care to residents who require rehabilitation following surgery; therapy to relearn an activity of daily living; nursing care and assisted living	Skilled care Assisted living Long-term care Consults 16 hours per month to provide assistance implementing JCAHO standards and to review documentation to various health care providers
Home Health	Organization that provides medical care for patients with either acute or chronic conditions in the patient's home via the supervision of a physician and registered nurse	Consults 16 hours per month to provide support designing forms and computer screens to collect health information
Hospice	A facility that provides palliative care and support to patients who are terminally ill and the families of the terminally ill	Home health Consults eight hours per month teaching volunteers how to collect health information on terminally ill patients; works with nurses regarding proper documentation of patient assessments, care plans, and progress notes

SETTING	DESCRIPTION	SYNONYMS/EXAMPLES
Dialysis Center	A facility that provides renal dialysis services to patients with end-stage renal disease or other conditions requiring dialysis	Renal dialysis Consults eight hours per month teaching nurses what documentation must occur in order to meet reimbursement from Medicare regulations
Behavioral Medicine	Facility that provides medical supervision, therapy, and a therapeutic environment to clients who are chemically dependent or mentally ill or both	Mental health agency Chemical dependency, substance abuse, addiction medicine Consults 25 hours per month providing support with quality improvement and various health information documentation issues
Managed Care	Manages monies expended for health care services	Health maintenance organization (HMO) Consults 40 hours per month to review documentation against patients' bills and reports findings to managed care executives
Insurance Company	Reimburses health care providers for services rendered	Third-party payer Consults 25 hours per month providing coding support and reviewing health information submitted via claims to ensure proper reimbursement
Physician's Office or Physician Group Practice	Provides health care services to the acutely and chronically ill with nonemergent conditions	Doctor's office Consults 16 hours per month providing coding support regarding current procedure terminology (CPT) codes and Centers for Medicare and Medicaid Services (CMS) coding methodologies
Legal Practice	Provides legal advise and service	Lawyer's office Law firm Consults 20 hours per month reviewing health information in records where negligence or malpractice is alleged

SETTING	DESCRIPTION	SYNONYMS/EXAMPLES
Health Information System Vendor	Develops, sells, and implements computerized health information software	Vendor Consults 40 hours per month providing support regarding software development

Introduction to Setting

Health information management (HIM) consultants may work in any setting where health care is provided or for organizations that reimburse or bill for health services. Examples of organizations that can potentially benefit from the services of an HIM consultant include acute care hospitals, ambulatory surgery centers, veterinary teaching hospitals, nursing facility corporate offices and/or multiple facilities, hospice, dialysis centers, home health, behavioral medicine (mental health and substance abuse), rehabilitation facilities, third-party billing companies, large and small physician group practices, governmental agencies, and technology vendors. Although this chapter is geared toward the independent consultant, there are also many job opportunities for HIM professionals in consulting firms.

Who Consultants Work With

Although the HIM professional is usually hired to provide expertise related to the HIM function, this function covers many diverse tasks. However, the most challenging and rewarding part of a consultant's job is working as a team member with key decision makers such as health care executives and administrators, physicians, nurses, clinical researchers, quality specialists and risk management professionals, accountants, attorneys, therapists (physical, occupational, and speech) as well as psychiatrists, psychologists, dietitians, social workers, and information technology professionals to name just a few.

The HIM consultant's knowledge of biomedical science, computerized databases, and privacy and compliance issues as well as the collection, storage, retrieval, and retention of health information in any medium makes him or her an asset in any facility designing and implementing an electronic medical record.

A consultant may be hired by an acute care hospital to provide Health Insurance Portability and Accountability Act (HIPAA) training, write a compliance plan and offer coding and classification system education, write policies and procedures, or assess physician documentation to ensure that it supports the diagnosis and procedure codes assigned. In this setting, the consultant could also serve as a member of the revenue cycle team that includes representatives from clinical, patient financial services, patient access, utilization review, HIM, managed care, billing, and collections departments.

In nursing, behavioral medicine, and rehabilitation facilities, the consultant's focus may be quality improvement efforts that focus on improving documentation and the collection of statistics. For example, in a nursing home the consultant may compute the following: percentage of residents who have decreased independence in their ability to perform activities of daily living, percentage of residents with a new infection, percentage of residents with a moderate level of pain occurring every day, percentage of residents with one or more pressure sores, and percentage of residents who are restrained daily. The consultant may be a member of a team that designs care paths aimed at improving treatment outcomes or an educator who provides in-service education regarding privacy and documentation requirements.

A large or small physicians' group practice or individual physician who wishes to improve efficiency may seek an HIM consultant to provide coding and billing expertise as well as to select, implement, and manage an electronic medical record that streamlines the appointment, clinical data collection, and billing processes.

As noted in Chapter 15, some veterinary teaching hospitals are utilizing the Systematized Nomenclature of Medicine (SNOMED) coding methodology for research purposes, and all require health information systems for animal records that are similar to those maintained by acute care hospitals for human records.

As the elderly population increases, the demand for health care services and health information technologists and administrators will also increase. Today's fragmented health care system, the federal government's prospective inpatient and outpatient payment methodologies, the complexity of third-party payers' billing requirements, and computerization of clinical data are providing numerous challenging employment opportunities for HIM professionals.

Regulatory Issues

Federal health care regulations continue to increase in number and complexity. Two examples are the *Health Insurance Portability and Accountability Act (HIPAA)* and the National Correct Coding Initiative (NCCI). All health care facilities must comply with HIPAA regulations. Hospitals must comply with Medicare's Prospective Payment System for hospital inpatients and the Outpatient Prospective Payment System for hospital outpatient services. Physicians must comply with Medicare billing regulations as well and a multitude of different insurance companies' requirements. Thus, there is a high demand for individuals possessing expertise as a privacy and/or compliance officer. HIM consultants must stay abreast of governmental regulations by being active members of the American Health Information Management Association (AHIMA), reading professional trade journals, and researching the *Federal Register* as well as licensing and accrediting standards that apply to health care facilities in which they consult. In the future, continuous surveying by the Joint Commission for the Accreditation of Healthcare Organizations (JCAHO) will make preparation for a survey an ongoing process. To help the client organization accomplish its goals with regard to regulatory requirements, the consultant may need to facilitate the development of an action plan (see Figure 16-1).

- Determine all steps necessary to attain goal.
- Assign responsibility for each step.
- Set deadlines for each goal.

Figure 16-1   Steps to develop action plans.

Documentation

If the client organization has contracted with the consultant to evaluate the quality of documentation, the consultant may need to develop an **audit** sheet to facilitate the review of the organization's documentation. To accomplish this task, the consultant will need to research the regulations, standards, and best practices that apply to the documentation in that type of facility. The key documentation points can be incorporated into an audit sheet, which the consultant can use to review a random sample of the client organization's records. The consultant then analyzes, interprets, and presents a summary of the audit results to the facility's administrative team. Completion of the audit cycle involves educating those who document in the records and then conducting a follow-up audit to determine improvement (see Figure 16-2).

Reimbursement and Compliance

There are many consulting opportunities in the area of reimbursement and compliance. The issues of documentation, reimbursement, and compliance are often linked. If the client organization believes its code-based reimbursement is not what it should be, the organization may contact a coding consultant for assistance. Sometimes the consultant may find that the organization's coders are coding properly, but that inadequate documentation is the true cause of missed revenue. Sometimes the consultant may find that both coding and documentation are in need of improvement. Whatever the finding, the consultant must be careful to be as objective as possible when auditing for reimbursement purposes. The consultant should not enter into a "contingency" contract with a client in which the consultant's fees are based on increasing reimbursement (e.g., the client pays the consultant a percentage of the increased revenue). The **Office of the Inspector General** (**OIG**, the agency charged with protecting the integrity of the Medicare and Medicaid programs) considers such contingency arrangements to provide an incentive for increasing revenues in an unethical manner, such as "upcoding." If the consultant has conducted a post-billing audit, he or she should instruct the client organization to resubmit any bills in which the codes or other

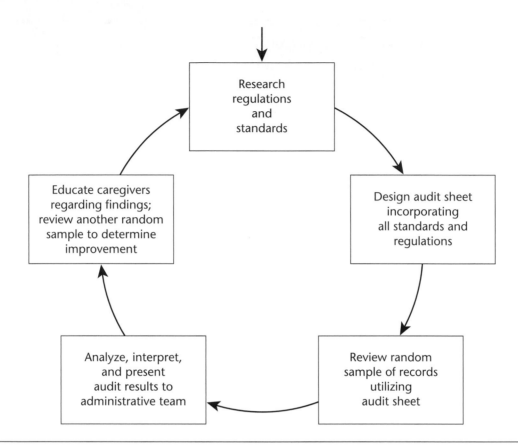

Figure 16-2 Documentation audit cycle.

items reported were found to be in error, regardless of whether the resubmission results in a higher or lower payment.

On the other hand, the OIG may have audited the provider and subsequently required it to enter into a **corporate integrity agreement** (**CIA**, an agreement that a health care provider or health plan reaches with the OIG as part of a settlement agreement when allegations of improper reimbursement have been made). In this circumstance, the provider may contract with the consultant as an independent reviewer to meet the OIG's requirements for ongoing monitoring and training in appropriate coding. Again, it is important for the consultant to be as objective as possible in auditing the coding and billing procedures of the client.

Finally, all health care providers who receive payments under Medicare or Medicaid are expected to establish compliance programs. A small provider may not have the resources to conduct its own compliance audits and may contract with a consultant for these services.

Role of the Health Information Management Professional

Choosing to be an independent consultant is synonymous with starting a new business and being self-employed. A successful health information consulting practice requires an RHIT or RHIA credential, relevant work experience, and careful research and planning. One should start by performing a rigorous self-assessment of interpersonal communication skills. Individuals who possess these skills often already have a strong network of professional contacts in place, making it easier to market themselves. Many independent consultants start by consulting on a part-time basis. Health care facilities often seek consultants because they do not wish to hire a full-time credentialed HIM professional. They want an individual who can provide certain services for a few hours each month. Satisfied clients often provide referrals. It may take a while to build a client base that provides an income that permits giving up the benefits associated with a full-time job.

Expertise in a particular profession or skill is a small part of being a consultant—the larger issue is the ability to run a business. Although a health information consulting business may be launched with a minimum of capital expense, perhaps only a computer and a telephone, it is critical to formalize the business by developing certain key documents. The consultant should formally document a mission statement, marketing plan, and a list of services to be offered. It is also helpful to compile a list of strengths and weaknesses, measurable personal and business objectives that can serve as an annual plan. Other documentation should include an objective statement of the percentage by which the client base will increase yearly, a list of clients who need these services, the demographics of potential clients, a list of competitors, equipment and office space requirements, and the number of employees now and in the future. Finally, the consultant should develop both monthly and yearly revenue and expense budgets. Later if the consultant needs to develop a **business plan** (a formal document summarizing the operational and financial objectives of a business), the basics of one are in place.

Formulating business plans (see Figures 16-3, 16-4, and 16-5) as well as annual plans is a good idea. Because HIM consulting is a knowledge-based business, very few funds should have to be raised to get started. However, a business plan is necessary if the consultant seeks capital (e.g., a loan from a bank). Some consultants have found it helpful to utilize business plan software in developing their business plans. A quick search of the Internet or of a company that sells software packages will yield numerous business planning programs to evaluate. In 2004, the following were examples of business planning Web sites:

- http://www.bplans.com
- http://www.planware.org/bizplan.htm
- http://www.sba.gov/starting_business/planning/basic.html
- http://www.businesstown.com/planning/creating.asp
- http://www.soyouwanna.com/site/syws/bizplan/bizplan.html

Objective Number	*Description of Objective*	*Date Completed*
#1	Make decision regarding whether to evaluate feasibility of becoming self-employed consultant.	Week 1
#2	Analyze professional competence by assessing strengths and weaknesses.	Week 2
#3	Conduct research to determine market demand for HIM consultants.	Week 3
#4	Project: The potential number of consulting contracts one could acquire and within what time frame.	Week 4
#5	Choose a site for home office.	Week 5
#6	Develop insurance plan (what insurance is required).	Week 6
#7	Develop legal plan (contracts).	Week 7
#8	Develop financial plan (expenses/revenue).	Week 8
#9	Develop accounting plan (what taxes are required).	Week 9
#10	Develop marketing plan.	Week 10
#11	Determine consulting practice organizational goals.	Week 11
#12	Develop action plans.	Week 12
#13	Prepare business plan.	Week 13
#14	Present plan to bank.	Week 14
#15	Secure loan.	Week 15
#16	Start practice.	Week 16

Figure 16-3   Steps to develop a business plan.

Leadership Ability

A consultant should have extensive previous experience, be an excellent communicator, possess leadership skills, and have the appropriate credentials and above all a good reputation. Being of good repute means that others believe an individual is trustworthy, hard working, and honest. Leadership has been defined as an influence

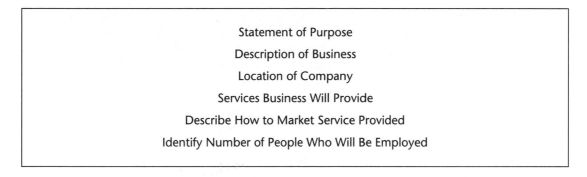

> Statement of Purpose
>
> Description of Business
>
> Location of Company
>
> Services Business Will Provide
>
> Describe How to Market Service Provided
>
> Identify Number of People Who Will Be Employed

Figure 16-4 Typical business plan format.

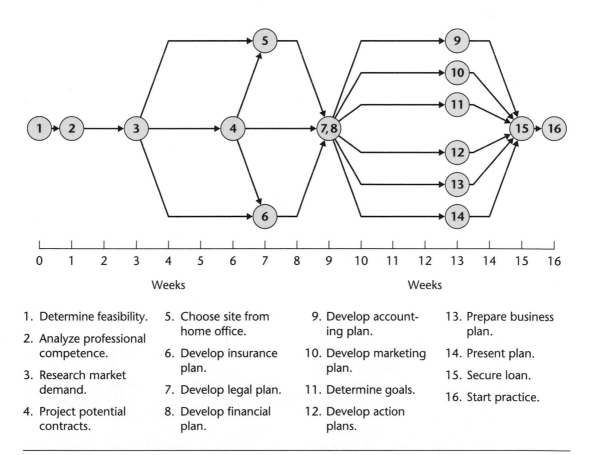

Figure 16-5 Sequence of steps and possible time frames for beginning a business.

1. Determine feasibility.
2. Analyze professional competence.
3. Research market demand.
4. Project potential contracts.
5. Choose site from home office.
6. Develop insurance plan.
7. Develop legal plan.
8. Develop financial plan.
9. Develop accounting plan.
10. Develop marketing plan.
11. Determine goals.
12. Develop action plans.
13. Prepare business plan.
14. Present plan.
15. Secure loan.
16. Start practice.

process. Any time an individual attempts to persuade others toward goal accomplishment, he or she is practicing leadership. A key role of the consultant is to work with others to ensure organizational and departmental compliance with laws, regulations, standards, polices, and procedures. In addition, consultants must be able to write proposals, solve problems, train staff, perform research (qualitative and quantitative), deal well with complexity and chaos, and be self-confident, self-reliant, disciplined, resilient, and financially astute. A consultant must be able to read between the lines to assess potential clients' needs and to negotiate mutual expectations about the consultant's role in that process. The consultant must be able to see the big picture and to communicate it clearly to others.

Leaders have high standards. When leaders lack character, they also lack integrity. Good leaders show no discrepancy between what they appear to be and who they are. They take responsibility and are credible, transparent, honest communicators with nothing to hide. Good leaders follow through to the final detail.

According to Harvard psychologist and professor, Howard Gardner, who specializes in the theory of multiple intelligence, a high cognitive intelligence (IQ) does not ensure success. What is more important in the business world today than knowing one's own strengths and weaknesses is the ability to get others to think about their abilities positively and in a way that maximizes their potential. Gardner states that the difference between success and failure is not taking courses to sharpen technical skills, but figuring out how, given one's abilities, to adjust to a given situation. An astute businessperson has interpersonal intelligence, which is the ability to understand other people, what motivates them, how they work, and how to work cooperatively with them (Koch, 1996).

As the paper medical record gives way to an electronic health record (EHR), the HIM professional must understand the technical requirements of the change. To prepare, the consultant might consider the American Health Information Management Association's (AHIMA) new e-HIM initiative that highlights the skills needed for electronic health information management, such as knowledge of data standards and project management skills (AHIMA, 2003, February). However, more important is gauging the attitude and ability of others to accept that change. Be prepared to listen and allow the individuals most affected by the change to provide ample input regarding decisions that affect them. Howard Gardner states that the organization must "think about how people's abilities can be rearranged or stretched or reconfigured or combined with other people's" (Koch, 1996, Online). Doctors and nurses who currently use an EHR report that it can take up to three months to fully learn and adapt to using a computer to document clinical information, but that a well-implemented system is worth the transition (Rollins, 2003; Wager et al., 1999).

One leadership challenge that a consultant faces is that the consultant's power is based on influence and expertise, not on organizationally mandated authority. The consultant makes recommendations to the client, and the client can choose to follow those recommendations or not. The consultant may have good ideas to help the client with many challenges, such as getting work done with imperfect people, setting clear goals and direction, training, development, and delegation. However, on occasion, the consultant may meet with resistance and conflict, intense competition, or rejection and criticism by others, and find that as a result the client discards the consultant's ideas or terminates the consultant's contract. Learning to nurture, mentor, and encourage oneself can help the consultant handle failures and continue to be willing to take risks. Also, developing a supportive personal and professional network assists the consultant in maintaining a positive attitude when difficulties arise.

Being responsible for influencing others requires acting ethically. Consulting involves a personal struggle based on acting on self-interest versus acting for the benefit of others. Individuals who are self-serving are arrogant, withhold information, seek power and recognition, are poor listeners, spend a great deal of time protecting their own status, and are unable to accept criticism. Recently, newspapers have reported numerous incidences of businesses' financial failures because of the illegal and unscrupulous acts of individuals in high-level management positions. In these situations, unbridled greed, the improper use of power, and a sense of entitlement replaced integrity. A consultant must guard against conflicts of interest and maintain high ethical standards.

What Fees Do HIM Consultants Charge?

The consultant must carefully assess future needs as well as current financial needs. The following questions list factors to consider when determining what to charge: What will it cost the consultant to provide services? What will the market bear? What is the consultant's reputation based on the testimony and referrals of others? What lifestyle does the consultant desire? Robert S. McGee in *The Search for Significance* (1998) defines self-worth as equal to performance plus the opinion of others. What an independent consultant charges is determined by each individual's abilities, prior experience, and what the market will bear. Success depends upon generating enough revenue to cover all expenses. Often the most successful consultants are those who can minimize expenses.

First, managing any business requires meticulous record keeping and careful analysis of current as well as future expenses. It is helpful to prepare a personal income statement that includes all current revenue and expenses. An individual considering self-employment should have adequate cash reserves to cover expenses for a three-month period. Consultants may have to wait for payment for periods longer than 90 days.

When an employer pays a salary, it often includes holidays, personal or vacation leave, medical leave, health insurance plans, and the employer portion of FICA tax. Benefits the employer provides are estimated at between 20 and 30 percent of the employee's gross salary. In addition, the employer provides office space, furniture, computer equipment, telephone, travel and training. A person who is in the process of making a decision to give up the benefits of working for someone else in order to establish his or her own business should realize that business revenue must be high enough to cover more than just the consultant's salary.

As a case study, consider a consultant who desires to earn a salary of $75,000 per year. The consultant adds 38 percent to this gross salary figure for fringe benefits and

$20,000 for operating expenses. This totals $123,500 that the consultant must bill per year to maintain the consultant's desired income level. Dividing this figure by 220 working days indicates that the consultant must charge around $561 per day or roughly $70 per hour at a minimum. Because it is common for an independent consultant to experience gaps in workload, it isn't realistic to expect to be engaged in billable consulting work 220 days per year. Therefore, to be able to pay oneself a salary of $75,000 may require charging a higher daily or hourly fee to allow time for seeking new clients and other activities for which no revenue is earned directly. Failure to plan and count the cost of being self-employed can lead to failure. Individuals who are interested in consulting should seek wise counsel and learn from others how they made the transition from being employees to being self-employed, attend professional meetings and conferences, as well as utilize AHIMA's Communities of Practice to network. Many have been deceived and failed because of the assumption that high hourly charges by consultants mean self-employment will be financially lucrative and provide more personal freedom. In addition, not considering the importance of a balanced lifestyle that provides adequate time with spouse, children, family and friends can lead to great personal loss as well as financial failure. In establishing an independent consulting practice, it is advisable to proceed cautiously and conservatively.

Seeking Clients

Individuals whom the consultant knows professionally and personally are the best source of referrals. The consultant should keep in regular contact with these individuals. AHIMA membership is also very valuable. Volunteer to speak at professional meetings and write articles for professional publications to build credibility. Send out a quarterly newsletter to your clients as well as potential new clients. Provide free seminars. Hold a block party and attend and support community events. Satisfied clients are an excellent source of referrals. Create a home page to market services on the World Wide Web, perhaps hiring another consultant to achieve the desired Internet image. Develop a logo and color scheme and use it consistently on stationery, business cards, and the Web page. Perform public service activities to network with individuals in your community. To decide whether to advertise in a trade journal, assess how previous or current clients were obtained.

Working at Home

Consulting requires an ability to develop a container for oneself, to stay focused, to work unsupervised, and to have healthy boundaries. A container refers to the place in which focused work is performed both physically and mentally. A physical workspace container needs to be planned in the home—a place recognized and respected as the office space of the new business.

This space can be a guest room planned in such a way that a sofa or futon in the room provides an extra bedroom when necessary, yet serves most of the time as an attractive, efficient office. Explore the tax laws with an accountant if you plan to use this office space as a tax deduction because this limits other uses of the space. Plan a space that meets work needs. A countertop around the periphery of a room with shelves above it and file cabinets under it provides a lot of desktop and storage space inexpensively. It is difficult to find furniture at a reasonable price that utilizes all your current physical space perfectly.

The consultant should utilize ergonomic techniques that facilitate comfort and convenience. For example, a computer with an adjustable screen, so the screen is at eye level, should be purchased. An adjustable keyboard tray for the keyboard, so the fingers, wrists, and elbows remain in a straight line to reduce the risk of cumulative trauma disorder, is needed. The chair should have adjustable arms, back, and seat. The seat should be capable of being lowered or raised so the knee and hip bone are in a straight line, with the feet sitting firmly placed on the floor or a foot rest. A space for the computer that allows work materials to be placed on both sides so that everything needed for work is within arm's reach is a part of the office plan. The workspace and desktop should be free of glare and shiny objects. A window as the backdrop for a computer is not advised. Miniblinds to regulate outside light can be utilized. Paint, furnishings, and countertops that have a matte finish, utilizing soft colors to create a space that facilitates calmness, clarity, and simplicity, are advocated. Fabric and carpet can be utilized to reduce noise and create an ambiance of comfort and softness.

Computer software can be utilized to accomplish many tasks such as word processing for resume and form design, spreadsheets for quality assurance reports, database software for tracking client data, and presentation software for professional presentations.

Being focused mentally requires setting boundaries. Work at home is conducted in the same fashion as one would act as an HIM department director in a health care facility. The integrity of the home office must be respected. Let the answering machine handle personal calls or unwanted telephone marketing ploys. To minimize interruptions, educate friends and family about work hours and ask not to be disturbed. Working at home does not mean a baby-sitter is no longer necessary. Being focused and productive means devoting full attention to the task at hand with minimal interruptions. If small children are at home, hire a baby-sitter and set clear boundaries, preferably in writing, regarding minimizing the use of the telephone, television, noise levels, what activities children are permitted, where, and with whom, how to handle minor emergencies, instructions about any medications a child routinely takes, which neighborhood children are permitted in the house or yard, and instructions for caring for household pets. (Crate train all pets while they are still young so they can be willingly and quietly confined in the event it is necessary.)

It is not unusual that family members find it difficult to accept and respect an individual's professional role at home. Generally it is not known what an individual really does at work, and family might not recognize activities conducted in a home office as work. Relatives can present multiple disruptions and expect work to cease so that their personal needs are met. A consultant must set firm boundaries and limits with family members in addition to baby-sitters and friends.

Home Office Equipment

To have an efficient operation at home, consultants need to have certain equipment to conduct business. Following is a checklist of suggested items:

- Computer with Internet access (high-speed if possible)
- Phone (two lines suggested)
- Answering machine or voice mail
- Fax machine
- Copier and printer

Computer

Computers have become an integral part of day-to-day business for consultants. Once considered a luxury, they now are often a necessity. Computers can be used in so many ways that it would be futile to attempt to list them all. To determine what type of computer setup is best for an individual's needs, a few questions need to be answered:

- Is access to the computer needed when traveling to clients?
- Are heavy graphics involved?
- What type of software will be used (e.g., word processing, database, spreadsheet, graphics)?
- Is there enough desktop space in the office for the monitor, printer, keyboard, and computer?

Thinking these questions through will help in determining the type of computer that will best fit one's needs. In most cases, it is not necessary to purchase the very latest model with the fastest speed available. Those who do will generally pay a premium for the privilege.

A dilemma for many consultants is deciding whether to invest in a laptop or desktop computer. The big advantage with a laptop is its portability. While in a hotel room, restaurant or flying to an appointment, work can be readily accessed. Many laptop models are just as capable as their desktop counterparts. As useful as a laptop can be, however, there are still some areas in which the smaller version is inferior to a desktop model. For one, the keyboard can be awkward and the mouse is usually relegated to a touchpad on which the user maneuvers his or her fingers to direct the cursor. When using a laptop in a location where space permits, the laptop can be connected to a regular keyboard and monitor for better ergonomics. Considering cost factors, laptops are generally more expensive than comparable desktop systems (see Figure 16-6).

Because of the fast pace of technological advances in the computer field, no specific speeds, memory sizes, or other attributes will be suggested here. However, current models available in any large electronics store can easily handle most consultant applications. It is generally not necessary and not prudent to procure the most

Laptops	Desktops
Pros	**Pros**
• Portable/compact	• More power for the money
• Notes can be taken on site	• Easy to upgrade
• Access to wireless networks	• More audio/video options
	• Normal keyboard and mouse
Cons	**Cons**
• More expensive	• Requires more space
• Small display	• Not portable
• Higher maintenance costs	

Figure 16-6   Advantages and disadvantages of laptop and desktop computers.

advanced system in the store. Buying a model that has been on the market for six months will cost considerably less and be more than adequate.

Having Internet access is fairly standard in the consulting arena today. E-mail is a way of life in business. In many cases a consultant would not be considered credible without an e-mail address. E-mail accounts can be set up at no cost on such sites as Yahoo.com and Hotmail.com. For a fee, one can also obtain an e-mail domain name using the name of the consultant's business. There is a wealth of information on the Internet that can often be beneficial in consulting work. Consultants should consider having their own Web page that describes their expertise and services available. Usually, a simple Web site can be built for a nominal fee. A consultant who uses the Internet extensively may need high-speed Internet access, such as cable or DSL.

Telephone and Wireless Services

Consultants definitely need at least one telephone and probably should have two. A new consultant may be surprised to learn that charges for a standard business line generally are higher than charges for a residential line. However, to attempt to share one line with family members, a fax machine, or the Internet could lead to busy signals and missed calls that would be detrimental to business. Consultants who visit various clients in different locations will likely need a cell phone in order to be reached easily.

Answering Machine or Voice Mail

Consultants need to be able to receive messages at any time. An answering machine or voice mail is critical. Answering machines need to have a very good sound quality. Remember, consultants always need to present a good image, and having an answering machine that has a garbled message does not make a good impression. Also, if the consultant will need to check messages while away from the office, an answering machine that provides this feature should be selected. Voice mail is simply an automated answering service provided by a local phone company or wireless communications provider. Voice mail messages generally can be checked from any telephone. Most providers charge a small monthly fee for voice mail services.

Fax Machines, Copiers, and Multipurpose Devices

Documents often need to be sent back and forth between a consultant and a client. Fax machines allow for rapid transmission of printed documents that cannot be easily e-mailed. Some consultants fax newsletters to their clients who request them as a means of keeping in touch. Fax machines are affordable and easy to use.

If copies need to be made on a regular basis, then a copy machine should be bought or leased. There is a vast array of copiers ranging in price from the hundreds to tens of thousands of dollars. If purchasing or leasing a copier, also consider the cost of toner and other supplies, which can add quite a bit to the operating costs of some machines. If copies are not made that often, using a local copying service may be more feasible.

An alternative to buying several different pieces of office equipment would be to purchase a multipurpose machine that acts as a printer, fax machine, scanner, and copier. Prices for these devices are very reasonable, and they can save substantial office space.

Negotiating Contracts

The HIM consultant should take an active role in designing a work contract. He or she should seek the help of an attorney in designing a contract that clearly spells out his or her needs regarding pay, authority, responsibility, and so forth. A written contract may outline the number of hours to be worked in a specific health care facility and the fee charged per hour by the consultant. Some contracts may include reimbursement for mileage and other travel expenses. The contract outlines responsibilities on the part of both participants. It often states that the contract employee (consultant) is responsible for all payroll deductions such as taxes, health insurance, and retirement. If the consultant is going to charge for information provided to the facility via phone consultation, or if some projects are going to be completed in the consultant's home office (such as preparing a policy and procedure manual or designing forms), clarify how to bill for this time. Most consulting contracts are for a one-year period, and a new contract is signed annually or is self-renewing. Most health care facilities want the contract to read that it can be voided at any time with 30 days' advance notice. Usually it is not possible to negotiate a termination clause. Clients often require the consultant to maintain professional liability insurance coverage. Figure 16-7 is only an outline of possible contract elements and should not be considered a model for contract development. A consultant should seek legal advice and assure that any contract is HIPAA-compliant and appropriate to the legal and business environment of the state and community.

CONSULTING AGREEMENT

This Agreement is made effective as of July 1, 20XX, by and between **Agency** and **Consultant**.

Consultant has a background in Health Information Systems Management and is willing to provide services to **Agency** based on this background.

Agency desires to have services provided by **Consultant**.

Therefore, the parties agree as follows:

1. DESCRIPTION OF SERVICES. Beginning on July 12, 20XX, **Consultant** will provide the following services (collectively the "Services"):

   a. Provide education for personnel regarding appropriate documentation for medical records.

   b. Provide information and other technical assistance for compliance with Ohio Department of Mental Health regulations.

   c. Provide technical assistance with quality assurance plans, activities, and reviews.

   d. Provide technical assistance to ensure compliance of Medical Records with Ohio Department of Mental Health regulations.

   e. Other duties within the scope of Health Information Systems Management expertise as requested by the Executive Director.

2. PERFORMANCE OF SERVICES. The manner in which the Services are to be performed and the specific hours to be worked shall be determined by **Consultant**. **Agency** will rely on **Consultant** to work as many hours as may be reasonably necessary to fulfill **Consultant's** obligations under this Agreement, not to exceed six and one-half hours per month unless approved in advance by the board of directors of **Agency**.

3. PAYMENT. **Agency** will pay a fee to **Consultant** of $XX.00 per hour for the Services. This fee shall not be payable until receipt of third party revenues.

4. LICENSURE/CERTIFICATION. **Consultant** shall at all times maintain all licensure and certifications required of a medical records technician and shall be responsible for any costs associated with such licensure and certification.

5. TERM/TERMINATION. Either party may terminate this Agreement upon giving 30 days written notice to the other party. This Agreement shall terminate automatically on June 30, 19XX.

6. RELATIONSHIP OF PARTIES. It is understood by the parties that **Consultant** is an independent contractor with respect to **Agency** and not an employee of **Agency**. **Agency** is not responsible for withholding and shall not withhold FICA or taxes of any

Figure 16-7   A sample contract (not to be used as a model).

kind from payments made to **Consultant**. **Consultant** shall not be entitled to receive any benefits that employees of **Agency** may be entitled to receive, and shall not be entitled to workers' compensation, unemployment compensation, medical insurance, life insurance, paid vacations, paid holidays, pension or social security on account of her work under this Agreement.

7. EMPLOYEES. **Consultant's** employees, if any, who perform services for **Agency** under this Agreement shall also be bound by the provisions of this Agreement. At the request of **Agency**, **Consultant** shall provide adequate evidence that such persons are **Consultant's** employees.

8. INJURIES. **Consultant** acknowledges **Consultant's** obligation to obtain appropriate insurance coverage for the benefit of **Consultant** (and **Consultant's** employees, if any). **Consultant** waives any rights to recovery from **Agency** for any injuries that **Consultant** (and/or **Consultant's** employees) may sustain while performing services under this Agreement.

9. INDEMNIFICATION. **Consultant** agrees to indemnify and hold **Agency** harmless from all claims, losses, expenses, fees including attorney fees, costs and judgments that may be asserted against **Agency** that result from the acts or omission of **Consultant**, **Consultant's** employees, if any, and **Consultant's** agents. If professional liability insurance is available to cover her acts or failure to act as a health information manager, **Consultant** shall obtain such insurance, at her own expense.

10. CONFIDENTIALITY. **Consultant** recognizes that **Agency** has and will have the following information:

   — client information and other proprietary information (collectively, "Information") which are valuable, special and unique assets of **Agency**. **Consultant** agrees that **Consultant** will not at any time or in any manner, either directly or indirectly, use any Information for **Consultant's** own benefit, or divulge, disclose, or communicate in any manner any Information to any third party without the prior written consent of **Agency**. **Consultant** will protect the Information and treat it as strictly confidential. A violation of this paragraph shall be a material violation of this Agreement.

11. CONFIDENTIALITY AFTER TERMINATION. The confidentiality provisions of this Agreement shall remain in full force and effect after the termination of this Agreement.

12. RECORDS AND RETURN OF RECORDS. Upon termination of this Agreement, **Consultant** shall deliver all records, notes, data, memorandum, models and equipment of any nature that are in **Consultant's** possession or under **Consultant's** control and that are **Agency's** property or relate to **Agency's** business.

Figure 16-7   *(Continued)*

13. NOTICES. All notices required or permitted under this Agreement shall be in writing and shall be deemed delivered when delivered in person or deposited in the United States mail, postage prepaid, addressed as follows:

> Company: name/address

> Consultant: name/address

Such address may be changed from time to time by either party by providing written notice to the other in the manner set forth above.

14. ENTIRE AGREEMENT. This Agreement contains the entire agreement of the parties and there are no other promises or conditions in any other agreement whether oral or written. This Agreement supersedes any prior written or oral agreements between the parties.

15. AMENDMENT. This Agreement may be modified or amended if the amendment is made in writing and is signed by both parties.

16. SEVERABILITY. If any provision of this Agreement shall be held to be invalid or unenforceable for any reason, the remaining provisions shall continue to be valid and enforceable. If a court finds that any provision of this Agreement is invalid or unenforceable, but that by limiting such provision it would become valid or enforceable, then such provision shall be deemed to be written, construed, and enforced as so limited.

17. WAIVER OF CONTRACTUAL RIGHT. The failure of either party to enforce any provision of this Agreement shall not be construed as a waiver or limitation of that party's right to subsequently enforce and compel strict compliance with every provision of this Agreement.

18. APPLICABLE LAW. This Agreement shall be governed by the laws of the State of (name of state).

> Consultant

> By:

> Agency

> By:

Figure 16-7   (*Continued*)

The privacy standards of HIPAA have specific requirements regarding the business associates of a covered entity. (Recall from Chapter 1 that a covered entity may be a health plan, a health care clearinghouse, or a health care provider. In this discussion we will use a health care provider as an example of a covered entity.) A **business associate** is a person who is not a member of the health care provider's workforce, but performs work on behalf of the provider that involves the use or disclosure of protected health information (Definitions, 2002). Because a consultant is not considered to be a member of the health care provider's workforce, the HIPAA privacy rule would dictate that the consultant have a written business associate agreement or contract with the facility. One example of the types of issues covered by the business associate agreement would be a provision for safeguards to prevent inappropriate use or disclosure of protected health information on the part of the consultant. The U.S. Department of Health and Human Services Office for Civil Rights provides sample business associate contract provisions on its Web site, which the HIM consultant may want to review (OCR, 2002).

Trends

Data released by AHIMA (2003, March) indicates that 13.3 percent of its members work as consultants or vendors. The Bureau of Labor Statistics projects a 49 percent growth in HIM employment during the decade ending in 2010. This makes HIM one of the fastest growing professions in the United States (Hecker, 2001). The overall increase in demand for HIM services should also increase the need for HIM consultants. Other factors contributing to the need for consultants are an increased emphasis on compliance activities, the complexity of new regulations and new payment systems affecting various health care settings, and health care providers' need to operate effectively and efficiently in an ever-changing environment.

Summary

Starting a new business as a consultant is challenging and requires careful research and planning. Once consulting contracts are obtained, success depends on the ability to gain administrative support and rapport. It is important to develop long-range goals and money management skills. Obtain the help of an attorney and an accountant to ensure compliance with tax code.

It is a good idea to seek and gain employment in various health care settings, volunteer, read professional journals, attend workshops and seminars, take college courses, and pursue additional credentials to ensure personal marketability.

The ability to set healthy boundaries and provide a container where focused work can be performed both mentally and physically is necessary. Design a home office space that incorporates ergonomic techniques to facilitate comfort and convenience.

The HIM consultant should take an active role in negotiating a contract that meets needs and spells out clearly the fee charged, what is covered, what is not covered, and when payment is expected.

To get started after obtaining a new contract for a health care facility, review all the regulations that apply to that facility regarding documentation requirements, develop an assessment tool, and conduct random audits on records to determine overall documentation compliance. Copies of all audits available to the health care facility administration should be kept.

Key Terms

audit   retrospective review of selected health care records or data documents to evaluate the quality of care, services provided, documentation, or coding compared with predetermined standards.

business associate   under HIPAA, a person who is not a member of the covered entity's (e.g., the health care provider's) workforce, but performs work on behalf of the covered entity that involves the use or disclosure of protected health information.

business plan   a formal written document summarizing the operational and financial objectives of a business. The business plan also includes the details of how the objectives are to be attained, including budgets and other financial forecasts. Lenders and investors generally require a business plan as one of the documents that they study when making a decision whether to lend to or invest in a business.

corporate integrity agreement (CIA)   an agreement that a health care provider or health plan reaches with the Department of Health and Human Services' Office of the Inspector General (OIG) as part of a settlement agreement when allegations of improper reimbursement have been made.

Office of the Inspector General (OIG)   a subdivision of the U. S. Department of Health and Human Services. "The mission of the Office of Inspector General is to protect the integrity of Department of Health and Human Services (HHS) programs, as well as the health and welfare of the beneficiaries of those programs. . . . The OIG's duties are carried out through a nationwide network of audits, investigations, inspections and other mission-related functions performed by OIG components" (OIG, No date, Online).

REVIEW QUESTIONS

Knowledge-based Questions

1. Name four professional interpersonal strengths of a health information consultant.
2. Define leadership.
3. List five character traits of a leader who exhibits integrity.
4. Describe why a consultant should not enter into a "contingency" contract with a client.
5. Summarize the privacy standards of HIPAA regarding business associates.
6. Explain why expertise in a particular profession or skill is a small part of being a consultant.

Application-based Questions

1. A health information consultant desires a gross salary of $50,000 per year. Operating expenses are estimated at $20,000 (which include payroll taxes such Social Security) and fringe benefits are 25 percent. Compute the total dollar amount the consultant must bill per year to maintain the desired gross salary of $50,000. If the consultant works 220 days, what must the consultant charge per day or per hour at a minimum?

2. Describe the key elements of a business plan for an independent consultant.

Web Activity

Find the *Conditions of Participation* or *Conditions for Coverage* for one of the settings discussed in any previous chapter. (One Web source for locating these documents is http://cms.hhs.gov/cop/1.asp at the Centers for Medicare and Medicaid Services.) Within the *Conditions*, locate the medical record standards for the selected setting. Develop an audit form that a consultant could use to audit the documentation in the selected setting based on the medical record standards found in the *Conditions*.

Case Study

Identify the problem areas for the facility described below and prepare a written recommendation addressing a plan of correction for each site.

You have been hired as a consultant for a behavioral health care facility that is comprised of 11 client service sites. They are JCAHO accredited and the next survey is two months away. After initial visits to each site your analysis of deficiencies includes:

Site 1—Residential Chemical Dependency Program for Adolescents

The medical records are well organized and in good order, but after closer inspection you find that the physician responsible for completing physical exams does not assess clients' motor skills, which is a requirement for adolescent admissions. You also find that though the history and physical is performed and dictated by the physician within twenty-four hours, the typed report does not appear in the chart for weeks.

Site 2—Residential Chemical Dependency Program for Adult Women

JCAHO and state standards require that a master treatment plan be completed within fourteen days of admission. A representative sample review of the facilities' charts reveals no treatment plans. Upon closer scrutiny you learn that none of the clients admitted in the past three months have treatment plans in their charts either.

Site 3—Outpatient Mental Health Clinic with 600 Active Clients

After conducting a study to determine the record retrievability rate, it is learned that 75 percent of the records are inaccessible. The day the study was completed, only forty clients had been scheduled for appointments. This location only has two health information clerks and one has been pulled frequently to answer the phone at the intake desk.

Site 4—Outpatient Chemical Dependency Site with 125 Active Clients

A quantitative analysis process has been set up and the record clerk trained. However, no quantitative analysis has occurred. Upon a return visit to analyze the situation, it is found that the records clerk is also the office manager with responsibilities to answer the phone, schedule appointments, conduct financial intakes, maintain time sheets for clinicians, and complete general correspondence.

Site 5—Outpatient Chemical Dependency Site with 40 Active Clients

The clinical supervisor is unwilling to follow the organization's policies. Upon receiving a subpoena duces tecum and a court order, she fails to notify the organization's clinical director, health information manager, or an administrator. Instead she takes the records home and asks her husband, who is an attorney, for advice.

Site 6—Outpatient Chemical Dependency Site with 50 Active Clients

A client who is enrolled in a government program that requires compliance with addiction treatment in order to maintain financial benefits begins to miss scheduled appointments. The government agency is notified that the client is noncompliant and the client's benefits are terminated. The client calls very irate and review of the record indicates the client has not signed an authorization to release information. The client threatens a lawsuit charging that his rights to confidentiality have been violated.

References and Suggested Readings

Abdelhak, M., Grostic, S., Hanken, M.A., and Jacobs, E. (2001). *Health Information: Management of a Strategic Resource* (2nd ed.). Philadelphia: W. B. Saunders.

[AHIMA]. American Health Information Management Association. (2003, February). AHIMA mobilizes to meet the e-HIM call. *AHIMA Advantage,* 7 (1) [Online]. http://library.ahima.org/xpedio/groups/secure/documents/ahima/pub_bok1_017431.html [2003, July 18].

[AHIMA]. American Health Information Management Association. (2003, March). New member profile data reveals rapid growth expansion. *AHIMA Advantage,* 7 (2), 2–7.

Adams, B., and Kintler, D. (1998). *Independent Consulting.* Avon, MA: Adams Media Corporation.

Bennett-Woods, D. (1997). Team facilitation skills: A step beyond running a good meeting. *Journal of AHIMA,* 68 (1), 20.

Blanchard, K., and Hodges, P. (2003). *The Servant Leader.* Nashville, TN: Thomas Nelson, Inc.

Brandt, M., Fletcher, D., Fenton, S., Richards, L.A., and Johnston, S.L. (1997). Practice brief— developing information capture tools. *Journal of AHIMA, 68* (3).

Definitions. (2002). *Code of Federal Regulations.* Title 45, Part 160, Subpart A, §160.103.

Economy, P., and Nelson, B. (1997). *Consulting for Dummies.* New York: Hungry Minds, Inc.

Hecker, D. E. (2001). Occupational employment projections to 2010. *Monthly Labor Review, 124* (11), 57–84. [Online]. http://www.bls.gov/opub/mlr/2001/11/art4full.pdf [2003, July 19].

Jones-Burns, M. (1997). Seeing your way through to AHIMA's Vision 2006. *Journal of AHIMA, 68* (1), 30.

Koch, C. (1996, March 15). The bright stuff. *CIO Magazine.* [Online]. http://www.cio.com/archive/031596/qa.html [2003, July 18].

LaTour, K. M., and Eichenwald, S. (2002). *Health Information Management: Concepts, Principles, and Practice.* Chicago: American Health Information Management Association.

Maxwell, J. C. (1993). *Developing the Leader Within You.* Nashville, TN: Thomas Nelson, Inc.

McGee, Robert S. (1998). *The Search for Significance.* Nashville, TN: Word Publishing.

McWay, D.C. (2003). *Legal Aspects of Health Information Management.* Clifton Park, NY: Delmar Learning.

Mitchell, S. (2003). Taking the initiative with nursing home quality. *Journal of the American Health Information Management Association, 74* (3), 56.

Nagel, S. (2003, February 10). HIM's role in the revenue cycle. *For the Record,* pp. 31–33.

[OCR] Office for Civil Rights (2002, August 14). Sample business associate contract provisions. *Medical Privacy—National Standards to Protect the Privacy of Personal Health Information.* [Online]. http://www.hhs.gov/ocr/hipaa/contractprov.html [2003, July 19].

Office Design for Comfort, Safety and Efficiency. *Bureau of Workers' Compensation Division of Safety and Hygiene*, Division of Safety and Hygiene Training Center Publication #0503.

[OIG] Office of the Inspector General. (No date). *OIG Mission.* [Online]. http://oig.hhs.gov/organization/OIGmission.html [2003, July 21].

Reed, J. (No date). Those who can, consult, part 1: What do I offer? [Online]. http://www.ivillage.co.uk/workcareer/findjob/careerchoice/articles/0,,182_161293,00.html [2003, July 21].

Reed, J. (No date). Those who can, consult, part 2: What is a consultant? Myths v realities. [Online]. http://www.ivillage.co.uk/workcareer/findjob/careerchoice/articles/0,,182_161291,00.html [2003, July 21].

Rollins, G. (2003). Turning a physician practice on its head. *Journal of the American Health Information Management Association, 74* (3), 32.

Seeking credibility: JCAHO revamps its survey process. (2003, January 27). *For the Record,* p. 39.

Siropolis, N. (1994). *Small Business Management: A Guide to Entrepreneurship.* Boston: Houghton Mifflin Company.

Squazzo, J. (2003). Doctors not ready for HIPAA. *Journal of the American Health Information Management Association, 74* (2), 10.

Wager, K. A., Lee, F. W., Glorioso, R. and Bergstrom, L. (1999). Working smarter, not harder, in a family practice. *Journal of AHIMA 70* (6), 44-46.

Key Resources

American Health Information Management Association
(See Chapter 1 for contact information.)

Internal Revenue Service
U.S. Treasury Department
(See local phone directory for contact information)
Federal Tax Information
Phone: 800-829-1040 (for individuals)
Phone: 800-829-4933 (for business)
http://www.irs.ustreas.gov

Index

A

AA. *See* Alcoholics Anonymous
AAAHC. *See* Accreditation Association for Ambulatory Health Care
AAHA. *See* American Animal Hospital Association
AAMR. *See* American Association on Mental Retardation
AAMR Adaptive Behavior Scales (ABS), 304
AAP. *See* American Academy of Pediatrics
AAVMC. *See* American Veterinary Medical Colleges
Abnormal test results, 91
ABS. *See* AAMR Adaptive Behavior Scales
ACA. *See* American Correctional Association
Accounting, dental care, 504
Accreditation
    correctional facilities, 177–78, 188
    facility for mentally retarded, 295–96
    freestanding ambulatory care, 63–64
    health care organizations, 10, 11
    home health care, 422–24
    hospice, 450
    hospital-based ambulatory care, 27
    long-term care, 334–36, 342–43
    managed care organizations, 111–12, 113
    mental health services, 212–13
    rehabilitation, 380–84
    substance abuse treatment, 255–56
    veterinary care, 522–24
Accreditation Association for Ambulatory Health Care (AAAHC), 111, 112
Accreditation Handbook for Ambulatory Health Care, 112

ACHSA. *See* American Correctional Health Services Association
Acquired Immune Deficiency Syndrome (AIDS), 165, 448
ACS. *See* American College of Surgeons
Active phase of dying, 450
Active treatment services, 292
Activities, long-term care, 332
Activities of daily living (ADL), 328, 429
Acute care hospital
    consultants, 551
    dental care, 486–87
Acute diseases, 173
Acute mental health services, 200
Acute rehabilitation, 371, 407–8
ADA. *See* American Dental Association
Addictions, 14, 202–3
Addiction Severity Index (ASI), 272
Addressable implementation specifications, 8–9
ADL. *See* Activities of daily living
Administrative information, correctional facilities, 182–83
Administrative simplification (HIPAA), 6–7
Administrative staff, facility for mentally retarded, 295
Adolescents
    dental care, 487–88
    mental/emotional illness, 206–9
    substance abuse treatment, 250–51
Adults
    dental care, 488
    mental/emotional illness, 201–6
Adverse effects, dental care, 493, 509
Affiliates, 422
Aftercare plans, mental health services, 219
After-hours crisis services, mental health services, 206
Age, 114, 172
Aggregate data, dialysis, 145

AHA. *See* American Hospital Association
AHIMA. *See* American Health Information Management Association Aides
AIDS. *See* Acquired Immune Deficiency Syndrome
Alcoholics Anonymous (AA), 245, 246, 249–50
Alcoholism, 245–46
AMA. *See* American Medical Association
Amalgam, 509
Ambulation aids, 379
Ambulatory care, freestanding
    caregiver types, 61
    coding and classification, 82–83
    computer systems, 86–88
    data and information flow, 83–85
    data sets, 88
    documentation, 65–78
    health information management, 91–92
    Medicare certification, 62–65
    patient types, 61
    quality improvement, 88–89
    record linkage, 85–86
    regulatory issues, 61–62
    reimbursement, 4, 79–82
    risk management, 89–91
    settings, 59–61
    trends, 92
    utilization management, 89
Ambulatory care, hospital-based
    accreditation, 27
    caregiver types, 26
    coding and classification, 40–41
    computer systems, 41–42
    data and information flow, 41
    data sets, 42–43
    documentation, 28–31
    federal regulations, 27
    health information management, 46–48

information management, 40–43
licensure, 27
patient types, 26
quality improvement, 44
reimbursement, 4, 33–40
risk management, 45–46
setting types, 24–26
trends, 48
utilization management, 45
Ambulatory payment classification
(APC), 33, 35–36, 38, 80–81
Ambulatory surgery, hospital-based,
24–25
Ambulatory surgery centers (ASCs)
documentation, 71–72, 90
growth, 60
Medicare reimbursement, 80
AMCRA. *See* American Managed Care
and Review Association
American Academy of Pediatrics (AAP),
250–51
American Animal Hospital Association
(AAHA), 524
American Association on Mental
Retardation (AAMR), 302–3
American College of Surgeons (ACS), 1
American Correctional Association
(ACA), 177, 178, 181
American Correctional Health Services
Association (ACHSA), 190
American Dental Association (ADA),
501–2
American Health Information
Management Association
(AHIMA)
consultants, 554, 560, 562, 570
E&M code assignment, 35
EDI standards, 7–8
home health care, 425
mental health services, 211
security issues, 9
American Hospital Association (AHA),
35
American Managed Care and Review
Association (AMCRA), 111
American Medical Association (AMA),
83, 118, 178
American Psychiatric Association (APA),
203, 269–70
American Public Health Association
(APHA), 177, 178, 179, 181
American Society of Addiction Medicine
(ASAM), 272
American Veterinary Health Information
Management Association
(AVHIMA), 542
American Veterinary Medical
Association (AVMA), 521, 522–24,
525–26, 535, 536, 539
American Veterinary Medical Colleges
(AAVMC), 524
Ancillary services, 26, 176
Anesthesia, 71
Animal cruelty, 540
Animal health technician. *See* Veterinary
technicians
Animals, 520–21
Animal welfare advocates, 540

Annual staffing, 297, 307
APA. *See* American Psychiatric
Association
APC. *See* Ambulatory payment
classification
Apgar score, 72
APHA. *See* American Public Health
Association
Appointments, patient
computer scheduling, 86–87
documentation, 90
scheduling, 83–85
ASCs. *See* Ambulatory surgery centers
ASI. *See* Addiction Severity Index
Assessment
facility for mentally retarded,
304–5
home health care, 425, 427–28
hospice care, 464
inmates, 174–75
long-term care, 337–42
mental health services, 213–14, 225
mentally retarded persons, 293, 297
rehabilitation, 392
substance abuse treatment, 257–63,
275, 276–79
Auditing
consultant role, 555
home health care, 431
long-term care, 359–60
Authorizations
care for mentally retarded, 304
managed care organizations, 121
AVHIMA. *See* American Veterinary
Health Information Management
Association
AVMA. *See* American Veterinary
Medical Association

B
Baby bottle tooth decay (BBTD), 487
Balanced Budget Act (1997), 451, 462
BBTD. *See* Baby bottle tooth decay
BCIS. *See* Bureau of Citizenship and
Immigration Services
Bed allocation, 230
Bed days, 124
Behavioral medicine, 552, 553
Benefit levels, 121
Bereavement assessment, 459–60, 471
Billing
managed care organizations, 121
Uniform Bill 92, 38–40
Bipolar disorder, 202
Birth centers
accreditation, 63–64
ambulatory care, 60–61, 72
Bite wing, 498
"Birthday rule," 116–17
Blood donors, veterinary care, 541
Bovines, 521
Bridge, dental, 491
Bureau of Citizenship and Immigration
Services (BCIS), 170
Bureau of Immigration and Customs
Enforcement (ICE), 170–71
Business associate, 570
Business plan, 557–58, 559

C
Calculus, 492
CAMBHC. *See* Comprehensive
Accreditation Manual for
Behavioral Health Care
CAMH. *See* Comprehensive
Accreditation Manual for Hospitals
Canines, 521
CAPD. *See* Continuous ambulatory
peritoneal dialysis
Capitation
correctional facilities, 183
features, 4
freestanding ambulatory care, 81
managed care organizations, 114
Caprines, 521
Caregivers
ambulatory care, freestanding, 61
ambulatory care, hospital-based, 26
correctional facilities, 173, 176–77
dental care, 508
dialysis, 138
facilities for mentally retarded,
293–95
home health care, 421–22
hospice, 449
long-term care, 330–34
managed care organizations, 109
mental health services, 209–11
rehabilitation, 372–75
substance abuse treatment, 252–54
veterinary care, 521–22
Care paths, rehabilitation, 407, 409–12
Care plans
dialysis, 140, 142
home health care, 425
hospice care, 458–59, 465
long-term care, 337, 339–40
CARF. *See* Commission on Accreditation
of Rehabilitation Facilities
Caries, dental, 487
Case management
hospice care, 458–59
managed care organizations, 121
mental health services, 206, 210–11
substance abuse treatment, 254
Case Mix Assessment Tool (CMAT), 222
Case-mix groups (CMGs), 345, 396–97
CASSP. *See* Child and Adolescent Service
System Program
CCHP. *See* Certified Correctional Health
Professional Program
CCI. *See* National Correct Coding
Initiative
CCPD. *See* Continuous cycling peritoneal
dialysis
CDM. *See* Charge description master
CDR. *See* Clinical data repository
CDT-4. *See* Current Dental Terminology
CE/CEs. *See* Covered entities
Census data, hospice care, 471
Center for Mental Health Services
(CMHS), 207
Centers for Medicare and Medicaid
Services (CMS)
ambulatory care, hospital-based,
38, 40

ambulatory care, freestanding, 81–82, 83
dialysis, 140
home health care, 422–23, 424
hospice care, 462
managed care regulations, 110
mental health services, 217
rehabilitation, 380, 382–84
Centralized health information services, 46–47
Certification
home health care, 425
hospice care, 451
Certified Correctional Health Professional (CCHP) Program, 190
Certified medication technicians (CMTs), 331
Certified nurse midwives (CNMs)
ambulatory care, 61
reimbursement, 79
rural health clinics, 63
Certified veterinary practice manager (CVPM), 522
CHAP. *See* Community Health Accreditation Program
Charge description master (CDM), 34
Chargemaster, 34
Chargemaster coordinator, 48
Charting, dental, 495, 496–97, 498–99
Chemical restraints, 217–18, 220–21
Chief information officer (CIO), 128
Child and Adolescent Service System Program (CASSP), 207
Children
dental care, 487–88, 501
mental/emotional illness, 206–9
Children's Health Act (2000), 218–19
CHIN. *See* Community health information network
Chronic diseases, 173
Chronic renal failure, 136
CIA. *See* Corporate integrity agreement
CIO. *See* Chief information officer
Civil money penalties, 335–336, 362–363
Claims audits,
retrospective/prospective, 64–65
Claims, managed care organizations, 120, 121, 128
Claims production, managed care organizations, 121
Claims tracking, dental care, 504
Classification. *See* Coding and classification
CLIA. *See* Clinical Laboratory Improvement Amendments
Client fees, substance abuse treatment, 266
Clients
facility for mentally retarded, 292
mental health services, 201–9
substance abuse treatment, 250–52
Clinical assessment, substance abuse treatment, 257–63
Clinical data repository (CDR), 13–14
Clinical data specialist, 128
Clinical depression, 202
Clinical documentation, substance abuse treatment, 257–66

Clinical Laboratory Improvement Amendments (CLIA), 110
Clinical professionals, 173, 176
Clinic outpatient, 26
Clinics. *See* Hospital clinics
Clinics, dental, 486
CMAT. *See* Case Mix Assessment Tool
CMGs. *See* Case-mix groups
CMHC. *See* Community mental health center
CMHS. *See* Center for Mental Health Services
CMS. *See* Centers for Medicare & Medicaid Services
CMS 1450. *See* Uniform Bill 92
CMS 485, 486, and 487 forms, 425, 426
CMS Common Procedural Coding System, 40
CMTs. *See* Certified medication technicians
CNMs. *See* Certified nurse midwives
COB. *See* Coordination of benefits
Code of Federal Regulations
ambulatory care documentation, 31–33
mental health services, 214, 216
rehabilitation, 380
section 42, 139–40, 144, 151, 254, 273–74
substance abuse treatment, 254, 273–74
Coding and classification
consultant role, 555
correctional facilities, 185
dialysis care, 144
facilities for mentally retarded, 301–3
freestanding ambulatory care, 82–83
home health care, 432–33
hospice care, 465, 468–69
hospital-based ambulatory care, 40–41
long-term care, 348–49
managed care organizations, 117–19
mental health services, 228
rehabilitation, 397, 401–4
substance abuse treatment, 269–70
veterinary care, 530–32
Coinsurance, 107
Color coding, 85
Commission for the Accreditation of Birth Centers, 63–64
Commission on Accreditation of Rehabilitation Facilities (CARF), 255, 380, 381–82, 385–90, 391–92
Common working file (CWF), 43
Communicable diseases, 173
Communities of practice (CoP), 15
Community Health Accreditation Program (CHAP), 422, 423–24
Community health centers, dental care, 487
Community health information network (CHIN), 13
Community mental health center (CMHC), 199, 222, 225, 230

Community Support Program (CSP), 203–4
Compliance
consultant role, 555–56
freestanding ambulatory care, 64–65, 89
managed care organizations, 110
Compliance officer, 47, 65
Composite rating, 114
Comprehensive Accreditation Manual for Behavioral Health Care (CAMBHC), 212, 296
Comprehensive Accreditation Manual for Health Care Networks, 112
Comprehensive Accreditation Manual for Hospitals (CAMH), 212, 255
Comprehensive Alcohol Abuse and Alcohol Prevention, Treatment and Rehabilitation Act (1970), 273
Comprehensive outpatient rehabilitation facilities (CORFs), 380, 382
Comprehensive resident assessment, 337–42
Computer-stored ambulatory record (COSTAR), 88
Computer systems
correctional facilities, 185
dental care, 502, 503, 506
dialysis care, 145
facilities for mentally retarded, 303–4
freestanding ambulatory care, 86–88, 92
home health care, 433
home office, 564–66
hospice care, 469–70
hospital-based ambulatory care, 41–42
long-term care, 352–353
managed care organizations, 120–22
rehabilitation, 380, 401, 408–9
substance abuse treatment, 271
veterinary care, 535
Concurrent review, 125
Conditions for Coverage of Suppliers of End Stage Renal Disease (ESRD) Services, 139–40
Conditions of Participation (Conditions of Coverage), 10
facility for mentally retarded, 295
freestanding ambulatory care, 62–63
home health care, 423, 424–25, 431
hospice care, 450–52, 454, 460–63, 473
mental health services, 213
rehabilitation, 380
Conditions of Participation for Hospitals, 27
Confidentiality
care for mentally retarded, 304, 317–18
correctional health record, 181–82, 184, 186–87
mental health services, 230–232
privacy rule, HIPAA, 7, 8–9
substance abuse treatment, 254, 272–74, 273–74

Consent for treatment
    ambulatory care, 71, 90–91
    care for mentally retarded, 304
    correctional facilities, 181–82
    hospice care, 453, 474–76
    managed care organizations, 125
Consolidated billing, 345
Constitutional Amendments, 164
Consultants/contractors
    computer systems, 564–66
    contract negotiation, 566–70
    correctional facilities, 166
    dialysis care, 155
    documentation, 555
    fees, 561–62
    home, working at, 562–64
    home office equipment, 564
    long-term care, 333–34, 360–61
    overview, 551–54
    regulatory issues, 554–55
    reimbursement, 555–56
    roles, 557–61
    seeking clients, 562
    setting, 553–54
    trends, 570
Consumers, mental health services, 201–2
Continuity of care, 203, 219, 227–28
Continuous ambulatory peritoneal dialysis (CAPD), 137
Continuous care, 461
Continuous cycling peritoneal dialysis (CCPD), 137
Continuous quality improvement (CQI), 229–30, 271
Contract management, 127
Contract negotiation, 566–70
Contractors. *See* Consultants/contractors
Contracts (insured units), 108
Coordination of benefits (COB), 115, 122
Coordination of care, 125
CoP. *See* Communities of practice
Copayments, 114, 183–84
Core team summary sheet, 305–6, 308–9
CORF. *See* Comprehensive outpatient rehabilitation facilities
Corporate integrity agreement (CIA), 556
Correctional facilities, 163–64
    caregiver types, 173, 176–77
    coding and classification, 185
    computer systems, 185
    data and information flow, 184
    documentation, 179–83
    health information managers, 190–91
    HIPAA, 185–87
    patient types, 171–75
    quality improvement, 188
    regulatory issues, 177–78
    reimbursement, 183–84
    risk management, 189–90
    setting, 164–71
    trends, 191–92
    utilization management, 188
Correctional health record, 179–82
Correctional institutions, 14
Cost accounting, managed care organizations, 122

COSTAR (computer-stored ambulatory record), 88
Council on Quality and Leadership in Support for People with Disabilities, 296
Counselors, substance abuse treatment, 253
Court-ordered treatment
    mental health services, 232–33
    substance abuse treatment, 274–75
Court-referred clients, 252
Covered entities (CEs), 6, 8–9, 152
CPM. *See* End-stage renal disease (ESRD) Clinical Performance Measures
CPT. *See* Current Procedural Terminology
CQI. *See* Continuous quality improvement
Credentialing, managed care organizations, 126–27
Crowns, prosthetic, 488
CSP. *See* Community Support Program
Curative therapy, 448
Current Dental Terminology (CDT–4), 501
Current Procedural Terminology (CPT)
    ambulatory care, 83
    home health care, 433
    hospice care, 468–69
    long-term care, 349
    managed care, 118
CVPM. *See* Certified veterinary practice manager
CWF. *See* Common working file

D

D.A.R.E. *See* Drug Abuse Resistance Education
Data and information flow
    correctional facilities, 184
    dialysis care, 144–45
    facilities for mentally retarded, 300–1
    freestanding ambulatory care, 83–85
    home health care, 433
    hospice care, 464–65, 466–67
    hospital-based ambulatory care, 41–43
    long-term care, 349–52
    managed care organizations, 119–20
    mental health services, 225–28
    substance abuse treatment, 267–69
Data Assessment and Verification (DAVE), 356
Databases, rehabilitation, 401
Data collection and transfer
    hospital-based ambulatory care, 42–43
    managed care organizations, 119
Data Infrastructure Grants (DIGs), 223–24

Data sets
    dialysis care, 145, 147
    facility for mentally retarded, 304–15
    freestanding ambulatory care, 88
    home health care, 433
    hospice care, 470–71
    long-term care, 353–55
    managed care organizations, 122–23
    mental health services, 228–29
    substance abuse treatment, 270–71
    veterinary care, 532–35
Data Standards for Mental Health Decision Support Systems (FN 10), 223, 229
DAVE. *See* Data Assessment and Verification
Day programming, mental health services, 206, 207–8
DEA. *See* Drug Enforcement Agency
Death, hospice patient, 459–60, 476
Decision-making process, managed care organizations, 122
Decision Support 2000+, 223
Decision-support systems, 87
Deductibles, 107
Deemed status, 10, 422–23
Delivery records, 72
Delusions, 202
Denial, Medicare payment, 431
Dental assistants, 492
Dental care
    documentation, 493–99
    health information managers, 510
    information management, 501–6
    patient types, 487–90
    practice management software, 502–6
    provider types, 490–92
    quality improvement, 507–8
    regulatory issues, 492–93
    reimbursement, 499–501
    risk management, 508–9
    settings, 484–87
    trends, 510–12
    utilization management, 507–8
Dental examination and charting, 495, 496–97
Dental history, 494–95
Dental hygienists, 492
Dental informatics, 512
Dental records, identification and, 509
Dental specialties, 490–92
Dentists, 490
Departments of corrections (DOCs), 163–64
Dependents, 108
Designated standards maintenance organization (DSMO), 43
Detainee, 168
Developmental disabilities, 202, 292, 489–90. *See also* Intermediate care facility for the mentally retarded (ICF/MR)
Diagnoses, postoperative/preoperative, 71
Diagnosis related group (DRG)
    ambulatory care, 34, 92

hospice care, 468
managed care organizations, 118–19
mental health care, 222
rehabilitation, 382, 392, 396
Diagnosis related group (DRG)
prospective payment system (PPS), 347
Diagnostic and Statistical Manual of Mental Disorders, Fourth Revision (DSM–IV), 228, 244, 269–270, 302
Diagnostic and Statistical Manual of Mental Disorders-IV-Text Revision (DSM-IV-TR), 203, 228, 269
Dialysate, 137
Dialysis
caregiver types, 138
coding and classification, 144
computer systems, 145
data and information flow, 144–45, 146
data sets, 145, 147–50
defined, 136
documentation, 140, 142–43
health information management, 155
patient types, 136–38
quality improvement, 151–52, 153–54
regulatory issues, 139–40, 141
reimbursement, 143
risk management, 152, 155
setting, 136
types, 137
utilization management, 152
Dialysis center, 136, 552
Dialysis unit, 136
Diet evaluation, dental care, 499
Dietitians, 138, 333–34
Digital cameras, 506
Digital imaging devices, 506
DIGs. *See* Data Infrastructure Grants
DIHS. *See* Division of Immigration Health Services
Direct care staff, 307
Disability, 376–77
Discharge summary
long-term care, 340–41
mental health services, 219
rehabilitation, 391, 393–95
Disciplines, home health care, 421–22
Discounted charges, 115
Discounted procedure, 35
Division of Immigration Health Services (DIHS), 171
DME. *See* Durable medical equipment
DOCs. *See* Departments of corrections
Documentation
consultant role, 555
correctional facilities, 179–83
dental care, 493–99
dialysis care, 140, 142–43
facilities for mentally retarded, 296–97, 298–99
freestanding ambulatory care, 65–78, 89–91
home health care, 424–28
hospice care, 455–60, 474–76

hospital ambulatory care, 27–33, 45, 46
long-term care, 336–43
managed care organizations, 112–13
mental health services, 213–21
rehabilitation, 384, 391–92, 409, 412
rural health clinics, 63
substance abuse treatment, 256–66
veterinary care, 524–28
Documentation by exception, 409, 412
Donations, animal, 541
Draft referral to staffing, 305
DRG. *See* Diagnosis related group
Drug Abuse and Treatment Act (1972), 273
Drug Abuse Resistance Education (D.A.R.E.), 249
Drug Enforcement Agency (DEA), 493
DSM-IV. See Diagnostic and Statistical Manual of Mental Disorders, Fourth Revision
DSM-IV-TR. See Diagnostic and Statistical Manual of Mental Disorders-IV-Text Revision
DSMO. *See* Designated standards maintenance organization
Dual diagnosis, mental illness, 202–3
Dual insurance coverage, 116–17
Dually diagnosed persons, 202, 252
Durable medical equipment (DME), 377–80, 422, 425, 432
Duty to warn, 231–32

E

E&M coding. *See* Evaluation and management coding
EAPs. *See* Employee assistance programs
Early and Periodic Screening, Diagnostic, and Treatment (EPSDT), 81
Economic credentialing, 127
ECUs. *See* Environmental control units (ECUs)
ED. *See* Emergency department
EDI. *See* Electronic data interchange
Education, dental care, 499
Educational model, mental health services, 203
Educational programs, substance abuse, 249
EHR. *See* Electronic health record
Elderly, dental care for, 488–89, 501
Election, hospice care, 450, 452, 462
Electronic data interchange (EDI), 7–8, 43, 87
Electronic dental record, 505–6
Electronic health information management, 13–14
Electronic health record (EHR)
capabilities, 14
consultant role, 560
correctional facilities, 191
freestanding ambulatory care, 77, 87, 92
hospital-based ambulatory care, 42
managed care organizations, 122
veterinary care, 542

Eligibility, managed care organizations, 120
E-mail, 88
Emergency department (ED)/emergency services
correctional facilities, 176
dental care, 511
hospitals, 25
mental health services, 208
risk management, 45–46
visit classifications, 35, 36
Emergency Medical Treatment and Active Labor Act (EMTALA), 46
Emergency outpatient, 26
Emotional illness, 201
Employee assistance programs (EAPs), 251–52, 280
Employer-specific data sets, 123
EMTALA. *See* Emergency Medical Treatment and Active Labor Act
Encoding, 397
Encounter data (data set), 88, 119
Encounter form, 68, 69
Endodontists, 491
End-Stage Renal Disease (ESRD) Program Management and Medical Information System (PMMIS), 145
End-stage renal disease (ESRD), 136
End-stage renal disease (ESRD) Clinical Performance Measures (CPM), 151, 153–54
End-stage renal disease (ESRD) facility, 136
End-stage renal disease (ESRD) Facility Survey, 145, 146
End-stage renal disease (ESRD) networks, 140, 141, 145, 151, 152, 155
Enrollment database, 120
Enrollment management, 128
Environmental control units (ECUs), 380
Episode of care, 222
EPSDT. *See* Early and Periodic Screening, Diagnostic, and Treatment
Equines, 521
Equipment, home office, 564
Equipment, medical
home health care, 422, 425, 432
rehabilitation, 377–80
Escorts, physical, 218–19
ESRD. *See* End-stage renal disease
Ethical issues, 155
Euthanasia, 541
Evaluation
hospice care, 474
mental health, 206, 207, 209–10
Evaluation and management (E&M) coding, 35–38
Experience rating, 114
External data reporting, 352

F

Family numbering system, 78
Family planning centers, 60–61
FBP. *See* Federal Bureau of Prisons
Federal Bureau of Prisons (FBP), 167
Federal False Claims Act, 64

Federal grants, mental health services, 223–24
Federal health programs, 2
Federal surveys
    dialysis care, 139, 145, 146
    long-term care, 334–42
Fee-for-service payment
    correctional facilities, 183–84
    freestanding ambulatory care, 79
    Medicare, 3
Fees, consultant, 561–62
Fee schedule, managed care organizations, 115
Felines, 521
FI. *See* Fiscal intermediary
Filing methods
    correctional health record, 180
    freestanding ambulatory care, 77–78, 85
FIM. *See* Functional independence measure
Financial indicators, 124
Financial stability, home health care, 430–31
Financial systems, 87
Fiscal intermediary (FI), 40
Fixed costs, 431
Flexner Report, 1
FN 10. See Data Standards for Mental Health Decision Support Systems
42 Code of Federal Regulations, 139–40, 144, 151, 254, 273–74
Forum of ESRD Networks' Quality Assurance Committee, 142–43
Foster care, 208
Freestanding ambulatory care. *See* Ambulatory care, freestanding
Freestanding dialysis facilities, 137
Freestanding home health care institutions, 422
Freestanding rehabilitation hospitals, 371–72
Functional history, 384
Functional independence measure (FIM), 405, 406
Funding. *See also* Reimbursement
    correctional facilities, 183–84
    facilities for mentally retarded, 297
    home health care, 428–31
    hospice care, 460–63
    long-term care, 343–47
    mental health services, 222
    rehabilitation, 392, 396–97
    substance abuse treatment, 266–67

G

Gatekeeper, 104
General inpatient care, 461
Gingiva, 491
Glasgow Coma Scale, 403, 404
Government funding
    mental health services, 222, 223–24
    substance abuse treatment, 266–67, 280
Grievance process, 189
Group dental practice, 485–86
Grouper, 119
Group Health Cooperative, 106

Group homes, mental health services, 208
Group model, managed indemnity plans, 113
Group model health maintenance organization (HMO), 106
Growth and development charts, 72, 74

H

Habilitation, 294
Habilitative staff, 294
Hallucinations, 202
Handheld computers, 87
Handicap, 376–77
HAVEN. *See* Home Assessment Validation and Entry
HCBS. *See* Home and Community Based Services Waiver
HCCs. *See* Hierarchical Condition Categories
HCFA. *See* Health Care Finance Administration
HCPCS. *See* Healthcare Common Procedural Coding System
Head and neck examination, 495
Healthcare Common Procedural Coding System (HCPCS), 35, 40, 79–80, 83, 118, 502
Health Care Finance Administration (HCFA), 217
Healthcare Information and Management Systems Society (HIMSS), 9
Health information management (HIM)
    ambulatory care, 46–48
    changes affecting role, 15
    consultants, 557–61
    correctional facilities, 190–91
    dental care, 510
    dialysis care, 155
    facilities for mentally retarded, 319–20
    freestanding ambulatory care, 91–92
    HIPAA standards, 7
    home health care, 437, 439–40
    hospice care, 451, 453, 476–77
    long-term care, 359–61
    managed care organizations, 127–128
    mental health services, 233–34
    patient care, 2
    prospective payment system, 3, 4
    rehabilitation, 407, 412
    substance abuse treatment, 275, 280
    veterinary care, 542
Health Insurance Portability and Accountability Act (HIPAA)
    ambulatory care, 43, 47, 64, 83
    consultants, 553, 554–55, 570
    correctional facilities, 181, 185–87
    dialysis care, 152
    home health care, 432
    hospice care, 478
    long-term care, 342
    mental health services, 230–32
    overview, 6–10
    substance abuse treatment, 254

Health Insurance Prospective Payment System (HIPPS), 430
Health Level 7 (HL7), 535
Health maintenance organizations (HMOs)
    capitation model, 4
    dental care, 500
    health information management, 127–28
    home health care, 421
    long-term care, 346–47
    models, 105–7
    rise of, 3–4
    staff model, 112–13, 114
Health Plan Employer Data and Information Set (HEDIS), 111–12, 122–23
Health services director (HSD), 166
Heavy care, 329
HEDIS. *See* Health Plan Employer Data and Information Set
Hemodialysis, 137, 144
Herd health, 526
HHRG. *See* Home Health Resource Group
Hierarchical Condition Categories (HCCs), 118
Hill-Burton Act (1946), 2
HIM. *See* Health information management
HIM-11 coverage guide, 424
HIMSS. *See* Healthcare Information and Management Systems Society
HIPAA. *See* Health Insurance Portability and Accountability Act
HIPPS. *See* Health Insurance Prospective Payment System
History. *See* Patient history
HL7. *See* Health Level 7 (HL7)
HMOs. *See* Health maintenance organizations
Home, working at, 562–63
Home and Community Based Services (HCBS) Waiver, 321
Home Assessment Validation and Entry (HAVEN), 428
Home-based services, mental health, 208
Homebound patient, 420
Home care visits, 421
Home health aides, 421, 449, 458
Home health care
    caregiver types, 421–22
    coding and classification, 432–33
    computer systems, 433
    consultants, 551
    data and information flow, 433
    data sets, 433, 434–35
    documentation, 424–28
    health information management, 439–40
    legal issues, 438–39
    patient types, 420–21
    quality improvement, 433, 436, 437
    regulatory issues, 422–24
    reimbursement, 428–31
    risk management, 437–38
    setting, 420
    trends, 440

utilization management, 436–37
Home health care rehabilitation, 372
Home Health Resource Group (HHRG), 429–30
Homeless population, 200
Home office equipment, 564
HOPPS. *See* Hospital Outpatient Prospective Payment System
Hospice care, 468–69
    caregiver types, 449
    coding and classification, 465, 468
    computer systems, 469–70
    consultants, 551
    data and information flow, 464–65, 466–67
    data sets, 470–71
    documentation, 455–60
    health information management, 476–77
    patient types, 448–49
    quality improvement, 472–73
    regulatory issues, 450–54
    reimbursement, 460–63
    risk management, 474–76
    setting, 447–48
    trends, 477–78
    utilization management, 473–74
Hospice inpatient unit, 457
Hospital-based ambulatory care. *See* Ambulatory care, hospital-based
Hospitals
    ambulatory care records, 68
    clinic reimbursement, 25, 38
    payment changes, 3–4
Hospital outpatient, 26
Hospital Outpatient Prospective Payment System (HOPPS or OPPS), 35–38
HSD. *See* Health services director
Hybrid covered entity, 185

I

ICAP. *See* Inventory for Client and Agency Planning
ICD-10-CM. See International Classification of Diseases, 10th Revision, Clinical Modification
ICD-9-CM. See International Classification of Diseases, 9th Revision, Clinical Modification
ICE. *See* Bureau of Immigration and Customs Enforcement
ICF/MR. *See* Intermediate care facility for the mentally retarded
ICPC. *See* International Classification of Primary Care
Identification, early, 207
Identification data, facility for mentally retarded, 307, 311
IDS/Ns. *See* Integrated delivery systems/networks
Illness-related care, 109
Immunizations, 72, 73
Impacted wisdom teeth, 491–92, 508
Impairment, 376–77, 396
Implant, dental, 491, 512
Incident, home health care, 438
Incident report, 91, 536–38

Incident to services, 79
Indemnity insurance, 107–8
Independent living, 408
Independent practice association (IPA), 106–7
Individualized treatment plan (ITP), 257, 264–66
Individual program plan (IPP), 305, 306–7
Industrial health services, 72–73, 76
Information flow, rehabilitation, 397. *See also* Data and information flow
Information management. *See also* Coding and classification; Data and information flow; Data sets
    dental care, 501–6
    mental health services, 222–29
Information release record, 304
Informed consent. *See* Consent for treatment
Initial baseline assessment, 425
Inmate population, 163–64
Inpatient hospitalization, mental health services, 208–9
Inpatient prospective payment system (IPPS), 4
Inpatient psychiatric facility prospective payment system (IPF PPS), 222
Inpatient rehabilitation facility patient assessment instrument (IRF-PAI), 396–97, 398–400, 405
Inpatient rehabilitation facility prospective payment system (IRF PPS), 382–84
Inpatient treatment, substance abuse, 248–50
Inpatient unit, hospice care, 457
Institute of Medicine (IOM), 41–42
Instructions, patient, 72, 90
Insurance
    dental, 500
    dental care billing, 504
    home health care, 429
    hospital outpatient care, 38
    long-term care, 346
    pet health, 529–30
    substance abuse treatment, 266
Insurance company, consultants at, 552
Insured units, 108
Intake process, substance abuse treatment, 267–68
Integrated delivery systems/networks (IDS/Ns), 129
Integrated records, 76, 427
Intensive outpatient treatment, substance abuse, 247–48
Interdisciplinary teams
    care for mentally retarded, 292, 293, 297
    dialysis, 138, 142, 152
    hospice care, 449, 458, 460, 465, 476
    rehabilitation, 372–75, 391, 392, 406, 409, 412
Intermediate care facility for the mentally retarded (ICF/MR)
    caregiver types, 293–95
    coding and classification, 301–3
    computer systems, 303–4

data and information flow, 300–1
data sets, 304–15
documentation, 296–97, 298–99
health information management, 319–20
individuals served, 292
legal issues, 317–19
quality improvement, 316
regulatory issues, 295–96
reimbursement, 297
risk management, 316–17
settings, 291, 295
trends, 320–21
utilization management, 316
International Classification of Diseases, 9th Revision, Clinical Modification (ICD-9-CM)
    ambulatory care, 40, 82–83
    care for mentally retarded, 301
    correctional facilities, 185
    dental care, 502
    home health care, 432
    hospice care, 468
    long-term care, 348–49
    managed care organizations, 117–18
    procedure codes, 118
    rehabilitation, 396, 397
    substance abuse treatment, 269–70
International Classification of Diseases, 10th Revision, Clinical Modification (ICD-10-CM), 83
International Classification of Primary Care (ICPC), 83
International Species Information System (ISIS), 532
Internet, 88
Intervention, early, 249
Intraoperative documentation, 71
Intraoral cameras, 506
Intraoral examination, 495
Inventory for Client and Agency Planning (ICAP), 297, 304
Inventory management, dental care, 505
Involuntary commitment, 200, 275, 276–79
IOM. *See* Institute of Medicine
IPA. *See* Independent practice association
IPF PPS. *See* Inpatient psychiatric facility prospective payment system
IPP. *See* Individual program plan
IPPS. *See* Inpatient prospective payment system
IRF-PAI. *See* Inpatient rehabilitation facility patient assessment instrument
IRF PPS. *See* Inpatient rehabilitation facility prospective payment system
ISIS. *See* International Species Information System
ITP. *See* Individualized treatment plan

J

Jails, 164, 169. *See also* Correctional facilities

JCAHO. *See* Joint Commission on Accreditation of Healthcare Organizations
Joint Commission on Accreditation of Healthcare Organizations (JCAHO), 2, 10
    ambulatory care, 28–31, 41, 46
    consultant role, 554–55
    correctional facilities, 178
    dialysis care, 136, 139, 140
    facility for mentally retarded, 296
    freestanding ambulatory care, 63–64
    home health care, 422–23, 428
    hospice care, 450
    long-term care, 336, 342–43
    managed care, 111, 112
    mental health services, 212, 230
    quality improvement programs, 44
    rehabilitation, 380, 381
    substance abuse treatment, 254–55, 271
Juvenile detention facilities, 169–70

K
Karnofsky scale, 474, 475
Kidney transplants, 147, 152, 155
Kinesiotherapist, 375

L
LA. *See* Loss of attachment
Laboratory services
    correctional facilities, 176
    freestanding ambulatory care, 66, 68, 85
    long-term care, 333
Labor records, 72
Leadership ability, 558, 560–61
Legal issues
    correctional facilities, 189–90
    dialysis, 152, 155
    facility for mentally retarded, 317–19
    freestanding ambulatory care, 89–91
    home health care, 438–39
    hospice care, 474–76
    hospital-based ambulatory care, 45–46
    managed care organizations, 125–27
    mental health services, 230–33
    substance abuse treatment, 256, 272–75
    veterinary care, 539–41
Legal practice consultants, 552
Legislation. *See* Balanced Budget Act; Children's Health Act; Clinical Laboratory Improvement Amendments (CLIA); Comprehensive Alcohol Abuse and Alcohol Prevention, Treatment and Rehabilitation Act; Drug Abuse and Treatment Act; Emergency Medical Treatment and Active Labor Act (EMTALA); Federal False Claims Act; Health Insurance Portability and

Accountability Act (HIPAA); Hill-Burton Act; Mental Health Act; Omnibus Budget Reconciliation Act; Professional fee schedule (PFS)
Level of care evaluation, 351
Licensure. *See also* Accreditation
    correctional facilities, 177
    dental care, 493
    freestanding ambulatory care, 62
    health care organizations, 10
    hospital-based ambulatory care, 27
    long-term care, 336, 342
    surveys, 334–35
Life care plan, rehabilitation, 406–7
LMRPs. *See* Local Medical Review Policies
Local Medical Review Policies (LMRPs), 81–82
Locum tenens, 79
Logical Observations, Identifiers, Names, and Codes (LOINC), 535
LOINC. *See* Logical Observations, Identifiers, Names, and Codes
Longitudinal patient record, 13–14
Long-term acute care hospital (LTCH), 327–28
Long-term acute care hospital (LTCH) patients, 329
Long-term acute care (LTAC), 371
Long-term care
    caregiver types, 330–34
    coding and classification, 348–49
    computer systems, 352–53
    data and information flow, 349–52
    data sets, 353–55
    documentation, 336–43
    health information management, 359–61
    importance, 14
    patient types, 328–30
    quality improvement, 356, 357–58
    regulatory issues, 334–36
    reimbursement, 343–47
    settings, 327–28
    utilization management, 356, 358–59
Long-term care hospital (LTCH) prospective payment system (PPS), 347
Long-term mental health care hospitals, 200
Loss of attachment (LA), 491
Low utilization payment adjustment (LUPA), 430
LTAC. *See* Long-term acute care
LTACH. *See* Long-term acute care hospital
LTCH. *See* Long-term acute care hospital
LUPA. *See* Low utilization payment adjustment

M
M+C. *See* Medicare+Choice
Mainframe computer systems, 122
Major diagnostic categories (MDC), 119
Malpractice, dental care, 508–98

Managed behavioral health care organization (MBHO), 212
Managed care organizations (MCOs), 3–4
    care for mentally retarded, 297, 299
    caregiver types, 109
    coding and classification, 117–19
    computer systems, 120–22
    consultants, 552
    coordination of benefits, 115–17
    correctional facilities, 183
    data and information flow, 119–20
    data sets, 122–23
    dental care, 510, 511
    documentation, 112–13
    health information management, 127–28
    long-term care, 346–47
    mental health services, 212, 222
    organization types, 105–8
    patient types, 108
    provider reimbursement, 114–15
    quality improvement, 123–24
    regulation/government, 110–12
    revenue, 113–14
    risk management, 125–27
    setting, 104–5
    substance abuse treatment, 281
    trends, 129
    utilization management, 124–25
Managed indemnity plans
    characteristics, 107–8
    group model, 113
Manic depression, 201–2
Manual on Terminology and Classification in Mental Retardation, 302–3
MAR. *See* Medication administration record
MBHO. *See* Managed behavioral health care organization
MCOP. *See* Conditions of Participation (Conditions of Coverage)
MCOs. *See* Managed care organizations
MDCs. *See* Major diagnostic categories
Meals on Wheels, 422
Medicaid
    dental care, 501
    EPSDT, 81
    fee payments for teaching physicians, 31–33
    long-term care, 343–47
    mental health services, 203–4, 212
    provisions, 2
    substance abuse treatment, 255–56, 266
Medical directors, rehabilitation, 384
Medical history, dental care, 494–95
Medical indicators, 124
Medically managed intensive inpatient treatment, 248, 249
Medical necessity, 212, 225, 256
Medical record librarians, 2
Medical record model, dialysis, 142–43
Medicare+Choice (M+C), 110, 118
Medicare carrier, 31
Medicare Carriers Manual, 31
Medicare ESRD Network Organizations Manual, 151

Medicare Managed Care Manual, 110
Medicare Physician Fee Schedule
    (MPFS), 79–80
Medicare PPS Assessment Form (MPAF),
    353, 355
Medicare
    ambulatory care, 35–36, 38, 60,
        62–63, 79–80
    common working file, 43
    Conditions of Participation. See
        Conditions of Participation
    dental care, 501
    diagnosis related groups, 34
    home health care, 429–31
    hospice care, 450–52
    long-term care, 343–47
    managed care regulations, 110
    mental health services, 204, 212–13
    partial hospitalization definition,
        25
    prospective payment system,
        35–38, 429–30
    provisions, 2, 3, 4–5
    substance abuse treatment, 266
Medication administration record
    (MAR), 315
Members, managed care organization,
    108
Mental Health Act (1965), 199
Mental health services
    caregiver types, 209–11
    client types, 201–9
    coding and classification, 228
    consumers, 201–2
    data and information flow, 225–28
    data sets, 228–29
    documentation, 213–21
    health information management,
        233–34
    information management, 222–29
    quality improvement, 229–30
    regulatory issues, 211–13
    reimbursement and funding, 222
    risk management, 230–33
    settings, 199–200
    trends, 234–35
    utilization management, 230
Mental Health Statistics Improvement
    Program (MHSIP), 223
Mental illness
    adolescents and children, 206–9
    adults, 201–6
    dental care, 490
    dual diagnosis, 202–3
Mental illness with chemical addiction
    (MICA), 202–3
Mental retardation, 202, 292. *See also*
    Intermediate care facility for the
    mentally retarded (ICF/MR)
Mental Retardation: Definition,
    Classification, and Systems of
    Supports, 302, 303
Mentoring, mental health services, 209
Metropolitan Statistical Area (MSA), 462
MHSIP. *See* Mental Health Statistics
    Improvement Program
MICA. *See* Mental illness with chemical
    addiction

Military bases, 487
Minimum data set, 354
Minimum data set (MDS), 337–39,
    349–51, 352–53, 357–58
Mixed model health maintenance
    organization (HMO), 107
Modified wave scheduling, 84–85
Mortality insurance, 529
Motor vehicle accidents, 117
MPAF. *See* Medicare PPS Assessment
    Form
MPFS. *See* Medicare Physician Fee
    Schedule
MSA. *See* Metropolitan Statistical Area
Multidisciplinary teams, 138, 142, 152.
    See also Interdisciplinary teams

N
NA. *See* Narcotics Anonymous
NAHC. *See* National Association for
    Home Care
Narcotics Anonymous (NA), 249–50
National Association for Home Care
    (NAHC), 424
National Commission on Correctional
    Health Care (NCCHC), 165, 177,
    178, 181, 184
National Committee for Quality
    Assurance (NCQA), 111–12, 122,
    212
National Committee on Vital and Health
    Statistics (NCVHS), 42–43
National Correct Coding Initiative
    (NCCI or CCI), 41
National Facility Register (NFR), 270
National Hospice and Palliative Case
    Organization (NHPCO), 448–49,
    470, 473
National Institute of Alcohol Abuse and
    Alcoholism (NIAAA), 270
National Institute of Dental Research,
    487
National Institute of Drug Abuse
    (NIDA), 270
National Institute of Mental Health
    (NIMH), 203
National Survey of Substance Treatment
    Services (N-SSATS): 2000, 245
National Uniform Billing Committee
    (NUBC), 38, 40
NCCHC. *See* National Commission on
    Correctional Health Care
NCCI. *See* National Correct Coding
    Initiative
NCQA. *See* National Committee for
    Quality Assurance
NCVHS. *See* National Committee on
    Vital and Health Statistics
Necropsy, 525
Negligence, dental care, 508–98
Neighborhood health centers, 60
Network model health maintenance
    organization (HMO), 106
Network of Animal Health (NOAH), 535
Newborn assessment, 72
NFs. *See* Nursing facilities
NHPCO. *See* National Hospice and
    Palliative Case Organization

NIAAA. *See* National Institute of Alcohol
    Abuse and Alcoholism
NIDA. *See* National Institute of Drug
    Abuse
NIMH. *See* National Institute of Mental
    Health
NOAH. *See* Network of Animal Health
Nonintegrated records, 455
Nonphysician documentation, 455
Notice of privacy practices (NPP), 8
NPP. *See* Notice of privacy practices
NPs. *See* Nurse practitioners
N-SSATS. *See* National Survey of
    Substance Abuse Treatment
    Services
NUBC. *See* National Uniform Billing
    Committee
Number of accessions, 523
Nurse practitioners (NPs)
    ambulatory care, 61
    managed care organizations, 109
    reimbursement, 79
    rural health clinics, 63
    substance abuse treatment, 253
Nurses/nursing
    ambulatory care, 26
    consultants, 551, 553
    correctional facilities, 173, 176
    dialysis, 138
    hospice, 449, 455–59, 464
    long-term care, 327, 330–31
    rehabilitation, 375
    substance abuse treatment, 253
Nursing assistants, long-term care, 331
Nursing data
    facilities for mentally retarded, 311,
        315
    hospice care, 468
Nursing facilities (NFs), 327, 551, 553
Nursing home minimum data set, 352
Nursing Home Quality Initiative, 356
Nursing visit note, 455, 456

O
OASIS. *See* Outcome and Assessment
    Information Set
OBQI. *See* Outcome-based quality
    improvement
OBQM. *See* Outcome-based quality
    management
OBRA. *See* Omnibus Budget
    Reconciliation Act
Observation services, 25
Occupational industrial health centers,
    60
Occupational Safety and Health
    Administration (OSHA), 439
Occupational therapists (OTs)
    home health care, 421
    mental health services, 211
    rehabilitation, 373, 392
Occurrence reports, 91
OCE. *See* Outpatient Code Editor
OFA. *See* Orthopedic Foundation for
    Animals
Offense, inmate, 172
Office of the Inspector General (OIG)
    ambulatory care compliance, 64–65

consultant role, 555–56
DRG work plan, 34
hospice care, 477–78
records audits, 32
OIG. *See* Office of the Inspector General
Omnibus Budget Reconciliation Act
(OBRA), 60, 140, 337
Operational indicators, 123–24
OPPS. *See* Outpatient prospective
payment system
Oral and maxillofacial surgeons, 491
Organ Procurement and Transplantation
Network (OPTN), 147
Orthodontists, 491
Orthopedic Foundation for Animals
(OFA), 535
Orthotic devices, 377–78
OSHA. *See* Occupational Safety and
Health Administration
OTs. *See* Occupational therapists
Outcome and Assessment Information
Set (OASIS), 427–28, 432, 433,
434–35, 436
Outcome-based quality improvement
(OBQI), 433, 436, 437
Outcome-based quality management
(OBQM), 433, 436
Outcome measures, 124
Outcomes, patient, 423
Outliers, 430
Out-of-pocket payment, veterinary care,
529
Outpatient Code Editor (OCE), 40–41
Outpatient prospective payment system
(OPPS), 4
Outpatients
ambulatory care, 47
clinic, 26
commitment, 200
emergency, 26
hospital, 26
mental health services, 207
referred, 26
rehabilitation, 372, 408
statistics, 24
substance abuse, 247–48
Oversight committees, 123
Ovines, 521
Ownership change, veterinary care, 541

P

Palliative care, 448, 478
Panel, provider's, 114
Panoramic radiograph, 498
Partial episode payment (PEP), 430
Partial hospitalization program (PHP),
25, 247–48
PAs. *See* Physician assistants
Pass-through payments, 38
Pathology report, 71–72
PATH (Physicians at Teaching
Hospitals), 32
Patient data sets, 88, 144–45, 470
Patient-focused care, 13
Patient history, freestanding ambulatory
care, 66
Patient identifier, ambulatory care,
77–78, 85

Patient information, dental care, 494
Patient transportation services, 422
Patient types
ambulatory care, 26, 61
correctional facilities, 171–73,
174–75
dental care, 487–90
dialysis, 136–38
home health care, 420–21
hospice, 448–49
long-term care, 328–30
managed care organizations, 108
rehabilitation, 375–77
veterinary care, 520–21
Payer mix, 430
Payment issues
affecting hospitals, 3–4
affecting other settings, 4–5
federal and state programs, 2–3
managed care organizations, 121
PCEs. *See* Potentially compensable
events
PCPM. *See* Per contact per month
PCPs. *See* Primary care providers
PDAs. *See* Personal digital assistants
Pediatric preventive health services, 72,
73–75
Pediatric rehabilitation, 376
PEP. *See* Partial episode payment
Per contact per month (PCPM), 120
Per diem payments, 3
hospice care, 461–62, 465, 477
long-term care, 343, 345
managed care organizations, 115
Performance Partnership Grants (PPGs),
224, 228
Periodontal examination, 495, 497
Periodontists, 491
Peritoneal dialysis, 137
Permanent residents, long-term care,
328–29
Per member per month, 114, 120
Per service reimbursement, hospice care,
461–62
Personal digital assistants (PDAs), 87, 91,
506
Personal health record (PHR), 14
Personal injury, 117
Person-centered information systems,
224
Person-first philosophy, 201–2, 294
Pet health insurance, 529–30
PFS. *See* Medicare Physician Fee
Schedule; Professional fee schedule
Pharmacists, 334, 449
PHI. *See* Protected health information
PHP. *See* Partial hospitalization program
PHR. *See* Personal health record
Physiatrists, 373, 406
Physical abuse reports, 493
Physical escorts, 218–19
Physical examinations
freestanding ambulatory care, 66
industrial health services, 72
rehabilitation, 391
Physical restraints, 217–18, 220–21
Physical therapists (PTs), 373–74, 392,
421

Physician assistants (PAs)
ambulatory care, 61
correctional facilities, 173
managed care organizations, 109
reimbursement, 79
rural health clinics, 63
substance abuse treatment, 253
Physician data, facilities for mentally
retarded, 311, 312–14
Physician extenders, 330
Physician Fee Schedule (PFS), 79–80
Physician private practices, 59–60
Physicians
ambulatory care, 26
correctional facilities, 173, 176
dialysis, 138
hospice care, 449, 457
long-term care, 330
rehabilitation, 391
substance abuse treatment, 253
Physicians at Teaching Hospitals
(PATH), 32
Physician's office, consultants at, 552, 554
PIP-DCG. *See* Principal In-Patient
Diagnostic Cost Group
Place of residence, 448
Plaque, 492
PMPM. *See* Per member per month
Point-of-service plans, 108
POMR. *See* Problem-oriented medical
record
Pontic, 491
Porcines, 521
Postacute rehabilitation, 371
Postoperative diagnoses, 71
Potentially compensable events (PCEs),
45–46
Poverty of thought, 210
PPG. *See* Performance Partnership
Grants
PPOs. *See* Preferred provider
organizations
PPS. *See* Prospective payment system
Preauthorization, medical procedures,
108, 125
Precertification, 89
Preferred provider organizations (PPOs)
characteristics, 107
dental care, 499, 500
home health care, 421
Pregnant females, dental care for, 488
Premiums, managed care organizations,
105, 113–14
Prenatal documentation, 72
Preoperative diagnoses, 71
Prepurchase examinations, 540
Prescriptions, 90, 91
Primary caregivers, 449
Primary care providers (PCPs), 104,
112–13, 120
Primary teeth, 487
Principal In-Patient Diagnostic Cost
Group (PIP-DCG), 118
Prisoner, 168
Prisons, 164, 166–68, 487. *See also*
Correctional facilities

Privacy rule, HIPAA, 7, 8–9. *See also*
    Health Insurance Portability and
    Assurance Act
Private pay, long-term care, 347
Problem list, ambulatory care, 68, 70
Problem-oriented medical record
    (POMR), 76–77, 427, 526
Procedure codes, *ICD-9-CM*, 118
Production medicine, 526
Professional fee schedule (PFS), 4
Program evaluation, rehabilitation, 406
Program manuals, Medicare and
    Medicaid, 81
Program memoranda, 81
Program transmittals, 81
Progress notes
    ambulatory care, 68, 91
    dialysis, 143
    hospice care, 455, 461, 465
    mental health services, 216
Prophylaxis, 498
Prospective payment system (PPS)
    home health care, 429–30
    hospital care, 3
    inpatient services, 5
    long-term care hospitals, 347
    mental health services, 222
    nursing facilities, 5
    overview, 5
    skilled nursing facilities, 345
Prospective review/precertification, 89
Prostheses, 379, 491
Prosthodontists, 491
Protected health information (PHI), 8–9,
    254
Provider data (data set), 88
Provider Self-Disclosure Protocol, 65
Provider's office evaluation, 126
Psychiatric medication management,
    206, 209–10
Psychiatrists, correctional facilities, 173,
    176
Psychologists, rehabilitation, 374
Psychosis, 199
Psychosocial rehabilitation, 204
Psychotropic medications, 189, 199–200,
    202
PTs. *See* Physical therapists
Public health departments, 60

Q

QI. *See* Quality improvement
QIO. *See* Quality Improvement
    Organization
QMRP. *See* Qualified mental retardation
    professional
Qualified mental retardation
    professional (QMRP), 293, 294
Quality assurance, hospice care, 453–54
Quality Improvement Organization
    (QIO), 436
Quality improvement (QI), 44
    consultant role, 553–54
    correctional facilities, 188
    dental care, 507–8
    dialysis, 151–52
    facility for mentally retarded, 316

freestanding ambulatory care,
    88–89
home health care, 433, 436
hospice care, 472–73
long-term care, 356, 357–58
managed care organizations,
    123–24
mental health services, 229–30
rehabilitation, 406
substance abuse treatment, 271
veterinary care, 535–36
Quality indicators, 123–24
Quality management, 128
Quality of care, federal regulations, 340,
    357–58
Quality of life, federal regulations, 341,
    357–58, 406

R

Radiography, dental, 498, 506
Radiology services
    correctional facilities, 176
    long-term care, 333
Rancho Los Amigos Levels of Cognitive
    Function Scale, 403
RAP. *See* Request for Anticipated
    Payment
RAP summary form, 338
Rational Recovery (RR), 250
RBRVS. *See* Resource-based relative
    value scale
RCT. *See* Root canal therapy
Recall reminders, dental care, 505
Recertification, home health care, 425
Record format
    ambulatory care, 76–77
    managed care organizations, 126
Record linkage, ambulatory care, 85–86
Record retention
    care for mentally retarded, 319
    correctional health record, 180
    dialysis facilities, 155
Record review, 126
Recovery, mental health, 234
Recovery period, 71
Recreational therapists, 211, 254
Recredentialing, 127
Reference laboratory services, 26
Referrals, 26, 119–20, 121, 505
Registered health information
    administrator (RHIA), 139, 359
Registered health information technician
    (RHIT), 139, 359
Registration
    ambulatory care, 65–66, 67
    computer system, 87, 121
    dental care, 502
Regulatory issues
    consultants, 554–55
    correctional facilities, 177–78
    dental care, 492–93
    dialysis, 139–40
    facilities for mentally retarded,
        295–96
    freestanding ambulatory care,
        61–65
    home health care, 422–24, 427–28
    hospice, 450–54

hospital-based ambulatory care, 27
    licensure, 62
    long-term care, 334–336
    managed care organizations,
        109–12
    Medicare certification, 10, 62–63
    mental health services, 211–13
    overview, 61–62
    rehabilitation, 380–84
    substance abuse treatment, 254–56
Rehabilitation
    caregiver types, 372–75
    classification system, 401–5
    coding, 397, 401
    computer systems, 401
    consultants, 553
    documentation, 384, 391–92,
        393–95
    importance, 14
    information flow, 397
    long-term care, 333
    medical equipment, 377–80
    national databases, 401
    patient types, 375–77
    quality improvement, 406
    regulatory issues, 380–84, 385–90
    reimbursement, 392, 396–97,
        398–400
    risk management, 406–7
    settings, 370–72
    trends, 407–12
Rehabilitation impairment categories
    (RICs), 396
Rehabilitation nurse, 375
Rehabilitation social workers, 374–75
Rehabilitation team, 372–75, 391, 392, 406,
    409, 412
Reimbursement
    consultant role, 555–56
    correctional facilities, 183–84
    dental care, 499–501
    dialysis, 143
    facility for mentally retarded, 297
    freestanding ambulatory care,
        79–82
    home health care, 428–31
    hospice care, 460–63
    hospital-based ambulatory care,
        33–40
    long-term care, 343–47
    managed care organizations,
        113–17
    mental health services, 222
    rehabilitation, 392, 396–97
    substance abuse treatment, 266–67
    veterinary care, 529–30
Relational and object-oriented
    technology, 229
Relational data-based technology, 228–29
Relative value unit (RVU), 80
Renal replacement therapy (RRT), 136,
    155
Request for Anticipated Payment (RAP),
    430
Resident assessment instrument (RAI),
    337–39
Resident assessment protocols (RAPs),
    337–39

Residential/inpatient treatment, substance abuse, 248
Residential living, mental health services, 206
Resident rights, long-term care, 341–42
Residents, 31
Medicare fee payments, 31–33
Resource-based relative value scale (RBRVS), 79–80, 115, 118
Resource data sets, hospice care, 471
Resource Utilization Groups III (RUGs), 345–46
Respiratory therapists, 333, 422
Respite care, 330, 422, 461, 462
Restraints, physical and chemical, 217–18, 220–21
Retrospective review, 89
Return-to-work physicals, 72
Revenue codes, ambulatory care, 40
Reviews, managed care organizations, 126
Revocation, hospice care, 451, 452, 463
RHC. *See* Rural health clinic
RHIA. *See* Registered health information administrator
RHIT. *See* Registered health information technician
RICs. *See* Rehabilitation impairment categories
Risk contracts, 346
Risk management (RM)
    correctional facilities, 189
    dental care, 508–9
    facilities for mentally retarded, 316–17
    freestanding ambulatory care, 89–91
    health information management, 128
    home health care, 437–38
    hospice care, 474–76
    hospital-based ambulatory care, 45–46
    managed care organizations, 125–27
    mental health services, 230–33
    substance abuse treatment, 272–75
    veterinary care, 536–39
RM. *See* Risk management
Root canal therapy (RCT), 488
Routine home care, 460
RR. *See* Rational Recovery
RRT. *See* Renal replacement therapy
RUGs. *See* Resource Utilization Groups III
Rural health clinic (RHC), 63
RVU. *See* Relative value unit

S

SAMHA. *See* Substance Abuse and Mental Health Services Administration
SAPT grants. *See* Substance abuse prevention and treatment grants
Satisfaction committee, 438
Scales of Independent Behavior—Revised (SIB-R), 304
Scheduling

    computer systems, 86–88, 121
    dental care, 503–4
    modified wave, 84–85
    standard, 83–84
    walk-ins, 85
    wave, 84
SCHIP. *See* State Children's Health Insurance Program
Schizophrenia, 201, 202
SCIC. *See* Significant change in condition
Screening
    correctional facilities, 168
    mental health services, 206
    substance abuse treatment, 275, 276–79
SCUs. *See* Special care units
Sealants, dental, 492, 508
Security risks, 8–9, 232
SED. *See* Serious emotional disturbance
Self-assessment, rehabilitation, 403
Self-help recovery groups, 245, 246, 249–50
Self-pay
    correctional facilities, 183–84
    dental care, 500, 508
Serious emotional disturbance (SED), 206–7
Seriously mentally ill (SMI), 201
Severity indexes, 272, 474, 475
Sex, health services required and, 172
Sex rating, 114
Shared Decision-Making in the Appropriate Initiation of and Withdrawal from Dialysis, 155
Short-term patients, 329
Short-term psychiatric care, 200
SIB-R. *See* Scales of Independent Behavior—Revised
Signficiant others, 448–49
Significant change, 350–51
Significant change in condition (SCIC), 430
Single point of entry (SPOE), 230
Skilled nursing facilities (SNFs)
    long-term care, 327
    per diem reimbursement, 115
    physicians, 330
    rehabilitation, 372
    reimbursement, 343, 345
    versus acute rehabilitation, 407–8
Skilled nursing services, home health care, 421, 422, 425
SMI. *See* Seriously mentally ill
SNFs. *See* Skilled nursing facilities
SNOMED. *See* Systematized Nomenclature of Medicine
SNVDO. *See* Standard Nomenclature of Veterinary Diseases and Operations
Social history, 384
Social Security Act, 2
Social Security Disability Income (SSDI), 203–4
Social services
    dialysis, 138
    home health care, 422
    hospice, 449
    long-term care, 331–32
    rehabilitation, 374–75

Societal changes, 14
Solo dental practice, 484–85
Source-oriented record, 76, 425, 427
Special care units (SCUs), 328–29
Special requirements, ambulatory care, 68, 71
Specialty services
    correctional facilities, 176–77
    home health care, 421–22
Speech and language pathologist, 374, 421
Spinal cord injury, 376, 402–3
SPOE. *See* Single point of entry
SSDI. *See* Social Security Disability Income
SSI. *See* Supplemental Security Income
Stabilization, mental health, 234
Staff model health maintenance organization (HMO), 106, 112–13, 114
Standard Nomenclature of Veterinary Diseases and Operations (SNVDO), 530–32, 533
Standards, JCAHO, 423
Standard scheduling, 83–84
Standard surveys, 334
State agencies
    Medicare, 2, 10
    substance abuse treatment, 255–56
State Children's Health Insurance Program (SCHIP), 2–3
State departments of corrections (DOCs), 163–64
State funding, mental health services, 222, 223
State Children's Health Insurance Program (SCHIP), 2
State licensure
    correctional facilities, 177
    dental care, 493
    long-term care, 336, 342
    managed care organizations, 111
State Operations Manual (SOM), 10, 12
Statistical data, 120
Status indicator, 35–37
Stray animals, 541
Strengths treatment model, 214–16
Structured review, 126
Subacute care, 329, 330
Subscribers, managed care organization, 108
Substance abuse
    caregiver types, 252–54
    care settings, 246–50
    client types, 250–52
    coding and classification, 269–70
    computer systems, 271
    confidentiality, 272–74
    court-ordered treatment, 274–75
    data and information flow, 267–69
    data sets, 270–71
    documentation, 256–66
    health information management, 275, 280
    introduction, 244–46
    involuntary commitments, 275, 276–79
    quality improvement, 271

regulatory issues, 254–56
reimbursement, 266–67
service provisions, 202–3
trends, 280–81
utilization management, 272
Substance Abuse and Mental Health
Services Administration (SAMHA),
267
Substance abuse prevention and
treatment (SAPT) grants, 267
Substandard quality of care, 334, 336
Superbills, 83
Supplemental Security Income (SSI),
203–4, 219
Surgery. *See* Ambulatory surgery,
hospital-based
Surveys
dialysis, 139, 145, 146
long-term care, 334–42
*Systemized Nomenclature of Medicine
(SNOMED)*, 530–32, 542, 554

T

TBI. *See* Traumatic brain injury
TDP. *See* TRICARE Dental Program
Teaching hospitals, 31–33
Technology. *See also* Computer systems
correctional facilities, 191–92
dental care, 506, 512
rehabilitation, 408–9
service delivery, 13–14
TEDS. *See* Treatment Episode Data Set
Telemedicine, 13
Terminal digit filing, 85
Terminally ill, 448
Therapeutic recreation, 332
Therapists
mental health services, 210, 211
substance abuse treatment, 253, 254
Theriogenology, 521
Third-party organizations, dental care,
486
Time-outs, 219
Total quality management (TQM),
229–30
TPO. *See* Treatment, payment, or
operations
TQM. *See* Total quality management
Training data, facilities for mentally
retarded, 305–7, 308–10
Training programs, compliance, 65
Transfer records
dialysis facilities, 144–45
inmates, 180–81
long-term care, 340–41
Transplantation surgeon, 138
Traumatic brain injury (TBI), 376, 403,
404
Treatment, payment, or operations
(TPO), 8
Treatment Episode Data Set (TEDS), 270
Treatment notes, dental care, 498–99
Treatment plan. *See also* Care plan
dental care, 498
hospice, 448–49
mental health services, 214–16

substance abuse treatment, 267–68
Trends
consulting, 570
correctional facilities, 191–92
dental care, 510–12
facilities for mentally retarded,
320–21
freestanding ambulatory care, 92
home health care, 440
hospice, 477–78
managed care organizations, 129
mental health services, 234–35
rehabilitation, 407–12
substance abuse treatment, 280–81
veterinary care, 542–43
TRICARE Dental Program (TDP), 501
24-Hour Active Treatment Schedule,
306–7, 309–10

U

UACDS. *See* Uniform Ambulatory Care
Data Set
UB-92. *See* Uniform Bill 92
UFDS. *See* Uniform Facility Data Set
UM. *See* Utilization management
Uniform Ambulatory Care Data Set
(UACDS), 42–43
Uniform Bill 92 (UB-92 or CMS 1450),
38–40, 119, 120, 397
Uniform Facility Data Set (UFDS), 270
United Network for Organ Sharing
(UNOS), 147
University health centers, 60
Unusual events, identification of, 125
Unusual occurrence, home health care,
438
Updating worksheet, 305
Urgent care centers, 60
Utilization management (UM)
ambulatory care, 45, 89
correctional facilities, 188
dental care, 507–8
dialysis facilities, 151, 152
facility for mentally retarded, 316
home health care, 436–37
hospice care, 473–74
long-term care, 356, 358–59
managed care organizations, 121,
124–25
mental health services, 230
substance abuse treatment, 272
veterinary care, 535–36
Utilization of supplies and services, 352

V

Validation surveys, 139
Variable costs, 431
Variance, 409, 412
Veterans Affairs (VA) hospitals, 487,
488–89, 501
Veterinarians, 521–22
Veterinary Hospital Managers
Association (VHMA), 522
Veterinary Medical Data Base (VMDB),
530, 532–35
Veterinary profession, 520

Veterinary settings
caregiver types, 521–22
coding and classification, 530–32
computer systems, 535
consultants, 551
data sets, 532–35
documentation, 524–29
health information management,
542
introduction, 520
legal issues, 539–41
patient types, 520–21
quality improvement, 535–36
regulatory issues, 522–24
reimbursement, 529–30
risk management, 536–39
trends, 542–43
utilization management, 535–36
Veterinary technicians, 521–22
Veterinary technologists, 522
VHMA. *See* Veterinary Hospital
Managers Association
Videotelemedicine, 191–92
Vineland Adaptive Behavior Scales, 304
Vision records, 72
VMDB. *See* Veterinary Medical Data Base
Voluntary accreditation
facility for mentally retarded, 296
managed care organizations,
111–12, 113
Voluntary hospital admission, 225, 227
Volunteers, hospice care, 449, 454, 459,
471

W

Walk-in appointments, 85
Wave scheduling, 84
Weed, Lawrence, 76
Wellness care, 109
Wheelchairs, 379–80
WHO. *See* World Health Organization
Wildlife management, 540
Wisdom teeth extraction, 508
Women, 251, 488
Workers' compensation, 117
World Health Organization (WHO), 401
Wrap-around services, 209
Written policies and procedures
care for mentally retarded, 318–19
correctional facilities, 180, 182
home health care, 439
Written utilization protocols, 125

X

X-ray reports
ambulatory care, 66, 68, 85
pregnant females, 488